**American College of
Foot Surgeons**

Complications in Foot Surgery

Prevention and Management

SECOND EDITION

American College of Foot Surgeons

Complications in Foot Surgery

Prevention and Management

SECOND EDITION

EDITOR

Stuart A. Marcus, D.P.M., F.A.C.F.S.

Diplomate, American Board of Podiatric Surgery
Past President, American College of Foot Surgeons

ASSOCIATE EDITOR

Barry H. Block, D.P.M., A.A.C.F.S.

Medical Arts Center
New York, New York
Astoria General Hospital
Astoria, New York

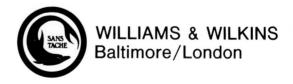

WILLIAMS & WILKINS
Baltimore/London

Editor: Jonathan W. Pine, Jr.
Copy Editor: Perry Ewell
Design: Jim Mulligan
Illustration Planning: Wayne Hubbel
Production: Carol Eckhart

Copyright © 1984
Williams & Wilkins
428 East Preston Street
Baltimore, MD 21202, U.S.A.

Accurate indications, adverse reactions, and dosage schedules for drugs are provided in this book, but it is possible that they may change. The reader is urged to review the package information data of the manufacturers of the medications mentioned.

Made in the United States of America

First Edition, 1976
Reprinted 1984

Library of Congress Cataloging in Publication Data

Main entry under title:

Complications in foot surgery.

Includes index.
1. Foot—Surgery—Complications and sequelae. I. Marcus, Stuart A. II. Block, Barry H. III. American College of Foot Surgeons.
RD563.C655 1983   617'.58501   83-7438
ISBN 0-683-05550-X.

Composed and printed at the
Waverly Press, Inc.

Foreword

The concept of a practical textbook devoted to the complications of foot surgery was initially considered by the Executive Board of the American College of Foot Surgeons in 1976, and led to their first publication, *Complications in Foot Surgery, Prevention and Management.*

Since that time, there have been a considerable number of new techniques and advances in the field of foot surgery, particularly in the areas of sports-related foot surgery, microsurgery, surgery on the diabetic patient, joint implant procedures and internal fixation. Of course, with the advent of new procedures comes the inevitable onslaught of post-operative complications.

The objective of the second edition is to review an adequate number of clinical cases from the many years of experience of the contributing authors, with practical insights and observations on newer procedures.

We hope this second edition will not only be a helpful adjunct for practicing surgical podiatrists and orthopaedic surgeons performing foot and ankle surgery, but also for residents and students of both podiatry and orthopaedic disciplines.

A sincere thank you is forwarded to the contributors, manuscript reviewers, and to the members of the Editorial Board. A special thank you goes out to Dr. Stuart A. Marcus, Editor and Dr. Barry H. Block, Associate Editor, for their help, advice and sustained effort in making this textbook a reality.

Donald W. Hugar, D.P.M., F.A.C.F.S.
Immediate Past President
American College of Foot Surgeons

Preface

I am grateful that I have had the opportunity to edit the second edition of *Complications in Foot Surgery* for it allows me to publicly thank my teacher, Dr. Earl G. Kaplan, who taught me the principles of podiatric surgery and showed me how to integrate and apply this training in the surgical care of the foot.

The basic organization and main objectives of this edition have been changed to adhere more closely to the title *Complications in Foot Surgery*. Every effort has been made to bring its content up to date and to improve the appearance of the illustrations. Every chapter has been altered and some have been rewritten. Others have been eliminated and still others expanded. Although it is, of course, not possible to give immediate recognition to every important advance in foot surgery, a considerable fund of new material has been included with completely new chapters. Some of the areas are: 1) microsurgery, where the use of the microscope and other new techniques have been so effective; 2) implants, where an in-depth review over a great number of years has allowed the author to pin-point the problems and their prevention; 3) ankle repair, with special emphasis to AO fixation techniques; and 4) sports-related injuries, where the rage in running and increase in participation of physical fitness programs by the public have created a host of lower extremity difficulties.

Attention has also been given to the quality of the photographs and illustrations, and to strengthening the ties between these and the text. This edition includes more than 200 new photographs and many of the drawings have been clarified and improved.

This is not a "how-to-do-it" textbook. We have attempted to discuss in detail the prevention and treatment of the complications that occur during the pre-operative, intra-operative, and post-operative phases of the patient undergoing foot surgery. Of special note is the fact that most of our authors have vast practical experience in addition to their current teaching and clinical positions in residency programs and schools of podiatric medicine. They have bridged the gap between research and clinical application so that the information presented will enable foot surgeons to treat surgical complications with a higher degree of understanding and therefore more successfully.

Appreciation is due first to my Associate Editor, Dr. Barry Block, whose invaluable aid and editorial advice helped revise and compile this book in an orderly fashion. One of the real privileges is the right to acknowledge those authors who have made this book possible. A special thank you must be said to all who, without exception, have full-time occupations as practitioners, clinicians, and teachers. As a novice editor, I am especially indebted to the professional skill and patience of Alice Reid, Jonathan Pine, and Carol Eckhart of Williams & Wilkins. Lastly, to my wife, Miriam, and to my daughters, Donna and Heather, who really paid the price, I express my love for their understanding and patience.

Stuart A. Marcus, D.P.M., F.A.C.F.S.

Contributors

Steven J. Berlin, D.P.M., F.A.C.F.S.
Bel Air, Maryland
Chief, Podiatry Section, Fallston General Hospital
Fallston, Maryland

Barry H. Block, D.P.M., A.A.C.F.S.
Medical Arts Center
New York, New York
Astoria General Hospital
Astoria, New York

Theodore H. Clarke, D.P.M., F.A.C.F.S.
Westview Osteopathic Medical Hospital
Indianapolis, Indiana

Victor E. Gambone, Jr., M.D.
Mease Hospital
Dunedin, Florida

Ronald Green, D.P.M., F.A.C.F.S.
Chief of Staff—Highlands Center Hospital
Denver, Colorado

Charles J. Gudas, D.P.M., F.A.C.F.S.
Associate Professor of Surgery
University of Chicago Hospitals & Clinics
Chicago, Illinois

Donald W. Hugar, D.P.M., F.A.C.F.S.
Elmwood Park, Illinois
Chairman, Department of Podiatry
Director, Podiatric Education
St. Anne's Hospital West
Chicago, Illinois

Allen M. Jacobs, D.P.M., F.A.C.F.S.
Director, Department of Podiatric Medicine & Surgery
Director, Residency Training in Podiatric Medicine & Surgery
Lindell Hospital
St. Louis, Missouri

Marla Jassen, D.P.M.
Surgical Consultant
Podiatry Residency Program
Fallston General Hospital
Fallston, Maryland

G. Wayne Jower, D.P.M., A.A.C.F.S.
Clinical Instructor for Off-Campus Education
California College of Podiatric Medicine
San Francisco, California

Stanley R. Kalish, D.P.M., F.A.C.F.S.
Jonesboro, Georgia
Doctors Hospital
Tucker, Georgia
Atlanta Hospital & Medical Center
Atlanta, Georgia

James H. Lawton, D.P.M., F.A.C.F.S.
Riverside, Illinois
Assistant Clinical Professor
University of Illinois—Abraham Lincoln School of Medicine
Associate Professor of Surgery
Dr. William Scholl College of Podiatric Medicine
Chicago, Illinois

Gary M. Lepow, D.P.M., M.S., F.A.C.F.S.
Harris County Podiatric Medical Residency Program
Houston, Texas

Jack Levitt, D.O.
Monsignor Clement Kern Hospital For Special Surgery
Warren, Michigan

Stuart A. Marcus, D.P.M., F.A.C.F.S.
Clearwater, Florida
Past President, American College of Foot Surgeons
Mease Hospital
Dunedin, Florida

Lawrence M. Oloff, D.P.M., F.A.C.F.S.
Director, Podiatric Clinical Services
Co-Director, Lindell Hospital Podiatry Residency Program
St. Louis, Missouri

Elliott H. Rose, M.D.
Plastic and Reconstructive Microsurgeon
Peninsula Hospital Medical Center
Burlingame, California

Steven I. Subotnick, D.P.M., M.S., F.A.C.F.S.
Hayward, California
Professor, Biomechanics & Surgery
California College of Podiatric Medicine
San Francisco, California
Chief of Podiatry
Eden Hospital
Castro Valley, California

Zoltan Szabo, Ph.D.
Director, Microsurgical Research Institute
San Francisco, California
Associate Director
Oregon Microsurgery Center
Portland, Oregon

Contents

SECTION 1: **PRE-OPERATIVE**

SECTION 2: **INTRA-OPERATIVE**

SECTION 3: **POST-OPERATIVE**

PRE-OPERATIVE

CHAPTER 1

Pre-operative Evaluation of the Surgical Patient

VICTOR E. GAMBONE, JR., M.D.

INTRODUCTION

It is our intent in this chapter to familiarize the reader with the more common conditions predisposing the surgical patient to increased risk of complications. A conscientious effort to identify potential problems pre-operatively is the cornerstone to their prevention post-operatively. Once risk factors are identified and proper intervention taken, most sequelae can be eliminated or substantially reduced.

HISTORY AND PHYSICAL EXAMINATION

A thorough history and physical examination should be undertaken in all patients undergoing surgery. The substantial information obtained will be the basis for assessing operative risk. History should include an account of previous hospitalizations, surgeries, transfusions, anesthetics, and complications. Adverse reactions to medications must be detailed. A meticulous review of systems is critical to the detection of pre-existing disease. Use of medication (with or without prescription), tobacco, and alcohol should be quantified and documented.

PRE-OPERATIVE INVESTIGATIVE STUDIES

Most textbooks of surgery and anesthesia recommend certain specific laboratory tests for pre-operative evaluation. These screening tests include: a complete blood count, platelet count, prothrombin time, partial thromboplastin time, urinalysis, and chest x-ray for presumably healthy young people. Blood chemistry analysis and an electrocardiogram are additionally recommended for those over 45 years of age. Bear in mind that these studies are not all-inclusive. If the history and physical examination detects specific significant abnormality, then further investigation may be necessary. In such an instance, surgery might need be postponed and an appropriate medical specialist consulted.

AGE AND NUTRITION

In the adult, surgical risk steadily increases with age. In younger patients, this risk may be inconsequential. However, after age 70, operative mortality increases by a factor of 4 to 8, depending on the surgical procedure. In part, this increased risk results from the presence of co-existing disease. Nevertheless, the elderly patient has a decreased cardiopulmonary reserve and is less likely to survive post-operative complications.

NUTRITIONAL DEFICIENCIES

It is well known that nutritional deficiencies result in impaired wound healing and increase susceptibility to infection. For this reason alone, it is no wonder that surgical risk is increased in chronic alcoholics and the malnourished. Elderly patients, as well, are likely to be malnourished due to marginal income and limited resources. In such patients, a 1- to 3-week nutritional preparation has been shown to substantially decrease the risk of complications in elective surgery.

MEDICATIONS

Because the interactions among drugs used peri-operatively can have an adverse effect on the patient, it is essential to know a patient's current medications and history of drug reactions before surgery. Most adverse reactions to medications are not true drug allergies. A careful description of the nature of any reaction should be obtained.

If true drug allergy is suspected, then the causative drug and structural congeners must be avoided. When a reaction can be attributed to a side-effect, often the medication can still be administered at a reduced dose without adverse effect. An accurate accounting of drugs recently taken and their dose can be best obtained by requesting patients to bring in their medications, including empty containers.

The use of corticosteroids for 2 or more weeks may cause enough adrenal suppression, so that the stress of surgery may precipitate an adrenal crisis.

Aminoglycoside antibiotics can substantially potentiate the action of non-depolarizing muscle relaxants used during surgery. This could result in profound muscle weakness requiring mechanical ventilation in the immediate postoperative period.

Digitalis may interact with anesthetics and enhance the tendency of the drug to produce serious cardiac arrhythmias. Hypokalemia will increase the likelihood of digitalis toxicity. For this reason, all patients taking diuretics and digitalis concomitantly should have their serum potassium checked pre-operatively. Any depletion of potassium storage should be corrected before surgery is contemplated.

ALCOHOL SEDATIVES

Excessive respiratory depression may follow the use of narcotic analgesics as pre-operative medications. This is more likely to occur in patients with liver or lung disease. Acute alcohol intoxication produces enhanced depressive effects of barbiturates used to induce anesthesia. Chronic alcohol use, however, leads to resistance to the effects of barbiturates. Quantification of the patient's alcohol intake daily must always be made. Knowledge of chronic use pre-operatively should always alert one to the potential for withdrawal symptoms post-operatively.

HYPERTENSION

Approximately 10% of surgical patients have hypertension. For some, this may be the first awareness of blood pressure elevation. For others, adequate treatment has been achieved with multiple medications. Earlier medical literature expressed the concern over the interaction of antihypertensive medications with anesthetic agents and implied that these drugs were major hazards to the surgical patient. However, in recent years, proper attention to the choice of anesthetic agent, its concentration, and rate of administration have minimized these risks. Except in the case of malignant hypertension, most would agree that moderate elevation in diastolic blood pressure (less than 120 mm of mercury) poses no contraindication to surgery. However, it is prudent to achieve normotension prior to surgery whenever possible.

In the context of this discussion, it is also noteworthy that patient compliance with antihypertensives (and for that matter any medication regimen) is far from ideal. Do not be surprised if a patient's blood pressure drops dramatically when given his "usual medications" during hospitalization.

CARDIOVASCULAR RISK

Coronary atherosclerosis represents the single largest cause of death in the United States. Unfortunately, coronary disease does not usually appear clinically evident until multiple vessel obstruction develops. When such patients are identified by history, physical examination, or electrocardiographic findings, it must be realized that they are at risk for post-operative myocardial infarction. The incidence of myocardial infarction in this group of patients is 6% in contrast to about 0.4% in patients without clinical evidence of cardiac disease. When a myocardial infarction occurs peri-operatively, 50–70% of the patients die.

Prior history of myocardial infarction appears to be the most lethal risk factor. If the infarction occurred within 6 months, the chance for reinfarction peri-operatively ranges from 18–20%. Operations performed within 3 months of a myocardial infarction attend an incidence of 30% reinfarction. Therefore, elective surgery should be delayed if at all possible when a myocardial infarction has occurred in the prior 6 months.

Patients who have undergone coronary artery bypass grafting (CABG) increasingly present for non-cardiac surgery. Recent reports suggest that these patients can undergo subsequent non-cardiac surgery with trivial cardiac risk.

The presence of stable angina pectoris has not been identified as predictive of increased risk of peri-operative cardiac complications. However, patients with unstable angina, impaired ventricular function, and ventricular irritability (more than five premature ventricular contractions per minute) are at high risk for cardiac complications. Elective surgery in such patients should be deferred until further investigation of these problems has been made and appropriate treatment administered. In many instances, coronary artery bypass surgery may be necessary before elective, non-cardiac surgery can be undertaken with safety.

Patients with valvular, congenital, and other forms of heart disease, if well compensated, can usually undergo anesthesia without excessive risk. Prophylaxis against bacterial endocarditis is extremely important in these patients.

Drugs used to control cardiovascular disorders should not be withdrawn before surgery. Usually they can be given intravenously or with a sip of water on the day of surgery. Abrupt withdrawal of some drugs (e.g., propranolol or clonidine) can be particularly hazardous.

Patients with prosthetic heart valves are often receiving anticoagulants. The incidence of severe bleeding and post-operative hematoma is 13% in these patients. This risk can be minimized without thromboembolic complications by discontinuing anticoagulant therapy 1–3 days before operation and reinstituting therapy within the 1st week after surgery. Patients taking large dose aspirin therapy for any reason should have the drug withdrawn for 2 weeks before elective surgery if the operation is a major one.

PULMONARY CONSIDERATIONS

All patients undergoing anesthesia and surgery are at some risk of developing pulmonary complications. Risk is increased in smokers, those with acute or chronic lung disease, and obese patients. When taking the medical history, attention should be paid to the presence of productive cough, shortness of breath with minimal to moderate activity, or knowledge of wheezing or asthma. A chest x-ray, spirometry, and arterial blood gases should be performed on all patients with a history of pulmonary symptoms, heavy smoking, cough, as well as the markedly obese. Accurate identification of pulmonary impairment allows one to institute appropriate measures pre-operatively which will reduce the chance of post-operative complications. In those at high risk, prophylactic maneuvers have been shown to decrease morbidity by 50%.

All smokers should be instructed to stop smoking at least 1 week (preferably 3 weeks) prior to elective surgery. Patients with bronchospasm should be treated with bronchodilators. Those with chronic bronchitis as manifest by chronic cough should additionally receive humidified inhalation therapy, chest physiotherapy, and antibiotics before surgery.

Many physicians share the common misconception that spinal anesthesia is safer than general anesthesia, particularly for the patient with lung disease. However, general endotracheal anesthesia may offer distinct advantages to some patients with compromised pulmonary status; and choice of anesthesia must be individualized. With endotracheal general anesthesia, ventilatory support can be continued as long as necessary to ensure smooth convalescence.

HEMATOLOGIC EVALUATION

A complete blood count is an essential part of the pre-operative evaluation. It should include a white blood cell differential count, blood smear review, and a platelet count or estimate. If anemia is present and can be corrected, it is wise to postpone surgery. Although it is customary to require a hematocrit of at least 30% before surgery, a patient with ischemic heart disease may require a hematocrit of 40% or more to ensure adequate coronary blood flow under the increased demands of surgical stress. In such patients, the benefits of transfusion, however, must be weighed against the risk of cardiac decompensation from volume overload.

The cause of polycythemia should always be determined when detected. If polycythemia vera is present, surgical complications from infection, hemorrhage, or thromboembolism can approach 50% in untreated patients.

Hemostatic competence is best assessed pre-operatively by history taking, measurement of the activated partial thromboplastin time (APTT), and a platelet estimate from the blood smear. A coagulation disorder should be suspected in all patients with a past history of hemorrhage (requiring transfusion or lasting more than 24 hours) after dental work, trauma, or prior surgery. Recurrent nose bleeds, hematuria, unexplained bruising, and a family history of bleeding tendency are additional clues to diagnosis.

HEPATIC AND RENAL DISORDERS

Because most anesthetic agents reduce liver blood flow and many are metabolized by the liver, patients with liver dysfunction must be identified to prevent further liver damage. If a patient presents with jaundice or abnormal liver enzyme studies, a diagnosis must be made pre-operatively if at all possible. For instance, a patient with a previous history of jaundice who now appears well may have chronic liver disease from persistent hepatitis B antigenemia. He is clearly at risk of infecting others and appropriate precautions must be taken.

In patients with renal disease, surgical risk increases with decrease in the glomerular filtration rate. In patients with moderate renal insufficiency (creatinine clearance less than 25–50 ml/min), if close attention is paid to fluid and electrolyte balance and the choice of peri-operative drugs, an increased risk of complications will not be a problem. However, the management of patients with more advanced disease will require the expertise of a medical specialist.

Bear in mind that significant reduction in renal function can be present without symptoms. Therefore, if screening laboratory studies (blood urea nitrogen, creatinine, electrolytes, or urinalysis) suggest renal dysfunction, elective surgery should be postponed until further investigation can be made and appropriate measures taken.

ENDOCRINE DISORDERS AND DIABETES

The recognition of altered function of the thyroid and adrenal gland is often difficult but imperative to the prevention of serious intra-operative complications.

Patients with untreated thyrotoxicosis are at risk of thyroid storm during surgery. Those with hypothyroidism or hypoadrenocorticism are very sensitive to sedatives and anesthetic agents. Severe hypotension can develop during induction of anesthesia.

Be alert to complaints of fatigue, weight loss, palpitations, heat or cold intolerance, tremor, constipation, hoarseness, and dry skin. The free T-4 index (T-7) is the best screening test when thyroid dysfunction is suspected. Surgery should be postponed until any thyroid hormone imbalance is corrected.

Symptoms of adrenal insufficiency include weight loss, fatigue, loss of appetite, diarrhea, and weakness. On examination, hyperpigmentation (particularly of the palmar creases) is present, and laboratory studies will reveal elevated serum potassium and low serum sodium levels. Proper replacement of adrenal corticosteroids peri-operatively will prevent complications.

A diabetic patient should be well controlled prior to surgery. Some patients may be newly diagnosed because of an elevated blood glucose at the time of admission. In such an instance, elective surgery should be delayed until appropriate treatment can be administered and blood sugar control achieved.

Diabetics treated with oral hypoglycemic agents will usually require insulin peri-operatively. Because of the prolonged half-life of some of these drugs (e.g., chlorpropamide), 3 days may be required before insulin therapy can be safely undertaken.

Patients on long-acting insulin products need not be switched to regular insulin if the operative procedure is minor and oral intake can be resumed early. Surgery on these patients should be scheduled early in the morning. Prior to surgery, one-half of the patient's usual insulin dose should be administered. After surgery, the remainder of the insulin dose can be given if adequate oral intake has been reestablished.

THROMBOEMBOLIC DISEASE

The risk of thromboembolic disease should be considered in the evaluation of every pre-operative patient. Post-operative deep vein thrombosis occurs in 30% of patients over 40 years of age, and pulmonary embolism is the single most common cause of post-operative death. Unfortunately, there is no prophylactic agent to prevent these dreaded complications which is both safe and effective. Obese individuals, women on oral contraceptives, and patients with a prior history of venous insufficiency, thrombophlebitis, or congestive heart failure are at the greatest risk of developing thromboembolic complications. If elevation of extremities is not possible or post-operative immobilization is necessary, thromboembolic risks are amplified. Under such circumstances, the need for low dose heparin therapy should be considered. Five thousand units of heparin is given subcutaneously before surgery and then every 8–12 hours after surgery until discharge. External pneumatic compression can be used alternatively and has been proven to be effective in patients who cannot tolerate heparin.

ANTIBIOTICS

The prophylactic use of antimicrobials in clean bone and joint surgery is controversial except in procedures involving total joint replacement where pre-operative administration of antibiotics has been shown to reduce the incidence of post-operative infection. These considerations are discussed in detail later in this text.

PSYCHOLOGIC FACTORS

Everyone has heard the saying, "I'm scared to death," and many physicians can recount examples of patients who apparently died under psychological stress. Therefore, it is of great importance to relieve as much of the nervousness surrounding surgery and anesthesia as possible. Patients who are apprehensive should be briefed about surgical procedure and related matters as fully as possible. A visit by the anesthesiologist the evening before surgery has been clearly shown to be of great value in alleviating the patient's fears and anxiety. Informed patients generally require less pre-operative sedation, require lighter planes of anesthesia, have an uneventful recovery period, and require less narcotics post-operatively. Extra time spent reassuring and informing the patient will markedly contribute to a decrease in a number of post-operative complications.

ANESTHESIA

Many anesthesiologists are convinced that local anesthetics can be as hazardous and dangerous as other forms of anesthesia. The capability and experience of the persons administering the anesthetic often determine the successful outcome of the procedure. The American Society of Anesthesiologists has adopted a classification for assessing anesthetic risk. This scale has been widely used for several decades:

Class I: A normally healthy individual.

Class II: A patient with mild systemic disease.

Class III: A patient with severe systemic disease that is not incapacitating.

Class IV: A patient with incapacitating systemic disease that is a constant threat to life.

Class V: A moribund patient who is not expected to survive 24 hours with or without operation.

E: Added to any class patient with emergency surgery.

In practice, it may be difficult to classify a particular patient because of many variables and overlapping of categories. However, it is helpful to translate the evaluation of the patient's surgical and anesthetic status into a quantitated measure of risk. Stating that the patient is an adequate or inadequate risk for contemplated surgery without a quantitated judgment is of limited value. It also makes little difference when estimating the physical status of the patient, whether the contemplated surgery will be performed using local anesthesia or other techniques.

The major key to decreasing the incidence, both in degree and number, of intra- and post-operative complications is to use every means possible to anticipate them before they occur. This can only be done through a conscientious and determined effort to examine and evaluate the pre-surgical patient, and to exercise preventative measures.

Suggested Readings

Corman, L. C., and Bolt, R. J. *Symposium on Medical Evaluation of the Preoperative Patient.* Med. Clin. North Am. 63:1129–1351, 1979.

Gracey, D. R., Divertie, M. B., and Didier, E. P. Preoperative pulmonary preparation of patients with chronic obstructive pulmonary disease. *Chest* 76:123–129, 1979.

Tinker, J. H., Noback, C. R., Vlietstra, R. E., et al. Management of patients with heart disease for noncardiac surgery. *JAMA* 246:1348–1350, 1981.

CHAPTER 2

The Practice of Communication

THEODORE H. CLARKE, D.P.M.

In this century, podiatric medicine and podiatric surgery are unique in surfacing as health care needs. Podiatry's scientific and technical advancement could not have come about without communication.

Most of the undesirable circumstances that can happen in medical practice may be traced to the lack of communication. Good in-depth communication can engender but never guarantee an easy, comfortable, successful practice experience. Likewise, the antithesis can be chaos! (Figure 2.1).

The ability to communicate is one of the most important skills a physician can master. It helps to get ideas across effectively and to get results in interrelationships.

REASONS FOR COMMUNICATION

In order that foot surgical services can result in the best of all relationships, a situation of understanding should be initiated as soon as possible and maintained throughout the experience. This supplies the surgeon with pertinent information necessary to arm and support his best judgment for decision-making.

COMMUNITY IMAGE

Oftentimes, the surgeon's community image and profile dictate a demand for a high level of communication. The community relationship is the initial stage of communication. The referral sources, the receptionist and the assistants involved with the practice, and the history and physical examination, must present the level of communication most desirable to the philosophy of the practice.

PRACTICE IMAGE

Once a patient has been initiated into the "modus operandi" of the practice, the thrust must be toward a well-attended, well-functioning method of maintenance of practice communication. The nucleus of this cell must be the podiatric physician. The attitudes, habits, and mannerisms of the doctor will supply the necessities of this system.

Such attributes as "ivory towerism," tardiness, hurriedness, preoccupation, assumptiveness, lack of friendliness, confusion, disenchantment, lack of positiveness, unkindness, and certainly many others on the part of the doctor are untenable and destructive. Perhaps it is more simply stated: we should practice the golden rule and pray to see ourselves as others see us.

ESTABLISHING CREDIBILITY

Good communication is based on credibility. No one wants to openly discuss with nor listen to anyone who does not present an image of believability. Anything communicated that is unbelievable or misunderstood should well be left unsaid.

DETERRENTS TO POSITIVE COMMUNICATION

Belief patterns
Myths, tales
Experience
Hopes
Short-cuts
Lack of reinforcement
Fear
Misinformation, no information
Third-party reimbursement
Advertising: unethical, improper, inac-

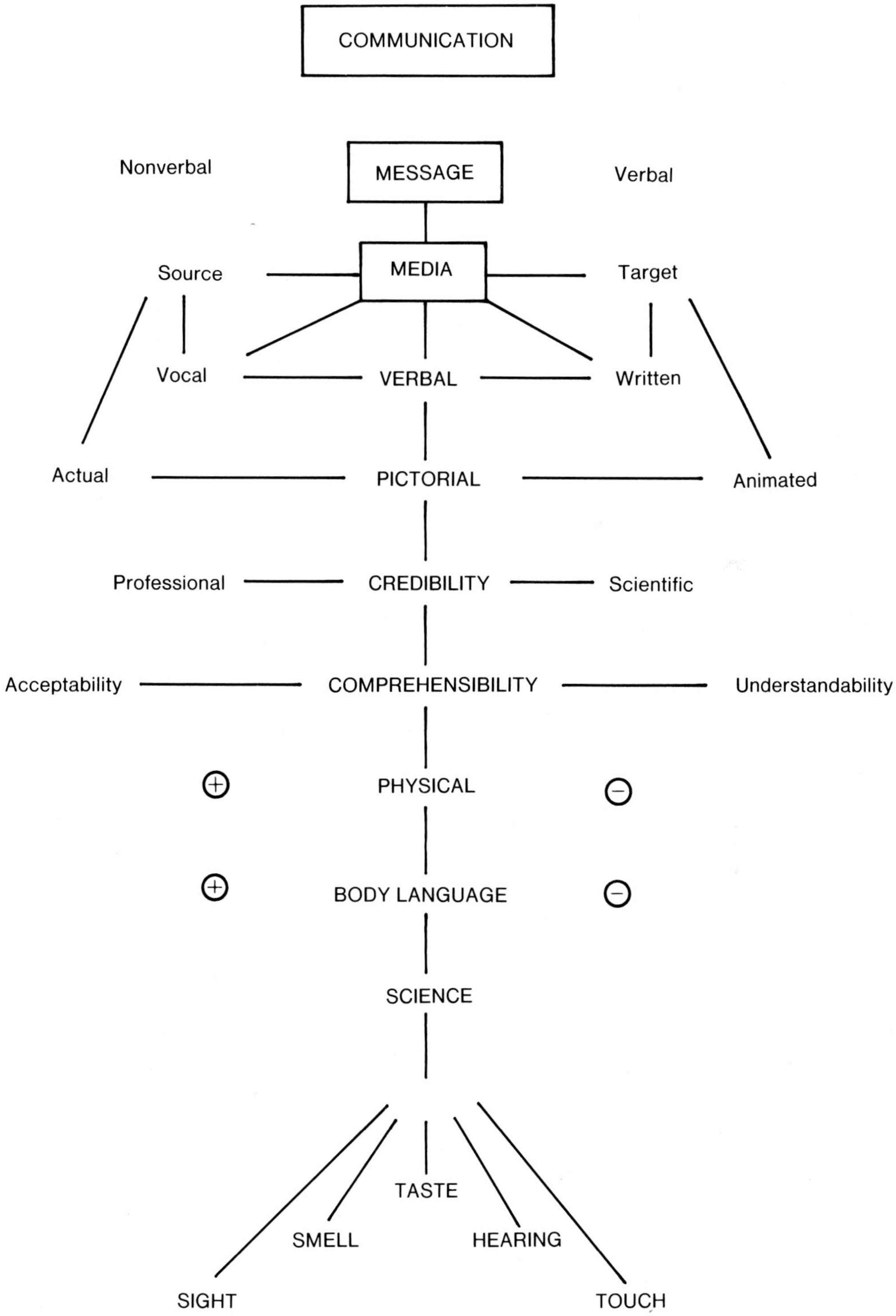
COMMUNICATION
Nonverbal
MESSAGE
Verbal
Source
MEDIA
Target
Vocal
VERBAL
Written
Actual
PICTORIAL
Animated
Professional
CREDIBILITY
Scientific
Acceptability
COMPREHENSIBILITY
Understandability
+
PHYSICAL
−
+
BODY LANGUAGE
−
SCIENCE
TASTE
SMELL
HEARING
SIGHT
TOUCH

Figure 2.1.

curate, inappropriate (by professionals and commercials)

Spoken and written presentations should include:

Patient's pain, cost, and time

Diagnosis in lay terminology

What can be done about it?

How will it be done?

Where will it be done?

Why?

Communication should include:

What is wrong in relationship to symptoms?

What is wrong in relationship to etiology?

What are the alternative programs of care?

What are the assessed prognoses in each circumstance?

What are the patient's responsibilities?

What are the responsibilities of the practice?

INFORMED CONSENT

A pre-surgical consultation should include information in terminology that the patient can understand. For instance, patients usually do not understand the term "arthroplasty;" however, they would understand "surgical remodeling of the small bones in the toe in an attempt to overcome the chronic discomfort and disability associated with the bony deformity and any lesion that is present." It may only take 15 minutes to perform the surgical procedure, but a much longer time to help your patient comprehend. This is why "informed" consent is so entitled.

Many patients do not understand anesthesia as local or general. It is usually understood as asleep, awake, or paralyzed from the waist down. Patients need to be given an idea of how long they will be disabled with regard to their domestic responsibilities, occupational responsibilities and social functions.An estimate of healing time and occupational disability should also be included in the presentation, always allowing for complications. It goes without saying that no guarantees, warranties, promises, or unrealistic commitments should be offered.

FEES

Surgical patients should be informed prior to their surgery as to the cost of the procedure being performed and extra incidentals as accurately as possible. These fees should be itemized and a statement should be made concerning responsibility for payment of the account whenever there is a discrepancy between what the third party pays and what the physician charges.

MEDICAL TERMINOLOGY

Although patients cannot understand podiatric medical terminology, it is a good practice to write down the diagnosis and the procedure for them so that they can consult their insurance company or take it with them for a second opinion.

PRE-ADMITTANCE AUTHORIZATION

In circumstances of hospital surgery, it is a good idea to have the patient sign the authorization in the office prior to admittance to the hospital. This does not mean that the patient is not obliged to sign one in the hospital as well.

DANGER SIGNS

The entering notes that state "this thing is *killing me*" and "I don't care *what* has to be done or what it costs" may be a danger signal to self-assessment and self-assignment. The author of such an entering statement may not know "what is wrong," "what can be done about it," and may *really* not care what it costs because they do not have any intention to pay the cost. They may be mislocated and need to be in the hands of a "higher healer."

Whenever this type of deterrent presents itself, auxiliary personnel should use the surgical presentation chart to reinforce patient understanding and attest to the same to assure the worthiness of the program.

FORENSIC MEDICINE

At this point something should be said concerning forensic medicine. This is a great and broad subject and this chapter should not really infringe on the subject. It will suffice to say: anything performed by hand, conceived in mind, and supported by heart should be documented in chart.

PRE-SURGICAL COMMUNICATION

Communication should not be utilized and directed toward convenience, to coerce the patient, or to urge the patient to leap to the OR table. It must be remembered that communication is mandated in order that patients understand and elect the program presented.

Properly communicated patients will then properly inform other referrals. "Like refers like." All patients should wish to become knowledgeable concerning diagnosis, treatment plan, and prognosis.

From time to time, patients seem to be "turned off," displeased, disenchanted, confused, and hostile. This is the time the doctor should ask the salient question, "Is there a reason that I am not pleasing you?" To ignore a communication "breakdown" is to flirt and dance with tragedy.

The *earliest* stages of practice communication which may be pre-surgical are vital to the communication level of the surgical program. Somehow, good surgical discipline is enhanced by understanding and reinforced by compliance and co-operation. There is no set method that we can use to measure the accuracy of the outcome of foot surgery with regard to this formula.

When the outcome of the surgeon's judgmental investigation has dictated procedural choice, and the outcome of the historical and physical examination have attested to the patient's physiological adequacies, then the surgical experience and the post-surgical responsibilities must be reinforced in communication with the patient.

On the day of the surgical presentation or admission, committed concern should be communicated to the patient and the family without any suggestion of overdramatization or risk of heightening anxiety. The day of surgery is a personal, private, and possibly a lonely day for the patient.

Tender loving care and concern should not only be the responsibility of family and loved ones. But, obtuse, and unbelievable "fuss-budgeting" can be so unusual in the program of care at this point that it can interrupt the smooth flow of reinforcing believable communication.

The podiatric surgeon must indoctrinate his hospital staff to the profile of communication that he has established with his office staff. Any break in the consistency of kindness, knowledgeability, and concern is easily noticeable, remembered, and remarked about by patients and loved ones.

In hospital surgical protocol, there may be other physicians involved who will affect the communication arena through history and physical examination, general anesthesia, surgical assistance, and/or resident. It is the responsibility of the podiatrist to define and maintain the consistency of communication and care that is optimum and ideal for his doctor-patient relationships. The night before surgery or the day of surgery is the proper time for the surgeon to examine the communication flow and consistency.

Whether the surgery is performed in or outside of the hospital setting, a post-surgical telephone call or visit from the office staff is never out of order. Very frequently, when telephoned, patients will feel more open and comfortable discussing their symptoms and asking normal questions or registering complaints (or pleasure) that they would not reveal to the surgeon or hospital staff during hospital or office visits. Most offices exercise this function for in-office, outpatient surgery and find it most reinforcing; but not all extend it to hospital experiences.

Family members and loved ones who sit in office reception rooms and hospital rooms and/or waiting rooms may be anxious, worried, or frustrated. This should be anticipated and relieved by the surgeon, the assistant, or resident. A staff member may prearrange to do this creditable service. This "all things went well" message may help to establish a post-operative experience that will reduce confusion and questionable rumors. It may even minimize discomfort.

AMBULATORY SURGERY

Even though many programs are identified as "ambulatory," no thought of tennis or kickball should be inaugurated. Showering in an unprotected bandage or cast should not be permitted. Taking for granted that patients can self-program optimum post-surgical care is frequently chaotic. Distribution of printed lists of "dos and don'ts" is advisable to avoid confusion.

QUESTIONS

As the ability of the podiatric surgeon to communicate is considered, several questions are raised. Some of these questions *need* communication while others *request* communication; but then there are those questions that *demand* communication.

Need Communication

Who is my patient?
What is wrong with my patient?
What can be done about the problem?
What are the alternatives?
Does my patient understand?
Why did the patient make this choice?
What are the necessities for recall and reassessment?
Is my patient of sound mind and body?:
What are my patient's responsibilities and desires?

Note: Be aware of the question that turns out to be a statement.

Request Communication

What is wrong with me, doctor?
What is the disability time?
What can be done about my problem?
What is apt to be the outcome?
Will it recur?
How much will it cost?
What about anesthesia?
What about post-op pain?
What about future disabilities?

Demand Communication

Were you available, doctor?
Did you provide coverage?
Was there *informed* consent, identifying the risks and hazards?
Did you justify your sound medical and surgical judgment?
Were there any promises or guarantees?
Did you entice this patient?
Who wanted the surgery most, you or the patient?
Did you discuss palliative care, repair, rehabilitation, correction, and/or salvage?
Is there evidence of competence, experience, and is this within the standard of care?
Would this situation have come to a different result if the patients had been adequately informed of their responsibility to support what you did to them or for them?

NETWORK OF PRACTICE COMMUNICATION

The network of practice communication may seem complex (Fig. 2.2), but it can become a practice of automaticity with awareness, attention, and commitment. Among many other things, the golden rule applies.
There must be communication with:
Third party and prior approval
Peer review request
Appeals and controls
Critique committees
Patterns of practice
Scope of practice
Integrity committees
Always communicate an "open door" policy for reassessment and for follow-up!
There is no terminal contact for the podiatric surgeon nor the podiatric patient. There is, indeed a wholistic concept of "family practice."

WHAT IS NEEDED?

Intra-office communication (all staff members being responsible for every patient):
1. Staff meetings
2. Practice pattern assessments

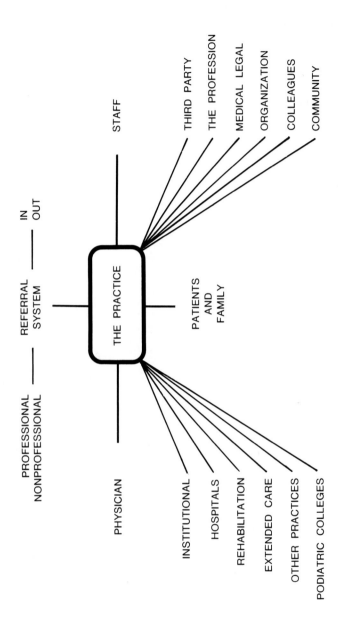

PROFESSIONAL ——— REFERRAL ——— IN

NONPROFESSIONAL SYSTEM OUT

THE PRACTICE

STAFF

PHYSICIAN

PATIENTS AND FAMILY

THIRD PARTY

THE PROFESSION

MEDICAL LEGAL

ORGANIZATION

COLLEAGUES

COMMUNITY

INSTITUTIONAL

HOSPITALS

REHABILITATION

EXTENDED CARE

OTHER PRACTICES

PODIATRIC COLLEGES

Figure 2.2. The network of practice communication may seem complex, but it can become a practice of automaticity with awareness, attention, and commitment.

3. Auxiliary personnel meetings

Inter-office communication:
1. Community colleagues
2. Inter-disciplinary relationship

SURVEY/PRE-SUMMARY

One method of measuring your success in communicating is to send out a questionnaire to your patients. The survey should ask several questions:

1. Did you know what was wrong with your feet when you entered our service?
2. Did you understand the service alternatives that were offered to you and the consequences you could expect?
3. Did the practice fulfill the expectations presented to you?
4. Do you still have foot problems of pain and dysfunction? Were these anticipated?
5. Have you followed all patient responsibilities and discipline programs of rehabilitation?
6. Have you registered your dissatisfaction or pleasure with your doctor or a member of the staff?

The information obtained will help you determine any communication weaknesses.

The primary patient concerns should always be foremost in the mind of the physician and staff when confronting the patient at all levels of communication, whether the problem is a *neuroma* (which gives no external visual evidence of its existence); *paronychia* (previously mistreated by another discipline); *bunion* (which mother and grandmother had and lived with); or *hammertoe* (which does not really need amputation).

REPORTS

As early as possible in a professional referral circumstance, a report should be made to the source. It may be as brief as a "Thank you for the professional confidence," or it may be as comprehensive as a reflection of history and examination notes and itemized program of care. The highest quality of professional special health care services also communicates a *post-service report*. These reports are best rendered in writing. The scientific depth of these reports are individual and artistic. They should honor the patient's personality, health circumstance, and cooperation. They should be honest in prognosis and follow-up program. By all means, the reports should reflect mechanisms of assessments and decisions regarding judgmental choices of procedures.

SUMMARY

The unique message of podiatric surgery should be spread to all in need of foot care. Possibly the most opportune vehicle is the *well-communicated* patient.

Suggested Readings

Altman, M. I., ed. *Modern Therapeutic Approaches to Foot Problems.* Futura, New York, 1973.

Berman, E. *The Solid Gold Stethescope.* Ballentine, New York, 1974.

Berne, E. *The Games People Play.* Grove, New York, 1964.

Berne, E. *What Do You Say After You Say Hello?* Bantam, New York, 1973.

Bernstein, M. Z. *Auxilliary Personnel in Podiatry.* Futura, New York, 1977.

Bird, B. *Talking with Patient.* Lippincott, New York, 1955.

Clarke, T. H. *The Professional Podiatry Assistant.* Indiana State Podiatry Association, Indianapolis, 1968.

Clarke, T. H., ed. *The Yearbook of Podiatry 1978/1989.* Futura, Mt. Kisco, New York, 1979.

Clarke, T. H. ed. *The Yearbook of Podiatry 1970/1981.* Futura, Mt. Kisco, New York, 1981.

Cotton, H. *Medical Group Practice.* Medical Economics, Oradell, New Jersey, 1965.

Cotton, H. *Medical Practice Management.* Medical Economics, Oradell, New Jersey, 1970.

MacBryde, C. M. *Signs and Symptoms.* Lippincott, New York, 1964.

Donick, I. I. *Podiatry for the Assistants.* Futura, New York, 1977.

Egeter, B. C. *The Professional Practice Management.* Pageant, New York, 1957.

Enget, O., and Morgan, O. *Interviewing the Patient.* Saunders, Philadelphia, 1973.

Gibran, K. *The Prophet.* Knopf, New York, 1923.

Harris, T. A. *I'm OK-You're OK.* Avon, New York, 1969.

Hassard, H. *Medical Malpractice Risks: Risks, Protestion, Prevention.* Medical Economics, Oradell, New Jersey, 1966.

Kinn, F. *The Office Assistant in Medical Practice.* Saunders, Philadelphia, 1969.

Levoy, R. P. *The $100,000 Practice and How to Build It.* Prentice-Hall, New Jersey, 1966.

Levoy, R. P. *The Successful Professional Practice.* Prentice-Hall, New Jersey, 1970.

Marx, O. *How to Practice Successful Dentistry.* Lippincott, Philadelphia, 1963.

Miller, B. M. *Medical Secretaries and Assistants Handbook.* Prentice-Hall, New Jersey, 1963.

Nirenberg, L. *Getting Through to People.* Prentice-Hall, New Jersey, 1963.

Nourse, A., and Marks, G. *Management of a Medical Practice.* Lippincott, New York, 1963.

Physician's Management. *Office Procedural Manual for the Medical Assistant.* Harbrace, New York, 1968.

Powell, J. *Why Am I Afraid to Tell You Who I Am?* Argus Communications, Niles, Illinois, 1969.

The Random House Dictionary of the English Language, 1969–1970.

Berg, D. L. *Doctor-Aide Program.* Medical Economics, Oradell, New Jersey, 1971, vols. I and II.

CHAPTER 3

Vascular Considerations

BARRY H. BLOCK, D.P.M.

VASCULAR EVALUATION

The presurgical vascular examination should include a history, palpation, inspection, auscultation, and tests to assure adequate pedal circulation. A careful review of the signs, symptoms, and management of common peripheral vascular disease is essential to minimize post-operative complications.

Arterial Pulsations

Pulsations in the arteries are graded from 0 to 4, reflecting the following parameters: 0–Non-palpable; 1–trace, minimal; 2–weak to mild; 3–moderate pulse; 4–strong pulse. The dorsalis pedis pulse may not be palpable in about 15% of normal subjects, since the vessel may take an anomalous course or be congenitally absent. The posterior tibial pulsations may not be palpable in a number of cases. This, along with the absence of the dorsalis pedis pulse, suggests occlusive vascular disease. If both the pedal pulses are unresponsive, palpate the popliteal artery and the femoral artery to estimate the level of occlusion.

A palpable pulse may be noted in the foot with a stenotic or obstructive lesion in the aortoiliac or femoral artery. If the individual exercises the involved limb, there will be no palpable pulse for 5 minutes or longer distal to the vascular obstruction. Exercising a healthy limb, however, would decrease the pulse amplitude for about 30 seconds.

Elevation Dependency Tests

Place the patient in a supine position in a comfortably warm room to avoid vasospasm. Raise the lower extremities at least 45° and flex the knees slightly. After 30 seconds, mild pallor is evidence of a normal arterial supply. With the legs elevated, have the patient exercise the toes vigorously. This will produce pallor. At the end of the exercise, pink color normally returns when there is adequate circulation. Extreme blanching to white on elevation indicates arterial impairment and inadequate collateral circulation. Extreme pallor may be uniform or may affect one or two toes, depending on the degree and location of arterial impairment or occlusion.

With a patient sitting with his legs in a dependent position, the color normally returns to the feet in about 10 seconds. If the return of color takes 30 seconds or more, impaired arterial circulation is indicated. Cyanosis and rubor are signs of severe ischemia. The elevation and dependency tests do not differentiate between spastic and organic arterial disease.

Venous Filling Time

The venous filling time test is performed concurrently with the previous tests. It measures the time it takes for blood to flow from the arterial to the venous system. Elevate the legs for 1 minute until the dorsal veins of the feet are drained, and then place the feet in a dependent, non-weight-bearing position. Normally the dorsal veins fill in 15 seconds. If the filling time is delayed, arterial obstruction is suspected. In severe obstruction, a filling time of 90 seconds is not unusual. It should be noted that the presence of varicose veins invalidates this test.

Subpapillary Venous Plexus Filling Time

Elevate the legs above the heart level and apply digital pressure to the end of the toe to produce blanching. When digital pressure is removed, pink color returns within 2 or 3 seconds. Delay indicates decreased arterial blood flow, which may be due to spasm, occlusion, reduced or absent tone in the subpapillary venous plexus or venous stasis.

Varicose Veins

Except for angiomas, the term varicose veins is used for dilated and/or tortuous veins. While primary varicosities develop spontaneously, secondary varicosities are caused by proximal obstructions such as compressing tumors, pregnancy, portal obstruction (esophageal only), thrombophlebitis and arteriovenous fistulas. Pulsations are often present in the dilated veins with arteriovenous fistula.

Sufficient blood pooling occurs in the lower extremities if the varicosities are extensive enough to cause orthostatic hypotension.

Percussions

To check for valvular competence in the great saphenous vein, the subject stands and the vein is allowed to fill. Palpate a segment of the vein in the leg and strike the vein above the knee with the tips of the fingers. If the impulse of the sharp percussion in the leg is felt by the examiner, incompetence of the intervening valves is indicated.

Brodie-Trendelenburg Test

This test is for competency in the saphenofemoral complex. With the subject supine, elevate the leg vertically so that the veins are drained. Apply a tourniquet at the midthigh to occlude the superficial veins. Have the patient stand and record the time for venous filling from below. It should take 35 seconds. Release the tourniquet within 60 seconds. Normally, no further venous filling should occur. If there is slow filling of the great saphenous vein upon release of the tourniquet, the result is positive, and incompetence of the great saphenous vein is indicated (Fig. 3.1, *A* and *B*).

A double positive test shows rapid filling of the great saphenous vein during compression and quick filling of the vein from above when the compression is released. This indicates incompetence in both the saphenous vein and its femoral communication.

Perthe's Test

This test evaluates obstruction of the deep veins and the valvular competence of the deep femoral vein and its communications.

Have the patient ambulate, and examine the existing varicosities. Apply a tourniquet to the midthigh with the patient standing and allow the veins to fill with blood. After the patient walks for 5 minutes, examine the veins. With competent valves and patent lumens in the deep veins, the size of the superficial veins should reduce with exercise as blood flows into the deep veins. If the varicose veins remain engorged following exercise, both saphenous and communicating veins are incompetent. If the lumen of the superficial veins increases in diameter and pain occurs, the deep veins are occluded. Determine the level of the deep vein occlusion by applying the tourniquet at different levels and repeating the test.

Oscillometry

This procedure measures the total pulsatile blood flow in the limb segment and detects small volume changes, but it does not record nonpulsatile collateral blood flow. Oscillometry provides useful information when comparing extremities. Variations in readings depend on the placement of the cuff and the positions of the limb. Repeat the test and correlate the findings with clinical observations in questionable cases.

Arteriography

Visualization of the arterial tree of the lower extremities usually requires an injec-

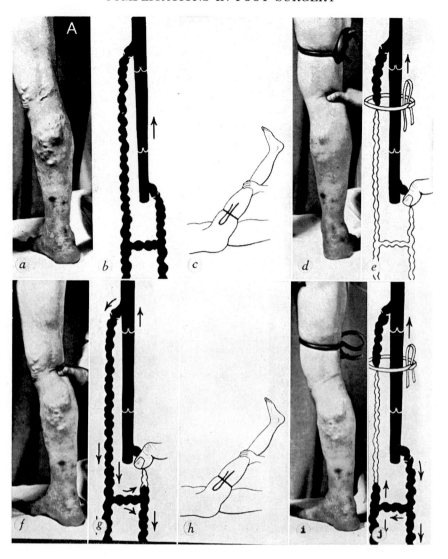

Figure 3.1. *A,* retrograde filling test (modified Brodie-Trendelenburg) showing incompetency of great and small saphenous veins. *a* and *b,* patient standing; both saphenous veins filled. *c,* veins emptied; tourniquet applied; thumb over small saphenous vein. *d* and *e,* patient standing; tourniquet occludes great saphenous vein; thumb occludes small saphenous vein. *f* and *g,* tourniquet is released after 15 seconds of standing. Prompt filling of veins proves incompetency of great saphenous vein. *h,* veins emptied again; tourniquet and thumb applied. *i* and *j,* patient standing; thumb removed in 15 seconds. Filling of veins proves incompetency of small saphenous vein. *B,* retrograde filling test (modified Brodie-Trendelenburg) showing competency of the great saphenous vein and incompetency of the small saphenous vein. *a* and *b,* patient standing; both systems are filled. *c,* veins emptied; tourniquet applied; thumb over small saphenous vein. *d* and *e,* patient standing; tourniquet occludes great saphenous vein; thumb occludes small saphenous vein. *f* and *g,* tourniquet released after 15 seconds of standing. No filling of veins proves competency of great saphenous veins. *h,* veins emptied again. *i* and *j,* patient standing; thumb removed after 15 seconds of standing. Filling of veins indicates incompetency of small saphenous vein. (*a, d, f* and *i* of both *A* and *B* from Meyers, T. T., and Cooley, J. C. Surg. Gynecol. Obstet. 99:733–744, 1954. Reprinted in Allen, E. V., Barker, N. W., and Hines, E. A., Jr. *Peripheral Vascular Diseases,* ed. 3. W. B. Saunders, Philadelphia, 1900, pp. 647–648. Reprinted by permission of *Surgery, Gynecology & Obstetrics* and W. B. Saunders Company.)

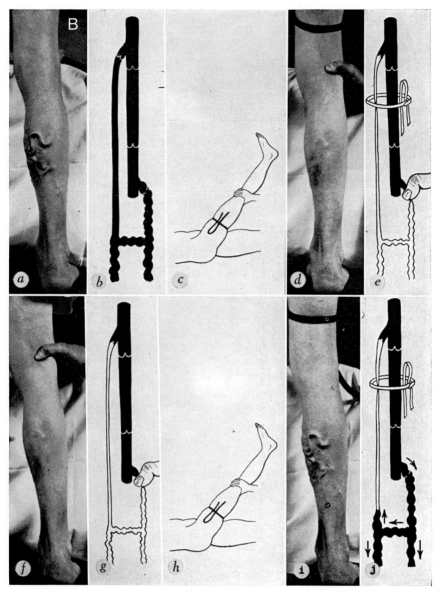

Figure 3.1. (*B*)

tion of radiopaque dyes (Hypaque®) into the vascular system. These dyes can have an effect on the smooth muscles of the blood vessels so that the actual state of the vascular tree may not be represented. However, the technique is valuable in establishing location and extent of obstruction, aneurysm, or gross abnormalities in the vascular tree.

Visualization of the lymphatic channels may also be achieved with radiopaque dyes. Venography and lymphangiography may also be performed in indicated cases.

Other Tests

Other tests include thermography, colorimetry, isotope clearance, and vibrometry. The reader is referred to the texts on peripheral vascular tests.

Plethysmography

Plethysmography reflects blood volume changes in the extremities, gives qualitative and quantitative information, and assesses the circulation of an involved area. Blood volume changes, which correspond to the pulsations of arteries, are represented as waves by the recording system. For example, occlusive disease states or vasospastic disorders are reflected by decreased amplitude of the pulse wave. There are set means and extremes of normal values for amplitude of pulsation at different locations on the upper and lower extremities, as well as a set ratio of ankle to wrist and above knee to above elbow. These ratios provide a basis for qualitative comparison to a normal range within the body.

Digital plethysmography measures blood flow by recording the volume changes at the end of a finger or toe. Examining digital pulse waves is similar to examining segmental pulse waves. Along with pulse waves, crest time and dicrotic notch morphology are important.

Venous congestion is created with a cuff around the ankle or the wrist. When the cuff is inflated to 60 or 70 mm Hg, the cuff prevents venous drainage but allows the arterial blood to enter the extremity distal to the tourniquet. Resulting volume changes indicate the actual blood flow as represented by the swelling of the digit. The flow to the digit is measured in cubic millimeters per second per milliliter of tissue.

The pulse and flow tests are run before and after vasodilation in indicated cases. If the values for pulse and blood flow are below normal before and after vasodilation, surgery is contraindicated. If the plethysmographic values are within normal limits, vasodilation tests are not necessary for pre-surgical studies. Plethysmographic values that are normal only after vasodilation indicate the need for vasodilation therapy postsurgically.

Vasodilating Procedures

Vasodilation for plethysmographic procedures is induced with the oral administration of 2 ounces of alcohol or by a posterior tibial nerve block. Vasodilation is manifested by an increase in pedal skin temperature, erythema, or flushing. If vasodilation is deemed necessary post-operatively, a posterior tibial nerve block or an adrenergic blocking agent such as tolazoline HCl is advisable. Tolazoline HCl is contraindicated in patients with coronary or cerebral vascular disease and hyperchlorhydria. Dosage is 25 mg t.i.d., or one 80-mg Lontab® once or twice a day. Nausea and tachycardia are possible side-effects. In some cases, 2 weeks are required before the effects of the adrenergic blocking agent can be noted clinically. If there is a question as to the patient's ability to tolerate increased cardiac output, consultation with a cardiologist is advised.

Skin Color Changes

The volume of blood flow and the blood color determine skin color changes. The size of the arteries and arterioles determines the blood flow. If blood flow is obstructed, as in thrombophlebitis, the skin is often cyanotic. Localized cyanosis of the skin may be due to venous congestion or to an organic occlusive process proximal to the area. A violaceous tint may mean complete or almost complete cessation of blood flow. Pallor in Raynaud's disease indicates cessation of blood flow in the capillaries. Excessive blood flow, polycythemia vera, and methemoglobinemia produce rubor.

A normal skin temperature range is 75°–90°F and is usually 5°–6° above room temperature. Skin temperature lower than the environmental temperature indicates vasospasm or organic occlusive arterial disease. A cold or blue extremity warrants further work-up. Adequate time should be allowed for the patient to acclimate to examining room conditions.

Trophic Changes

Trophic changes occur as deformed, thickened, brittle toenails, decreased nail growth, loss of hair, shiny skin, atrophy of the subcutaneous tissue, and tapered digits.

In the diabetic, abnormal weight stress and diabetic neuropathy often produce ulcers at the metatarsal heads and on the digits. Venous ulcers are typically seen above the medial malleolus.

Sickle cell ulcers are caused by obstruction of the small vessels. These ulcers present a punched out appearance with a whitish base and are painful.

Hines' ulcer is a painful lesion at the lower lateral aspect of the leg. The ulcer, which is palpable, is believed to be secondary to an arteriolar occlusion.

Diabetes Mellitus

A diabetic patient considered for surgery should be cleared by the primary physician. An assessment of the patient's circulatory status before elective surgery is a necessity.

Uncontrolled diabetics are poor surgical candidates for elective surgery because of the possibility of delayed wound healing and increased tendency for infection. Patients with trophic skin and nails, hair loss, and delayed capillary filling time warrant further testing for diabetes.

Pain

Pain is common in peripheral vascular disease. In ulceration and gangrene associated with thromboangiitis obliterans, pain is acute, while in arteriosclerosis obliterans, the pain will probably be less. The discomfort in ischemic neuritis is severe while the pain from ischemic neuropathy is burning and lancinating. It is most likely caused by ischemic changes in the nerve trunks and endings affected by occlusive arterial disease. The pain occurs in paroxysms and lasts from a few minutes to hours. It begins in the toes and radiates proximally to the leg. Nocturnal pain is intensified (Table 3.1).

Intermittent Claudication

With intermittent claudication, pain and discomfort affect muscles being exercised. Rest relieves the pain. The relationship between pain and exercise is the major characteristic in the diagnosis.

Claudication occurs when narrowed or obstructed arteries fail to provide adequate blood to the muscles. The gastro-soleus complex is often affected since the femoral and popliteal arteries are subject to atherosclerosis and arterial occlusion. Obstruction in the arteries proximal to the foot may cause claudication in the foot and can be misdiagnosed as a strain.

The severity of pain from intermittent claudication varies with the rate of walking, the grade of the terrain and temperature changes. In mild claudication, the patient decelerates but continues walking. In severe cases the patient must stop walking because of intense ischemic pain. The condition of most patients afflicted with intermittent claudication remains unchanged.

Graduated walking exercises stimulate the development of collateral circulation. Proper diet and weight control reduce the burden of obesity, and proper podiatric treatment avoids trauma and infection. Wearing tight stockings and ill fitting footgear are forbidden.

Patients should not use hot water foot baths or hot water bottles. To prevent ischemic damage, the general surgeon may perform sympathectomy to improve collateral circulation in certain patients.

Plethysmography will indicate the extent of collateral circulation, and the patient's healing rate can be assessed.

Doppler Ultrasonic Flow Detector

The principle of the ultrasonic flow detector was first described by Doppler in 1843. Sound travels as waves of determined frequency (oscillations per second). When these waves are reflected from a moving object, their frequencies change.

Blood represents a moving anatomical structure which can be detected by Doppler ultrasound. In 1961, Franklin described the use of an ultrasonic flow detector in animals. In 1963, Watson and Rushmer dem-

Table 3.1.
Differential Diagnosis of Pain in the Extremities*

I. LOCATION IN EITHER UPPER OR LOWER EXTREMITIES OR BOTH

Clinical entities in which symptom is found	Etiologic factor or pathogenesis	Conditions under which symptom is experienced	Effect of other conditions	Description of pain	Location	Signs of arterial or venous impairment	Neurologic findings
AO and TAO; AV¹ fistula; postligation or occlusion of main arteries, coarctation of aorta, marked anemia	Transient muscle ischemia	Exercise of muscles	Standing, sitting, and lying down relieve symptom	Fatigue, ache, cramp, compression sensation, located in exercising muscles (intermittent claudication)	Muscles of upper and lower extremities	Arterial involvement invariably present in occlusive arterial diseases but not in other entities	Minor ones may be present
TAO, AO; Raynaud's disease; postarterial embolism; frostbite; thrombosis associated with cervical rib or infectious diseases	Trophic changes of arterial origin (ulcer of gangrene)	Rest	Pain aggravated by moving involved portion	Sharp, continuous or intermittent; at times excruciating, at other times mild	Vicinity of ulcer or gangrene	Arterial involvement, severe locally	Minor ones may be present
Sudden occlusion of main artery by embolism or thrombosis	Acute anoxia of tissues	Rest	Pain exaggerated by movement	Severe, continuous excruciating; numbness and paresthesia	Digits and foot or hand	Arterial involvement invariably present	Anesthesia; hypesthesia; in severe type, foot and wrist drop
Polyneuritis; toxic neuritis; posttrench foot and frostbite	Peripheral neuritis	Rest	Little change with activity	Paresthesia: numbness; sense of swelling	Fingers and toes	None	Hypesthesia; anesthesia; loss of vibration sense perception
Psychoneuroses; normal individuals	Maintenance of limb in one position for prolonged period of time	Lying down or sitting; in case of hands, holding an object for any period of time	Activity relieves symptoms	Uncomfortable sensation, difficult to describe; numbness; paresthesia (restless hands and feet)	Digits and hand, forearm, foot, and leg	None	None
Causalgia; neuroma; occupational pressure on nerves	Injury of or pressure on peripheral nerves in limb	Rest	Slightest activity markedly exaggerates pain	Severe, excruciating, lancinating, burning	Hand or foot	Signs of increased sympathetic tonus	Signs of partial destruction, peripheral nerves
Posttraumatic vasomotor disorders	Injury of other tissues in limb	Rest	Activity exaggerates pain	Severe, continuous	Hand or foot	Signs of increased sympathetic tonus	None

Rheumatoid arthritis; osteoarthritis; acute rheumatic fever	Local changes in joints	Movement of involved joint; also present at rest	Rest relieves pain to some extent	Dull or sharp	Vicinity of involved joint(s)	Signs of increased sympathetic tonus in some instances	None
Glomus tumor	Dilated vascular channels with pressure on nerves in vicinity	Local heat, trauma, dependency	Elevation of normal environment relieves pain	Excruciating, burning	Around nailbed of digits	None	None
Dermatomyositis; non-specific myositis; myositis associated with systemic infections; polyarteritis nodosa	Myositis	Movement of muscle group; local pressure	Rest and heat relieve pain	Dull ache, at times severe	Involved muscle group	No gross findings	None
Erythromelalgia; early state of trenchfoot and frostbite	Exposure to heat	High environmental temperature or rise in body temperature	Dependency accentuates pain; elevation and immersion in cold water relieve it	Severe burning	Hands, fingers, feet, toes	None	None
Normal individuals; sequel, iliofemoral thrombophlebitis; AO and TAO: calcium deficiency; sudden loss of fluids and salt; varicosities	Stretching of muscles of limb	Lying on bed or sitting	Standing, walking, or massage relieves pain	Severe, cramp-like; pain, generally while in bed (night cramps)	Generally in calves; less often in feet, hands, thighs, forearms	Definite signs of arterial impairment in AO and TAO; signs of venous stasis in postphlebitic syndrome	None
AO; TAO: polyarteritis nodosa	Ischemic neuritis	Rest; lying in bed	Dependency usually relieves pain, occasionally exaggerates it; standing or walking relieves it	Paresthesia, lancinating pain; burning sensation; sensation of extreme coldness	Toes, fingers	Signs of arterial involvement in AO and TAO	Mild changes: reduction or absence of vibratory sense perception in digits
Superficial benign thrombophlebitis; superficial migratory thrombophlebitis	Acute occlusion of superficial veins	Movement of involved part or pressure over it	Rest relieves pain	Moderate, dull or sharp	Legs, thighs, forearms	Signs of superficial venous thrombosis	None
Axillary vein thrombosis; thrombosis of popliteal or iliofemoral vein	Acute occlusion of main venous channels	Rest	Movement exaggerates symptom	Severe, constant, dull at times	Along course of vein	Swelling; vasospasm; distention of superficial veins	None

* From Abramson, D. I.: Vascular Disorders of the Extremities, ed. 2, Table 3, Chap. 1. Hagerstown Md.: Harper & Row, Publishers, Medical Department, 19 00. Reprinted with permission of the author and publisher.

† AO, arteriosclerosis obliterans; TAO, thromboangiitis obliterans; AV, arteriovenous.

Clinical entities in which symptom is found	Etiologic factor or pathogenesis	Conditions under which symptom is experienced	Effect of other conditions	Description of pain	Location	Signs of arterial or venous impairment	Neurologic findings
Herpes zoster; neurofibroma; radiculitis; fracture of vertebra; Paget's disease; displaced disk; osteoarthritis	Pressure on nerve root at intervertebral foramen; irritation of posterior root ganglion	Rest	Movement may exaggerate pain	Burning	Entire extremity	No gross changes other than vasospasm at times	Present in some instances
Erysipelas; cellulitis associated with dermatophytosis	Acute cellulitis	Rest	Movement exaggerates pain	Intense	Site of lesion	None	None
II. LOCATION IN LOWER EXTREMITIES ONLY							
Shortening of Achilles tendon and gastrocnemius; paralysis of a group of muscles; tetany; extrapyramidal tract involvement	Paralysis or shortening of muscles; alterations in neuromuscular junctions	Exercise	Sitting or lying down relieves symptoms	Cramplike pain or sense of exhaustion	Calf	None	Signs of extrapyramidal tract involvement may be present
Sciatica; lumbrosacral disease	Pressure on nerve plexus or root	Change in position from lying down to standing	Activity does not particularly affect pain	Radiating	Along course of sciatic nerve	None	Absent Achilles tendon reflex and loss of sensation in toes may be noted
Sciatica; lumbrosacral disease	Pressure on nerve plexus or root	Change in position from lying down to standing	Activity does not particularly affect pain	Radiating	Along course of sciatic nerve	None	Absent Achilles tendon reflex and loss of sensation in toes may be noted
Pes planus metatarsalgia	Alterations in the dynamics of the foot	Standing	Walking may increase pain somewhat; lying down or sitting relieves it	Dull	Foot	None	None
Varicosities; postphlebitic syndrome	Trophic changes of venous origin (ulceration)	Rest	Activity exaggerates pain	Sharp pain or dull ache	Generally around medial malleolus	Signs of venous stasis	None
Severe varicosities; postphlebitic syndrome	Venous stasis	Standing; dependency	Elevation relieves pain; walking reduces it somewhat	Aching; heaviness; tiredness	Leg and foot	Signs of venous stasis	None

III. LOCATION IN UPPER EXTREMITIES ONLY

Cervical rib, scalenus anticus, hyperabduction, and costoclavicular syndromes; pressure of glands or tumors	Pressure on brachial plexus and subclavian artery and vein	Movement of arms and shoulders in different positions	Return to resting position relieves pain	Numbness; paresthesia	Fingers, hands, forearms	Temporary obliteration of pulse on assumption of responsible position; at times, permanent occlusion	Hyperesthesia; anesthesia
Angina pectoris; myocardial infarction; shoulder-hand syndrome	Referred pain	Physical activity; also at rest	Rest causes relief in case of angina	Numbness	Inner surface of arm and forearm; ulnar side of hand	Vasomotor alterations in shoulder-hand syndrome	None

onstrated that blood flow could be detected by pulsed ultrasound through intact skin. In 1966, Strandness proved the efficacy of ultrasound in the elevation of occlusive arterial disease.

The Doppler sound of arterial blood flow is easily recognized by its systolic and diastolic components. When a stenotic area is approached, the frequency of the Doppler signal increases. This is caused by the temporary increase in blood velocity caused by the narrowing of the lumen. In the case of complete occlusion, no sound will be heard distal to the site of blockage.

The Doppler unit (see Figure 3.2) consists of a transducer head connected to a frequency detector. A doppler is also capable of detecting venous pulses.

Ankle/Arm Systolic Blood Pressure Ratio

Normally, the blood pressure at the ankle is greater than at the arm. Travis Windsor, in 1950, reported that in cases of occlusive vascular disease, this ratio was often reversed. Baron and Heisler, in 1979, established a grading system for arterial occlusive disease bases on the ankle/arm systolic blood pressure ratio (see Table 3.2).

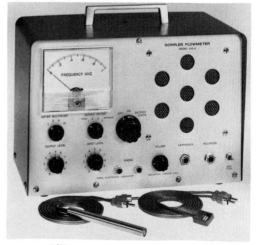

Figure 3.2. Doppler ultrasonic flowmeter, model 810-A (photo courtesy of Parks Electronic Laboratory, Beaverton, Oregon, with permission).

Table 3.2.
Grading System for Arterial Occlusive Disease[a]

Grade	Ankle/Arm Systolic Blood Pressure Ratio	Degree of Claudication
I	0.9–0.6	Mild to stable
II	0.6–0.4	Moderate to severe
III	0.4–0.2	Severe, with rest pain, and ischemic changes
IV	Less than 0.2	Severe rest pain, distal necrosis

[a] From Baron, H. C., and Heisler, E. Significance of ankle blood pressure in diagnosis of peripheral vascular disease. Am. Surg. 45: 289–292, 1979.

The ankle systolic blood pressure is best obtained using a Doppler ultrasonic flow detector in conjunction with a sphygmomanometer and a pneumatic occlusion cuff. This test should be performed prior to and following exercise.

Hypertension

Essential hypertension is indicated by a blood pressure reading greater than 140/90, with qualification for systolic change with age. The etiology of essential hypertension is generally unknown. A high degree of correlation exists clinically between hypertension and poor arterial perfusion in the lower extremities. Hypertension with peripheral edema and dyspnea, as well as arrhythmia, systolic or diastolic murmur, or irregular pulse, should be referred immediately to the primary physician. Left-sided congestive heart failure stimulates pulmonary signs of dyspnea and orthopnea. Pure right-sided failure is rare, but a right-sided failure due to left-sided failure is common. The lower extremity edema secondary to hypertension occurs in patients who are not in failure but who have venous insufficiency and/or stand for long periods of time.

Smoking

Nicotine may induce vasospasm and put stress on the cardiopulmonary system. Nicotine seriously affects the lower extremities by constricting cutaneous blood vessels, which in turn decreases skin blood flow as much as 40% in the foot. After smoking, the decrease in blood flow may last 20 to 50 minutes. Smoking affects the cutaneous blood vessels through the sympathetic nervous system.

Arteriovenous Fistulas

Arteriovenous fistulas are abnormal communications between an artery and vein. Arteries and veins arise from the embryonic vascular plexus, and only late in embryonic development do they divide into distinct structures.

Arteriovenous anastomoses develop normally in certain parts of the body, and they are numerous in the nailbeds and on the soles. The number of arteriovenous anastomoses is not fixed, but new anastomoses are formed with increased blood flow to an area. Arteriovenous shunts also occur in muscles, forming a short circuit through which blood flows during periods of metabolic inactivity.

Diagnosis of Congenital Arteriovenous Fistula

Varicose veins are generally present. The varices can occur early in life and be unilateral, or they may occur in an unusual location. Varicose veins may be associated with ulceration or elongation of the limb. In some cases, the enlarged varicosed veins may be tortuous. In about 50% of cases affecting the extremities, there are port wine stains, cavernous hemangiomas, or diffuse hemangiomas. There may also be increased hair growth and perspiration in the involved area. The temperature of the skin of the affected extremity is higher than the contralateral extremity. Usually, bruits and thrills are not evident in congenital arteriovenous fistula since the abnormal communications between artery and vein may be very small. Arteriography is of limited value when small vessels are involved and the fistulas are small.

Treatment

Management in the extremity is difficult when the arteriovenous communications are numerous. If the communications are single or a few communications are close together, surgical procedures can correct the condition.

TRAUMATIC ARTERIOVENOUS FISTULA

This fistula is produced by a penetrating wound that lacerates an artery and the adjacent vein. A communication develops between the traumatic openings in the involved vessels, or an aneurysmal sac is interposed between the artery and the vein.

Diagnosis

The primary diagnostic signs are the presence of a continuous systolic and diastolic bruit that is accentuated during systole. A thrill is often present. The thrill and bruit can be eliminated by compression of the artery proximal to the fistula, or by pressure over the site of communication. This completely or partially closes the fistula and the pulse rate falls (Branham's sign). Branham's sign is pathognomonic of arteriovenous fistula. Other signs are: the pulsatile mass of an associated false aneurysm, increased skin temperature at the site, varicosities, skin ulcerations, decreased arterial perfusion in the distal part, increased pulse rate and pulse pressure, accelerated limb growth in children, gangrene of the digits and the distal portion of the extremity as a result of ischemia, and cardiac enlargement with or without decompensation.

Arteriography may locate the fistula, determine its size, and indicate the mechanism of circulation below the fistula.

Treatment

A few fistulas close spontaneously as a result of thrombosis, but the majority must be repaired by excising the abnormal communication and adjacent vessels and reestablishing arterial continuity with a graft. If after 3–6 months, venous congestion occurs, a venous continuity must also be established.

Atherosclerosis

This is an organic occlusive disease that changes the intima of the arteries, producing focal accumulation of lipids, complex carbohydrates, blood and blood products, fibrous tissue, and calcium deposits. This condition of the vascular structure not only leads to arterial occlusion but causes loss of elasticity, thrombus formation, aneurysm, decreased blood flow and decreased or absent pulse distally, and anoxia of tissue.

Ulceration of the fatty plaques and embolization of cholesterol crystals or atherosclerotic debris are also manifested in the intima.

Atherosclerosis affects the main arteries in a patchy manner. Small arteries usually are not affected. It is the commonest cause of peripheral vascular disease; it narrows the lumen and promotes eventual vascular occlusion from thrombosis.

A loose correlation exists between age and the degree of degenerative arterial disease. Fluid dynamic stress leads to damage on the intima walls promoting the formation of fibrotic tissue. The degree of involvement seems to be related to family patterns, diet, race, sex, stress, and hypertension. It is not uncommon for younger males (25–30 years) to have severe coronary artery disease. Mönckeberg's sclerosis may occur in the diabetic at an earlier age, just as it does in hyperparathyroidism, and hypervitaminosis D from unknown causes.

Patients with diabetes mellitus develop more diffuse arteriosclerosis obliterans in the tibial and peroneal arteries and a more rapid progression of this disease than do nondiabetics.

Patients with femoropopliteal arteriosclerosis are generally in their 70's. The vast majority of patients in their 60's with aortoiliac obstructive disease are victims of atherosclerosis.

Atherosclerosis must be suspected in patients with weak or absent pulses and intermittent claudication of the buttocks, calf muscles, or feet. Many patients complain of cold feet, paresthesias, and nonhealing lesions of the foot. Rest pain may occur if the collateral blood supply to the limb is not adequate. When the tibial and peroneal arteries are obstructed, ischemic changes are absent and the popliteal pulse may be exaggerated because of increased distal resistance.

Clinically, there is also a decreased subpapillary venous plexus filling time, absence of, or minimal hair growth, thick nails and blanching upon elevation of the lower extremities, and an increased time (more than 30 seconds) for the color to return to the feet in a dependent position.

Plethysmography should be used to determine the vascular status. Both the volume and volume flow should be studied to determine the patient's ability to heal. A peripheral vascular consultation is in order if the occlusive disease is advanced. In such cases foot surgery should not be performed.

Aneurysms

Most aneuryms are associated with atherosclerosis, and they weaken or damage the media of the artery. Those not related to atherosclerosis are generally the result of injuries, penetrating wounds, or surgical trauma.

The most common peripheral aneurysm is a popliteal aneurysm, an important cause of ischemic symptoms in the lower extremities. Popliteal aneurysm can produce intermittent claudication, and the clot can cause distal embolization of the arteries.

Thromboangiitis Obliterans (TAO) (Buerger's Disease)

This is an organic inflammatory disease of the small and medium-size arteries and veins in which the walls of the vessels are infiltrated with lymphocytes and plasma cells. Red thrombi form in these vessels, and sterile microabscesses and multinucleated cells are found within the thrombi.

Males from the age of 20–40 are more commonly affected by this disease than are females. The typical TAO patient smokes heavily. Migratory superficial thrombophlebitis occurs in about 30–40% of TAO patients. The patient complains of intermittent claudication and extreme pain. There is a lack of pulse distal to the occlusion, signs of vasospasm, and a cyanotic rubor. Thrombus in the acute stage and inflammatory fibrosis in the chronic stage decrease the diameter of the arteries peripherally. Treatment consists of vasodilating drugs and steroids. For acute attacks, anticoagulant therapy is indicated. The patient should be advised to discontinue smoking.

The surgical risk is high. A thorough examination, including plethysmographic evaluation, is required, and consultation is recommended.

Raynaud's Disease

Raynaud's disease is a relatively benign idiopathic disorder seen most commonly in women in the 20–40 age group. Bilateral or symmetrical involvement occurs, causing pallor or cyanosis of the digits on exposure to cold or emotional stress. There is no concomitant disease in the main arteries and no association with primary systemic disease. The prognosis is good and, although attacks persist, they do not increase in severity. Patients who are candidates for surgery should protect the extremities from cold and stop smoking. Post-operatively, vasodilators and/or posterior tibial nerve blocks may be utilized to assure tissue perfusion. When emotional disturbance and nervous tension bring on the attacks, tranquilizers should be considered.

Raynaud's Phenomenon

Bilateral intermittent attacks of pallor or cyanosis of the digits may occur at any age.

Raynaud's phenomenon is linked to peripheral arterial disease. It may be secondary to trauma, atherosclerosis, thromboangiitis obliterans, and collagen disease, particularly scleroderma, or blood dyscrasias.

The intermittent ischemic episodes of the digits, which last from several minutes to several hours, are the result of loss of circulation from the closure of digital arterioles. Circulation in the capillary loops of the nailbed stops during the attack, and the fingers may not bleed when pricked. Plethysmography will not record blood flow to the digits during the attack.

Raynaud's phenomenon has a more serious prognosis than does Raynaud's disease. Gangrene may occur in small patches on the fingertips. Patients should avoid exposure to the cold and stop smoking. Some cases may require sympathectomy.

Erythromelalgia

Erythromelalgia is a bilateral, painful, erythematous disease of the extremities. The lower extremity is more commonly involved. The symptoms are analogous to extreme vasodilation: heat, redness, and swelling. Increased pulse amplitude can be demonstrated with plethysmography. Loss of vasomotor tone usually occurs when a certain temperature is reached (31°C or more). Erythromelalgia affects the male more frequently than the female. Although the etiology is unknown, the disease may be a phenomenon secondary to polycythemia or hypertension.

Patients complain of tingling, pain, burning, pressure, and sometimes pruritis. The condition, which occurs more commonly in the summer or in a warm environment, is aggravated by placing the legs in a dependent position. Painful attacks are relieved by elevation and by cooling the environment. Vasoconstrictors (e.g., ergotamine tartrate, ephedrine, nicotine) may prevent or relieve symptoms. Antihistamines can reduce swelling.

Acrocyanosis

Acrocyanosis is a relatively benign vasospastic condition in which the hands and feet are cyanotic, cold, and sweaty. Cyanosis disappears with elevation of the limb. Cool or cold environment and mental anxiety may be aggravating factors. The cyanosis, which is intensified by cold, is produced by arteriolar constriction, plus capillary and venous dilation.

Acrocyanosis is most prevalent in young women, and the hands are more affected than the feet. The condition is bilateral and symmetrical. Warm clothing and tranquilizers are indicated. When the patient is warm, the involved extremities are red or reddish blue in color. Some patients exhibit signs and symptoms of Raynaud's phenomenon.

Plethysmographic studies are indicated presurgically to determine the circulatory status.

HEMORRHAGIC DISORDERS

A careful history before surgery may reveal the existence of prior hemorrhagic disorders. Healing rate and the probability of post-operative complications must be ascertained.

Bleeding Disorders

Congenital coagulation disorders are usually discovered in infancy. The illnesses accompanying bleeding disorders include leukemia, liver disease, macroglobulinemia, and carcinomatosis. A tendency for ecchymosis may be indicative of thrombocytopenia or hemophilia. Hemarthrosis is associated with hemophilia and, if it recurs, may be pathognomonic of severe hemophilia. Clotting difficulties experienced with dental extractions and tonsillectomies or from past trauma should be ascertained. Menorrhagia is occasionally the result of a hematologic disturbance.

HEMOSTASIS

Knowledge of the mechanisms of hemostasis continues to grow at a fast pace. Technological development has allowed for the discovery of new substances involved in the complicated picture of the various clotting pathways. Three basic mechanisms are thought to be involved in hemostasis.

Vasoconstriction

When damage occurs to the endothelium of vascular tissue, a localized spasm of the vessel results, decreasing the size of the lumen. This spasm is thought to be neurogenic and of short duration, followed by a more sustained localized muscular contraction. This localized reaction depends in part upon the release of serotonin and other vasoconstricting substances. The overall effect of this initial slowing of blood flow is the activation of the other clotting mechanisms.

Platelet Function

The combination of diminished blood flow and exposed epithelial surfaces serves to activate the passing platelets by 1) changing their shape from round or ovoid to irregular. This change in platelet shape makes it far easier for their rupture to occur; 2) causing the platelets to adhere to the damaged epithelium forming a "loose plug" and 3) releasing still more serotonin.

Coagulation

EXTERNAL PATHWAY

Activation of the external mechanism occurs when vascular tissue is damaged. The function of this mechanism is thought to be primarily the rapid formation of a clot. Damaged tissue releases tissue thromboplastin, which reacts with factors IV, V, VII, and X to result in prothrombin activator. Prothrombin activator serves to catalyze the conversion of prothrombin to thrombin (see Figure 3.3).

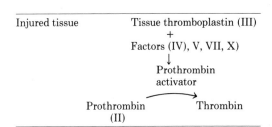

Figure 3.3. Activation of thrombin via external pathway.

INTRINSIC PATHWAY

The intrinsic pathway is initiated within the blood itself. The key difference between the activation of this system by platelet factor versus the activation of the extrinsic system (by tissue thromboplastin) is time. The extrinsic system occurs rapidly over the course of a few minutes. Activation of the intrinsic system can occur when blood is exposed to collagen or damaged epithelium. Platelet factor III is released and reacts with factors V, VII, IX, X, XI, and XII, resulting in the formation of prothrombin activator.

Common Blood Factors

  I. Fibrinogen
 II. Prothrombin
III. Tissue thromboplastin, platelet factor, thrombokinase
IV. Calcium
  V. Proaccelerin
 VI. Not assigned
VII. Stable factor
VIII. Anti-hemophilic factor (AHF)
 IX. Christmas factor
  X. Stuart-Prower factor
 XI. Plasma thromboplastin antecedent (PTA)
XII. Hageman factor
XIII. Fibrin stabilizing factor (FSF)

CLOTTING

Prothrombin activator from either hemostatic pathway catalyzes the transformation of prothrombin to thrombin. Thrombin in turn acts enzymatically to convert fibrinogen to fibrin. The resulting meshwork traps adjoining red blood cells, plasma, and platelets into a clot.

SYNERESIS

The final stage of hemostasis is known as syneresis. This shrinking of the clot occurs as the entrapped blood serum is secreted from the clot leaving the fibrinogen and clotting factors within the tightly structured clot.

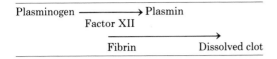

Figure 3.4. Activation of plasmin.

FIBRINOLYSIS

Dissolution of a blood clot is accomplished by enzymatic hydrolysis mediated by plasmin (fibrinolysin). Activation of plasmin requires factor XII and is illustrated below (Fig. 3.4).

ANTI-COAGULATION PLATELET FUNCTION

The smooth nature of the endothelial lining of blood vessels prevents platelet activation. Protein absorbed on this lining tends to be negatively charged and actively repels nearby platelets, preventing their activation. Any disease or drug which decreases the platelet count will serve to decrease coagulation.

COUMADIN

Prothrombin production occurs in the liver and requires vitamin K. Coumadin acts competitively with vitamin K and is thus an anticoagulant. Because of the competition between vitamin K and coumadin, vitamin K is administered when an overdose of coumadin causes prothrombin time to rise excessively, and is utilized as an anticoagulant when long-term therapy is required. It is a slow-acting drug in comparison with heparin and is taken orally (dosage, 1–20 mg daily). The most commonly prescribed coumadin drug is sodium warfarin. Indications for utilization of this drug include deep venous thrombosis, repeated episodes of thrombophlebitis, pulmonary embolisms, as well as long-standing arterial occlusive disease.

Use of coumadin-type drugs requires careful daily monitoring and prothrombin times. The patient and physician must be aware of other drugs which interact with coumadin, including phenylbutazone, chloralhydrate, and barbiturates.

HEPARIN

Heparin was first isolated by McLeon from the liver in 1916. Heparin must be used parentally and is most commonly available in doses of 5000 units per milliliter. The use of heparin requires hospitalization. Periodic assessment of clotting time and activated prothromboplastin time is necessary. Heparin is the drug of choice in acute arterial occlusion or venous thrombosis and after pulmonary embolism. The usual dosage is 5000 units administered intravenously every 4 hours.

Heparin is a powerful anticoagulant that is secreted by mast cells and tissue basophils. It prevents clotting by: 1) preventing activation of factor IX (Christmas factor); 2) accelerating the reaction of thrombin with anti-thrombin, neutralizing any thrombin formed; 3) inhibiting the action of thrombin on fibrinogen.

CALCIUM

Calcium is essential to the activation of many stages in the clotting process. Hypocalcemia results in a breakdown of the clotting mechanism at both the extrinsic and intrinsic levels and is required again in the activation of prothrombin to thrombin.

Delayed Clotting

Delayed clotting is caused by anticoagulant therapy that decreases liver synthesis of prothrombin (factor II) and other clotting factors produced by the liver, and interferes with the action of vitamin K in clotting factor synthesis (factors X, XII).

Several therapeutic agents cause a relative or absolute thrombocytopenia, either by direct effects upon the platelets or by marrow depression. Long-term therapy with salicylates increases the bleeding time because of decreased platelet agglutination. This can be reversed with vitamin K. Chloral hydrate, penicillin, and quinine cause purpura in some patients. ACTH, adrenalin, and cortisone drugs are procoagulants. Capillary fragility can be traced to vitamin C deficiency.

Laboratory Tests

CLOTTING TIME

This is an *in vitro* test in which a sample of blood is placed in a clean glass tube and tilted every 30 seconds until coagulation occurs. Normal clotting time is 5–9 minutes. This test is of limited value, being most useful in monitoring the action of heparin therapy.

BLEEDING TIME

This is an *in vivo* test of clot formation. An earlobe or fingertip is pierced and the time for stoppage of bleeding is noted. Clinically this test is not of great value because it does not differentiate what factors are responsible for clotting failure.

PROTHROMBIN TIME (PT)

This test provides a measure of the activity of the extrinsic pathway by measuring the total quantity of prothrombin present. A blood sample treated with oxalate to remove Ca^{++} is rapidly mixed with the blood and the clotting time measured. Normal time is 10–14 seconds. This test is commonly used to monitor coumadin therapy.

PARTIAL THROMBOPLASTIN TIME (PTT)

This provides a measure of the formation of intrinsic thromboplastin. If an abnormal result is obtained, normal plasma (factors I, V, VIII, XI, and XII) and normal serum (factors IV, VII, X, XI, and XII) are substituted, one at a time to determine which corrects the patient's defect. Therefore, deficiencies of factors VIII, IX, XI, or XII can be detected. This test is commonly used to monitor heparin therapy.

TOURNIQUET

The use of a tourniquet is widespread and considered to be a safe, accepted practice. The obvious advantage is the creation of a dry field that affords better visualization. The necessity of frequent sponging is reduced, and all structures are easily identified.

A digital tourniquet compresses both nerves and arteries. Wrap several layers of gauze sponge around the base of the toe before applying a tourniquet in order to protect the underlying structures.

When using an ankle or midthigh tourniquet, elevate and drain the leg for approximately 3 minutes to prevent thrombosis of stagnated blood. Apply padding under the cuff. At midthigh, the pneumatic cuff can be inflated from 250–450 mm Hg for adults, depending upon the girth. A cuff pressure of 175–275 mm Hg or lower is used for children. When a Martin's bandage is placed above the ankle, avoid excessive pressure on the superficial nerves, because tourniquet paralysis can ensue. If the tourniquet occludes the venous return without stopping arterial flow, there is danger of Volkman's ischemic contracture.

When operating under a dry field, avoid prolonged exposure to a hot spotlight, so that tissues do not dry out. Frequent irrigation keeps the tissues moist and viable. The tourniquet time limit is approximately 1½ hours for the healthy adult and approximately 1 hour for children and geriatric patients. At midthigh, it is recommended to release the tourniquet slowly to offset the sudden surge of blood into the extremity. This slow release prevents hypotension and tissue congestion. If reactive hyperemia does not bring full color return to the feet including the toes within 3–4 minutes after release, place the involved extremity in a dependent position. If only one digit is involved, check for a tight or poorly placed suture. In cases of vasospasm, tranquilizers may be required. Following reactive hyperemia, have the patient equilibrate and allow the surgical wound to bleed out before applying dressings.

Complications

Tourniquets compress tissue, causing injury to the musculature, vascular structures, and peripheral nerves. Injury to the vascular structure may enhance thrombus and embolus formation, and injury to the peripheral nerves can cause transient or permanent paralysis. Superficial nerve damage by compression may bring paresthesia, burning, or exaggerated pain postoperatively. Edema may be more pronounced as a result of anoxia.

If tourniquet paralysis of a peripheral nerve does not improve after several months, surgical exploration may be necessary to determine the presence or absence of fibrosis around the neural sheath or to rule out a neuroma formation. In most cases, tourniquet paralysis of the lower extremities is transient and spontaneous recovery occurs within a few days to a few weeks.

A tourniquet should not be used in a patient with a history of arteritis, phlebitis, or extensive varicosities.

Before final closure is made, release the tourniquet and ligate bleeding vessels.

Tissue Effects

With a tourniquet, the complete arrest of circulation encourages acidosis within the tissue, depending on the tourniquet time. An excess of 2 hours causes ischemia of the limb and a markedly elevated pCO_2 with a severely decreased pH. Prolonged tourniquet time can produce irreversible tissue damage and changes in the coagulability of the blood. Clotting time may be as long as 16 minutes.

Proper clotting time prevents hematoma in the operative area, so blood coagulability must be close to normal at the end of surgery. Tourniquet ischemia lasting over 2 hours encourages severe muscle fatigue. Some surgeons use pneumatic tourniquets for up to 3 hours with no ill effects, but it is recommended that surgery with a tourniquet should be limited to 2 hours to avoid ischemia.

THROMBOPHLEBITIS

Thrombophlebitis is an acute inflammatory disease in which there is partial or complete occlusion of the vein by a thrombus. Three primary etiologic factors contribute to thrombophlebitis, whether it is deep or superficial. They are lesions of the endothelium, venous stasis, and hypercoagulability of the blood. When two or more of these factors are present, a thrombophlebitis episode is imminent.

Sclerosing agents injected into the veins, vascular trauma from local anesthesia, surgical trauma, tourniquet hemostasis, tight dressings and casts, and severe stretching of superficial venous structures can produce thrombophlebitis. Infectious processes and ischemia may damage the endothelial lining of the veins and cause thrombus formation. Patients with varicose veins have stasis and endothelial pathology and consequently are susceptible to thrombophlebitis. Contraceptive drugs have also been implicated in the development of thrombophlebitis. Thrombophlebitis of the large superficial vein of the leg is marked by a slow onset of 12 hours or more, with mild symptoms. Tenderness over the vein is usually the first symptom and is accompanied by a slight elevation in temperature. Swelling is generally limited to a small area and is difficult to measure in the early stage. The skin over the involved area is red and swollen, and tenderness may persist for several weeks.

Thrombophlebitis can be confused with cellulitis or infection. Differentiation is imperative when directing appropriate therapy. The superficial veins may dilate and incapacitate the valves, depriving the subcutaneous tissue of nutrition and causing ulceration.

Involvement of the deep veins is characterized by a sudden onset and pain in the calf, popliteal area, inner side of the thigh or the groin. A febrile state of 100°–102°F may persist for several weeks. There is usually a positive Homan's sign. With deep vein thrombophlebitis, there may be associated reflex arterial and venous spasm. If obstructive deep thrombophlebitis occurs in the femoral or iliac veins, edema will be pronounced.

Differential Diagnosis

Thrombophlebitis must be differentiated from plantaris tendon injuries, which exhibit a positive Homan's sign and edema. Ecchymosis may appear along the tendo achilles within 24 hours of trauma. Homan's sign is positive in traumatic myositis of the calf also. The foot and leg may become edematous and the calf muscles tender. The presence of edema due to thrombophlebitis must be differentiated from edema caused by lymphadenitis, cardiac decompensation, arterial occlusion, and lymphatic obstruction.

Prevention

Preventive measures are based on the patient's history. In patients with varicose veins, tight garters and shoes should be avoided. Gradient elastic stockings should be prescribed, and a tourniquet should be avoided in surgery. When using a local anesthetic, a small-bore needle with minimal anesthetic volume is advised. Avoid traumatizing the dorsal venous arch, the small and great saphenous veins, and the deeper veins accompanying the arteries. In surgery, identify the neurovascular structures and retract instead of ligating them. If the small vein must be transected, ligate it to prevent thrombus.

In patients with histories of pulmonary embolism, phlebitis, and varicose veins, the lower extremities should be wrapped with elastic bandages. If edema persists, application of a rubber bandage over a stocking is recommended. The elastic bandage should be applied in the morning and kept on except when the patient is in bed at night. This measure should be continued for several months.

Encourage early ambulation to prevent venous stasis and frequent exercise of the leg muscles through movement of the ankles, feet and toes while the patient is in bed or sitting in a chair.

A patient with a history of several episodes of deep vein thrombophlebitis is a high surgical risk since thrombophlebitis often recurs.

Complications

With infectious or septic thrombophlebitis, a thrombus may form with many pathologic organisms. An embolus from the infected thrombus can get into general circulation, lodge in the lungs and produce a pulmonary abscess. If emboli get into the portal circulation, there is danger of multiple abscesses occurring in the liver. Abscesses in the lungs or the liver cause general pyemia, and acute endocarditis may result, serving as a focus for disseminating bacteria.

In addition, chronic venous insufficiency, postphlebitic syndrome, and post-phlebitic neuropathy may develop.

Hematogenic thrombophlebitis has been noted with polycythemia vera, pernicious anemia, and lymphatic leukemia.

Treatment

Consider the following therapeutic course post-operatively.

1. Reassure the patient, and prescribe tranquilizers and analgesics.
2. Consult an internist and initiate anticoagulant therapy.
3. Instruct the patient to elevate the limb, and place a comfortably warm, moist towel over the area. Cover the towel with plastic and use an Ace bandage to hold these in place.
4. Anti-inflammatory agents such as phenylbutazone may be helpful.
5. Oral enzymes may be helpful.
6. Elevate the foot of the bed to attain gravitational venous drainage.
7. Appropriate antibiotics are advised if suppurative thrombophlebitis is suspected.
8. Prescribe a low-fat diet since lipids have an increased clot accelerating effect.
9. Eliminate smoking.
10. Control hyperuricemia because this condition increases the platelet adhesive index.
11. For superficial thrombophlebitis, use a mild compression elastic bandage or elastic stocking up to the knees. As soon as possible, the patient should exercise and walk moderately to pre-

vent postphlebitic ulcerations. Encourage periods of rest and elevation.

12. In thrombophlebitis of the foot, use appropriate appliances to assist in aligning the component parts and to promote improved function and circulation.
13. Put obese patients on a low-calorie diet to minimize stress and strain on lower extremities.
14. Use diuretics as needed.

ARTERIAL EMBOLUS

Emboli contain blood clots (thrombi), atherosclerotic debris, cholesterol crystals, and fat emboli from bone injuries. Emboli that originate in the heart may derive from myocardial infarction with thrombus forming over the infarcted area, rheumatic heart disease with mitral stenosis with or without atrial fibrillation, subacute or acute bacterial endocarditis, chronic congestive heart failure, and myxomas of the heart. An arterial embolus rarely originates from a peripheral vein thrombus. Arterial emboli usually lodge at the aortic bifurcation, femoral bifurcation, and popliteal trifurcation. The sudden obstruction of arterial blood flow causes excruciating pain and paresthesia. The pulses distal to the occlusion are lost and the veins collapse. If atheromatous microemboli obstruct the vascular tree, they can cause spontaneous painful and dusky discoloration of one or more toes.

If a collateral circulation is not present or adequate, ischemia and loss of the limb may ensue. Gangrene is common after the age of 60, since collateral vessels also become arteriosclerotic. The larger the artery involved with the embolus, the worse the prognosis. Aortoiliac saddle emboli are linked to a high incidence of limb loss unless the emboli are removed quickly. Recurrent embolization, especially in atrial fibrillation with mitral stenosis, has a mortality rate in excess of 20%. When emboli affect the large vessels such as the aorta, nausea, vomiting, and shock may ensue.

Patients suspected of incurring arterial emboli should be referred promptly for emergency care. Anticoagulation therapy with intravenous heparin prevents propagation of the thrombus distal to the embolus. If the foot and lower extremities show no ischemic rest pain and have normal sensation and motion, continue conservative care. With acute pain, hypesthesia, and loss of motor function, surgical removal of the embolus is indicated. Most femoral emboli and nearly all emboli to the aortic bifurcation require surgical removal to prevent ischemia and limb amputation. A method widely accepted involves a Fogarty balloon catheter, which is introduced through a small arteriotomy into the vessel containing the embolus and the propagated thrombus. When the inflated balloon presses against the arterial wall and the catheter is withdrawn, the intervening thrombus and embolus are extracted.

HEMATOMA

A hematoma is a sharply demarcated, well-localized extravasation of blood into tissues or dead space. It may be caused by trauma, inadequate hemostasis, failure to obliterate dead space and poor ligation during surgery. Hematoma delays wound healing and can cause wound sloughing and occasionally localized infection. There is no circulation within a hematoma until it becomes organized and therefore tissue apposition is prevented and a culture medium for bacterial growth is afforded. A hematoma puts pressure on neurovascular structures, decreases circulation and creates pain. If it is still connected to the lumen of the vessel where it originated, a pulsating hematoma or a false aneurysm may be formed. If it becomes calcified in its later stages, it must be differentiated from myositis ossificans.

Treatment depends on the stage of development. A fresh hematoma can be aspirated followed by a compression dressing. If it is extensive and hemorrhage persists with a pressure dressing, the wound must be opened, bleeding vessels identified, ligated, and the wound reclosed with a compressive bandage.

With a fibrotic hematoma, the recommended procedure is surgical removal, ligation of bleeding vessels and closure of the dead space.

Hematoma causes blood accumulation in the tissue spaces and exerts pressure on the capillaries and veins. Stagnation and clotting within the lumen of the vessel result, affecting venous and lymphatic drainage and causing gross edema. There is marked proliferation of fibroblasts and capillary endothelium, which develops granulation tissue and fibrous connective tissue.

Tendency towards calcification exists because blood components have an affinity for calcium. Therefore, ossifying hematoma in muscles and myositis ossificans are frequently confused. In myositis ossificans the aberrant bone is usually adjacent or attached to a nearby bone, and it is frequently parallel to a long bone.

Subungual hematoma occurs when there is free blood between the nail and nailbed. Elevation of the nail or drainage through the nail plate relieves the pressure and pain.

GANGRENE

Gangrene is the putrefaction of necrotic tissue as a result of insufficient blood supply. Dry gangrene indicates arterial occlusion, and the etiology can be traced to any peripheral vascular disease, be it spastic or nonspastic in etiology.

Moist gangrene suggests some degree of venous congestion, with the bacterial putrefaction in the involved area being dark blue, swollen and painful. It may be seen with severe, uncontrolled diabetes mellitus, thromboangiitis obliterans and osteomyelitis. Gas gangrene can be a sequela.

X-rays will rule out osteomyelitis. Culture and sensitivity tests are recommended. Systemic antibiotic therapy should be initiated if infection is present. Keep the local area dry and clean. If no evidence of active or spreading infection with pyrexia, cellulitis or leukocytosis exists, have the patient ambulate to stimulate collateral circulation and prevent venous thrombosis. Work with a peripheral vascular specialist to determine any additional therapy.

Gangrene post-operatively is not a common sequela. Multiple surgical procedures in a small area can compromise circulation and cause gangrene.

Patients with scleroderma have a peripheral vascular disease that produces intermittent vasospasm. Sclerosis of the skin is often seen, and the toes may become pointed and shrunken. Occasionally, subcutaneous nodules of calcium may be palpable. Gangrene may appear at the end of the toes.

In arteriosclerosis obliterans, thrombosis in the femoral and popliteal region is common. Tissue ischemia causes atrophy and thinning of the skin, loss of subcutaneous fat, and muscle atrophy. In the digits, fat is replaced by fibrous tissue and osteoporosis, and ischemic neuropathy may be noted. The tissue ischemia can lead to gangrene and such patients are best treated palliatively.

LYMPHEDEMA

Lymphatic vessels are much like modified veins with valvular components. They are found accompanying primary blood vessels. The superficial and deep lymphatic vessels have a primary communication only at the popliteal and inguinal lymph nodes. The primary superficial lymphatics in the lower extremities accompany the small and great saphenous veins. The deep lymphatic vessels accompany the deeper vascular structures.

The lymphatic vessels remove approximately 50% of the circulating tissue protein to the general circulation and are essentially noncontractile, and movement of the lymphatic fluids is dependent on muscle contraction and filtration of fluid from tissue spaces into its capillaries. If a lymphatic vessel is obstructed, lymphatic pressure will increase, which dilates the vessels. Lymph fluid then progresses to other communicating channels. If stasis persists, the fluid's protein level will increase fibroblastic activity. This further increases fibrosis and stasis, so that the cycle becomes self-perpetuating.

The etiology of secondary lymphedema is most often related to trauma of surgery and infection, which causes lymphangitis and cellulitis.

Early symptoms of lymphedema affect the foot, ankle and the lower extremity. As it progresses, the entire extremity increases in soft tissue size and density.

Treatment depends upon the etiologic factor. The following measures are recommended.

1. Bed rest, with the affected extremities elevated about 30 degrees above body level.
2. Diuretics to reduce the edema.
3. Intermittent compression unit and premeasured elastic stockings with proper gradient pressures.
4. Determination of any infection with appropriate tests, and selection of a suitable antibiotic if necessary.

It is imperative that lymphedema be treated rapidly following pedal surgery to prevent extensive fibrotic development and subsequent chronicity.

SYMPATHECTOMY

The mechanisms controlling blood flow to the skin are vasoconstriction on the one hand and inhibition of vasoconstrictive mechanisms on the other hand. Active vasodilation is almost entirely lacking. Vasoconstrictive mechanisms from the sympathetic system are in a tonic state of activity. The influence of the system is primarily upon the skin of the soles and palms of the hands. Blood flow is reduced by restriction of the size of the terminal arteries and arterioles. Blood flow is increased by passive dilatation of the vessels which follows inhibition of the chronically active vasoconstrictive impulses. Sympathectomy cannot be relied upon to augment blood flow to muscles. Its major effect is upon the nutrition of the skin.

Two to 3 months following sympathectomy, blood flow to the extremity is approximately double that of the pre-operative level. Generally, there is no clinical deterioration of the sympathectomized limb unless a major extension of the arterial occlusion has occurred.

Sympathectomy works best with patients whose main symptom has been intermittent claudication of a mild to moderate nature. Superficial or localized necrosis of the toes will often improve, but ischemia of the entire forefoot, severe rest pain, atrophy of skin or muscle or other advanced arterial insufficiencies cannot be arrested or improved solely by sympathectomy. Advanced arterial insufficiencies may require arterial reconstruction.

Sympathectomy may be helpful in Buerger's disease, if the patient stops smoking. It is useful in Raynaud's disease and other vasospastic diseases that do not respond to medical therapy. It aggravates lymphedema.

Patients who are to benefit from lumbar sympathectomy must have a demonstrable lumbar sympathetic activity. Patients with diabetes mellitus may have an absence of sympathetic nervous tone, especially in the lower limbs.

Suggested Readings

Abramson, D. I., ed. *Circulation in the Extremities.* Academic Press, New York, 1967.

Abramson, D. I., *Vascular Disorders of the Extremities,* 2nd ed. Harper, New York, 1974.

Adams, F. D. *Physical Diagnosis.* Williams & Wilkins, Baltimore, 1958.

Altman, M. L. Use of the pneumatic tourniquet for hemostasis in foot surgery. J. Foot Surg. 8:25, 1969.

American College of Surgeons. *Manual of Pre-operative and Post-operative Care.* W. B. Saunders, Philadelphia, 1967.

Baron, H. C., and Purdy, R. T. The Ischemic Lower Extremity. *A Scientific Exhibit.* U. S. A.

Baron, H. C., and Hiesiger, E. Ankle-arm blood pressure ratio. N. Y. St. J. Med. 78:1072–1076, 1978.

Baron, H. C., and Hiesiger, E. Significance of ankle blood pressure in diagnosis of vascular disease. Am. Surg. 45:289–292, 1979.

Bateman, J. E. *Trauma to Nerves in Limbs.* W. B. Saunders, Philadelphia, 1961.

Beninson, J. Six years of pressure-gradient therapy. Angiology 12:38–45, 1961.

Bertelsen, D. Reaction of the venous wall to experimentally induced thrombi. Acta Chir. Scand. 135:491–494, 1969.

Birnstingl, M. *Peripheral Vascular Surgery,* Philadelphia, Lippincott, 1974.

Block, B. H. Doppler ultrasonic diagnosis of vascular insufficiency of the lower extremity. Arch. Podiatr. Med. Foot. Surg. 4:45–54, 1978.

Borgeas, A. T. Avascular necrosis following plantar condylectomy. J. Foot Surg. 10:21–24, 1971.

Boyd, W. C. *A Textbook of Pathology.* Lea & Febiger, Philadelphia, 1961.

Brainerd, H., Margen, S., and Chatton, M. I. *Current Diagnosis and Treatment.* Lanfe, Los Altos, 1968.

Britton, R. C. Management of peripheral edema, including lymphedema of the arm, after radical mastectomy. Cleve. Clin. Q 26:53–61, 1959.

Brodie, B. C. *Pathology and Surgery.* Longman, Brown, Green & Longman, London, 1846.

Brush, B. E., Wylie, J. H., and Beninson, J. Some devices for the management of lymphedema of the extremities. Surg. Clin. North Am. 39:1493–1498, 1959.

Bunnell, S. *Bunnel's Surgery of the Hand,* 5th ed. J. B. Lippincott, Philadelphia, 1970.

Cecil, R. D., and Loeb, R. F. *A Textbook of Medicine,* 10th ed. W. B. Saunders, Philadelphia, 1959.

Christopher, F. *Minor Surgery.* W. B. Saunders, Philadelphia, 1944.

Collens, W. S., et al. Conservative management of gangrene in the diabetic patient. JAMA 181:690–698, 1962.

Crawley, J. J. *Vascular Surgery, Vol. 2: Peripheral Venous Diseases.* Harper, New York, 1975.

Davis, L. *Christopher's Textbook of Surgery,* 7th ed. W. B. Saunders, Philadelphia, 1960.

Dible, H. *Pathology of Limb Ischaema,* Green, St. Louis, 1967.

De Takats, G., and Vaithianathan, T. Bodily defenses against thrombosis. Am. J. Surg. 120:73–76, 1970.

Doppler, C. *Veber das Farbige Licht der Doppelstern.* Vienna, Austria, 1842.

D'Souza, M. F. Generalized lymphedema with yellow nails, pleural effusions and macroglobulinaemia. Proc. R. Soc. Med. 63:24, 1970.

Edwards, E. A. Nail changes. N. Engl. J. Med. 239:362–365, 1948.

Evans, D. S. The diagnosis of the deep vein thrombosis by ultrasound. Nursing Times 65:1319, 1969.

Ferguson, L. K. *Surgery of the Ambulatory Patient,* 4th ed. J. B. Lippincott, Philadelphia, 1966.

Fish, P. J., Corrigan, T., and Fakkar, W. Arteriography using ultrasound. Lancet 1:1269–1270, 1972.

Fox, I. M., et al. The pneumatic tourniquet in extremity surgery. JAPA 71:5, 237–242, 1981.

Franklin, D. L., Schlegel, W. A., and Rushmer, R. F. Blood flow measured by Doppler frequency shift of backscattered ultrasound. Science 134:564–568, 1961.

Friedman, S. A., and Rakow, R. B. Osseous lesions of the foot in diabetic neuropathy. Diabetes 20:1971.

Giannestras, N. J. *Foot Disorders, Medical and Surgical Management.* 2nd ed. Lea & Febiger, Philadelphia, 1973.

Goldberg, B., et al. *Diagnostic Uses of Ultrasound.* Grune & Stratton, New York, 1975.

Goodman, L. S., and Gilman, A. *The Pharmacological Basis of Therapeutics,* 5th ed. Macmillan, New York, 1975.

Greenfield, G. B. *Radiology of Bone Diseases.* 2nd ed. J. B. Lippincott, Philadelphia, 1975.

Gross, C. M., ed. *Gray's Anatomy of the Human Body,* 29 ed. Lea & Febiger, Philadelphia, 1973.

Haller, J. A., Jr. *Deep Thrombophlebitis, Pathophysiology and Treatment,* vol. 4. W. B. Saunders, Philadelphia, 1967.

Haller, J. A., Jr. Pathophysiology and management of postphlebitic venous insufficiency. South. Med. J. 63:177–182, 1970.

Halmovic, H. *Vascular Surgery.* McGraw, New York, 1976.

Hokanson, D. E. Mozensky, D. J., and Sumner, D. S. Ultrasonic arteriography: A non-invasive method of arterial visualization. Radiology 102:1435–436, 1972.

Holling, H. E. *Peripheral Vascular Diseases: Diagnosis and Management.* Lippincott, Philadelphia, 1972.

Holzknecht, F., Spottl, F., Constantini, R., Knapp, E., Herbst, M., and Braunsteiner, H. Platelet adhesion before and after venous occlusion. Atherosclerosis 2:105–117, 1970.

Hugo, N. E. Recent advances in the treatment of lymphedema. Surg. Clin. North Am. 51:111–123, 1971.

Jackson, B. T., and Kinmonth, J. B. Pes cavus and lymphedema. J. Bone Jt. Surg. 52B:518–520, 1970.

Johnson, W. B., and Golda, K. R. Venous thromboembolic disease. JAPA 71:254, 1981.

Juergens, J. L., et al. Peripheral Vascular Diseases, 5th ed. W. B. Saunders, Philadelphia, 1980.

Kanof, N. M. Gold leaf in the treatment of cutaneous ulcers. J. Invest. Deratol. 43:441, 1964.

Kelikian, H. *Hallux Valgus: Allied Deformities of the Forefoot and Metatarsalgia.* Saunders, Philadelphia, 1965.

Kramer, D. W. *Manual of Vascular Disorders.* Blakiston, Philadelphia, 1940.

Kruse, R. D., Kruse, A., and Britton, R. C. Physical therapy for the patient with peripheral edema: Procedures for management. Phys. Ther. Rev. 40:29–33, 1960.

Lambie, J. M., Mahaffy, R. G., Barber, D. C., Karmody, A. M. Scott, M. M., and Matheson, N. A. Diagnostic accuracy in venous thrombosis. Br. Med. J. 2:142–143, 1970.

Landau, J., and Stanley, J. JAPA 53:434–438, 1963.

Lapayowker, M. S., Cliff, M. M., and Tourtelotte, D. D. Arthrography in the diagnosis of calf pain. Radiology 95:319–323, 1970.

Leopold, S. Perifheral disorders. *Footprints* July, 1968, p. 5.

Lewin, P.: *The Foot and Ankle.* Lea & Febiger, Philadelphia, 1947.

Lewis, T. *Vascular Disorders of the Limbs.* Macmillan, New York, 1936.

Lieberman, J. S. Region III lecture, Gullman Laboratory, New York Hospital. Cornell University Medical Center, April, 1970.

Little, O. M. *Major Amputations for Vascular Disease.* Churchill, London, 1975.

Lofgen, K. A. Kustler, G., and Hollinshead, W. H. Anatomy of the veins of the foot. Surg. Gynecol. Obstet. 127:817–823, 1968.

Lofgren, K. A., and Lofgren, E. P.: Extensive ulcerations of the post-phlebitic leg. Arch. Surg. 103:554–560, 1971.

Lord, J. W., Jr.: Varicose veins: A surgeon's view. Hosp. Med. 5:61–77, 1969.

MacCaughey, A. M., and Welch, J. *Instructions for Pressure Therapy Management.* Pamphlet from Physical Therapy Department, St. Francis Hospital, Evanston, Ill. April, 1963.

Makin, G. S. A clinical trial of "Tubigrip" to prevent deep venous thrombosis. Br. J. Surg. 56:373–375, 1969.

Mann, R. A. *DuVries' Surgery of the Foot,* 4th ed. C. V. Mosby, St. Louis, 1978.

Mannich, J. and Coffman, J. *Ischemic Limbs: Surgical*

approved & Physiological Principals. Grune, New York, 1973.

Margo, M. K. Surgical treatment of conditions of the forepart of the foot. J. Bone. Jt. Surg. 49A:1665–1674, 1974.

Martin, P. The failure of compression stockings (Tubigrip) to prevent deep thrombosis after operation. Br. J. Surg. 57:296–299, 1970.

Millberg, J. L., and Tolmach, J. A. Treatment of chronic leg ulcers with absorbable gelatin sponge (Gelfoam) powder. JAMA 156:12, 1954.

Miller, E. Role of lymphangiography in evaluating patients with lymphedema. Mod. Treat 6:375–380, 1969.

Modell, W. *Drugs of Choice.* C. V. Mosby, St. Louis, 1980.

Moyer, J. E., Rhoads, J. E., Garrott, A. S., and Harkings, H. N. *Surgery, Principles and Practices.* J. B. Lippincott, Philadelphia, 1970.

Mullick, S. C., Wheeler, H. B., and Songster, G. F. Diagnosis of deep venous thrombosis by measurement of electrical impedance. Am. J. Surg. 119:417–422, 1970.

Naide, M., and Naide, D. Management of thrombphlebotos and pulmonary embolism. Part II. In Leaman, W. G. Jr., ed. *Pennsylvania Medicine, Cardiovascular Briefs,* Jan, 1970, p. 71.

Ochsnor, A. Preventing and treating venous thrombosis. Postgrad. Med. 44:91, 1968.

Patterson, L. Surgical treatment of lymphedema and treatment of lymphangiosarcoma. Mod. Treat. 6:413–421, 1969.

Perthes, G. Deutsche Med. Wchnschr 21:253, 1895.

Pories, W. J., and Strain, W. H. Once upon a trace metal: The Zinc story. Med. Opinion Rev. 7:38–45, 1971.

Pugh, D. G. *Roentgenologic Diagnosis of Diseases of Bone.* Williams & Wilkins, Baltimore, 1950.

Richards, R. L. *Peripheral Arterial Disease: Physician's Approach.* Livingstone, Edinbourgh, 1970.

Rittenhouse, E. A., and Brockenbrough, E. C. A method of assessing the circulation distal to a femoral artery obstruction Surg. Gynecol. Obstet. 129:538, 1969.

Rosengarten, D. S., Laird, J. Jeyasingh, K., Silver, D. Gleysteen, J. J., Rhodes, G. R., Georgiade, N. G., and Anlyan, W. G. Surgical treatment of the refractory post-phlebitic ulcer. Arch. Surg. 103:554–560, 1971.

Siegel, B., Popsky, G. L., and Wagner, D. K. Comparison of clinical evaluation of confirmed lower extremity venous disease. Surgery 64:332–338, 1968.

Siegel, B., Popsky, G. L., et al. A Doppler ultrasound method for diagnosing lower extemity venous disease. Surg. Gynecol. Obstet. 127:339, 1968.

Spittell, J. A., Jr. Treatment of secondary lymphedema. Mod. Treat. 6:384–390, March 1969.

Steel, P. H. Boot-leg phlebitis. JAMA 218:739, 1971.

Stein, J. M., and Pruit, B. A., Jr. Suppurative thrombophlebitis. N. Engl. J. Med. 282:1452–1455, 1970.

Stillwell, G. K. Treatment of postmastectomy lymphedema. Mod. Treat. 6:396–412, 1969.

Strandness, D. E., Jr., and Sumner, D. S. *Ultrasonic Techniques In Angiology.* Hans Huber Publishers, Vienna, Austria, 1975.

Strandness, D. E., Jr., McCutcheon, L., E., and Rushmer, R. F. Application of a transcutaneous Doppler flowmeter in evaluation of occlusive arterial disease. Surg. Gynceol Obstet. 122:1039–1045, 1966.

Strandness, D. E., Jr., Schultz, R. D., Sumner, D. S., and Rushmer, R. F. Ultrasonic flow detection in the evaluation of peripheral vascular disease. Am. J. Surg. 113:311–320, 1967.

Tsadakas, E., Rigas, A., and Chrusanthkapoalos, S. New aspects in the surgical treatment of lymphedema of the extremities. Surgury 68:53–61, 1959.

Tsapogas, J. H., Miller R., Peabody, R. A., and Eckert, C. L. Detection of post-operative venous thrombosis and effectiveness of prophylactic measures. Arch. Surg. 101:149–154, 1970.

Tsapogas, M. J., Goussous, H., Peabody, R. A., Karmody, A. M., and Eckert, C. Post-operative thrombosis and the effectiveness of prophylactic measures. Arch. Surg. 103:561–567, 1971.

Watson, T., and Rushmer, R. F. Ultrasonic blood flow transducers. Proc. San Diego Symp. Bio. Med. Engl. 3:87, 1963.

Wheeler, H., et al. Bedside screening for venous thrombosis using impedance phlebography. Angiology 26:199–209, 1975.

Weinstein, F. *Principles and Practice of Podiatry.* Lea & Febiger, Philadelphia, 1968.

Weisbert, M. H. Wound disruption and ancillary measures. J. Foot Surg. 5:71, 1966.

CHAPTER 4

Neurological Considerations

GARY M. LEPOW, D.P.M.

The components of a full neurological assessment include: evaluation of the motor system, reflex assessment, coordination tests, and evaluation of the sensory system.

EVALUATION OF THE MOTOR SYSTEM

Three parameters are carefully examined to fully elucidate the extent of function of the motor system. They are 1) strength, 2) bulk, and 3) muscle tone. Strength of muscle contraction helps to evaluate upper motor neuron distribution versus lower motor neuron distribution. One attempts to localize a lesion of the brain and spinal cord that may manifest itself by reduced muscle contraction, atrophy of muscle, or paralysis. Gross muscle movements are produced by a multitude of neuronal innervations which when stimulated result in a gross muscular contraction. If a lesion exists in the brain and spinal cord, and the strength of muscular contraction is noted to be reduced, one may then attempt to determine if this lesion is of lower motor neuron or upper motor neuron origin. The measuring scale to standardize strength of muscle contraction is the degree of movement produced by the muscle against gravity and resistance. The determination of muscle bulk is another parameter used in the evaluation of the motor system. Through clinical, functional examination of the muscle involved and a well-detailed history, muscle atrophy is certainly a clear-cut signal of neurological deficit that needs to be investigated further. Abnormal muscle hypertrophy prompts further clinical examination as well. One must also differentiate in neurological assessment between muscle hypertrophy and increase in muscle mass; as in Duchenne's muscular dystrophy where the hypertrophy is an increase in muscle bulk due to fat accumulation and not an augmentation of muscle mass. The third clinical factor to be considered regarding a full examination of the motor system is muscle tone. Exaggerated muscle tone (hypertonia) may present itself in three forms; spasticity, rigidity, or paratonia. A clinical evaluation of the upper motor neuron distribution is suggested when hypertonic reflexes are noted. Decreased muscle tonus is associated with several neurological disorders such as myopathies, cerebellar disease, spinal shock syndrome, and lower motor neuron diseases. If, after careful evaluation of the motor system, a neurological deficit is determined, certain movement disorders otherwise known as dyskinesias should also be included in the differential diagnosis for the particular etiology in question. These include chorea, athetosis, asterixis, dystonia, hemiballismus, tics, myoclonus, tremors, and fasciculations.

REFLEX ASSESSMENT

In evaluating neurological function regarding the lower extremities, two particular deep tendon reflexes are evaluated. The quadricep extensor reflex and the tendo-achilles reflex. An attempt is made to determine the symmetry, as well as the quality. To standardize the quality of the reflex elicited, a grading system is employed. The extremes are absence of the reflex or clonus. There are diseases that are associated with both hypotonia or exaggerated reflex hypotonia. In addition, pathological reflexes to be noted are the Babinski and the frontal release signs.

COORDINATION TESTS

The cerebellum is the highest center of coordination. Hence, there are coordination tests, which are included in a full neurological evaluation. Gait testing, assessment of speech, rhythm, cadence and enunciation are included to assess cerebellar function. If lack of coordination and balance present themselves, it is important to examine inner ear function before such coordination loss can be noted to be a manifestation of cerebellar disease.

EVALUATION OF THE SENSORY SYSTEM

Sensation modalities of hot and cold, sharp and dull, and vibration and light touch are used to determine the extent of neurological sensory deficit. Sensation testing can localize lesions of the spinal column manifesting particular spinal track sensory impairment. In addition, spinal root lesions can be determined through evaluation of the sensorium. Peripheral nerve damage or neuropathies brought on by diabetes or alcoholism can also be thoroughly evaluated through the sensation modalities discussed. Likewise, sensory testing with particular attention to distribution and areas involved can give further insight into the clinical determination of particular diseases. For example, the Brown-Sequard, the commissural-type syndrome, as well as the thalamic syndrome produce transverse lesions of the brain and spinal columns. They can all be clinically assessed in part by a thorough examination of the sensorium (Figs. 4.1 and 4.2).

Interpretation of Medical, Family, and Psychosocial History

MEDICAL HISTORY

Investigation of the symptomatology experienced is of paramount importance in the medical history. Questions regarding type of symptoms experienced, duration, and particular location of each symptom must be determined. In addition, particular physical activity producing sensations such as pain, weakness, and paresthesia should be elucidated. Prior medical consultation and initiation of treatments for the presenting symptoms should be noted. Inquiries as to concurrent illnesses, including sexually transmitted diseases past and present, should be recorded. A knowledge of previous injuries, surgical procedures, endocrine disorders, congenital abnormalities, current medications, and a history of allergic reactions must be obtained.

FAMILY HISTORY

A detailed family history is also necessary to complete the profile of the presenting complaint. Inquiries regarding family members possessing congenital deformities, (e.g., talipes equino varus or calcaneal valgus), genetically transmitted diseases (e.g., syphilis), acquired myopathies (e.g., Duchenne's muscular dystrophy), and endocrine disorders (e.g., diabetes mellitus) are invaluable in an attempt to fully comprehend the problem at hand.

PSYCHOSOCIAL HISTORY

Psychosocial factors must also be investigated. Occupational factors, including the degree of physical activity, both past and present, along with recreational activities, can play a significant role in determining the etiology of the presenting disorder. Significant also are alcohol and drug use, as well as recent changes in stress and tension levels.

Specific Diagnostic Techniques

PHYSICAL EXAMINATION

Initially, the area in question should be explored. The skin should be inspected and observations recorded. Is the skin soft and moist, or dry and cracked? Is scar tissue present? Are the signs of potential ulcerations, including erythema, edema, ecchymosis, hematoma, blistering, increased local temperature, or heavy callous, present? The involved area should be palpated for

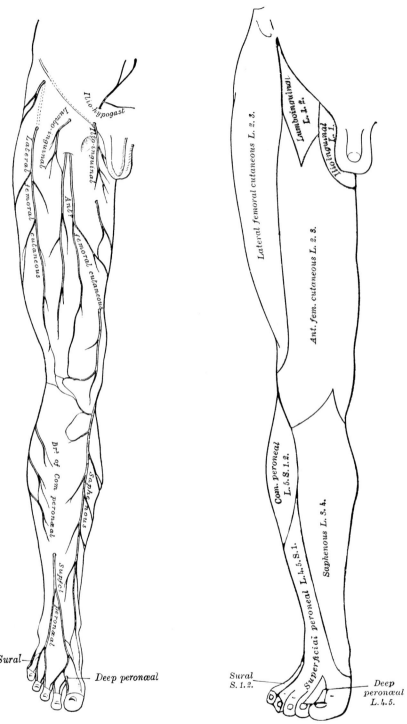

Figure 4.1. *Left,* cutaneous nerves of the right lower extremity, front view. *Right,* diagram of segmental distribution of the cutaneous nerves of the right lower extremity, front view. (From Goss, C. M., ed. *Gray's Anatomy of the Human Body,* 29th ed. Lea & Febiger, Philadelphia, 1973, with permission.)

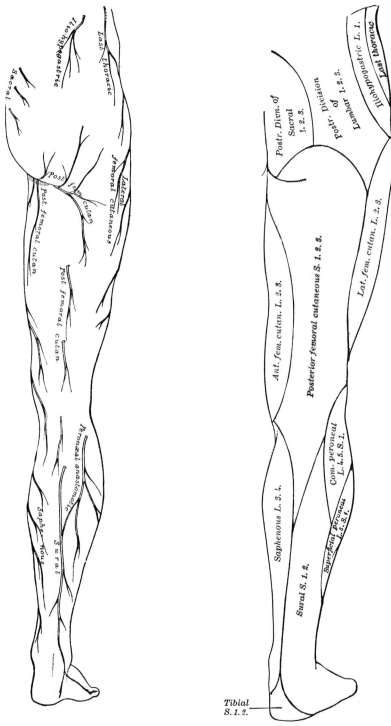

Figure 4.2. *Left,* cutaneous nerves of the right lower extremity, posterior view. *Right,* diagram of the segmental distribution of the cutaneous nerves of the right lower extremity, posterior view. (From Goss, C. M., ed. *Gray's Anatomy of the Human Body,* 29th ed. Lea & Febiger, Philadelphia, 1973, with permission.)

local pain or tenderness, as well as proximal and distal to the involvement. Lymphadenopathy of the groin may be indicative of an insensitive foot.

FOOTPRINT RECORDING

This can be used to indicate areas of pressure in the insensitive foot. Evidence of stressful high-pressure areas of the foot may suggest the need for modification in footgear. Footprint recording can contribute to evaluation, correction, and prevention of plantar surface problems in deformities resulting from diabetes and other diseases.

VOLUMETRIC MEASUREMENTS

In the presence of edema, this test is particularly useful in monitoring foot volume evidence by water displacement. It can be utilized to monitor treatment effectiveness and pre- and post-operative progress regarding swelling.

TEMPERATURE ASSESSMENT

This is particularly useful in the detection of damage in insensitive feet. Temperature measurements can reduce the incidence of injury and ulceration by functioning as a pain substitute. Differences of 2° may be detected by palpation. Thermocouples and infrared thermographic devices provide visual displays of plantar surface temperature. It is most important to note that injury or inflammation may result in differences of 6–8°C.

ELECTROMYOGRAPHIC AND NERVE CONDITION STUDIES

These are essential in the determination of peripheral nerve lesions. Such studies record electrical currents generated in an active muscle and have proven to be more sensitive in diagnosing peripheral neuropathy than other surface action potentials. These studies are also useful in the diagnosis of L4,L5 nerve plexus and lesions of the sciatic, posterior tibial, and medial plantar nerves.

NEUROGRAPHY

A means of tracing nerve trunk functions through an intraneural injection of radiopaque dyes. Neurography, however, is not commonly used because of the potential nerve damage which may result from needle penetration, as well as allergic reaction to the contrast medium utilized.

FOOT AND ANKLE PAIN SYNDROMES

Susceptibility to External Trauma

Superficial nerves are most readily palpable in the foot and ankle owing to their close proximity directly beneath the skin layer (Fig. 4.3). Specific nerves, such as the intermediate and medial dorsal cutaneous, are highly susceptible to external trauma. In addition, traumatic episodes can manifest injury to peripheral nerves of lower extremities. Complete ischemia associated with pressure can damage the peripheral nerve, as well as cause injury to such nerves

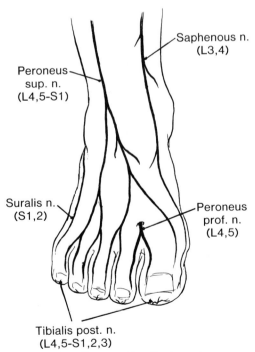

Figure 4.3. Sensory distribution of nerves to be divided. (From Arch. Surg. 111:558, 1976, copyright 1976, American Medical Association.)

from mild contusions. The most devastating of the external traumatic episodes would be complete severance of the peripheral nerve with an associated loss of substance from the actual nerve tissue.

Types of Nerve Injuries (Fig. 4.4)

NEUROPRAXIA

The injured nerve is severely contused. Transmission along the nerve is altered by impaired conductivity. Microscopically, there appears to be no significant alteration in the nerve tissue. Complete sensory loss does not occur and there does appear to be complete and rapid recovery from this injury within a few days to a few weeks.

AXONOTMESIS

In this type of injury the axon of the nerve is involved. Wallerian degeneration is evident at the injured site but the basic nerve cell or Schwann tubule is preserved. The recovery time in axonotmesis is complete in a few months.

NEUROTMESIS

Damage to the nerve is either partial or complete severance. A neuroma and glioma

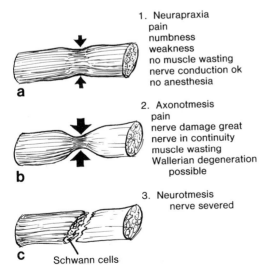

1. Neurapraxia
   pain
   numbness
   weakness
   no muscle wasting
   nerve conduction ok
   no anesthesia

2. Axonotmesis
   pain
   nerve damage great
   nerve in continuity
   muscle wasting
   Wallerian degeneration
   possible

3. Neurotmesis
   nerve severed

Schwann cells

Figure 4.4. Degree of nerve damage. (From Clin. Orthop. Relat. Res. 141, June, 1979, with permission.)

may form at the injured site. This particular type of injury is irreversible and recovery is rare.

The aforementioned injuries may present in a single nerve. Depending on the extent of the nerve trauma, symptomatology as well as recovery time will vary greatly.

Common Surgical Approaches to Correction of Nerve Damage

NEUROLYSIS

This approach is used in complicated first-degree injury if conduction has been interrupted by scarring or adhesions. The technique involves freeing the nerve from adhesions or scar tissue which are obstructing the growth of regenerating axons or blocking conduction of the nerve impulses. In second-degree nerve injuries, the procedure is difficult and risky. The nerve may appear to be intact and normal; however, scarring is evident on the interfunicular tissue. In addition, internal neurolysis may require the surgeon to split the nerve sheath and release the bundle from the interfunicular scar tissue. The surgical approach should be made interior and superior to the particular scar. This cautious attempt assures separation of the nerve and its branches, as well as preserving the vasculature of the nerve and surrounding tissues. Electrical stimulation can be used to monitor this procedure. Particular attention must be given to immature nerve fibers which may suffer from temporary conduction blockage when this procedure is employed. Likewise, if a nerve is entrapped in dense scar tissue, it is recommended to reroute the nerve to an area in which there is less risk of compression or relocate the nerve to avoid tension or friction stemming from fibro-osseous structures. If the patient's progress does not proceed favorably after surgery due to failure from constricting scar tissue preventing nerve regeneration, additional neurolysis is indicated.

NEURORRHAPHY (FIGURE 4.5)

This technique involves resection of the traumatized nerve tissue with end-to-end

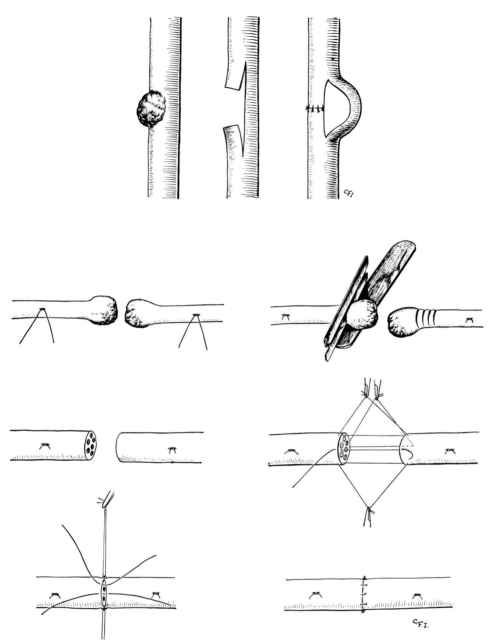

Figure 4.5. *Top,* technique of partial neurorrhaphy. *Bottom,* technique of nerve suture. The divided nerve is exposed, and the orientation sutures are inserted. The ends are mobilized, and sections of bulbous proximal and distal segments are removed successively until normal funiculi are encountered. Interrupted epineural sutures are inserted circumferentially. If silk is used throughout, two tantalum marker sutures permit subsequent roentgenographic determination of the suture line. (From Simmons, J. C. H. Early management of nerve injuries. In Crenshaw, A. H., ed. *Campbell's Orthopaedics,* 5th ed. C. V. Mosby, St. Louis, 1971, with permission.)

repair of the distal and proximal segments. Before this is employed, it should be determined if spontaneous recovery of the injured nerve is possible. Depending on the severity of the nerve lesion, the time interval between the injury and spontaneous recovery will vary greatly. If spontaneous recovery is possible, normal function most commonly will occur within 6 months and can be evidenced by the return of nerve function which is monitored by voluntary contraction of previous paralyzed muscles. In the instance of acute nerve trauma, debridement of the traumatized nerve tissue may be necessary to promote healing. Neurorrhaphy should certainly be delayed if contamination and infection are evident following nerve damage. The surgical technique involves special instrumentation such as magnification lenses, electrical or battery-operated nerve stimulators, rubber covered forceps, umbilical tape, a nerve hemostat, and swaged ophthalmic sutures. To avoid adhesions and skin scarring, the approach should involve incising the skin away from the course of the nerve. If extensive destruction has resulted from trauma or scarring of a nerve trunk, significant mobilization of the distal and proximal nerve segments are required with this approach. If disruption involves half of a large nerve, partial neurorrhaphy is advised. Once the traumatized nerve tissue has been resected, end-to-end repair of the distal and proximal segments is indicated. In addition, one must recognize that the transected nerve segments retract 4% of the normal length of the nerve between excision points. Once the procedure has been performed, the involved extremity must be immobilized 3–4 weeks for maximal surgical success. It should be understood that complete neurorrhaphy does not usually bring about full return of motor and sensory function. The extent of recovery depends upon the nature and extent of nerve involvement and the degree of damage to the motor and sensory apparatus.

Non-invasive Therapy for Control of Acute and Chronic Pain: Transcutaneous Nerve Stimulation (TNS)

Transcutaneous nerve stimulation is a modality employed to reduce the pain threshold. The technique of surface placement of carbon-impregnated silicone electrodes in the region of acute or chronic pain masks the awareness of the physical discomfort. TNS may be used in conjunction with pain medication and may be a supplement to primary pain therapy. The use of transelectrical nerve stimulation requires continuous assessment of the patient's response to the treatment and subsequent modification of the treatment plan. Prolonged usage of the modality may develop a physiological tolerance to the treatment similar to that seen in chronic opiate usage. To delay tolerance, one should limit the daily use of the treatment. One theory as to the success of this therapy is the belief that endogenous opioid substances are released by the body producing an analgesic effect.

COMMON NERVE PATHOLOGIES
Neuroma

The term neuroma refers to any neoplasm that affects the central nervous system's cellular structure. Neoplasms involving nerves of the foot are not uncommon; however, malignancies of nerves affecting the feet are significantly rare. Neuromas are considered lesions rather than true nerve tumors of the foot. The most clinically identifiable sign of an intermetatarsal neuroma is intense pain relieved only by removing the footgear and massaging the metatarsal region of the foot. The patient in addition may also complain of burning and cramping symptoms. Physical examination and radiological findings are usually negative. Mulder's sign (a clicking sound elicited by palpation of the adjoining metatarsal heads) eludes to a clinical neuroma. Morton's neuroma typically involves a localized degeneration and proliferation of the interdigital nerve in the web space that produces pain when palpated. The etiology of this particular condition is unknown. However, trauma and ischemia are often predisposing factors for this clinical entity. It is most commonly found in middle-aged women. The most common location is the third interspace. Traumatic neuromas present somewhat differently as a proliferative mass formed at a site of injury. They are usually small and less symptomatic, resulting from poor nerve apposition and increasing soft tissue interposition. The third class of neuroma is termed an amputation neuroma which follows the entanglement of a nerve in a mass of scar tissue. The differential diagnosis of a neuroma includes ganglionic cysts, as well as nerve entrapment syndromes.

The most common nerve tumor found on a foot is the neurofibroma (Fig. 4.6). This neoplasm is usually benign, not encapsulated, and presents as a solitary mass of Schwann cells. It commonly develops in the nerve fibers of skin and bones. Other solitary benign nerve sheet tumors include the neurilemoma and the neurofibroma with neurofibromatosis. The neurilemoma is otherwise called: neurinoma, solitary schwannoma, encapsulated neurilemoma, perineurofibroplastoma, and acoustic neuroma. The neurofibroma with neurofibromatosis is found in the literature as plexiform neurofibroma, elephantitis neuromatosis, and multiple neuroma. Malignant nerve tumors include the neuroblastoma and primary nerve sheath tumors. The neuroblastoma is a neuroectodermal tumor which is an immature embryonic-type neoplasm consisting of slightly differentiated nerve cells. The neuroblastoma is found in infants or children under 10 years of age in over 75% of identified cases. These primary malignant nerve tumors are likely located in the mediastinal and retroperitoneal regions. Primary nerve sheath tumors include the malignant schwannoma, malignant epithelioid schwannoma, malignant melanocytic schwannoma, nerve sheath fibrosarcoma or malignant mesenchynoma, and the neurofibrosarcoma otherwise termed neu-

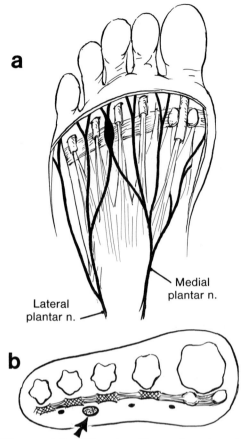

Figure 4.6. Diagrams illustrating that the neuroma lies on the plantar aspect of the deep transverse ligament; hence, below the level of the metatarsal heads and cannot be pinched by the flanking bones.

rogenic sarcoma. The neurofibrosarcoma is the most common neoplasm with fibromatosis. It is highly malignant and frequently reoccurs at the surgical incision. Most malignancies that affect the feet are usually associated with Von Recklinghausen's disease. Ten per cent of neurofibromas associated with this clinical entity show malignant changes in nerve tissue.

Treatment of these common nerve pathologies includes careful attention to such factors as mechanical or anatomical friction as a cause of chronic irritation since that may be of etiological significance. The differential diagnosis includes arthritis, March fracture, Freiberg's disease, bursitis, capsulitis, periostitis, subluxations, and tarsal tunnel syndrome. In addition to a radiological examination, laboratory tests should include a sedimentation rate, an arthritis panel, urinalysis, and random blood sugar for diabetes associated paresthesias, and plethysmography for the possibility of vasospastic disease or vascular insufficiency. Conservative therapy includes injections of vitamin B-12, xylocaine, and steroids, as well as sclerosing agents. In addition, physiomodalities may be employed. Surgical excision usually provides permanent relief and is the treatment of choice for alleviation of symptoms.

Associated tumors such as ganglionic cysts and rheumatoid nodules may be noted adjacent to or attached to a neuroma. Conservative surgical approaches to malignancies often result in reoccurrence. Microsurgery is effective in alleviating pain associated with peripheral nerve injuries as found in a stump neuroma. The nerve is sectioned and divided into two equal fasicles and then free ends of these two fasicles are atraumatically joined, thus constituting a closed circuit for outgrowing axons. The effectiveness of this technique in eliminating the phantom limb pain is not known.

Peripheral Nerve Entrapment Neuropathies

These neuropathies most commonly result from mechanical pathology to peripheral nerves by some impinging anatomic neighbor. Symptoms are common in the lower extremities. Body type and occupation have been associated with a predilection to these clinical entities. In addition, atraumatic etiological factors have been identified such as congenital abnormalities of bone and muscle resulting in nerve compression. Biomechanical factors may result in traction injuries to peripheral nerves. Spatial changes resulting from adjacent neoplasms such as ganglionic cysts, lipomas, fibromas, as well as collagen diseases may also manifest peripheral nerve entrapment neuropathies. Traumatic or post-traumatic etiological factors of these pathologies include: traction injury resulting from fracture or sprain, spatial alterations due to edema, hematoma or tenosynovitis, and poor post-reduction alignment of a fracture which may produce excessive callous formation or reactive fibrosis of the surrounding tissue. The symptoms presented may depend upon the extent of the involvement as well as the specific innervations of the three types of peripheral nerves that present as entrapment neuropathies. The entrapped nerve may be sensory, causing sharp pain, burning, and paresthesias. The end product may be an altered sensation in the area of distribution felt as a hypesthesia or dysesthesia. Trophic changes in the skin may also be noted. Motor nerves that are entrapped may cause a dull ache or a sharp tearing pain over a larger area including the innervated muscle. The muscle is usually tender and paresis and atrophy of muscle fibers may be present. A combination entrapment may cause any or all of the symptoms previously described. Pain related to sensory fibers usually appear earliest. Trauma may involve only one portion of the nerve, sensory and not motor, and consequently the symptoms of the related area of nerve damage will be noted. Symptomatic diagnoses include pain present at rest, but exacerbated by increased activity, or increased pain experienced at night. Most intense pain is usually experienced at the point of origin, though pain may spread both proximally and distally. Altered sensation may include intermittent burning, tingling, or numbness. The patient may experience muscle cramping or a sense of heaviness. Loss of two-point tactile discrimination is an early indicator of an entrapment neuropathy. Other diagnostic signs are: the possible palpation of fusiform swelling of the nerve; a positive Tinel sign, and a positive Vallieux phenomenon. These diagnostic indicators must be carefully evaluated for a complete assessment of a entrapment neuropathy.

There are several diagnostic methods that are employed in evaluating the extent of the nerve entrapment syndrome. One such technique is electrodiagnosis. This procedure documents delayed nerve conduction velocity by placing electrodes properly on the skin in the region of the particular entrapped nerve. If delays of more than 6.1 meters per second for the medial plantar nerve and 6.7 meters per second for the lateral plantar nerve are recorded, this is considered a qualitative indicator of a compression neuropathy. Of greater significance is the inequality between the symptomatic and the asymptomatic limb. Another diagnostic method is electromyography, which involves the placement of intramuscular electrodes to determine the relative motor unit potential.

Perineural injections of anti-inflammatory agents may produce prolonged relief if the pain stems from a post-traumatic neuroinflammation caused by acute trauma. Treatment measures include concurrent oral drug therapy consisting of anti-inflammatory drugs, as well as biomechanical devices to relieve stresses on the peripheral nerves. These treatments can be combined with physiologic rest, i.e., immobilization, to produce even greater relief. Surgery is considered if the conservative treatment measures have failed or if there is definite anatomic encroachment by the adjacent soft tissue structures which maintain the entrapment syndrome.

A complete assessment includes an extensive differential diagnosis. One such syndrome to be considered is strain or plantar fasciitis resulting from excessive pronation. Systemic diseases with pedal manifestations are those arising from rheumatoid arthritis or peripheral vascular disease. Peripheral neuropathies can also be associated with metabolic disease such as diabetes mellitus, chronic alcoholism, drug toxicity, and vitamin B-6 deficiency.

Specific Nerve Entrapment Neuropathies (Figure 4.7)

Tarsal tunnel syndrome (TTS) involves compression of the posterior tibial nerve. Symptoms of this condition include local edema, cellular infiltration, and a vacuolation of the myelin sheath. Paresthesias and pain are produced with numbness or burning radiating to along the plantar surfaces of the foot and the toes. The patient may demonstrate muscle weakness and muscle atrophy especially aggravated weight-bearing. Symptoms may become worse at night. Relief may be obtained temporarily by loose foot gear or going barefoot. If this condition has not been treated for some time, these later symptoms may simulate sciatica. The etiology of tarsal tunnel syndrome is most commonly related to a spontaneous entrapment following a fracture or dislocation involving the malleolus, talus, or calcaneus. Men and women are equally affected. Compression of the posterior tibial nerve may stem from a post-traumatic edema and result in fibrosis. Chronic compression may be a result of a space-occupying lesion such as a synovial cyst on the medial side of the ankle joint, ganglions, lipomas, neurofibromas, or neurolemmomas. Several systemic diseases are linked to the tarsal tunnel syndrome and include diabetes mellitus, myxedema, and rheumatoid arthritis. Though quite uncommon, spontaneous tarsal tunnel syndrome without specific trauma may be related to a rapid weight gain or fluid retention. Chlorothiazide, hydrochlorothiazide, and nitrofurantoin may produce a toxic drug response manifesting a spontaneous tarsal tunnel syndrome. Aging can produce changes in connective tissue that may result in spontaneous tarsal tunnel syndrome as well. Other causes of this condition may be a chronic foot strain, arthritic spurring, or stretching of the nerve over the medial malleolus in chronic foot strain.

Diagnostic aids utilized in evaluating this syndrome include two-point discrimination, which is diminished in tarsal tunnel syndrome. A tourniquet test is also used which, when applied to the lower extremity, may produce symptoms sooner on the affected limb. A Vallieux phenomenon previously discussed is also utilized in assessing this nerve entrapment syndrome. A

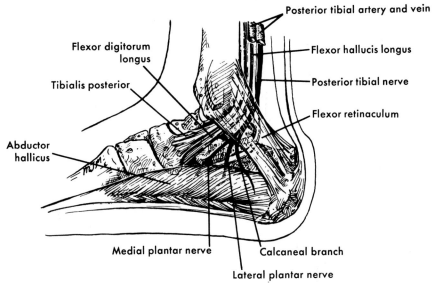

Figure 4.7. Anatomy of the tarsal tunnel. (From Inman, V. T., ed. *DuVries' Surgery of the Foot*, 3rd ed. C. V. Mosby, St. Louis, 1973, with permission.)

positive Tinel sign will be demonstrated. Palpation of the posterior tibial nerve may reveal fusiform swelling of the nerve trunk. Radiographs may demonstrate evidence of degenerative arthritis or old healed fractures. Electromyographic studies, including both motor and sensory conduction tests, are most useful in determining tarsal tunnel syndrome. An abnormal conduction velocity noted when compared with the asymptomatic extremity is most significant. Standardized values from medial and plantar nerve latency techniques have been developed by Fu et al. (1980). Prolonged latency measurements and delayed conduction time are indicators of the tarsal tunnel syndrome.

The differential diagnosis of the tarsal tunnel syndrome may include a host of clinical pathologies. A complete history and physical examination generally suggest a diagnosis that may be confirmed by electromyographic studies. However, other conditions to be considered include neuropathies associated with systemic and metabolic disease, as well as interdigital neuroma, and a radiculitis secondary to herniated intervertebral disc. Toxic drug response should be

ruled out, as well as a sciatic nerve irritation or peripheral neuritis. Tenosynovitis, plantar fibromatosis or fibrositis, intermittant claudication and erythromelalgia (rare) completes the list of possibilities in the differential diagnosis of tarsal tunnel syndrome.

Conservative treatment may include injections of corticosteroids locally into the region of the entrapment. Investigation of biomechanical abnormalities contributing to the syndrome and their correction through orthotic devices and other modalities may produce significant benefit and relief. Surgical decompression of the tarsal tunnel, having attempted conservative measures unsuccessfully, would then be the treatment of choice.

Another entrapment syndrome may present as an anterior tibial neuropathy with compression of the nerve near the point of termination on the dorsum of the foot. Depending on the portion of nerve involved, symptoms associated with this condition may include pain in the great toe, as well as sensory disturbances of the first web space. Aching discomfort of the mid-foot region may occur, along with atrophy of the dorsal muscle mass.

The etiology of this entrapment syndrome is related to the anatomic path of the nerve because of its proximity to the tibia. The nerve rests directly on the tibia and is easily injured due to its superficial position. An object dropped on the foot, as well as other direct trauma, are the primary causes of this neuropathy. Footgear or a tight cast may manifest repeated trauma to the nerve and therefore may also be a factor in the etiology of this condition. Following a violent backward force, a traction injury may occur manifesting this compression of the anterior tibial nerve. Less commonly, a ganglionic cyst or synovial pseudo-cyst in the tarsal area may cause a traction neuropathy.

Conservative treatment measures may, as with other neuropathies, include injections of anti-inflammatory agents directly into the region of the entrapment along with systemic anti-inflammatory medication. Rest and non-weightbearing may also contribute to the relief of symptoms, as well as change of footgear or removal of the aggravating factor such as a below knee cast. Surgical intervention involves decompression at the site of the involvement. If a neurectomy is required, the proper technique involves performing the surgery proximal to the extensor retinaculum to avoid neuroma formation in the tendons under this particular ligament.

Another compression neuropathy involves entrapment of the saphenous nerve at the exit from the subsartorial canal innervation to the medial aspect of the knee, leg, arch, or foot (Figure 4.8). The symptomatology usually involves the arch area of the foot. Adduction of the hip or extension of the knee will aggravate the already existing painful condition. The etiology of a saphenous neuropathy rarely involves trauma. Patients are usually over age 40 and present with excessively heavy thighs. In addition, a genu varus deformity with associated internal tibial torsion is a common complicating factor. Direct trauma to

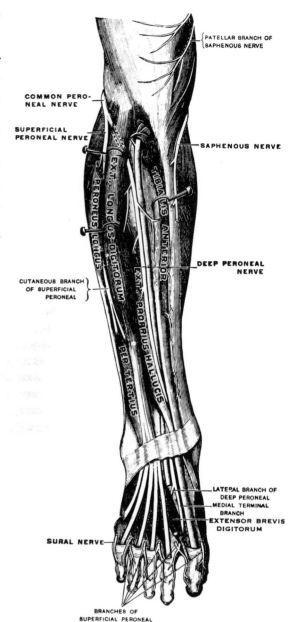

Figure 4.8. Deep nerves of the front of the leg. (From Goss, C. M., ed. *Gray's Anatomy of the Human Body*, 29th ed. Lea & Febiger, Philadelphia, 1973, with permission.)

the knee manifesting a saphenous neuropathy is an atypical etiological entity. More commonly, indirect trauma due to a torsional force at the knee joint may impinge the saphenous nerve near the medial meniscus. Treatment of this entrapment

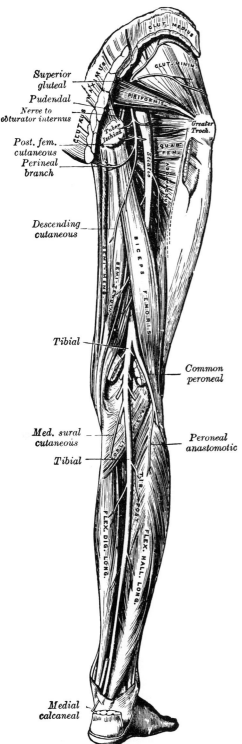

Figure 4.9. Nerves of the right lower extremity, posterior view. Note: In this diagram, the medial sural cutaneous and peroneal anastomotic nerves have been displaced from their normal positions by the removal of the superfi-

syndrome includes rest, physical therapy, and anti-inflammatory medications. Surgery for a saphenous neuropathy includes mobilization of the nerve and freedom from soft tissue adhesions.

A superficial peroneal neuropathy may present with burning pain and retrograde radiation of this pain to other areas of the leg, along with a palpable hyperesthesia of the involved area. There may also be a hyperesthesia of the adjacent areas of the skin. If patients have little subcutaneous fat, a nodular mass along the coarse of the nerve may be palpated. This neuropathy will present with a positive Tinel sign. The causal factors of a superficial peroneal neuropathy include forced plantarflexion, direct trauma, or repeated irritation from high boots (Figure 4.9).

Conservative measures for relief of symptomatology include local injections of anti-inflammatories, rest, immobilization, physical therapy, and a lateral sole wedge to the shoe gear to cause pronation. Surgical intervention involves local fascial release with possible resection of the involved nerve. This may result in cutaneous anesthesia of the region, as well as relief of symptomology.

Another entrapment syndrome may present as a common peroneal neuropathy (Figure 4.9). Pain and sensory alteration along the lateral aspect of the foot and leg may occur and be the presenting complaint. Motor dysfunction of the muscles innervated by the particular nerve involved may occur as well. Radiologic evidence of some osteoporosis may be noted. Inversion sprain is the most common etiological agent for this condition.

Conservative therapy involves protecting the foot with forefoot control or shoe wedging to limit the potential for excessive plantarflexion or inversion, as well as anti-inflammatory agents and physiomodalities. The surgical approach afterward includes sectioning of the peroneus longus muscle

cial muscles. (From Goss, C. M., ed. *Gray's Anatomy of the Human Body,* 29th ed. Lea & Febiger, Philadelphia, 1973, with permission.)

at the origin with a neurolysis of the nerve trunk.

Finally, the posterior tibial nerve may present as a compression neuropathy in other ways than a tarsal tunnel syndrome, depending on the area of involvement. Plantar divisions of the posterior nerve may become entrapped and its entrance into the plantar surface of the foot manifest a compression neuropathy (Figure 4.10). In addition, the intermetatarsal nerve at the bifurcation of the posterior tibial nerve to the plantar digital nerves may become compressed forming another entrapment syndrome. Symptoms include sensory alterations involving the plantar aspect of the foot and the end of the toes. There may be intermittent burning, tingling, numbness, and muscle cramps as well. Retrograde pain

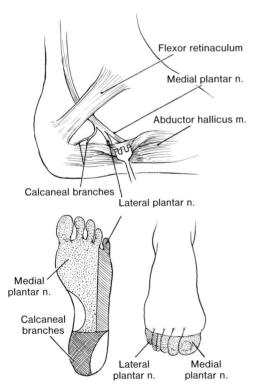

Figure 4.10. Plantar divisions of the posterior nerve may become entrapped and its entrance into the plantar surface may manifest a compression neuropathy. (From Goss, C. M., ed. *Gray's Anatomy of the Human Body,* 29th ed. Lea & Febiger, Philadelphia, 1973, with permission.)

along the sciatic axis to the gluteal region is not uncommon with this type of neuropathy. Owing to posterior tibial nerve entrapments, you might also find weakness, loss of flexion, stability, and clawing of the digits.

The etiology of a posterior tibial nerve entrapment syndrome may be related to traumatic effusion producing adhesions around the nerve or possibly a fracture resulting in soft tissue fibrosis which may adhere to the nerve. Non-traumatic spatial changes such as venous stasis or engorgement of the posterior tibial veins can cause pressure atrophy and thereby entrap the nerve. Repeated microtrauma that may be associated with biomechanical pathology such as severe pronation accompanying an accommodative forefoot varus foot type, as well as severe equinovarus deformity, may also result in a posterior tibial nerve entrapment. Diagnosis is based on clinical findings, as well as electrical conduction studies. The electrical conduction studies have been discussed previously. Once the clinical findings have been established to focus in on a posterior tibial nerve entrapment, other clinical entities must be ruled out. They are: plantar fasciitis, entrapment neuropathy of plantar nerves, interdigital neuroma, and peripheral neuropathy secondary to diabetes, alcoholism, or other systemic diseases.

Conservative treatment is aimed at reversal of the underlying pathological process if the entrapment syndrome is due to changes in spatial relationships as discussed above. If biomechanical pathology is the underlying etiology, accommodation of deformity must be achieved. Surgical intervention is directed toward mobilization of the nerve. Post-operatively, a short leg cast may be used. Relief from pain and paresthesia may result within 1 day following nerve decompression.

Another entrapment syndrome may involve the medial plantar nerve and or the lateral plantar nerve. The symptoms parallel those of the tarsal tunnel syndrome with the major complaint burning pain on the plantar aspect of the foot (Figures 4.10 and 4.11). The etiology of this entrapment syndrome may be trauma, such as landing flatfooted from a fall, or dropping a heavy object on the foot. Plantar nerves may also be subject to direct trauma in some situations, such as occupations where there are prolonged periods of working while standing on rungs of a ladder. Having enumerated the clinical findings, some other clinical pathologies to be ruled out in a differential diagnosis include: acute chronic foot strain, plantar fasciitis, or the inflammation of the spring ligament. In addition, tendinitis, bursitis at the intersection of the tibialis posterior or tibialis anterior muscles may present itself as a plantar nerve entrapment. A nerve entrapment proximal or distal to the plantar site involving the posterior tibial nerve or its branches may mask

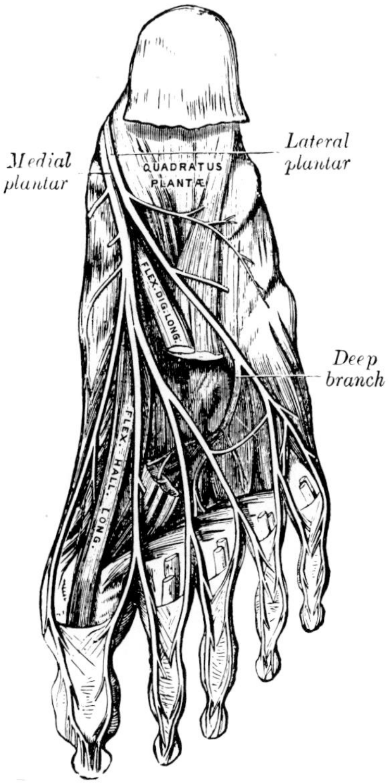

Figure 4.11. The plantar nerves. (From Goss, C. M., ed. *Gray's Anatomy of the Human Body,* 29th ed. Lea & Febiger, Philadelphia, 1973, with permission.)

as a medial plantar or lateral nerve entrapment syndrome.

One clinical entity that is associated with this particular plantar nerve compression is called "jogger's foot" which is a medial plantar neuropraxia related to long-distance running. The patient presents most commonly with burning heel pain, aching in the arch, as well as decreased sensation in the sole of the foot behind the great toe. Repeated trauma to this nerve results in intractable inflammation at the point of entrapment. A local anesthetic injection at the entrapment point is effective in relieving the discomfort. The patient should also be instructed that running shoes must be selected with greater care, especially the avoidance of artificial arch supports. A change in running posture should also be discussed with the patient. This should involve running on the lateral aspect of the foot. A slight "toeing-in" will take pressure off of the medial plantar structures.

Treatment of these syndromes conservatively can include supportive measures such as proper footgear, together with anti-inflammatory medication and physiotherapy. Surgery entails mobilization of plantar nerves. A neurolysis is undesirable for the plantar nerve entrapment unless the adhesiotomy and nerve release do not prove successful. However, in a chronic medial plantar neuropraxia, surgical neurolysis may be the eventual procedure of choice.

Causalgia

Causalgia is a term that refers to the sequelae of peripheral nerve injury. Nerve damage from minor trauma usually does not cause sensory or motor changes. However, more significant trauma may result in destruction of the entire nerve trunk. Most commonly, the nerves from the carpal and tarsal tunnel and their branches are affected. The etiology of causalgia is attributable to a traumatic episode that produces exaggerated activity in the spinal cord. Causalgia may also follow irritation of uncut sensory fibers, inflammation of peripheral sympathetic nerve fibers, or infection associated with a penetrating wound. Sustained pressure with a plaster cast may also manifest causalgia. Incorporation of a nerve trunk in a surgical or fracture scar can damage the peripheral nerve involved and thereby manifest symptoms. However, this can be avoided by thorough identification, mobilization, and retraction of nerves in the region of the surgical site. Care must certainly be taken to avoid placement of sutures around nerves that can cause strangulation, producing peripheral injury and causalgic symptoms.

The symptoms associated with this clinical entity are intense burning and acute disabling pain, which usually develop immediately following nerve trauma. Sensory and emotional stimuli intensify the pain. The patient will tend to demonstrate emotional instability and hyperirritability. The trophic changes in the skin and nails are due to increased sympathetic tonus and are evident by coldness in the involved extremity. An unusual moistness may be felt on the skin in the region of the nerve injury. In the early stages of causalgia, a vasodilation may cause a warm, dry, pink appearance to the skin. Radiologic evidence of bone changes can range from slight demineralization of bone to advanced osteoporosis. Fibrous changes may be apparent in involved muscles in the region. Small joints may appear to be stiff and ankylosed. The diagnosis of causalgia can be confirmed by an anesthetic blocking of the second or third lumbar sympathetic ganglia.

Treatment of this condition includes moist compresses which provide temporary relief of the disabling symptoms. If a hyperemia and/or edema are present, rest and elevation of the parts will also aid in the reduction of discomfort. An anterior and posterior tibial nerve block is of significant benefit in preventing the persistent pain and deformity that may be irreversible if prompt treatment is not instituted. If treatment is delayed, the intense pain associated with causalgia may become implanted in the central nervous system. Extreme measures may become necessary involving a cordotomy or lobotomy. Oral medication such as tolazoline, as well as tetraethylammonium, may be used in providing symptomatic relief. However, these medications can exacerbate the already intensely painful condition in the vasodilated type causalgia. Finally, a neurolysis may be the surgical approach indicated if a sensory nerve trunk is involved because of scar tissue adhesions from direct injury. If excessive scar tissue is present in the surgical site, the nerve may be excised if neurolysis is not possible. If a partial nerve lesion can be identified the residual pain, or paresthesia associated can be eliminated. The surgical approach if a nerve lesion is identified includes: neurolysis, neurorrhaphy, resection of a neuroma, and sympathectomy.

UNUSUAL NEUROLOGICAL DIAGNOSES IN FOOT SURGERY
Charcot Joint

Charcot joint involves a progressive degeneration of a joint, along with an abnormal sensory distribution. The etiological agents involved include many systemic diseases. Most common are syphilis and diabetes mellitus. Leprosy, syringomyelia, along with other spinal lesions and spinal tumors, are also causative factors.

Joint destruction of this magnitude can be manifested by chronic anemia as well as the repeated injection of intra-articular corticosteroids. Prerequisites to a Charcot joint include neuropathy and trauma to the joint. Most commonly, patients will present with this degeneration in the sixth decade of life. Weight-bearing joints such as the knee, foot, ankle, and hip are the joints most commonly affected.

Symptoms of Charcot joint disease include painless or painful swelling of the involved articulation. Joint effusion is a clinical finding. Ligament relaxation and capsular distention can also be noted in the involved articulation leading to instability, numbness, and/or weakness of the affected part. A chronic synovitis along with abnormal neurological findings are also present. Gross evidence of imbedded cartilage and bone debris within the synovium is clinically significant in diagnosing Charcot joint. Differential diagnosis includes osteoarthritis, tubercular joint manifestation, rheumatoid arthritis, pyogenic arthritis, gout, traumatic arthritis, gonorrheal arthritis, and arthritidies associated with neoplastic disease.

Treatment of a Charcot joint involves control of the underlying disease. In addition, if ulcers are present, debridement and appropriate therapy is indicated. In the early stages of a Charcot joint, molding the foot in a plaster cast and the manufacture of a molded shoe may be beneficial in reducing instability of the joint. Finally, if the joint progresses with extensive degeneration and destruction, a surgical approach involving joint resection or arthrodesis may prove to be highly successful in reducing symptomatology.

Charcot-Marie-Tooth Disease (CMT)

Charcot-Marie-Tooth disease is another neurologic condition with manifestations in the foot that is remedied by surgical intervention. CMT is characterized by progressive muscular atrophy, along with degeneration of a peripheral nerve. The causal factors of this debilitating pathologic condition is familial in that the heredity pattern determines the age of onset and severity of symptoms. The male female ratio is 3.5 to 1.

CMT disease generally occurs in the last portion of the first decade of life. The condition may follow an acute infection. CMT disease is characterized by difficulty in walking, along with intense muscle cramps, paresthesias, and spontaneous pains in the lower extremities. Deformities presented are a pes cavus deformity with very thin legs, producing a steppage gait and a foot drop. The deep tendon reflexes may be hypoactive or absent. Differential diagnosis of this condition are Friedrich's ataxia, Roussy-Levy syndrome, progressive muscular atrophy, polyneuritis, muscular dystrophy, and amyotrophic lateral sclerosis.

Treatment can include physical therapy applications, orthopaedic and biomechanical devices, and supportive braces. Osseous and soft tissue surgical procedures can be employed for a more permanent correction.

Other Neurological Disorders with Foot Involvement

These include: Friedrich's ataxia, the compartment syndromes, lumbar disc syndromes, spina bifida, and myelomeningocele.

Acknowledgments—I wish to thank Colleen Braun and Jeffrey Tannenbaum, D.P.M., for their assistance in the preparation of this chapter.

Suggested Readings

Bergtholdt, H. T. Temperature assessment of the insensitive foot. Phys. Ther. 59:18–22, 1979.

Berlin, S. J., Donick, I. I., Block, L. D., and Costa, A. J. Nerve tumors of the foot: Diagnosis and treatment. JAPA 65:157–166, 1975.

Caillet, R. Neurological disorders of the foot. *Foot and Ankle Pain.* F. A. Davis, Philadelphia, 1974, vol. 5.

Fisher, C. M. Plantar reflexes—elicitation by the patient. Trans. Am. Neurol. Assoc. 98:262, 1973.

Fu, R., DeLisa, J. A., and Kraft, G. H. Motor nerve latencies through the tarsal tunnel in normal adult subjects: Standard determinations corrected for temperature and distance. Arch. Phys. Med. Rehab. 61:243–248, 1980.

Gardner, E., and Gray, I. J. The innervation of the joints of the foot. Anal. Rec. 161:141–148, 1968.

Gersh, M. R., Wolf, S. L., and Rao, V. R. Evaluation of transcutaneous electrical nerve stimulation for pain relief in peripheral neuropathy. Phys. Ther. 60:48–52, 1980.

Grosack, M. A., Gibbons, R. W., and Cohen, G. Transcutaneous nerve stimulation: Its significance and applications in podiatry. J. Foot Surg. 20:127, 1981.

Guiloff, R. J., and Sherratt, R. M. Sensory conduction in medial plantar nerve. J. Neurol. Neurosurg. Psychiat. 40:1168–1181, 1977.

Jahss, M. H. Unusual diagnostic problems of the foot. Clin. Orthop. Relat. Res. 85:42–49, 1972.

Kaplan, E. B. Some principles of anatomy and kinesiology in stabilization operations of the foot. Clin. Orthopol. 34:7–13, 1964.

Kravette, M. A. Peripheral nerve entrapment syndromes in the foot. JAPA 61:457–472, 1972.

Lemont, H., and Hernandez, A. Recalcitrant pain syndromes of the foot and ankle: Evaluation of the lateral dorsal cutaneous nerve. JAPA 62:331–335, 1972.

McCutcheon, R. Regional anesthesia for the foot. Can. Anesth. Soc. J. 12:465–474, 1965.

Mullens, I., Spector, E. E., Subotnick, S. I., Sharpe, I. A. *Third Annual Residents Alumni Association Seminar: Neurological Diseases as They Relate to the Foot, March 8–10, 1974, San Francisco* (symposium).

Rask, M. R. Medial plantar neuropraxia (jogger's foot). Clin. Orthopol. 134:193–195, 1978.

Roth, R. D., and Harford, G. E. Peripheral nerve and dermatomal sensory innervation of the lower extremities. JAPA 70:215–223, 1980.

Shipley, D. E. Clinical evaluation and care of the insensitive foot. Phys. Ther. 59:13–18, 1979.

Sloof, A. C. J. Microsurgical possibilities in the treatment of peripheral pain. Clin. Neurol. Neurosurg. 80:107–111, 1977.

Strauch, B., and Tsur, H. Restoration of sensation to the head by a free neurovascular flap from the first web space to the foot. Plast. Reconstr. Surg. 62:361–367, 1978.

Terzis, J. K. Sensory mapping. Clin. Plast. Surg. 3:59–64, 1976.

Trafton, P. G. Jogger's foot (letter). Clin. Orthopol. 141:308, 1979.

Van Gijn, J. The Babinski sign and the pyramidal syndrome. J. Neurol. Neurosurg. Psychiatr. 41:865–873, 1978.

CHAPTER 5

Wound Healing

DONALD W. HUGAR, D.P.M.

In order to facilitate wound healing, the practitioner should understand the three phases of the process. The substrate phase is characterized by vascular, hemostatic, and cellular response and occurs from the 1st to the 4th day. During this lag period, hemorrhage is controlled and fibrin is deposited in the wound. Also, mucopolysaccharides and soluble protein precursors of collagen are produced.

In the proliferative or repair phase, there is epithelization, wound contraction, connective tissue repair, and healing in special tissue. The production of collagen fibers brings tensile strength. The estimated time period is the 5th to the 20th day.

The remodeling phase begins approximately 3 weeks after surgery. In this phase, remodeling, reorganization, and differentiation occur. The fibroblast acts in migration and realignment at this phase. Tensile strength is not fully regained for several months.

ATRAUMATIC SURGERY

A rapid rate of healing in surgical wounds is partly attributable to atraumatic surgery. The major factors to be considered are the following.

Instrumentation

—Use sharp blades to minimize tissue damage. Do not hack tissues, and avoid blunt dissection wherever possible.

—Retractors should be blunt to prevent penetration of nerves, blood vessels, and tissue. Avoid retraction that overstretches the wound; instead, gently lift the wound edges for maximal exposure. With self-retaining retractors, place them in the wound carefully and open it slowly to prevent tearing of tissue. Unnecessary tissue injury de-

lays healing and causes wound complications.

—Bone cutting instruments must be sharp to avoid fracturing or splintering the bone and to prevent the formation of bizarre callus.

—The size of the instrument should be appropriate for the operative area. Large instruments in a tiny area hinder free access and cause added tissue damage.

Skin Preparation

Home scrubbing with the prescribed cleanser should be instituted 3–4 days before surgery. Shave the hair on the day of surgery to avoid abrasions that may be colonized with bacteria. Thorough scrubbing of the feet and legs removes lipids, surface pathogens, and desquamated epithelium.

Asepsis

Strict asepsis must be observed by the surgical team. Sterilizer controls at several sites in the instrument or drape pack assure that the material is properly autoclaved.

The patient should be draped, with only the operative area exposed. Any team member with a respiratory infection should not attend. Personnel with septic lesions must be excluded. If there is an active rash, eruption, infection, or contaminated fissure at the surgical site, elective surgery should be postponed.

Anesthesia

Excessive amounts of local anesthesia in a confined area should be avoided in order to prevent tissue damage by distention and prolonged ischemia.

It has recently been reported that lidocaine and bupivicaine can inhibit the synthesis of collagenous proteins in tissue cultures when administered in very low concentrations. These findings suggest that local anesthetics might be avoided in poorly healing wounds, leg ulcers, or anywhere that fast healing is essential. On the other hand, they may prove a useful adjunct in the management of keloids or hypertrophic scars by inhibiting rapid protein synthesis.

Incisions

The incision should be made perpendicular to the skin. It should be placed where there will be minimal irritation from the shoe in order to avoid excessive tension on the wound margins. Do not make plantar incisions directly under bony prominences. Also, take into account the need for exposure of the underlying structure to bar excessive retraction of tissue.

Hemostasis

Adequate visualization of tissue is essential. In ligation of vessels, use fine sutures consistent with the need, and avoid strangulating the adjacent soft tissues. Whenever possible, operate without a tourniquet. If a tourniquet is used, elevate the limb to drain it and pad the extremity.

Flushing of Wound

Bone chips, bone dust, and debris should be flushed out with saline solution to promote normal healing. Use a cool flushing solution to discourage vasodilation. Bacteriocidal agents should not be placed within a wound since the cells that control infection and healing may be damaged. These are the polymorphonuclear leukocytes, macrophages, and lymphocytes. Most authorities agree that it is not as important to use a particular kind of flush (e.g., saline or kanamycin), as it is to actually irrigate and cleanse the wound of debris with the flush.

Dissection

Blunt dissection should be minimized. Extensive undermining or flagrant underscoring can rapidly devitalize the area and lead to tissue breakdown. Adhere to the guideline of minimal sharp dissection consistent with operative needs.

Closure

If a tourniquet is used, release it following proper closure of the deeper layers of the wound. This will make it possible to identify and ligate subcutaneous bleeding vessels prior to skin closure. Precise closure of any incision is necessary (Fig. 5.1). If a tissue space is left unclosed, scar tissue forms in direct proportion to the size of the space. It later contracts, pulling the tissue from side to side and drawing the skin downward, causing a scar. Correct layer closure and buried sutures allow the wound edges to fall together neatly before final skin edge closure is accomplished.

Dressings

The use of a compression dressing is an adjunct to good wound closure since it helps immobilize the surgical site, thereby limiting scar formation. It also controls postoperative hemorrhage. One must be careful not to apply a dressing too tightly or devitalization of the wound will occur. Always check the capillary filling time of all digits to insure adequate circulation after the dressing is applied.

Assistant Surgeon

An assistant must be able to perform surgery. Attempting extensive surgery alone is unwise because the surgical wound is exposed longer and is subject to airborne bacteria. If there are complications, an able assistant surgeon is essential. Surgery proceeds faster and is less traumatic when a seasoned assistant works in concert with the surgeon. A team approach also allows for ready consultation during the surgical procedure.

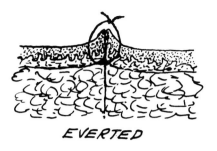

EVERTED

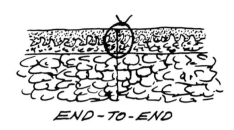

END-TO-END

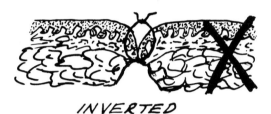

INVERTED

Figure 5.1. The wound edges are everted or sutured end-to-end. Avoid inversion of skin edges, which delays healing. (All drawings in this chapter by J. W. Hill, D.P.M.)

Consultation

Not all doctors are surgeons. For more extensive surgery, the practitioner should seek a competent consultant. The exercises of good judgment, skill, and the planning of procedures are essential.

SUTURES

Sutures obliterate dead space, stop hemorrhage, and approximate tissues at the wound site so that cells, capillaries, ground substance, and fibrin can contribute to tensile strength.

There are several characteristics of suture material. One of them is its rate of absorption by tissue. Slow-healing tissues such as tendon or bone require non-absorbable sutures since they must be maintained in good apposition for a long period of time before they heal. Non-absorbable sutures will also maintain tension better. The non-absorbable sutures include silk, dermal (twisted silk encased in protein), surgical cotton, linen, stainless steel wire (non-nickel-chromium alloy), and the synthetic materials, nylon (Ethilon®, Nurolon®),

polyester (Mersilene®, Ethibond®, Ethiflex®), and polypropylene (Prolene®). Surgical gut (plain or chromic) collagen, polyglactin 910 (Vicryl®) and polyglycolic acid (Dexon®) are absorbable sutures used in faster healing tissue like subcutaneous fat. (All sutures trademarks of Ethicon, Inc. Dexon® trademark of Davis & Geck.) Sutures are also monofilament or braided. Braided (or multifilament) sutures like silk, cotton, polyester, braided nylon (Nurolon®), steel, Vicryl®, and Dexon® are easier to handle and are more secure. However, braided sutures have "drag" which tends to cause friction burns in tissue and seems to harbor more bacteria, but the latter difference is insignificant. Monofilament sutures like catgut, Prolene®, monofilament nylon (Ethilon®), and steel cause less tissue trauma, but have "memory," that is, they "remember" they were once straight fibers in the manufacturing process and as the knots are subjected to stress, they tend to straighten and the knots slip.

Suture material varies tensile strength. Ideally, you want suture material to decrease in tensile strength as the wound's tensile strength increases. As a result, absorbable sutures have become very popular. Remember, though, that the rate of tensile strength loss and the rate of suture absorption are separate events. You also want to use a suture of the proper tensile strength. Dorsal incisions can be closed with 5-0 nylon, whereas plantar incisions, which are subjected to the stress of weightbearing, require 3-0 nylon for more strength. The number of aughts is inversely proportional to tensile strength.

Some sutures cause more tissue reaction than others. Surgical catgut causes the most reaction and should be avoided whenever possible. The new synthetics rarely cause a problem.

The most common suture material used in podiatric surgery for closure of capsule, fascia, and subcutaneous fat is Dexon. It is absorbed by hydrolysis and unlike surgical gut, which depends on enzymatic activity (which is why it causes little tissue reaction), can maintain its strength in the presence of infection. It handles well and forms secure knots. Recent literature has shown that Vicryl may be a better material to use than Dexon® because, in addition to having the same aforementioned characteristics of Dexon®, it is unlike Dexon® in that it has more tensile strength remaining after 2 weeks and is absorbed more quickly.

Monofilament nylon is the most commonly used suture for skin closure. It causes very little tissue reaction and only loses 20% of its strength in 60 days. It does have considerable "memory," however. The newer material, Prolene®, seems to be better than nylon. It causes less tissue reaction, has no tensile strength loss, and has plasticity. This allows it to accommodate for the edema that occurs during wound healing. Its major disadvantage is its considerable amount of memory.

Stainless steel should be used exclusively for closing infected wounds. 5-0 steel and Dexon® can be used for subcuticular closure.

Place sutures so that they do not cause tissue necrosis by strangulation, and check for superficial vessels before suturing layers together. For hemostasis, vessels should be tied with minimal surrounding tissue. Avoid tight skin sutures because normal post-operative edema adds tension (Fig. 5.2). If more than minimal post-operative edema occurs, it should be reduced rapidly with administration of a diuretic, elevation of the limb, elastic bandage, and reduced standing.

Retention sutures may carry surface contaminants deeper into the tissues. Also, good approximation of each layer of fascia, fat, and skin may not take place, and vertical malalignment may occur. If sutures are too tight, tissue ischemia is possible and healing may be delayed. Sutures passing through epidermis, dermis, and subcutaneous tissue can produce an epithelial-lined tract, which can cause inflammation and a scarred suture tract. Closure that proceeds layer by layer assures good approximation of tissues, minimizes dehiscence, promotes even surface planes, and avoids excessive tension on the skin sutures.

Use the simple interrupted suture technique whenever possible. When compared to the continuous technique, there is less edema, less sluggish afferent and efferent

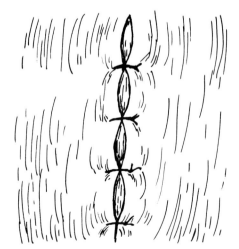

Figure 5.2. The sutures are too tight and inadequate in number. The wound is under tension.

microcirculation, and at 12 days, the burst strength is greater by 30–50%. This is especially important when impaired healing might occur due to vascular disease or old age, or when incisions are made across a moveable joint.

Skin Clips

Skin clips require special instruments and skill. The advantages are quick application and elimination of skin edge inversion. Apply with moderate tension to prevent tissue damage. Their major disadvantages are unsightly suture tracts and occasional discomfort upon removal.

Adhesive Strips

Adhesive strips close the wound but fail to bring the deeper tissues into approximation. The tape may not control bleeding from the wound edges, and hemorrhage can loosen the adhesive and cause dehiscence. A compromise would be a combination of sutures and tape. Early suture removal and replacement with adhesive is useful in certain procedures. Adhesive strips do not inflame the part, and they discourage the formation of suppuration and the development of sinus tracts.

Subcuticular Sutures

Subcuticular sutures are placed in the dermis and remain while scar remodeling is in progress. Proper placement requires practice. It must be superficial enough to hold skin edges in close approximation but deep enough so that epithelium will cover it. Butterfly sutures are helpful when the subcuticular sutures weaken during wound healing. Absorbable sutures obviate the necessity for removal, and their longer stay in the wound assures coaptation of tissue and prevents widening of a surgical scar.

Suture Removal

Early removal of sutures is not recommended because the scar at 6 days postoperatively is still weak, and there is not enough collagen to create tensile strength. A wound held only by fibrin and cells may be disrupted. The natural fibers must be synthesized and assembled. If the sutures must be removed because of abscess, adhesive strips may be substituted. Sutures should be removed when the wound has adequate tensile strength and can withstand tissue tension and ambulation. For slower healing areas or where stress is great, as in the sole, sutures should be retained for a longer period, using materials of proven low tissue irritation potential.

A continual leak of serum signals failure to heal or delay in healing. There may be deep layer dehiscence, and sutures should be left in place longer, if there is no sign of infection. Sutures must be removed before marks develop or before epithelium-lined sinus tracts and excessive scarring develop. Remove a few sutures and check the tensile strength of the wound, then proceed accordingly.

A significant gain in tensile strength occurs between the 15th and 20th days. Since the wounds in which collagen has been laid down are inelastic and weak, severe stress in the surgical area must be avoided postoperatively for a month or more, depending on the recovery.

DRESSING OF WOUNDS

The operative area is vulnerable to bacterial contamination and trauma, and the surgical dressing protects and keeps it clean. The wound should be immobilized during collagen synthesis and remodeling. The dressing also absorbs any suture abscess or viscous exudate at the surgical site. Use emollient-impregnated gauze so that the coagulating exudate will not seal the dressing to the wound surface. With an open wound, avoid direct application of large mesh gauze to prevent capillary or cellular growth in the interstices of the gauze. Removal of such dressings causes hemorrhage and detachment of surface cells, thus delaying healing. On a wound undergoing epithelization, the emollient-impregnated gauze may be left in place until the area becomes dry and there is no further evidence of infection.

One can also use betadine-soaked gauze on surgical wounds, provided it is in low concentrations. A 1% povidone-iodine solution appears best in reducing the incidence of post-op wound infections. Bear in mind that if wound antiseptics are to be used, they should be as low in concentration as possible without losing microbiocoidal properties and they should be as physiologic as possible so that normal wound healing is not impaired.

Do not use insoluble substances that coat the wound and limit wound healing. Protect the fresh wound from surface contamination, trauma, and mechanical and chemical irritants.

Fluff dressing is useful because it minimizes pressure on a fresh wound.

With a pressure dressing, gauze alone is not enough since the pressure is dissipated. A material such as elastroplast maintains the desired tension. The tips of the toes should be left exposed when possible so that sensation and microcirculation may be easily evaluated.

In cases of infection, wet dressings encourage capillary dilation and promote drainage. However, wet dressings can macerate tissues. They are also beneficial for wounds with viscous drainage, and they dilute the viscosity of the secretion. If the viscous exudate does not form a coagulum, dry dressing alone is sufficient. Wet dressings are not meant to debride the wound, but if debridement is desired, enzymatic preparations may be used or manual debridement may be necessary.

Splints should be kept in place beyond the time of the removal of cutaneous sutures since collagen synthesis and alignment are proceeding and tensile strength is limited. External splinting relieves tension across the wound during healing, thereby providing a countermeasure against the development of a wide scar.

WOUND DEHISCENCE

Dehiscence is the rupturing or gaping of an incision. Wound dehiscence may be par-

tial or complete, depending on the degree of separation of skin edges, post-operative herniation, and evisceration.

The predisposing factors for dehiscence include faulty closure, use of improper suture material, hematoma and seroma formation, infection, and the presence of necrotic tissue. Uncontrolled metabolic disorders, anemia, protein dietary deficiences, vitamin C deficiency, and vascular deficiencies are conditions that contribute to slow healing and wound breakdown. Rough handling and stretching of tissue, and pressure and irritation caused by the plaster cast or the shoe against the surgical site further encourage dehiscence.

If a strong surgical closure is desired, the wound should be closed in layers. Sutures in the fat and muscles do not contribute strength to the wound. Muscle and fat should be approximated by suturing their surrounding fasciae or connective tissue septae. To enhance a strong closure, make the incision parallel to the fibers of the fasciae so that the sutures pull at right angles to the fibers. If the incision divides the fibers, use mattress sutures. The wound has the greatest sutured strength when repaired with fine, interrupted sutures in the fasciae (Fig. 5.3).

Hematoma

Hematoma formation is minimized by ligating the bleeding vessels and closing the wound in layers to avoid dead spaces (Fig. 5.4). If a tourniquet is used, it should be released after the major work is done, and the bleeding vessels should be ligated before skin closure. This will avoid hematoma, which delays healing and provides a good culture medium for bacteria. Reliance upon pressure bandage to control internal bleeding is poor management. Hematoma also causes post-operative skin tension, pain, and even skin sloughing.

Seroma

Seroma may result from lymphatic drainage, excessive trauma to the tissue, and reaction to foreign bodies such as su-

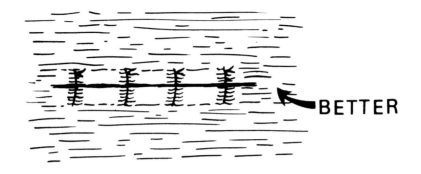

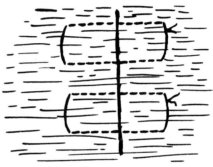

Figure 5.3. The surgical incision is best made parallel rather than at right angles to the fibers of the fasciae.

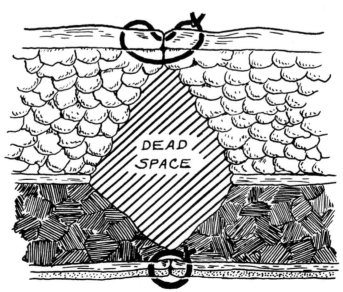

Figure 5.4. Dead space delays healing and permits the formation of fibrosis. The wound should be closed in layers.

ture materials and glove powder. An atraumatic technique and the use of less reactive suture materials lessen post-operative complications. Wash off glove powder with sterile water before surgery.

Edema

Edema should be controlled quickly since swelling delays healing and produces fibrosis. Elevate the extremities and employ elastic supportive bandages to prevent excessive tension and rupturing of the wound. Consider the use of a diuretic when swelling is excessive.

Dehiscence

Dehiscence involving separation of skin edges is often due to faulty suturing. The skin edges may be inverted, or excessive tightening of the sutures may strangulate tissue. Faulty suturing may also make skin levels uneven, causing improper apposition of the tissues. In such cases, there is wound dehiscence when the sutures are removed. If skin sutures are angulated and create skin puckering, proper healing will not result.

It is important to inspect the underside of the skin to determine whether there are vessels coursing along the path of the incision. If so, care should be exercised to avoid ligating those vessels during wound closure. Otherwise, local ischemia may result and superficial gangrene may develop along the wound incision. Failure to utilize square knots allows sutures to untie and the wound to gap. Similarly, with continuous sutures, dehiscence is permitted to occur when the final knot becomes untied.

If there is excessive skin tension, relaxation, or release incisions on one or both sides of the incision, or the use of perforated buttons can be utilized to reduce the tension (Figs. 5.5 and 5.6).

Avoid maceration by frequent changing of bandages with a suitable drying agent. For dorsal incision of the intermetatarsal space, incise the dorsum of the toe rather than the web space to minimize the possibility of interdigital maceration and fungus

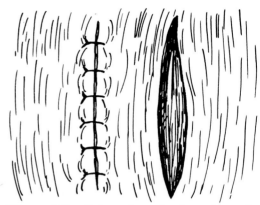

Figure 5.5. Release inversion is made parallel to the primary incision to prevent tension on the wound.

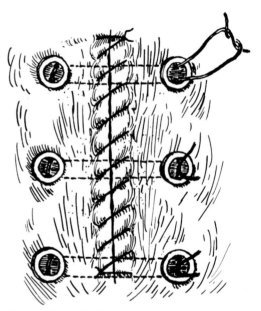

Figure 5.6. Buttons are used to support tension in a wound.

infection. Successive bandages should be less bulky for adequate aeration. With a removable cast, make numerous holes to provide ventilation.

Sutures should be left in place for approximately 3 weeks for many plantar incisions. Interdigital sutures, following syndactylism, for example, are generally not removed before 2 weeks. Dorsal sutures should be left in place for 10–14 days. A few sutures at a time may be removed as indicated. If sutures are removed prematurely, dehiscence frequently results. Check the wound strength by applying gentle side-to-side tension to the incision before any removal. At an appropriate time, suture removal and paper tape replacement are good safeguards. Generally speaking, the patient should refrain from full-time activities for approximately 1 month.

Many types of drains are available, the most common being rubber, plastic, and gauze. Gauze has limited value since it performs only as long as the capillary action in the fabric absorbs the fluid. Then the gauze becomes a plug rather than a drain. A Penrose drain serves as a conduit and should be fixed with a non-absorbable suture so that the drain emerges through the skin and will not be pulled out. Drains are then withdrawn bit by bit so that the cavity may close from the bottom up. The drain should be eliminated as soon as its use is unnecessary.

LOCAL FACTORS THAT DELAY WOUND HEALING

The major causes of retarded wound healing include the following.

—Surgical incisions made at an angle rather than perpendicular to the skin surface, thus preventing primary closure of wound edges.

—Severe traumatization of tissue. A higher incidence of suppurative infection even under aseptic conditions can occur from rough handling, inordinate blunt dissection, indiscriminate clamping and strangulation by sutures tied too tightly. Hand-held retractors or skin hooks are less traumatic than self-retaining retractors.

—Failure to flush out bone chips, bone dust, caked blood, and fragments of necrotic tissue and fat from the operative area. Irrigate thoroughly and flush the wound before closure.

—Inadequate hemostasis. This creates a pooling effect, distention of tissue, and a dead space. If temporary hypotension occurs before wound closure, wait until blood pressure is stabilized so that a collapsed vessel that bleeds may be identified and properly ligated.

—Post-operative hemorrhage. This results in pressure build-up and also increases pain. The involved area becomes edematous and firm or fluctuant. If there is hemorrhaging from a larger vessel, return the patient to the operating room, open the wound, and ligate the involved vessel.

—Drying out of tissue during surgery. Keep the tissue moist with sterile water or normal saline solution.

—Crushing the bone or causing minute fractures with bone rongeur or forceps. Swelling and increased pain result, and in the digits, sausage toes develop. Use an appropriate power tool when indicated.

—Infections cause purulent separation of wound edges. Clean wounds in elective surgeries limit complications to less than 2%. Contamination occurs in all wounds, but infection occurs if the dosage and virulence of the organism overcome the resistance of the host. The suppurating wound must be opened wide to allow for drainage and the release of backed-up pressure.

Specific antibiotics control systemic infections and prevent cellulitis, but antibiotics will not sterilize necrotic, devitalized tissue and blood clots. Nor will antibiotics neutralize the proteolytic enzymes in undrained pus. All abscesses must be drained and the necessary debridement performed before the wound begins to heal.

In a known contaminated wound, initiate and maintain specific antibiotic therapy prior to surgery, and establish a protective blood level.

—Prolonged dependent position of the extremity soon after surgery. Maintaining the limb at a lower elevation than the rest of the body can lead to edema, infection, and thromboembolism. Post-operative elevation of the lower extremities aids the venous return and promotes arterial flow. Elastic compression dressings prevent edema and venous stasis. Wound hypoxia must be avoided since it kills local cells and affects the egress of leukocytes into the damaged or contaminated tissues.

—Use of corticosteroids. Cortisone may delay the development of granulation tissue, depress the proliferation of capillaries, and retard healing when administered before and during surgery. In large amounts, cortisone suppresses fibroblast proliferation, and it can also mask an existing infection and postpone prompt management. However, injected around the surgical site, dexamethasone limits post-op pain by preventing excessive edema formation.

SYSTEMIC FACTORS THAT DELAY WOUND HEALING

Systemic factors that contribute to delayed wound healing are as follows:

—Uncontrolled diabetes mellitus.

—Alcoholism. In alcoholic patients there is decreased protein intake and protein metabolism is reduced. Hypoproteinemia prolongs the lag phase and slows the onset of the fibroblastic phase. A high protein diet does not shorten the lag period, but it does accelerate tensile strength gain. Protein deficiency can be corrected with high protein intake.

—Malabsorption by the gastrointestinal tract.

—Ascorbic acid deficiency. This deficiency inhibits the production of collagen and adversely affects the tensile strength of the healing tissue. The rapid synthesis of collagen and epithelial regeneration are dependent on ascorbic acid.

—Steroids. Prolonged high dosage of steroids administered prior to and at the time of surgery can inhibit the synthesis of collagen and mucopolysaccharides.

—Drugs inhibiting the "release reaction" of platelets and impairing platelet aggregation. These drugs include aspirin, phenylbutazone, sulfinpyrazone, antihistamines, indomethacin, chlorpromazine, a number of tranquilizers, and heparin.

—Anemia can lead to diminished oxygen availability. Hemoglobin below 10 gm/100 ml and hematocrit less than 33% are considered inadequate for successful wound healing.

—Hepatic disease can lead to a decrease in clotting factors and the production of albumin, and will cause altered metabolism of drugs.

—Obesity. Unsatisfactory oxygen saturation, diminished protection against microbial invasion, and hypercoagulability are associated with obesity.

—Delayed wound healing in the aged is related to an increase in the number of autoantibodies, the production of altered proteins, and a decrease in the production of connective tissues.

CYST AND FIBROMA

There are occasions when subsequent to podiatric surgery, an epidermal inclusion cyst or foreign body fibroma may develop.

Epidermal inclusion cysts develop secondary to the inadvertent implantation of an epidermal fragment. A "stab" type of surgical procedure or suture needle penetration could conceivably cause such a cyst formation.

The presence of a cyst is characterized by a round or oval swelling with reactive inflammation. The cyst contains a thick horny material and resolution is accomplished by complete resection of the encapsulated mass.

A post-surgical fibroma can develop secondary to the implantation of a foreign body such as a particle of nail tissue, glove powder, or a fragment of gauze. The body may encapsulate the material in a fibrous cover, as a means of isolation, or a reactive leucocytosis may take place in an effort to exude it.

If the foreign body is encapsulated and the fibrous wall thickens and hypertrophies to the point of positive subjective or objective symptomatology, the fibroma should be excised.

Keloid

A keloid is an irregular fibrous growth that appears subsequent to an injury or as a fibroplasia of a surgical scar. The mass, which occurs more frequently in the black race, may be red, pink, white, or black in color, and has an elevated, smooth, shiny surface. The lesion tends to extend beyond the limits of the original trauma. In the human foot, the ensuing inelasticity, bulk, and distortion caused by a keloid, present problems. A concomitant nerve entrapment or pressure due to keloid formation on a nerve trunk can produce intractable discomfort.

ETIOLOGY

The true etiology of keloid formation is not fully understood; however, the theories include hormonal influence, fibroplastic diathesis and chemotrophic effect of serum on fibroblasts. Trauma to skin and subcutaneous tissues as a result of burns, bacterial invasion, chemical, and mechanical irritants, as well as poor surgical technique and poor tissue handling, also can cause hypertrophic scar formation.

PATHOLOGY

Histopathologic sections reveal fibrous tissue hyperplasia with the fibroblasts arranged in randomly oriented parallel strands. The process is thought to start around blood vessels. The keloid is devoid of sebaceous and sudoriferous glands because of pressure atrophy.

SYMPTOMS

The subjective symptoms include itching, burning, paresthesia, anesthesia and pain if nerve entrapment occurs with fibrosis. A keloid, if subjected to weight-bearing or shoe pressure, can accentuate the aforementioned symtomatology and may at times restrict or disrupt joint motion.

TREATMENT

Available modes of treatment have produced only relative success and include physical, pharmacologic, and surgical approaches used singly or in combination.

Hypothermia (carbon dioxide snow and liquid nitrogen), ultrasonic therapy, and x-ray have been used with varying degrees of success. Surgical excision, followed by radiation, has proven beneficial. The use of topical, systemic, or intralesional approaches have afforded only minimal benefit. The injection of steroids intralesionally has been the most effective pharmacologic approach, but it is a slow and tedious process, used to soften and reduce the fibrosis. The surgical approach, after the tissue reaction has ceased, would be as follows: excise the mass, enclosing it in a pair of elliptical incisions, perform a subdermal adhesiotomy and a primary closure. Avoid the use of buried sutures to minimize tissue reactivity. This approach should be complemented with steroid injections or radiation therapy, or both.

Hypertrophic Scar

A hypertrophic scar results from abnormal collagenous proliferation with the bundles of connective tissue lying parallel to the surface of the skin. It can be differentiated from a keloid in that the hypertrophy stays within the margins of the original scar and it is less dense and less indurated than the keloid. This lesion can occur secondary to the trauma of mechanical, chemical, or bacterial etiology.

The symptoms can be similar to those of the keloid, as described above, because of the ensuing "pressure" discomfort.

In differential diagnosis, the mature keloid is rounded and circumscribed, but nonencapsulated, and is composed of fibers that are oriented in a random pattern, while in hypertrophic scar, the predominant fiber pattern is parallel to the surface of the skin. Also, the keloid tends to extend beyond the limits of the original scar while hypertrophic scar does not.

Prophylaxis

The best treatment is prophylaxis. This begins with obtaining an in-depth familial and personal history and conducting a thorough inspection of the integument for scars. Note skin furrows or lines in relationship to the size of scars and their linear axes. Surgical procedures on the human foot encourage hypertrophic scar or keloid formation. Therefore, the location and the direction of surgical incision should be chosen with care. In order to minimize fibrotic hyperplasia, the surgeon must handle tissue with care, avoiding tight sutures and tissue strangulation. Proper primary closure is essential. Some salient factors bear repetition:

—Keloid and hypertrophic scar are possible post-operative complications.

—They may result from improper techniques in sterility and the handling of tissues during surgery.

—They are better prevented than treated.

—Their presence can complicate foot function and comfort by restriction, constriction, and crowding of footgear.

—Since the key etiologic factor is the individual predilection or tendency toward collagenous hyperplasia, taking a thorough history is vital. Surgical judgment will dictate the wisdom of further surgical intervention.

Suggested Readings

Adams, R., and Fahlman, F. Sterility in operating rooms. Surg. Gynecol. Obstet. 110:360, 1960.

Adriani, J. Relationship of the absorption to toxicity of local anesthetics. Am. Surg. 28:45, 1962.

Amberry, T. *Scientific Illustrators.* Long Beach, California, 1960.

Artz, C. P., and Hardy, J. D. *Complications in Surgery and Their Management,* 2nd ed. W. B. Saunders, Philadelphia, 1967.

Baker, C. P. Tumors and cysts: Exostoses. In DuVries, H. L., ed. *Surgery of the Foot,* 2nd ed. C. V. Mosby, St. Louis, 1965.

Beck, E. A. Evaluation of the DuVries modification of the McBride hallux abducto valgus correction. JAPA 6:12, 1971.

Berson, D., Zauberman, H., Landau, L., and Blumenthal, M. Filtering operations in Africans. Am. J. Ophthalmol. 3:122–129, 1969.

Brennan, R. L. Delayed wound healing in foot surgery. J. Am. Coll. Foot Surg. 3:56–58, 1964.

Christopher, F. *Minor Surgery,* 6th ed. W. B. Saunders, Philadelphia, 1948.

Chvapil, M., et al. Local anesthetics and wound healing. J. Surg. Res. 27:367–371, 1979.

Coleman, G. Wound healing and wound hormones. Br. J. Surg. 51:448, 1964.

Cozen, L. *An Atlas of Orthopedic Surgery.* Lea & Febiger, Philadelphia, 1966.

Davis and Geck: *Suture Manual.* American Cyanamid Company, Danbury, 1968.

DuVries, H. L. *Surgery of the Foot.* C. V. Mosby, St. Louis, 1959.

Estersohn, H. S., and Fuerstman, R. The local use of antibiotics to prevent wound infection. JAPA 69:127–130, 1979.

Flowers, R. S. Unexpected post-operative problems in skin grafting. Surg. Clin. North Am. 4:331–348, 1970.

Fox, C. Infections as an impairment to wound healing. J. Trauma 11:156–168, 1979.

Frantz, V. K., and Harvey, H. D. *Introduction to Surgery,* 2nd ed. Oxford University Press, New York, 1951.

Freeman, B. S., Parry, J., and Brown, D. Experimental study of adhesive surgical tape for nerve anastamosis. J. Plastic Reconstr. Surg. 43:22–28, 1969.

Getzen, L. C., and Jansen, G. J. Correlation between allergy to suture material and post-operative wound infections. Surgery 60:824–826, 1966.

Giannestras, N. J. *Foot Disorders, Medical Surgical Management.* Lea & Febiger, Philadelphia, 1967.

Grabb, W. C., and Smith, J. W. *Plastic Surgery.* J & A Churchill, London, 1968.

Graham, J. R. Paper presented at Symposium on the Management of Infections. Instructional Course Lectures, Hopedale Medical Complex, 1971.

Harkins, H. M., Moyer, C. A., Rhoads, J. E., and Allen, J. G. *Surgery Principles and Practice,* 2nd ed. J. B. Lippincott, Philadelphia, 1961.

Hunt, T. K. Wound management and infection. J. Trauma 11:188–206, 1979.

Jones, C. L.: A surgical adhesive tape for wound closure. JAPA 53:5, 1963.

Kelikian, H. *Hallux Valgus, Allied Deformities of the Forefoot and Metatarsalgia.* W. B. Saunders, Philadelphia, 1965.

King, G. D., and Salzman, F. A. Keloid scars: Analysis of eighty-nine patients. Surg. Clin. North Am. 6:91–102, 1970.

Kopf, A. W., and Andrade, R. *Yearbook of Dermatology.* Yearbook Medical, Chicago, 1966.

Lacy, G. M., and Hemphill, J. E. Facial scar revision. Surg. Clin. North Am. 12:181–184, 1969.

Laurie, P., et al. The absorption of surgical catgut. Br. J. Surg. 46:639, 1959.

Lever, W. F. *Histopathology of the Skin,* 4th ed. J. B. Lippincott, Philadelphia, 1967.

Lewin, A. *The Foot and Ankle.* Lea & Febiger, Philadelphia, 1947.

Lilly, G. E., Armstrong, X., and Koucher, X. Reaction of oral tissue to suture materials. J. Oral Surg. Med. Oral Pathol. 26:592–599, 1968.

Orentreich, N. Dermabrasion. J. Am. Med. Women's Assoc. 4:212–217, 1969.

Peacock, E. E., and VanWinkle, W. *Surgery and Biology of Wound Repair.* W. B. Saunders, Philadelphia, 1979.

Pollack, S. V. Wound healing: A review. III. Nutritional factors affecting wound healing. J. Dermatol. Surg. Oncol. 5:615–619, 1979.

Rakow, R. A method of treatment of post-operative infection. J. Am. Coll. Foot Surg. 6:10–17, 1967.

Robbins, S. L. *Textbook of Pathology with Clinical Application.* W. B. Saunders, Philadelphia, 1962.

Rook, A., Wilkinson, D. S., and Ebling, S. J. G. *Textbook of Dermatology.* F. A. Davis, Philadelphia, 1968.

Sauer, G. D. *Manual of Skin Diseases,* 2nd ed. J. B. Lippincott, Philadelphia, 1966.

Scapinelli, R. Correlation between hyperplastic scars, hyperplastic callus, and heterotopic ossifications. Ital. J. Orthop. Traumatol. 5:207–212, 1979.

Schumann, D. Pre-operative measures to promote

wound healing. Nurs. Clin. North Am. 14:4–12, 1979.

Settler, J. Paper presented at Symposium on the Management of Infections. Instructional Course Lectures, Hopedale Medical Complex, 1971.

Speer, D. P. The influence of suture technique on early wound healing. J. Surg. Res. 27:385, 1979.

Suppan, R. Lecture notes. Ohio College of Podiatry and Medicine, April, 1967.

Suture Use Manual. Use and Handling of Sutures and Needles. Ethicon Corporation, Somerville, New Jersey, 1977.

Vallis, C. P. Intralesional injection of keloids and hypertrophic scars with the Dermo-Jet. Paper presented at the Annual Meeting of the New England Society of Plastic and Reconstructive Surgery, Worcester, Massachusetts April 15, 1967.

Wansker, B. A. *X-ray and Radium in Dermatology.* Charles C. Thomas, Springfield, 1959.

Weaver, R. R., and Berliner, D. L. The action of fluocinolone acetonide upon scar tissue formation. J. Urol. 10:253–260, 1970.

Weisberg, M. H. Wound disruption and ancillary measures. J. Am. Coll. Foot Surg. 5:33–38, 1966.

Wound Healing in Surgery. Abstract of a round table discussion (Chicago). Distributed by Ethicon, Inc., February, 1971.

Wrong, N. M. Post-operative keloids: Treat or ignore? Can. Med. Assoc. J. 8:39–44, 1969.

Yale, I. *Podiatric Medicine.* Williams & Wilkins, Baltimore, 1974.

CHAPTER 6

Pharmacology

RONALD GREEN, D.P.M.

PRE-OPERATIVE TREATMENT
Evaluation of Chronic Medical Conditions Requiring Medication

It is common for the podiatrist to consider surgical intervention in the patient with co-existing chronic medical conditions well controlled by medication. These conditions include: hypertension, cardiac and respiratory disease, collagen vascular disease, diabetes and endocrine disorders, asthma, convulsive seizure disorders, peptic ulcer disease, and many other disorders. Generally, there are no specific pre-operative guidelines for modifying the chronic medications the patients may be utilizing for these conditions. Each patient must be evaluated on an individual basis with appropriate evaluation of their general medical history and physical condition. The use of indicated laboratory investigation and consultation with the patient's family, physician, or internist and anesthesiologist are advisable. It may be necessary, for example, to administer potassium supplements to a hypertensive patient who is hypokalemic in response to diuretic therapy. Insulin-dependent diabetics obviously need special attention and may require adjustment of insulin dosage during the pre-, peri-, and post-operative period. When any doubts exist concerning the patient's co-existing medical condition and its effect on the operative course, medical consultation is always advised (Tables 6.1 and 6.2).

Pre-operative Evaluation of the Diabetic

It is vitally important that the patient's diabetes be well controlled pre-operatively; he should not be allowed to go to surgery in ketosis or with a very high blood glucose level. Even if the case is urgent, a few hours or a single day's delay may free the patient of acidosis, ketosis, and extreme hyperglycemia, thereby making the total operative procedure, including anesthesia management and the immediate post-operative period, safer for the patient (1).

For the insulin-requiring diabetic who must undergo surgery, one-half of the patient's usual dose of intermediate insulin subcutaneously on the morning of surgery is given. In addition, the patient should start receiving intravenous glucose in water or Ringer's lactate at the time the insulin is administered and continued for 24 hours. Short-acting crystalline insulin is added as needed to supplement the pre-operative insulin and to keep the blood glucose levels in a satisfactory range. In the diabetic patient undergoing foot surgery, spinal anesthesia is preferred. General anesthesia is not always necessary and has the added disadvantage of increasing insulin requirement, causing post-anesthesia nausea and vomiting, and delaying the intake of diet and oral medication. With spinal anesthesia, the patient is usually able to take oral fluids and food by the evening meal. When this is achieved, intravenous fluids can be discontinued (1).

Long-term Steroid Therapy

Patients who are on chronic long-term steroid therapy pre-operatively have adenohypophyseal and adrenocortical atrophy. Long-term steroid therapy is defined as a daily dosage of larger than the equivalent of 20 mg per day of cortisone for at least one week, in the year previous to the proposed operation. Although such a patient's response to a period of operative stress and healing is variable, patients with adrenal

Table 6.1.
Factors to Consider before Using Antimicrobial Prophylaxis (4)

1. The risk of infection, including the identification of special groups of patients at higher risk
2. The site of probable infection
3. The most likely bacterial pathogens and their drug susceptibility pattern for a particular hospital
4. The antibacterial spectrum of the antibiotic and expectation that it will be effective against the causative pathogens
5. The protein-binding ability and toxicity of the antibiotic
6. The adequacy of blood levels at the site of anticipated infection
7. The optimum timing and duration of drug administration
8. The adverse consequences to be expected from the interaction of the prophylactic drug with other medications
9. The cost of the drug relative to the benefit to be derived

Table 6.2.
High Risk Factors (7)

1. Previous history of thrombophlebitis or deep vein thrombosis
2. Previous history of pulmonary embolism
3. Previous history of myocardial infarction
4. Previous history of lower extremity fracture
5. Chronic bronchitis
6. Advanced age
7. Oral anti-ovulatory drugs or estrogen therapy
8. Varicose veins
9. Healed varicose ulcers
10. Varicose eczema
11. Obesity
12. Diabetes mellitus
13. Hypertension
14. Malignant disease

insufficiency may exhibit sudden and severe hypotension, progressing to anuria, shock, and coma leading to death (2). This usually takes place in the immediate postoperative period.

Pre-operatively, patients previously on steroids who exhibit weakness, fatigue, and excitability are especially vulnerable to the effects of adrenal insufficiency. Recommended treatment pre-operatively to prevent adrenal insufficiency is to double the normal daily dosage for the day prior to, the day of, and the day following the operation, and then to taper gradually back to the patient's normal dosage (2).

Prophylactic Antibiosis

Prophylactic antibiosis is valuable in preventing post-operative infection in selective circumstances. Is this patient an "at risk" patient with an increased chance of susceptibility to infection? The following circumstances may contribute to increased risk of post-operative infection.

1. Contaminated or dirty surgery
2. Surgery on open fractures
3. Large joint replacements
4. Patients with a previous history of post-operative infection
5. The patient with natural defense mechanism impairment, i.e., diabetics who are poorly controlled, patients on immunosuppressive therapy, including corticosteroids, the presence of alcoholism, anemia, or malnutrition
6. Poor vascularity to the affected limb
7. Procedures with prolonged operating room time, extensive tissue dissection, or increased chance of hematoma formation

DRUG SELECTION

The same factors that are used in selection of an agent for treatment of an infection are considered in the use of prophylactic pre-operative antibiotics. These factors include: the site of potential infection, the specific microorganisms that will tend to cause a potential infection, the status of the hosts defenses, and the pharmokinetics of the drug contemplated for use. Possible toxic effects must be weighed against the risk of infection. Potential harmful effects include: toxic or allergic drug reactions, bacterial or fungal superinfection, and altering the hospital environment in favor of bacterial strains resistant to antibiotics (3).

Most proposed regimens suggest a penicillin or cephalosporin for prophylactic use in musculoskeletal surgery. Cephalzolin, with its longer serum half-life, is the current cephalosporin of choice for prophylaxis. The dosage is 1 gm every 4–8 hours IV/IM starting 1–2 hours before surgery. An alternative is the penicillin derivatives nafcillin or oxacillin: 1 gm every 4 hours IV starting 1–2 hours before surgery (5). Effective use of prophylactic antimicrobials depends on the timing of administration. Antimicrobials should first be given 1–2 hours prior to operative procedures. This is enough time to achieve therapeutic drug levels in the wound during the procedure, but not enough time to select bacterial resistance to the drug. Prophylactic drugs should usually be stopped within 24 hours since continuing prophylaxis increases the risk of drug toxicity and bacterial superinfection but does not reduce the incidence of subsequent infection (6).

Prevention of Deep Thrombophlebitis

Some of the factors that predispose a patient to increased risk of post-operative deep vein thrombosis are: post-operative immobilization and decreased ambulation, use of tourniquet hemostasis, endothelial trauma due to injection of local anesthetics, careless surgical dissection, infection, tight dressings, and casts. All of these factors may be present in current podiatric surgical practice (7). There is also evidence to show that lower limb operations (exclusive of vascular procedures involving the thigh, leg, and foot) have a higher prevalence and incidence of venous occlusion than the average for the entire surgical population (8).

PHARMACOLOGICAL TREATMENT OF POST-OPERATIVE COMPLICATIONS

Treatment of Phlebitis (Superficial Phlebitis)

Phlebitis is a non-suppurative inflammation of a vein and is the most common problem involving the venous system. Following surgery, it may occur secondary through the initiation of the intravenous solution and needle used during the administration of general anesthesia. It may also occur in a lower extremity following pedal surgery during the immediate post-operative period (10). Treatment for phlebitis is:

1. Moist hot packs
2. Compression
3. Range of motion exercises and ambulation
4. Use of anti-inflammatory agents, i.e., phenylbutazone, 200 mg 3 or 4 times a day. Phenylbutazone is contraindicated in the presence of peptic ulcer disease and has many reported side effects (11)

Septic thrombophlebitis is most often due to the presence of indwelling intravenous catheters left in place at a single site. Patients on intravenous solutions for several days following surgery are at greatest risk. The critical time is between 36–72 hours post-operatively. It is generally recommended that catheters be removed and reinserted at a new site after 48 hours. The occurrence of septic thrombophlebitis may be insidious. When general signs of sepsis, including positive blood cultures without other identifiable infected sites, are present, the diagnosis is suggestive. Removal of venous cannula, heat, elevation, and appropriate antibiotics based on the blood cultures is the recommended treatment (12).

Deep Vein Thrombosis

The incidence of deep vein thrombosis is not precisely known since clinical signs and symptoms are notoriously unreliable. Reports vary with an incidence of 5% of all post-operative surgical patients to 88% of all patients undergoing knee replacement (13, 14). Diagnosis is dependent on previous history of deep thrombophlebitis and/or pulmonary embolism, clinical examination, and the use of the newer objective methods for assessment of venous circulation. These methods are; ultrasonic velocity detection, ascending phlebography, ^{125}I fibrinogen scanning, and impedance plethysmography (12).

The best treatment is prevention. When

the diagnosis of deep venous thrombosis has been established, then treatment should begin immediately and vigorously. The average adult should receive an initial intravenous aqueous heparin dose of 5000–7500 units, depending on size, and a dose of 5000 units is repeated every 6 hours. In addition, the leg should be elevated 30°–45° above the torso and compression wraps should be utilized from the toes to the mid-thigh. Local heat for the treatment of deep venous thrombosis is not recommended (15).

Heparin is a glycosaminoglycan whose major pharmacological property is impairment of blood coagulation. Because of its therapeutic efficacy, rapid onset, and short duration of action, it has been the drug of choice for deep venous thrombosis and its major sequelae, pulmonary embolism.

Heparin has a potent antithrombin effect and effectively prevents clots propagating and re-embolization. It does not have any fibrinolytic activity and is dependent on the endogenous lytic mechanism for clot dissolution (16, 17). To be effective, heparin therapy must increase partial thromboplastin time (PTT) to within two and one-half times the normal range. Obviously, an initial baseline PTT and subsequent PTTs must be performed to monitor anticoagulation effect. The major complication of heparin therapy is hemorrhage (18). Protamine sulfate is a specific antagonist for hemorrhage due to heparin therapy. A severe hemorrhage diathesis is the major contraindication to heparin therapy (16, 17).

Usually, 2 or 3 days after the initiation of parenteral heparin, the use of oral warfarin sodium is started. Warfarin is an anticoagulant which inhibits blood clotting by interference with the hepatic synthesis of the vitamin K-dependent clotting factors (II-VII-IX-X). There is a 1–3-day delay in maximum warfarin hypoprothrombinemic effect following oral administration (16). This necessitates the need for initiating warfarin therapy before cessation of the heparin. Warfarin therapy is monitored with the prothrombin time and daily doses of 5–7 mg are administered until the desired prothrombin level of 1.5–2.5 times the control are reached. Oral warfarin anticoagulation is usually continued for 6 to 12 weeks after the patient has become ambulatory and the signs of deep venous thrombosis have subsided (12). Warfarin's side effect is hemorrhage, and its specific antagonist is vitamin K. Drug interactions with warfarin are very common and can cause clinically serious effects of hemorrhage or inadequate lack of anticoagulation. Drugs most commonly taken that interact with warfarin are barbiturates, salicylates, and phenylbutazone (16).

Gout

An acute gouty attack in the immediate post-operative period can be precipitated by the stress-induced trauma of foot surgery. The joint most often affected is the first metatarsal-phalangeal joint (19).

In the post-operative period following bunion correction, an acute attack can be disastrous. It is important to be aware that other areas of the foot can also be the site of an acute gouty attack and the site is not always a joint (20–22) (Table 6.3).

The involved joint is acutely inflamed and has the characteristic signs of heat, rubor, pain, and swelling. These signs may be similar to those present in the normal post-operative period following surgery around a foot joint, and careful clinical examination is necessary to distinguish between a possible gouty attack or the normal post-operative appearing foot. Laboratory tests in acute gout may show a leukocytosis and elevated erythrocyte sedimentation rate. This may be helpful in establishing a diagnosis. The blood uric acid level may or may not be elevated during the acute attack (19). Treatment of a post-operative acute gouty attack is:

1. Tibial nerve block with 2% lidocaine or 0.5% marcaine. Contraindications to this procedure are: marked ankle edema, local infection, thrombophle-

Table 6.3.
Criteria for Diagnosis of Acute Gout[a]

Definite
  Demonstration of sodium urate crystals in
    affected joint
Suggestive (presence of six or more)
  More than one attack of arthritis
  Development of maximum inflammation
    within one day
  Oligoarthritis attack
  Redness over joint
  Painful or swollen first metatarsophalangeal
    joint
  Unilateral attack on first metatarsophalan-
    geal joint
  Unilateral attack on tarsal joint
  Tophus (proven or suspected)
  Hyperuricemia
  Asymmetric swelling within a joint
  Termination of attack

[a] Diagnosis is based on the criteria recently
developed by the American Rheumatism Association for acute gout (23).

bitis, and known sensitivity to the local anesthetic agent (19).

2. Use of oral anti-inflammatory agents
   such as phenylbutazone (800 mg/day),
   indomethacin (200 mg/day), or ibu-
   profen (2400–3200 mg/day). These
   drugs are highly effective and have a
   low incidence of short-term gastrointestinal toxicity. However, these drugs
   may not be tolerated for even a short
   course in the presence of significant
   intestinal disease, and other medical
   contraindications may preclude their
   use.

3. Intravenous colchicine is the recommended alternative therapy (21).

Therapy of Post-operative Pain

Post-operative pain may or may not be
considered a "complication" of foot surgery,
depending on its contributing causes. Post-
operative pain can be due to any of the
following factors, either singularly or in
combination: excessive tissue dissection,
prolonged surgical time, complex surgical
operations, edema, tight dressings, infection, hematoma, post-operative gouty or
arthritic attack, excessive post-operative
ambulation or dependency, low patient
pain threshold, inadequate post-operative
analgesia, phlebitis, allergic reaction, psychological attitude of the patient, and many
other factors. Obviously, primary attention
must be made by the surgeon to the cause
of the pain rather than treating all patients
who complain of pain with increased doses
of analgesics. If a dressing is too tight,
relaxing the dressing is the treatment. Surgeons must understand that excessive tissue handling and dissection will cause patients increased pain post-operatively.
Treating patients with pain following surgery is an art and requires a thorough
knowledge of surgical procedures and their
normal post-operative care. Knowledge of
the patient's background and psychological
status, and an understanding of the use of
all of the therapeutic weapons in the treatment of post-operative pain are imperative.

NON-PHARMACOLOGICAL THERAPY OF PAIN

When evaluating a patient who is complaining of pain, an assessment must be
made as to how much pain this patient has,
compared to the amount the surgeon would
normally expect *this* patient to have at this
point post-operatively. If the pain is excessive, then an attempt should be made to
diagnose and correct if possible the cause
of this excessive pain. Ice, elevation, and a
moderate compression dressing with limited appropriate weightbearing represent
the most important treatment for pain.
Calm reassurance on the part of the doctor
will help alleviate the often prominent anxiety component of pain.

Pharmacology of Analgesia

The type of analgesia used in a given
situation should be based on the intensity
of pain and degree of relief desired (22). In
the management of some post-operative patients, it may be necessary for the patient
to experience some discomfort to discour-

age excessive ambulation. Analgesics are broadly divided into two categories.

ASPIRIN-LIKE DRUGS

These agents have anti-inflammatory, analgesic, and anti-pyretic actions, and are a heterogenous group of compounds of which aspirin is the prototype (Table 6.4). They are effective by virtue of their property of inhibiting the biosynthesis and release of prostaglandins. Although often used for their anti-inflammatory properties, they are effective in post-operative pain of mild to moderate intensity, especially if the pain is chronic in nature. As a class, these drugs have a much lower maximum effect than do opioids, but they do not lead to addiction and are mainly free of the unwanted side effects of the opioids on the central nervous system. Aspirin-like drugs share several undesired side effects; the most common is gastric or intestinal

Table 6.4.
Aspirin-like Drugs: Inhibitors of Prostaglandin Biosynthesis

Drug	Oral Dose	Analgesic	Anti-in-flammatory	Anti-pyretic	Gastro-intestinal Side Effects	Unique Side Effects
Aspirin	600–900 mg q6h	Yes	Yes at higher doses	Yes	Yes	Increased bleeding time, multiple drug interaction
Pyrozolon derivatives phenylbutazone; oxyphenbuta-zone	300–600 mg daily	Yes	Yes	No	Yes	Agranulocytosis, aplas-tic anemia, many drug interactions, safe only for use of 1-week intervals
Para-aminophonol derivatives Acetaminophen	300–600 mg q4h	Yes	Very weak	Yes	No	Liver and kidney ne-crosis
Indomethacin deriva-tives Indomethacin	100–200 mg daily	Yes	Yes	Yes	Yes	Headaches, vertigo, confusion
Sulindac	400 mg daily	Yes	Yes	Yes	Yes	
Fenamates Mefenamic	100 mg daily	Yes	Yes	Yes	Yes	
Meclofenamate	200–400 mg daily	Yes	Yes	Yes	Yes, but less than other agents	Diarrhea, colitis
Tolmetin	600–1200 mg daily	Yes	Yes	Yes	Yes	Pseudoproteinuria
Propionic acid deriv-atives Ibuprofen	1200–2400 mg daily	Yes	Yes	Yes	Yes	
Naproxen	500–750 mg daily	Yes	Yes	Yes	Yes	Insomnia
Fenoprofen	600–250 mg daily	Yes	Yes	Yes	Yes	
Zomepirac	200–500 mg daily	Yes	Yes	Yes	Yes	

ulceration or accompanying symptoms. Hypersensitivity to aspirin is a contraindication to therapy with all drugs in this class. Patients who are sensitive to aspirin react to inhibitors of prostaglandin biosynthesis (16).

OPIOID ANALGESICS

Opioid drugs are those drugs which possess morphine-like properties. These drugs are essentially identical in producing analgesia by acting on specific narcotic (opiate) receptors located in the central nervous system. However, these agents differ from one another in terms of their relative potency, onset and duration of action, effectiveness by different routes of administration, and potential for producing dependence and adverse reactions (24). Their main therapeutic indication is for acute pain. The adverse reactions of opioid analgesics are dose-related. The common reactions are: sedation and drowsiness, respiratory depression, nausea and vomiting, constipation, hypotension, spasm of urinary and biliary tracts, and, rarely, hypersensitivity reactions.

Codeine and propoxyphene are widely used in combination with aspirin-like drugs. There is substantial evidence that codeine-aspirin combinations may provide a greater degree of pain relief than can be obtained with aspirin alone. These mixtures take advantage of the fact that aspirin and codeine produce their analgesic effects by different pharmacological mechanisms. The resultant analgesia is greater than the pain relief that could be achieved with the usual doses of either drug alone. This occurs when acetaminophen or other aspirin-like analgesics are combined with either codeine or propoxyphene (24).

The selection of a specific analgesic agent should be based on the degree of pain and the amount of relief desired. Initially, consideration should be given to a salicylate type agent, either alone or in combination with codeine or propoxyphene. If this is not sufficient, pentazocine or mixtures containing a stronger agent such as oxycodone

(Percodan®) should be utilized. Finally, a morphine-like analgesic may be used. It must be realized that the stronger the agent and the higher the dose, the greater the incidence of toxic reactions.

TREATMENT OF OVERDOSAGE OF ANALGESIC AGENTS

Overdosage can occur when a patient is exposed to excessive amounts of a narcotic agent or agents in combination. Most commonly in the post-operative patient, these agents are narcotics, barbiturates, and tranquilizers. These agents can also interact with recently given anesthetic agents to prevent central nervous system depression. The most dangerous effect of central nervous system depression is respiratory depression. Treatment for overdosage, once adequate ventilation and circulatory measures are taken, is intravenous naloxone. This agent reverses the pharmacological effects of narcotics, barbiturates, diazepam, and related drugs. It can be administered intramuscularly or intravenously and is effective within 1–2 minutes. The dosage is 0.4–0.8 mg and repeat doses may be necessary. Unlike nalorphine, naloxone has no specific narcotic-like actions of its own and, therefore, repeat doses are safe (16).

Antibiotic Treatment of Infection

The goal of antibiotic therapy is to select an appropriate antibiotic that will reach the infecting agent(s) at the site of the infection in a sufficient concentration so as to inhibit or kill this agent(s) with minimum adverse effect on the patient (25–27) (Tables 6.6 and 6.7).

FACTORS IN THE SELECTION OF AN ANTIBIOTIC

The initial choice facing the podiatrist is whether an antibiotic is indicated. Are the signs and symptoms exhibited by the patient consistent with infection and, if so, are other treatment methods such as incision and drainage, suction irrigation, or surgical intervention indicated primarily? Optimal initiation of antibiotic therapy requires the identification of the infecting agent. Since therapy may be required before bacteriological confirmation of identity is available, the physician must make a clinical judgement to identify the most likely organism responsible for this infection (see Table 6.5). A gram stain is a simple and helpful test that can be done immediately to help narrow the list of potential pathogens and permit rational selection of an appropriate antibiotic.

It is important, prior to the initiation of antibiotic therapy on a presumptive basis, to have cultures taken of the infected site (16).

In testing for microbial sensitivity, there are two tests now available that are widely used: the Kirby-Bauer or disc diffusion test is simple and inexpensive. A more reliable and quantitative test is one that uses serial dilutions of antibiotics in a suitable media containing the test microorganism. This test will provide minimum inhibitory concentration (MIC), and it has been found that serum antibiotic levels of 2–4 times the MIC of the drug has been correlated with success of treatment in infections (30).

PHARMACOKINETIC FACTORS

Although an antibiotic may be effective against an infecting organism in laboratory tests, there are several drug-related and host factors to be considered. These include (Table 6.9):

1. Can adequate multiples of the MIC be achieved at the anatomical site of this infection?
2. Does the antibiotic interact with other medications to make it less effective or more toxic?
3. Does the patient have the ability to metabolize and detoxify the drug? Patients with renal or liver impairment may need lower doses of the antibiotic to achieve the MIC and also avoid toxicity.

HOST FACTORS

Is the host defense mechanism impaired or intact? With inadequacy of the type, quality, and quantity of the immunoglobulins, alterations of the host cellular immune system, or defects in the quantity or quality of phagocytic cells may result in therapeutic failure, despite the use of otherwise effective and appropriate drugs (16). Patients with comprised immune systems such as diabetics, those with malignancy, and patients on corticosteroids pre-operatively may contribute to antimicrobial treatment failure. Local wound factors such as the presence of an abscess, chemical changes in pH, and oxygenation, decreased local

Table 6.5.
Opiate Analgesics (16, 24)

Analgesic	Trade Name	IM Dose (mg)[a]	Peak (hr)	Duration (hr)	Oral IM Potency Ratio
Morphine		10	¾–1	4–6	Low (1:6)
Hydromorphone	Dilaudid®	1.5	½–¾	4–5	Low (1:5)
Oxymorphine	Numorphan®	1–15	1	4–6	Low (1:6)
Oxycodone	Percodan®	10–15 (oral)	2–4	4–6	
Levorphanol	Levo-Dromaran®	2–3	¾–1	4–6	High (1:6)
Methadone	Dolophine®	7.5–10	¾–1	3–5	High (1:2)
Meperidine	Demerol®	80–100	½–1	2–4	Moderate (1:4 to 1:3)
Pentazocine	Talwin®	30–60	¾	4–5	Moderate (1:3)
Codeine		120	1–2	4–6	High (1:2)
Propoxyphene	Darvon®	60 (oral)	1–2	4–6	

[a] Equivalent to 10 mg of morphine.

Table 6.6.
Common Bacterial Agents in Post-operative Infection (28)

Gram-positive coccus
  Staphylococcus aureus: coagulase positive, either penicillinase producing or not
Gram-negative bacillus
  Pseudomonas aeruginosa
  Proteus species
  Escherichia coli
Gram-positive coccus
  Lancefield group A *Streptococcus pyogenes*
  Streptococcus faecalis (enterococcus)
  Streptococcus anaerobius (chronic infections)
Gram-negative bacillus
  Bacteroides species (chronic infections)
Gram-positive bacillus
  Clostridium welchii

Table 6.7.
Infecting Agents following Post-operative Foot Surgery Infections (29)

S. epidermidis	32%
S. aureus	34%
Streptococci	17%
Gram-negatives	12%
Other bacteria	5%

Table 6.8.
Bacteriocidal and Bacteriostatic Antibiotics

Primarily bacteriocidal antibiotics
Penicillins
Cephalosporins
Aminoglycosides
Polymyxins
Sulfamethoxazole
Trimethoprin
Primarily bacteriostatic antibiotics
Tetracyclines
Chloramphenicol
Erythromycin
Lincomycins and clindamycin

access of circulation to the abscess, presence of a foreign body, all affect the efficacy of an antibiotic (16). In addition, the effects of age on renal and hepatic biotransformation must be considered, as must genetic metabolic abnormalities, pregnancy, drug allergy, and the presence of other disease states which may make the patient more susceptible to antibiotic effects (16).

COMBINING ANTIBIOTICS

Combining two or more antibiotics can enhance or inhibit therapeutic and toxic effects of one another (16). A simple grouping of antibiotics into bactericidal and bacteriostatic helps determine whether two antibiotics can be used effectively together. Generally, there is frequent antagonism in mixing a bactericidal and bacteriostatic drug. This is because bactericidal antibiotics require active cell division and protein synthesis to function and bacteriostatic drugs inhibit these processes. However, combining bactericidal drugs is often therapeutically beneficial (31) (Tables 6.8 and 6.10).

Combinations of antibiotics may be justified in the following situation:

1. Treatment of mixed bacterial infections
2. Therapy of severe infections in which specific etiology is unknown
3. Enhancement of antibacterial activity in treatment of specific infections
4. Prevention of the emergence of resistant microorganisms (31)

MISUSES OF ANTIBIOTICS

The most common error in the use of antibiotics within the podiatric field are probably:

1. Erroneous dosage of agent: either underdosage or overdosage
2. Reliance on antibiotics with omission of surgical drainage
3. Lack of adequate bacteriological information

It is crucial that appropriate cultures and sensitivities are obtained and that the clinician be familiar with local resistance patterns of microbes to specific antibiotics.

Antimicrobial Agents (Penicillin-related Compounds)

  a. Penicillin compounds are bactericidal and act by inhibiting cell wall synthe-

Table 6.9.
**Potential Problems of Route of Delivery and Physiologic Actions Influencing
Antibiotic Levels in Blood and Tissue (32)**

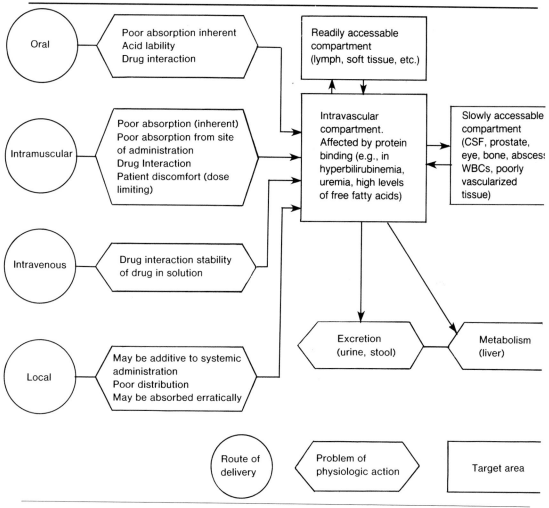

sis. Penicillin is effective against most gram-positive organisms except for penicillinase-producing stains. Penicillin is available in various parenteral dosages and as oral penicillin V.

b. Penicillinase-resistant penicillins. These drugs are not hydrolyzed by staphylococcal penicillinase. While they are less active than penicillin G against penicillin-sensitive microorganisms, they are the drug of choice for penicillin-resistant staphylococcal infections. These drugs are available orally and parenterally.

Broad Spectrum Penicillins

Ampicillin and amoxicillin have a similar antibacterial activity and a broader spectrum than the other penicillins. They are ineffective against penicillinase-producing microorganisms, but have some antibacterial action against gram-negative organisms.

Carbenicillin and Ticarcillin

These penicillins are active against most isolates of *Pseudomonas aeruginosa* and *Proteus* species.

Table 6.10.
Antimicrobial Drugs of Choice[a]

Infecting Organism	Drug of First Choice	Alternate Drugs
Gram-positive cocci		
Staphylococcus aureus		
Non-penicillinase-producing	Penicillin G or V	A cephalosporin; clindamycin
Penicillinase-producing	Penicillinase-resistant Penicillin	A cephalosporin; clindamycin
Streptococcus pyogenes (Group A) and groups C and G	Penicillin G or V	An erythromycin; a cephalosporin
Streptococcus, group B	Penicillin G	Chloramphenicol; erythromycin
	Ampicillin	A cephalosporin
Streptococcus, viridans	Penicillin G	A cephalosporin
Gram-positive cocci		
Clostridium perfringens	Penicillin G	Chloramphenicol; clindamycin; a cephalosporin
Clostridium tetani	Penicillin G	A tetracycline; a cephalosporin
Cornybacterium diphtherial	Erythromycin	Penicillin G
Enteric gram-negative bacilli		
Bacteroides	Clindamycin	Chloramphenicol; cefoxitan
Enterobacter	Gentamycin	Carbenicillin, ticarcillin
	Tobramycin	Amikacin; cefamandole
Escherichia coli	Gentamycin	Ampicillin; a cephalosporin
	Tobramycin	Kanamycin; a tetracycline
Klebsiella pneumoniae	Gentamycin	A cephalosporin; kanamycin
	Tobramycin	Amikacin; a tetracycline
Proteus mirabilis	Ampicillin	A cephalosporin; gentamycin; amikacin
Salmonella typhi	Chloramphenicol	Ampicillin
Other *Salmonella*	Ampicillin	Chloramphenicol
Serratia	Gentamycin	Amikacin; cefoxitan
Other gram-negative bacilli		
Pseudomonas aeruginosa	Tobramycin	Tobramycin
	Gentamycin with carbenicillin or ticarcillin	Gentamycin; amikacin

[a] From *The Medical Letter*, volume 22, No. 2 (Issue 549), January 25, 1980.

All penicillins cause hypersensitivity reactions. These reactions are in order of decreasing frequency; maculopapular rash, urticarial rash, fever, bronchospasm, vasculitis, serum sickness, exfoliative dermatitis, Stevens-Johnson syndrome, and anaphylaxis. The overall incidence of such reactions is between 0.7–10% (16, 32, 33).

Cephalosporins

This antibiotic group is bactericidal and has broad spectrum effectiveness, although gram-negative organisms are generally less susceptible. These drugs are effective against penicillinase-producing strains of *Staphylococcus.* Hypersensitivity reactions occur with these drugs and there is some cross-sensitivity of allergic reaction between the penicillin and cephalosporin groups (16).

Aminoglycosides

This group is used almost exclusively to treat gram-negative infection. They are bactericidal and act to interfere with protein synthesis in susceptible microorganisms. All drugs in this class have major oto- and nephrotoxicity. Generally, these drugs are used parenterally.

Tetracyclines

As a group, tetracyclines are considered to be bacteriostatic. Their site of action is the bacterial ribosome, and they are broad spectrum in action. The tetracyclines are no longer indicated for infections caused by staphylococci or streptococci due to a high incidence of resistant strains. Unless specifically indicated by culture and sensitivity, there is not much specific indication for this group of drugs in the treatment of post-operative foot infections. The toxicity of these drugs is usually gastrointestinal irritation, photosensitivity, and discoloration of teeth in children (34).

Chloramphenicol

Chloramphenicol is a broad spectrum antibiotic and is bacteriostatic. Since this drug can cause irreversible and fatal pancytopenia, its use is indicated only when other less toxic antibiotics cannot be used in its place.

Erythromycin

Erythromycin is an orally effective bacteriostatic antibiotic which is most effective against gram-positive cocci. Its use against *Staphylococcus aureas* is dependent upon sensitivity, and some strains are resistant to all but extremely high concentrations of erythromycin. It is not an active agent against most gram-negative aerobes. Erythromycin is a safe drug and serious side effects are rare. The estolate salt of erythromycin can cause a cholestatic hepatitis which is reversible.

Clindamycin

This antibiotic has replaced lincomycin. Its activity is similar to that of erythromycin but it is more active against anaerobic bacteria, especially *Bacillus fragilis*. It produces an incidence of diarrhea of approximately 8% and may cause pseudomembranous colitis which can be fatal. This disease is apparently due to the production of an exotoxin by clindamycin-resistant strains of *Clostridium difficile* (35). If significant diarrhea or colitis occurs with the use of this drug, therapy should be discontinued immediately. Vancomycin®, in oral doses of 2 gm per day, is effective in reducing the frequency of this diarrhea. Agents that inhibit peristalsis, such as opiates, are *not* indicated and may worsen the condition (16). The evidence that clindamycin has increased bone-binding properties over other antibiotics and therefore is especially useful in the treatment of osteomyelitis is equivocal and may have no basis in fact.

Reflex Sympathetic Dystrophy (RSD)

RSD can be a complication of foot surgery or of plaster immobilization following surgery (19, 36). RSD is characterized by persistent pain and tenderness of the affected limb. It is often described as a severe burning or aching that is out of proportion to the traumatic insult. A trigger area may cause exacerbation of pain and paresthesia, and dysesthesia may be present. Associated vasomotor disturbances are frequently found. In early stages, local temperature may be increased and hyperhidrosis and edema may appear. Later, vasospastic symptoms with persistent coldness of the affected extremity, pallor, or cyanosis, atrophy of the skin, and Raynaud's phenomenon may be prominent (37). Osteoporosis can be present on roentgenographic examination and it is often diffuse or spotty (38).

It is crucial to initiate treatment early since the degree of physical impairment depends to a large extent on the time that elapses between onset of sympathetic dystrophy and initiation of treatment (37). Physical therapy is indicated for mild cases. Periarterial blocks of 2% lidocaine or marcaine cause a "chemical sympathectomy" and are effective in treatment. These blocks may be repeated weekly to monthly in mild cases. In severe RSD, a periarterial catheter in the area of the tibial artery and nerve may be placed subcutaneously and a vasodilating anesthetic agent administered every few hours.

For more severe cases, the following treatment plan is recommended.

1. Hospitalization and initial continuous bedrest
2. Tranquilizers, i.e., diazepam 5 mg every 6 hours
3. Continuous elevation and compression dressings
4. Diuretics: furosemide intravenously may be initially indicated. Later, oral medication may be sufficient
5. Local nerve blocks with marcaine or xylocaine
6. Prednisone in the following dosage: day 1, 50–100 mg; day 2, 50–100 mg; day 3, 45 mg; day 4, 45 mg; day 5 and 6, 40 mg; day 7, 35 mg; thereafter decreasing the dose by 5 mg per day.

This plan can be modified and smaller starting doses of prednisone used in less severe cases (39).

Post-operative Edema

Post-operative edema is a "normal" result of surgical intervention. This edema is a symptom usually of lymphatic congestion secondary to surgical trauma. However, a distinction must be made in evaluating this "normal" post-operative edema from all other possible complications of surgery that can cause edema. These complications include: thrombophlebitis, infection, hematoma, reflex sympathetic dystrophy, electrolyte imbalance, lymphatic obstruction, hypertension, cardiac disease, diabetes, lipidema, arterial or venous insufficiency, and other various systemic disease processes.

If the diagnosis of post-operative edema can be made, the following therapeutic measures may be indicated:

1. Elevation of the extremity
2. Ice packs to popliteal fossa or dorsum of ankle
3. Limited ambulation
4. Furosemide 40 mg daily
5. Compression dressing
6. Limited ambulation may be helpful in restoring venous return

Table 6.11.
Classification of Adverse Drug Reactions (42)

Type	Definition
Allergic reaction	Immunologic response to drug
Idiosyncratic reaction	Qualitatively abnormal reaction unrelated to usual pharmacologic action of drug
Intolerance	Extreme of normal pharmacologic effect of drug
Secondary effect	Indirect effect that may result from drug use but is not inevitable
Side effect	Unavoidable and undesired effect of drug
Toxic reaction	Untoward effect directly related to amount of drug administered or to accumulation of drug because of decreased excretion or metabolism

7. Range of motion exercises; massage and isometric muscle exercises are also helpful (40, 41).

Treatment of Adverse Drug Reactions Post-operatively

Adverse drug reactions can occur to any of the myriad of chemical substances that the patient comes in contact with in the course of operative care. Adverse drug reactions can be classified as to type (Table 6.11). Only an allergic reaction produces an immunological response to a drug. Immune reactions can also be divided into type (Table 6.12). Knowledge of different types of adverse drug reactions is a major step to a proper diagnosis and management. Recognition that not all reactions stem from "allergy" allows the mechanistic approach to the problem and more specific diagnosis and treatment (42). Adverse drug reactions can affect all organ systems and, potentially, all drugs can cause them. The surgeon should possess knowledge of the most common reactions and should be familiar with the general pharmacological and adverse reactions of all drugs he utilizes.

Table 6.12.
Classification of Immune Reactions (42)

Type	Mechanism		Examples
	Specific	Effector	
I (anaphylactic, immediate)	IgE	Histamine, eosinophilic chemotactic factor, slow-reacting substance or anaphylaxis	Urticaria, asthma, anaphylaxis
II (cytotoxic)	IgG, IgM	Complement cascade	Hemolysis
III (immune complex)	IgG, IgM	Complement cascade	Serum sickness, lupus-like syndromes
IV (delayed)	T lymphocytes	Lymphokines	"Furadantin lung"

Table 6.13.
Common Adverse Drug Reactions (44)

Cutaneous	Contact dermatitis, eczema, erythema group reactions, exfoliation, fixed eruptions, urticaria
Collagen vascular	Lupus-like syndromes, polyarteritis, vasculitis
Hematologic	Agranulocytosis, eosinophilia, hemolysis, thrombocytopenia
Hepatic	Cholestatic and hepatocellular reactions
Neurologic	Headaches, peripheral neuropathy, pseudomotor cerebri, seizures
Pulmonary	Asthma, hypersensitivity lung disease, intestinal fibrosis, pulmonary vasculitis
Renal	Glomerulitis, nephrotic syndrome, tubular defects
Vascular	Circulatory collapse
Miscellaneous	Anaphylaxis, drug fever, serum sickness

Table 6.14.
Drugs or Drug Classes Commonly Causing Adverse Reactions (42)

Antibiotics
Anticonvulsants
Aspirin
Barbiturates
Corticosteroids
Diuretics
Local anesthetics
Radiocontrast agents
Tranquilizers
Vaccines

Treatment of All Adverse Drug Reactions

The drug history must be carefully reviewed, and since the frequency of drug reactions is related to the number of agents used, this number should be limited whenever possible. Next, the reactions associated with the prescribed drugs should be considered. These two steps often allow specific diagnosis and the offending drug can be discontinued. Most reactions begin to subside within 24 hours after termination of the causative drug (42) (Tables 6.13 and 6.14).

If after these steps no firm diagnosis is possible, all non-essential agents should be stopped. If therapy cannot be interrupted, an attempt should be made to switch to alternative drugs. The original medication then can be carefully re-introduced one at a time so that recurrence of symptoms is detected early and a diagnosis confirmed (42).

Aside from this, specific treatment of adverse reactions usually consists of minimal symptomatic treatment. Antihistamines, topical and systemic steroids, analgesics, and other appropriate agents may be used but should always be done so with caution.

Treatment of anaphylactic shock requires special attention. The inciting agent can be any drug, diagnostic agent, and contact media, insect bites, or even certain

Table 6.15.
Suggested Emergency Kit (43)

Drugs
  Aminophylline (generic)
  Amyl nitrate (generic)
  Aramine® (Merck Sharp & Dohme, West Point, Pennsylvania)
  Aromatic spirits of ammonia (generic)
  Atropine (generic)
  Benadryl (Parke Davis, Detroit, Michigan)
  Caffeine and sodium benzoate (generic)
  Calcium chloride (generic)
  Calcium gluconate (generic)
  Dextrose (generic)
  Diazepam (Valium®) (Roche Laboratories, Nutley, New Jersey)
  Diazoxide (Hyperstat®) (Schering, Kenilworth, New Jersey)
  Digoxin (Lanoxin®) (Burroughs Wellcome, Research Triangle, North Carolina)
  Diphenhydramine (Benadryl®) (Parke Davis, Detroit, Michigan)
  Epinephrine (Adrenalin®) (Parke Davis, Detroit, Michigan)
  Hydrocortisone Na succinate (Solu-Cortef®) (Upjohn, Kalamazoo, Michigan)
  Levarterenol (Levophed®) (Winthrop, New York, New York)
  Lidocaine (Xylocaine®) (Astra, Worchester, Massachusetts)
  Meperidine (Demerol®) or morphine sulfate (Winthrop, New York, New York)
  Metaraminol (Aramine®) (Merck Sharp & Dohme, West Point, Pennsylvania)
  Methoxamine (Vasoxyl®) (Burroughs Wellcome, Research Triangle, North Carolina)
  Methylprednisolone Na succinate (Solu-Medrol®) (Upjohn Kalamazoo, Michigan)
  Naloxone (Narcan®) (Endo, Garden City, New York)
  Nembutal® (Abbott, Chicago)
  Nitroglycerin (generic)
  Pentobarbital (Nembutal®, Abbott Laboratories) or secobarbital (Seconal®, Lilly, Indianapolis, Indiana)
  Phenytoin (Dilantin®) (Parke Davis, Detroit)
  Ringer's lactate (intravenous bottle) (generic)
  Seconal® (Lilly, Indianapolis)
  Sodium bicarbonate (generic)
  Trimethaphan (Arfonad®) (Roche, Nutley, New Jersey)
Equipment and Supplies
  Airway needle
  Cuffed endotracheal tubes (infant, child, and adult size)
  Hemostasis
  IV administration kit
  Laryngoscope and light source
  Needles and syringes (including needles for cardiac administration)

Table 6.15. (Continued)

  Oxygen alcohol sponges
  Resuscitube
  Scissors
  Sphygmomanometer
  Stethescope
  Stylet
  Tourniquet

foods. Signs and symptoms can appear immediately after challenge with the initiating agent or hours later. Usually, the patient will appear flushed with a rapid pulse and palpitations. Other symptoms can include urticaria, pruritis, edema, cyanosis, sneezing, choking, coughing, paresthesia, and unconsciousness. Incontinence and convulsions can follow with severe progressive respiratory symptoms and profound shock. Rapid recognition of the signs and symptoms and immediate treatment is necessary for patient survival (43) (Table 6.15).

Supportive immediate treatment for anaphylactic shock:
1. Stop exposure to inciting agent
2. Place patient in supine position with elevation of the lower extremities
3. Administer 0.3–0.5 cc of aqueous epinephrine 1:1000 sublingually or intramuscularly
4. Apply a tourniquet proximal to the injection site if appropriate
5. Maintain an open airway
6. Initiate cardiopumonary resuscitation if necessary

Supportive treatment consists of:
1. Elevation of blood pressure
   a. Trendelenburg position
   b. Use of vasopressor agents such as metaraminol, 0.5–5 mg IV or levarterenol, 4 ml in 500–1000 cc of dextrose 5% water IV
2. Control of convulsions utilizing 100–300 mg of pentobarbital, secobarbital, or diazepam 10–20 mg IV
3. Control of bronchospasm, utilizing aminophylline, 500 mg IV, over a 10-minute period (44)

References

1. Levin, M. E., and O'Neal, L. W. *The Diabetic Food,* 2nd ed. C. V. Mosby, St. Louis, 1977.
2. Durkin, J. F. Patients on long-term steroid therapy, JAPA 66:847–849, 1976.
3. Sack, R. P. N. Engl. J. Med. 300:1107, 1979.
4. Goldman, P. L., and Petersdorf, R. G. Prophylactic antibiotics: Controversy Give Way to guidelines. Drug Ther. Rev. 9:57–77, 1979.
5. Authors. Antimicrobial prophylaxis for surgery. *The Medical Letter.* Volume 21, No. 18 (Issue 539), September 7, 1979.
6. Stone, H. H., et al. Ann. Surg. 189:691, 1979.
7. Hatch, D. J., Magnusson, P. G., and DiGiovanni, J. E. Mini-dose heparin prophylaxis for high-risk patients in podiatric surgery. JAPA 70:73–81, 1980.
8. Siegel, B., Ispen, J., and Felix, W. R. The epidemiology of lower extremity deep venous thrombosis in surgical patients. Ann. Surg. 179:278, 1974.
9. Council on Thrombosis of the American Heart Association. Prevention of Venous Thrombosis in Surgical Patients by Low-Dose Heparin: Circulation 55:423, 1977.
10. Bogen, J. E. Local complication in 167 patients with indwelling venous catheters. Surg. Gynecol. Obstet. 110:112, 1960.
11. Wolf, E. W. Case records of the California Podiatry Hospital clinicopathologic exercise: Post-operative thrombophlebitis. JAPA 69:207–210, 1979.
12. Epps, C. H., Jr. ed. *Complications in Orthopaedic Surgery.* Lippincott, Philadelphia, 1978.
13. Barker, N. E., Nygaard, K. K., Walter, W., et al. A statistical study of post-operative venous thrombosis and pulmonary embolism: Incidence in various types of operations. Prog. Staff Meet. Mayo Clin. 15:769, 1940.
14. McKenna, R., Bachmann, F., Kausahal, S. P., and Galente, S. O. Thromboembolic disease in patients undergoing total knee replacement. J. Bone Jt. Surg. 58A:928, 1976.
15. Conn, H. F., ed. *Current Therapy.* Saunders, Philadelphia, 1977.
16. Gilman, A., and Goodman, L. S. *Pharmacological Basis of Therapeutics,* 6th ed. Macmillan, New York, 1980.
17. Guidice, J. C., Romansky, H. J., and Kaufman, J. Pulmonary thromboembolism: New trends in prophylaxis and therapy. Postgrad. Med. 67:81–89, 1980.
18. Salzman, E. W., Deykin, D., Shapriro, R. M., et al. Management of heparin therapy: Controlled prospective trial. N. Engl. J. Med. 292:1046–1050, 1975.
19. Steinberg, M. D., Steinberg, L. B., Fields, G. S., Fields, L. Sl: Gout and Sudeck's atrophy. JAPA 65:499–502, 1975.
20. Shaw, A. H. Acute gout in the soft tissue. JAPA 62:192–193, 1972.
21. Gomes, D. R. Acute gout of subtalar joint in the 56-year-old white female. JAPA 67:68–69, 1977.
22. Brynickzka, G. C., and Pascente, R. W. Gouty arthritis of the subtalar joint. JAPA 67:115–116, 1977.
23. Wallace, S. L., et al. Preliminary criteria for the classification of acute arthritis of primary gout. Arthritis Rheum. 20:895–900, 1977.
24. Inturrise, C. E. Targeting narcotic action to patients' needs. Drug Ther. 10:49–55, 1980.
25. Jawetz, E. Principles of antimicrobial therapy. Mod. Treat. 1:819, 1964.
26. Rangno, R. E. Antibiotics—An Overview. Infection, Orthopaedic Surgery Seminar, Montreal, May 1974.
27. Sokolowski, K., Smith, S. D., and Weil, L. S. Therapeutic approaches to major post-operative infections in podiatric surgery. JAPA 65:522–539, 1975.
28. Aaron, H., ed. *Handbook of Antimicrobial Therapy* p. The Medical Letter, New York, 1974.
29. Rubinlicht, J. R. Bacterial infections of the foot. JAPA 66:553–554, 1976.
30. Smith, J. K. Current criteria for selecting an antibiotic. Drug Ther. 11:115–119, 1981.
31. Rahal, J., Jr. Antibiotic combinations: The clinical relevance of synergy and antagonism. Medicine (Baltimore) 13:331–336, 1978.
32. Levine, B. B. Skin rashes with penicillin therapy: Current management. N. Engl. J. Med. 286:42–43, 1972.
33. Idsoe, D., Guthe, T., Willcox, R. R., and DeWeck, A. L. Nature and extent of penicillin side reactions, with particular reference to fatalities from anaphylactic shock. Bull. WHD 38:159–188, 1968.
34. Hatch, D. J., and Pagcente, R. N. Photo-onycholysis associated with tetracycline. JAPA 68:172–177, 1978.
35. Larson, H. E., and Price, A. B. Pseudomembraneous colitis: Presence of clostridial toxin. Lancet 2:1312–1314, 1977.
36. Papier, M. J., and Papier, M. J., II. Sudeck's atrophy. JAPA 66:327–331, 1976.
37. Juergens, J. L., Spittell, J. A., and Fairbairn, J. F., II. *Peripheral Vascular Diseases,* 5th ed. Saunders, Philadelphia, 1980, p. 616.
38. Gamble, F. O., and Yale, I. *Clinical Foot Roentgenology,* 2nd ed. Krieger, Huntington, New York, 1975.
39. Willenegger, H. A.S.I.F./A.O. Instructional Course, Aspen, February, 1981.
40. Grossman, H. S. Evaluation and treatment of pre- and post-operative edema: A symptom, not a disease. J. Foot Surg. 18:102–106, 1979.
41. Wood, W. A. Post-operative pedal edema. J. Foot Surg. 16:15–16, 1977.
42. Deweck, A. L. Drug reactions. In Samter, M., et al., eds. *Immunological Disease,* 3rd ed. Little, Brown & Co., New York, 1978, p. 413.
43. Gell, P. G., and Coombs, R. R., eds. *Clinical Aspects of Immunology,* 2nd ed. Blackwell, Oxford, England, 1968.
44. Webb, D. R. Drug allergy in clinical practice. Postgrad. Med. 65:62–72, 1979.
45. McCormick, C., Scapa, B., and Shea, T. Acute anaphylatic shock. JAPA 69:604–607, 1979.
46. Queng, J. T., and McGovern, J. P. Acute anaphylaxis. Hosp. Med. 12:13, 1976.

CHAPTER 7

General Anesthesia

JACK LEVITT, D.O.

The category of general anesthesia can be divided into inhalation and intravenous general anesthesia. The intravenous segment is further divided into neuroleptic, opiate analgesic, barbiturate, and agonist-antagonist.

In order for one to best understand the pitfalls, complications and their prevention, one should have a basic knowledge of the agents and their effect on the physiology and pharmacological status of the patient being anesthetized.

INHALATIONAL ANESTHETICS

The inhalational anesthetics are normally regarded as chemically stable. The anesthetic state results from the development of appropriate brain anesthetic partial pressure. Each tissue removes anesthetic coming through it via the bloodstream. The factors influencing tissue uptake are:

1. Tissue/blood partition coefficient
2. Tissue volume in relation to amount of blood flow
3. Partial pressure of anesthetic between arterial blood and the tissues

The cardiac output influences the anesthetic uptake; a larger output increases the uptake.

The recovery from anesthesia occurs by loss of anesthetic from blood to alveolar gas space. The factors controlling the recovery are: a) rate of fall in alveolar concentration, and b) increased ventilation speeds up recovery time.

The various parameters which must be considered in the decision as to the type of agent or agents used are:

Patient's history as to:
1. Previous surgery (type and date)
2. Type of anesthesia administered
3. Cardiac disease
4. Circulatory disease
5. Pulmonary disease
6. Renal disease
7. Neurological disease
8. Endocrine status (e.g., diabetes, thyroid)
9. Smoking habits
10. Alcohol intake and habits
11. Drug history

NITROUS OXIDE

This was first utilized in 1844. It is very soluble in the plasma and does not undergo any chemical combination in the body. Absorption and elimination are very rapid. It is not a very potent anesthetic, and is used as a secondary agent to supplement halothane, ethrane, etc., in its proper percentage. When used in proper, safe percentages, there are no complications.

HALOTHANE (FLUOTHANE®)

This halogenated hydrocarbon was investigated in 1956, and has become the most widely used inhalation anesthetic agent. The agent is potent, non-explosive, non-irritating, and easily controlled. It produces bronchodilatation, and is therefore especially suited as an anesthetic in patients suffering from pulmonary disorders.

METHOXY FLUORANE (PENTHRANE®)

This is a potent agent which produces excellent muscle relaxation and analgesia in the lighter planes of anesthesia. It causes a minimum of myocardial irritability. There is a lack of irritation, increased secretions, and very little post-operative nausea and vomiting. Penthrane has been found to maintain normal heart response, even in the presence of high concentrations of circulating catecholamines.

ENFLURANE (ETHRANE®)

This is a potent, non-flammable inhalational anesthetic agent which resembles Penthrane in chemical structure, but its physical characteristics are related to Fluothane. It has a low blood/gas partition coefficient and, therefore, produces an anesthetic level which is easily controlled and both the induction and recovery stages are rapid. There is very minimal myocardial depression.

MUSCLE RELAXANTS

There are two classes of muscle relaxants:
1. Depolarizing (succinylcholine chloride)
2. Non-depolarizing (Tubocurare®, Pavulon®, etc.)
These are mainly used in conjunction with inhalation anesthesia. Their purpose is to allow for better muscle relaxation during the surgical procedure, and to aid in the performance of endotracheal intubation.

Pitfalls, Complications, and Prevention

NITROUS OXIDE

The major concern is the possibility of diminished oxygenation leading to hypoxia. The hypoxic state is detrimental to persons having pulmonary or cardiovascular diseases in particular. When this does occur, oxygenation of the patient is of utmost importance and the discontinuing of the administration of nitrous oxide.

HALOTHANE

Some of its undesirable features are myocardial depression and irritability, both of which can produce or precipitate cardiac arrhythmias. There is some cardiac slowing, which becomes more pronounced as anesthesia deepens. These changes are mainly due to increased nasal activity and can be reversed by lightening of the anesthesia and utilizing atropine sulfate.

The myocardium is sensitized to the effect of catecholamines hypercarbia which may give rise to beginning or ventricular tachycardia. These must be treated immediately by correcting respiratory acidosis and oxygenating the patient well.

In patients with hepatic disease, Fluothane® is contraindicated due to fear of further damage to the liver. Repeated Fluothane® administrations within a short time span is not recommended.

METHOXY FLUORANE

Due to its high blood/gas partition coefficient, there is a prolonged recovery period. It is usually contraindicated in renal disease; may depress respirations.

ENFLURANE

The use of enflurane may lead to the occurrence of muscular twitchings of the face and limbs. It is contraindicated in patients with a history of convulsive disorders. When this occurs, a lightening of the level of anesthesia will return the patient back to normal. It may cause respiratory depression if the anesthetic level is too deep; if so, lighten anesthetic level and oxygenate well, also increasing minute volume ventilation.

MUSCLE RELAXANTS

The use of the relaxants in patients who have neuromuscular disorders is contraindicated. Patients on neomycin, streptomycin, etc., should not be given succinylcholine chloride due to the possibility of prolongation of the action of the depolarizing agents. This would require placing the patient on a mechanical ventilator until metabolism of the agent occurred.

Other contraindications to inhalation anesthesia are:
1. Inadequate airway before induction
2. Risk of loss of airway during anesthesia. Ensure a free airway before starting
3. Untreated adrenal-cortical insufficiency due to the inability to respond to stress

4. Unavailability of proper equipment to properly aerate the patient

INTRAVENOUS ANESTHETICS

BARBITURATES

It is of utmost importance and desirability that the induction agents be rapid in action and produce a loss of consciousness. The total dosage of the agent is usually titrated against a patient's requirements.

The drugs with a rapid onset usually have a shorter duration than the slower acting compounds. The rapid induction agents usually produce less side-effects than the slower induction agents.

The rapid induction agents are usually the thiobarbiturates. The slower acting are the basal hypnotics, e.g., tranquilizers (diazepam), phencyclidine (ketamine), neuroleptic drug combinations, intravenous analgesics, and agonist-antagonist combinations.

It is important to keep in mind that the release of consciousness following intravenous barbiturates occurs with a large amount of active drug remaining in the body.

Immediately upon injection, a large proportion of the barbiturate is rendered pharmacologically inactive by being bound to the non-diffusable ions of plasma. The thiobarbiturate is taken up by the brain and other vessel-rich tissues, the liver, and kidney. This causes a rapid decline in the concentration of the drug in the brain, which leads to a lighter plane of anesthesia.

The mechanisms of transport of the intravenous anesthetics are from vein to brain, as compared to the inhalation anesthetics, leads to a high concentration suddenly coming into contact with the heart, vasomotor, and respiratory centers.

Pitfalls, Complications, and Prevention during Intravenous Barbiturate Anesthesia

RAPID AND SLOWER ACTING AGENTS

There is a transitory cardiovascular and respiratory depression with the rapid induction agents. They should be given at a slower injection rate and not too large a bolus.

It must be reiterated that a larger amount of active drug remains in the body after the release of consciousness. Therefore, there is a tendency for the patient to lapse back to sleep if left undisturbed, and drugs given in the immediate post-operative period can lead to reinduction of anesthesia.

In patients with a decreased cardiovascular reserve, hypotension leads to a decreased venous return which in turn causes a further fall in cardiac output, and a decreased coronary blood flow.

The rapid onset of anesthesia with intravenous agents may lead to a relaxed cardiac sphincter which may lead to a loss of protective reflexes.

The above may be prevented by proper and adequate monitoring of the patient: adequate oxygenation, proper rate of injection of the agent, adequately trained personnel who are familiar with the pitfalls and complications of the agents, and knowing how to treat any complication which may arise.

It is important to keep in mind the following contraindications to the barbiturate agents, and therefore prevent any misadventure.

1. Severe cardiac decompensation or circulatory failure
2. Severe anemia
3. Hypersensitivity
4. Porphyria
5. Status asthmaticus
6. Bronchospasm on laryngospasm

KETAMINE® (PHENCYCLIDINE)

Effective when given intravenously or intramuscularly. The intravenous dose is effective between 30–60 seconds, intramuscular dose is effective in 2–4 minutes. Ketamine® has a cataleptic, analgesic, and anesthetic action, but lacks hypnotic properties. It does not produce muscle relaxation. Ketamine causes a stimlation of the cardiovascular system. Analgesia is extremely good. The agent is associated with hypertonus, purposeful movements of the extremities, and horizontal and vertical nystagmus. Respiratory depression is minimal, and the patient has the laryngeal reflexes intact.

Ketamine will cause severe hallucinations and emergence delirium. It has been found that these may be altered with the utilization of intravenous barbiturates or drugs such as diazepam given prior to Ketamine®. Ketamine® is contraindicated in the following:

1. Hypertension
2. Increased intracranial or intraorbital pressure
3. Psychiatric disorders
4. Congestive heart failure
5. Operations involving pharynx, larynx, or trachiobronchial tree
6. Alcoholics or thyrotoxic patients

VALIUM® (DIAZEPAM)

It exhibits an excellent tranquilizing effect. Potentiates the action of narcotics, agonist-antagonist agents, and general inhalational anesthetic agents.

TALWIN® (PENTAZOCINE)

It is a weak antagonist of morphine. There is a small abuse potential and it is non-addictive. Non-addictive. It works well in conjunction with Valium® or droperidol.

SUBLIMAZE® (FENTANYL)

Has excellent analgesic properties. Used well in conjuction with Valium® or droperidol. When in combination with droperidol is called Innovar®.

STADOL® (BUTORPHANOL)

This is an agonist-antagonist agent. It is five times more potent than morphine. Stadol® combines potent analgesic properties intravenously with sedative action and minimal euphoria. It does not lead to abuse.

The main pitfall of the above mentioned is being careful not to make the patients drug-dependent. This is especially true for diazepam. Proper dosage must be kept in mind at all times to prevent any misadventures pharmacologically. This is especially true when utilizing the agents in combination.

One must keep in mind all the complications of a particular agent and its contraindications.

SUMMARY

This has been an overview of general anesthesia, inhalation and intravenous, the types available, some of the agents' pharmacological actions, the pitfalls, complications, and prevention of possible mishaps. Another important factor which must be kept in mind at all times is that in order to use the agents, one must be well equipped and trained to resuscitate the patient, and treat all complications relating to the use of the agents mentioned.

Suggested Readings

Clarke, R. S. J. Newer intravenous anesthetics. Int. Anesthesiol. Clin. 7: No. 1, 1969.
Collins, V. J. *Principles of Anesthesiology.* Lea & Febiger, Philadelphia, 1972.
Gray, Nunn, and Utting. *General Anesthesia.* Buttersworth, London, 1980.
Hewer, C. L. Recent advances in AnesthoAnalgesia. Int. Anesthesiol. Clin. 11: No. 1, 1978.
Losstrom, J. B. Peripheral circulation anesthesia. Int. Anesthesiol. Clin. 7: No. 2, 1969.
Krantz-Carr's Pharm. Principles Med. Practice, 8th ed. Williams & Wilkins, Baltimore, 1972.
Neurolept anesthesia. Int. Anesthesiol. Clin. 11: 1973.
Philbin, D. M. Anesthetic mgt. patient with cardiovascular disease. Int. Anesthesiol. Clin. 17: No. 1, 1979.
Wylie, Churchill, and Davidson. *Practice of Anesthesia.* Yearbook, Chicago, 1966.

INTRA-OPERATIVE

CHAPTER 8

Microsurgery

ELLIOTT H. ROSE, M.D., ZOLTAN SZABO, Ph.D., and G. WAYNE JOWER, D.P.M.

A. Basic Microsurgical Principles and Skill Acquisition

Microsurgery is a quantum leap from macro- or conventional surgery. With the introduction of the surgical microscope or magnifying loupes, one is able to visualize finer details in tissues, providing visual clues and feedback for improved eye-hand coordination needed for delicate tissue handling and precision technique. Significant improvement in reconstructing and manipulating vital tissue or organ components is a consequence.

A microsurgical procedure involves the use of optical magnification, specifically designed microsurgical instruments, and appropriate microsurgical technique as required by each specialty. Microsurgery entails fine dissection or preparation (preceded by conventional or gross exposure), with the actual microsurgical operation involving the anastomosis of arteries, veins, lymphatics, and peripheral nerves. Postanastomotic evaluation, such as measuring flow via a magnetic flow meter, etc., follows. The post-operative period is mainly restricted to the monitoring of the anastomosis, directly or indirectly, during the critical phase, e.g., measuring capillary flow, temperature, etc., for approximately 5–7 days (Figs. 8A.1–8A.4).

BRIEF HISTORY: FROM VASCULAR TO MICROVASCULAR SURGERY

In tracing the history of microsurgery, it behooves one to look far into the past where the foundation was laid. Our concern mainly centers around the vascular tree and peripheral nerve network, which are relevant to podiatric microsurgery, and here the important milestones that led to the evolution of current surgical knowledge will be briefly traced.

In the 1500s, Ambrose Pare practiced the ligation of blood vessels for controlling hemorrhage. William Harvey was the first to describe the principle of blood circulation in the human body in 1628 (1). In the subsequent centuries, numerous contributions were made but it was not until 1905 that Carrel and Guthrie described standardized and consistently successful vascular surgical techniques that led to widespread acceptance (2). Between the 1940s and 1950s there was an added stimulus for successful management of vascular trauma resulting from various military conflicts. Although around the turn of the century the successful repair of smaller vessels was recognized, it was not until 1960 when Jacobson and Suarez reported success in repairing truly microvascular structures (3).

This development in microvascular anastomosis was preceded, paralleled, and followed by advances in other microsurgical techniques, such as those used in ophthalmology, ENT, neurosurgery, plastic and hand reconstructive surgery, and infertility surgery (male and female). After the 1960s these segmented efforts were combined into a multidisciplinary approach, creating a broad base from which progress became very rapid.

In the initial phases it was mainly the pioneering efforts of individual surgeons that advanced knowledge of microsurgical techniques. Today, this knowledge is widely disseminated and there are indeed few sur-

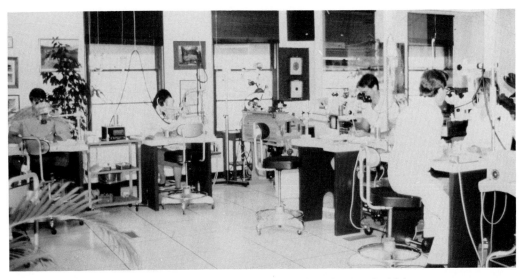

Figure 8A.1. Instruction and practice in the microsurgical laboratory.

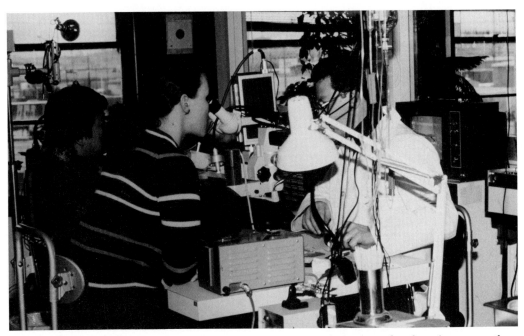

Figure 8A.2. As the instructor demonstrates suturing techniques under the microscope, these techniques can be observed via a diploscope extension and through a video monitor.

gical subspecialties able to resist exploring the possible benefits of the microsurgical approach.

DOMAINS OF MICROSURGERY

There are enough common denominators among the various subspecialties utilizing microsurgical techniques, such as similar equipment, instrumentation, and surgical strategy, to view microsurgery as a whole; however, for the individual surgeon there are more than enough variations and differences which will result in the surgeon focusing attention only on the narrow range of his specialty (Figs. 8A.5–8A.8).

It is helpful to classify the various areas

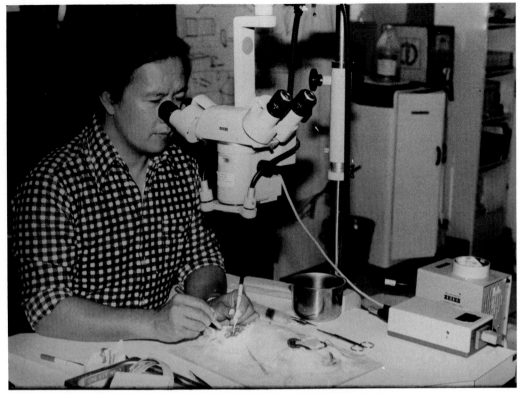

Figure 8A.3. The clinical microscope station allows a microsurgeon to work with the same microscope system in the laboratory that is used in the operating theater.

of microsurgery according to the variations and differences. With this in mind, the structures, tissues, and organs operated on can be used as a basis for this classification. These classifications are general as there may be some crossover and combinations in some specialties.

1. **Biomass microsurgery** pertains to various small components of individual organs that vary in shape, structure, and function, e.g., the cornea, stapes, minute cerebral aneurysms or tumors.
2. **Bioconduit microsurgery** involves structures that are involved with the transport of fluids, secretions, signals, or specific cells, e.g., the circulatory system, bile duct, peripheral nerves, vas deferens, and fallopian tube.

For podiatric surgery, microsurgical discussion will be limited to the vascular system and the peripheral nerves; the rest has been mentioned only for completeness.

BASIC PRINCIPLES OF MICROVASCULAR SURGERY

When examining the basic principles of microvascular surgery, attention is directed to: 1) the target tissues, structures, or organs, their physiology, function, pathology, and the healing process; and 2) the capacity of the surgeon to perform operations with the aid of magnification.

Microvascular Anastomosis

The domain of microvascular surgery is determined by the size of the vessels, measured in their fully dilated outer diameter. The smallest vessel that can be successfully repaired in the clinical setting is about 0.3–0.4 mm. Even smaller vessels can be successfully repaired but they require special techniques, considerable expertise, and increased operating time. At the other end of the spectrum are vessels which range from 1.2–2.0 mm. Undoubtedly, the repair of vessels larger than 2 mm can benefit from the use of microscopes and microtechniques; however, the marginal improvement rarely

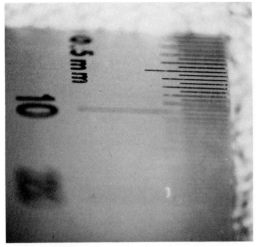

Figure 8A.4. Demonstrating the narrow depth of field of the operating microscope, which is the consequence of increased optical magnification.

justifies the increase in the operator's effort and time.

Within the domain of microvascular surgery there are three distinct areas that are determined by the diameters of the vasculature: regular, medium, and fine. Each category has its own ideal magnification, instrumentation, and technique: the smaller the structure, the finer the instrument tips, smaller diameter microneedles, and greater the effort is required from the surgeon to maintain control of the eye-hand coordination and consistently successful results.

The function and structural differences also have to be considered; for example, an artery 1 mm in diameter will have a higher blood pressure and thicker walls than a corresponding vein. On the other hand, the vein requires more delicate handling by the operator and the margin for error is narrower.

The important principles or requirements for consistently successful results can be listed as follows:

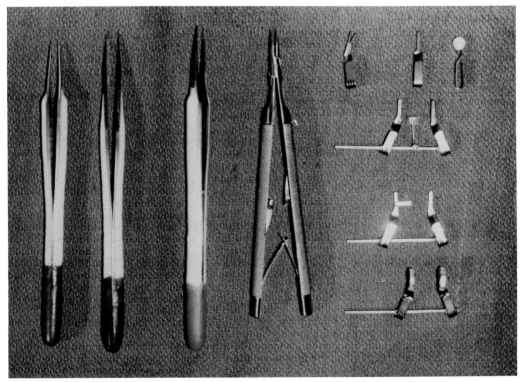

Figure 8A.5. Basic instruments are simple and few in number: various clamps, a dual-action needle driver, and color-coded, round-handled forceps.

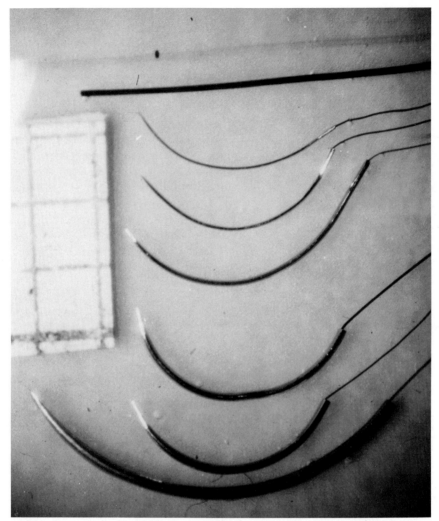

Figure 8A.6.   An array of microsurgical needles and suture material compared to a human hair and a millimeter scale. From *top* to *bottom*: a blond human hair, a black hair, 50-micron needle with 18-micron thread, 70-micron needle with 22-micron thread, 100-micron needle with 22-micron thread, 140-micron needle with 35-micron thread, 140-micron needle with 22-micron thread, 200-micron needle with 35-micron thread.

1. Taking an **adequate amount of bite** (the distance between the edge of the cut vessel and the point of needle penetration) and placing the **required number of stitches** into the circumference of the vessel ends to be coaptated (4, 5). This is necessary to achieve layer-to-layer approximation of respective tissue layers and proper hemostasis. It has been experimentally demonstrated that a completed anastomosis that persists in bleeding can develop a lumenal clot at the site of the gap, jeopardizing normal flow (4).

2. **Maintaining the original lumen diameter** is equally vital. Lumen narrowing at the anastomotic site hinders flow since this is profoundly affected by minute changes in the caliber of the vessel (Poiseuille's law).

3. **Turbulence at the anastomosis site should be avoided** since it slows the laminar flow. For this reason, the

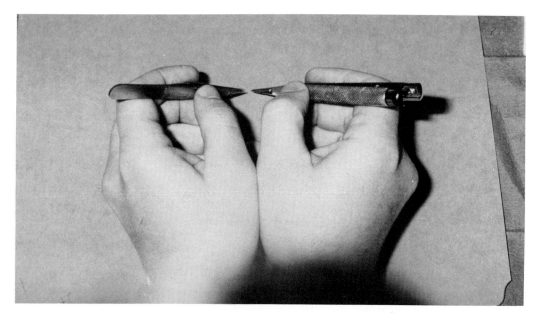

Figure 8A.7. Instruments should be held in a pencil grip and the hands should touch each other for mutual support and reduction of tremor: the so-called, "handcuff technique."

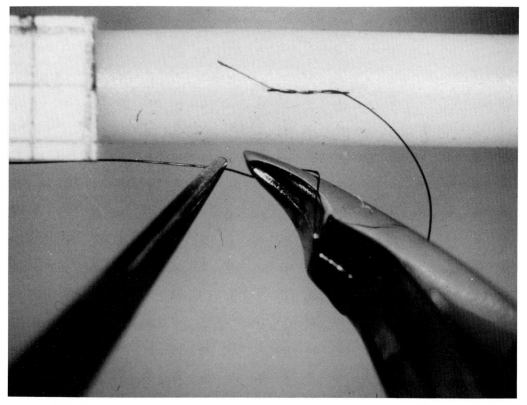

Figure 8A.8. Initially, the novice should practice improving eye-hand coordination under a microscope by tying various types of knots.

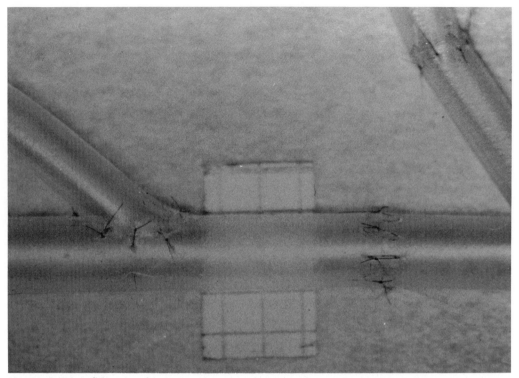

Figure 8A.9.   Silicone tubing is used to practice the end-to-end and end-to-side anastomoses.

end-to-end anastomosis should not exceed a 3:1 disparity and the end-to-side anastomosis should be angled for ideal flow (6).

4. **Use of heparin or other platelet stabilizing reagents prevent or reduce the chances of platelet clot formation** at the site of surgical trauma, and reagents that alter the blood viscosity to prevent sluggish flow.

5. **Vasodilators should be used to prevent or counteract vasospasm in the arterial segment.**

6. **Tension of the anastomosed segment should be avoided,** either by dissecting an adequate length of vessel, or by using interposed grafts.

TYPES OF ANASTOMOSIS

The most frequent types of coaptation are the end-to-end and end-to-side anastomoses (Figs. 8A.9–8A.13).

End-to-end

The end-to-end anastomosis technique varies with the diameter and wall thickness of the vessel. The ultimate aim is to place the minimum number of stitches that will provide hemostasis and tensile strength while preserving the original lumen size.

QUADRANGULAR SUTURE PLACEMENT

Semicircumferential suturing is an ideal technique where the first two stitches are placed 180° apart; one-half of the circumference is anastomosed first, then the other. This technique requires a precise order of suture placement (7).

The minimum number of stitches placed in a small vessel, 0.3 mm, which will prevent the collapse of the anastomosis, is four. As the size of the structure increases, the number of stitches also increases, main-

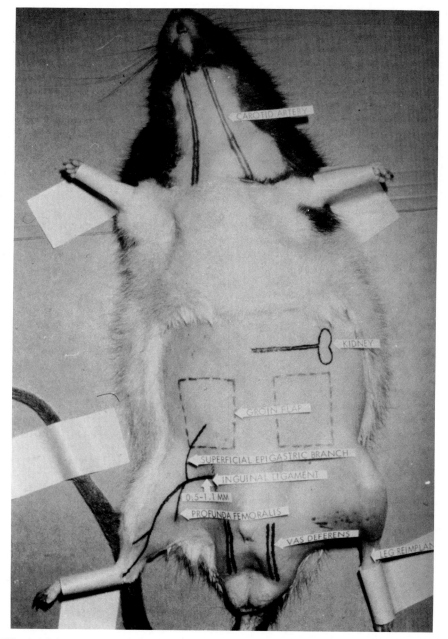

Figure 8A.10.   The rat provides a universal practice model for several specialties.

taining an even distribution of stitches around the circumference.

With larger diameter vessels, i.e., 1.2 mm or more, a triangular technique is more efficient. This entails placing the first three stitches at points 120° to each other, then completing the anastomosis with either interrupted or continuous sutures.

TYPE OF SUTURING

Continuous or running, and **interrupted** or button-hole. Each suturing technique has its pros and cons (8). In larger vessels, continuous suturing, executed carefully, is more rapid and the success rates are consistently within the surgeon's expectations. Furthermore, larger caliber,

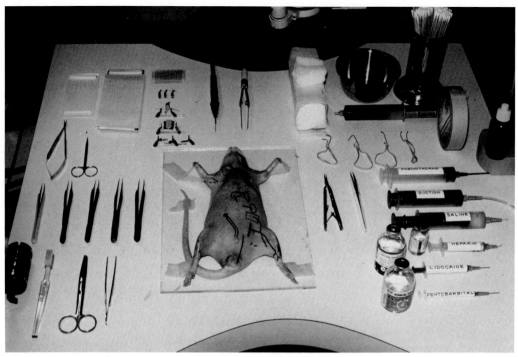

Figure 8A.11. The animal model with the necessary instrumentation and accessories are displayed on the microscope table.

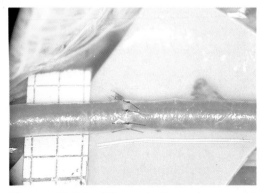

Figure 8A.12. The main femoral artery of the rat measures approximately 1 millimeter in outer diameter. Here it has been successfully anastomosed in the end-to-end fashion.

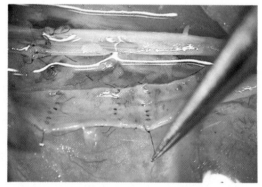

Figure 8A.13. Several anastomoses can be practiced in a relatively short segment of the essel. Upon completion, the structure can be opened longitudinally and the luminal surface of the suture line can be examined.

"hardened-walled" vessels are less apt to purse-string, and the margin for error in restoring the original caliber is considerably greater than with small vessels. Using only interrupted sutures on a large vessel would be rather time-consuming and not improve patency rates significantly. On the other hand, vessels less than 1.2 mm man-

dates interrupted suture placement even at the cost of increasing operating time. The margin for error is narrow and constriction of the caliber must be avoided at all costs.

It is worth mentioning that in the hands of a very experienced microsurgeon, such as a busy instructor with many hundreds of various anastomoses accomplished in the ideal laboratory setting, either technique can be employed with the same high success rate. For the clinical practitioner of infrequent practice, the interrupted suturing is a safer way to proceed when dealing with small vessels (Figs. 8A.14–8A.15).

End-to-side

Frequently, it is not feasible to perform an end-to-end anastomosis because of various factors; thus, an end-to-side anastomosis is required to provide a more favorable blood flow. Conditions requiring an end-to-side anastomosis, include:

1. A need for both proximal and distal perfusion, e.g., in the superficial temporal bypass.
2. A situation where the end-to-end anastomosis would compromise distal blood supply, e.g., free island flap to the lower leg area.
3. When the disparity between the diameters of the donor and recipient vessels exceed a 3:1 ratio.
4. When there is a great likelihood of vessel spasm at the anastomosis site in the case of end-to-end anastomosis.

The end-to-side anastomosis suture placement is similar to the end-to-end quadrangular semi-circumferential suturing, except that the first two stitches that are placed 180° lies parallel with the main axis of the recipient vessel. These "toe and heel" stitches that align the cut surfaces are very important. First, one-half, then the other half is sutured with the in-between stitches placed in a radial configuration.

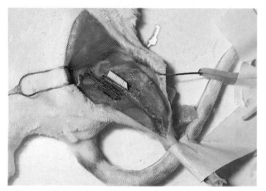

Figure 8A.14. The rat leg reimplantation model: preparation of the donor site.

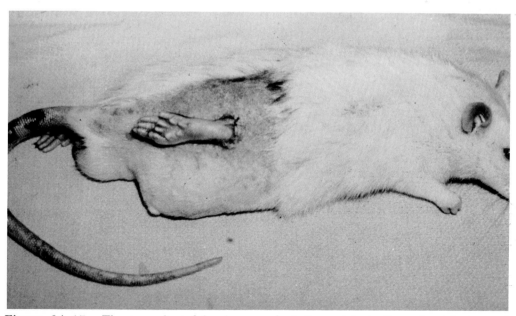

Figure 8A.15. The transplanted leg is secured at the recipient site and nutrient vessels anastomosed.

In cutting the recipient window, it is of paramount importance to create an oval-shaped fenestration, with the resulting window one-third greater than the diameter of the donor vessel end. If a longitudinal slit is made, rather than an oval opening, the spasm of the donor vessel end may reduce the orifice significantly. The junction should be made somewhat of a bell shape to minimize flow turbulences at the anastomotic site. At times the donor vessel end may be fish-mouthed to form this bell shape and create a better hemostasis. The angling of the recipient and donor vessels in relation to each other can further improve the flow of the anastomosis.

Interposed Grafts

At times, due to loss or damage of the original vasculature, an interposed graft is

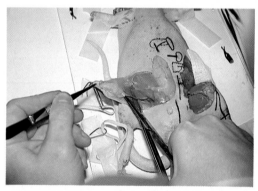

Figure 8A.16. Free groin patch transplant to the neck: elevation of the donor tissue.

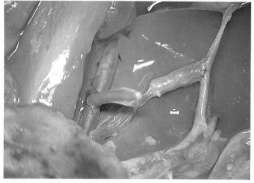

Figure 8A.17. Arterial and venous end-to-side anastomoses at the recipient site.

used to bridge the gap and avoid tension. In the microvasculature, though synthetic graft materials are being continuously improved, the autogenous vein graft is still the material of choice. When interposing between arterial segments, it is important to select a donor graft whose diameter is somewhat narrower than the recipient vessel so that upon completion of the anastomosis, undue dilation of the vein graft is avoided (due to the higher arterial pressure of the restored blood flow) (Figs. 8A.16–8A.18).

Peripheral Nerve Microsurgery

Once adequate microvascular suturing technique has been attained, the peripheral nerve is anastomosed using the perineural suturing technique. Three or four interrupted stitches are used to provide adequate tensile strength for the anastomosed nerve ends. Of utmost importance is that the anastomosis should not be subjected to any longitudinal tension (9). If there is a large enough gap between the nerve endings, an interposed nerve graft is used.

TECHNIQUES AND SKILL ACQUISITION

The learning of microsurgical skill begins in the training and practice laboratory with the student participating in an organized and standardized course under the supervision of a skilled instructor.* This initial course consists of 40 hours of basic instruction, followed by another 40 hours of advanced laboratory training.

During the basic course (10), the surgeon learns about the operating microscope, instrumentation, suturing techniques, strategy, and mental concentration. This initiation is, perhaps, the most important part of the training since it offers the student self-evaluation and stimulation necessary

---

*"...throughout his career he promoted—in principle and in practice—the idea that freshmen needed to be taught by the very best teachers on the faculty." (From "Hildebrand: The First 100 Years," *California Monthly,* published by the California Alumni Association. Copyright 1981.)

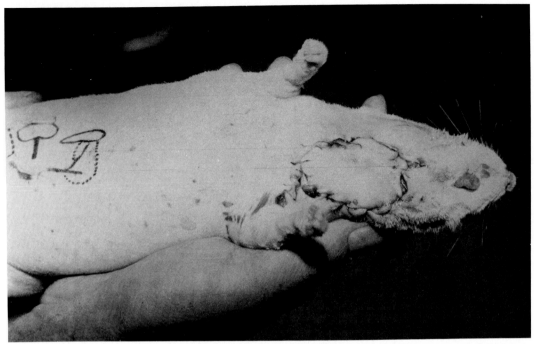

Figure 8A.18.   The transplanted groin patch.

for charting his future involvement with microsurgery.

The advanced course reinforces the basic skills and expands into small scale tissue or organ transplantation. During this time, various research models can be practiced in anticipation of the participant's special interest. Even though the laboratory and clinical situations are quite different, the foundations are laid in the laboratory, enhancing and expediting the learning of the clinical technique.

The next phase is observing and assisting a practicing microsurgical clinician in the operating room. The final phase of the learning process is gaining experience through the surgeon performing his own clinical cases.

References

1. Harvey, W. An anatomical treatise on the motion of the heart and blood in animals, 1628.
2. Harbison, S. P., and B. Fisher. *The contributions of Dr. C. C. Guthrie to Vascular Surgery.* University of Pittsburgh Press, Pittsburgh, 1959, p. 9.
3. Jacobson, J. H., and Suarez, E. L. Microsurgery in anastomosis of small vessels. Surg. Forum 11:243–245, 1960.
4. Weinstein, P. R., Mehdorn, H. M., and Szabo, Z. Microsurgical anastomosis: Vessel injury, regeneration, and repair. In *Microsurgical Composite Tissue Transplantation*, edited by D. Serafin and H. J. Buncke. C. V. Mosby, St. Louis, 1979, pp. 111–114.
5. Colen, L. B., Gonzales, F. P., and Buncke, H. J. The relationship between the number of sutures and the strength of microvascular anastomoses. Plast. Reconstr. Surg. 64:325–329, 1979.
6. Buchler, U., and Buncke, H. J. Experimental microvascular autografts. In *Microsurgical Composite Tissue Transplantation*, edited by D. Serafin and H. J. Buncke. C. V. Mosby, St. Louis, 1979, pp. 83–89.
7. Szabo, Z. Microvascular surgical technique today. In *Microsurgery in Gynecology*, edited by J. M. Phillips. American Association of Gynecologic Laparoscopists., Downey, California, 1977, pp. 213–227.
8. Man, D., and Acland, R. D. Continuous-suture technique in microvascular end-to-end anastomosis. J. Microsurg. 2:238–243, 1981.
9. Millesi, H., Meissl, G., and Berger, A. Further experiences with interfascicular grafting of the median, ulnar, and radial nerves. J. Bone Jt. Surg. 58A:209–218, 1976.
10. Buncke, H. J., Chater, N. L., and Szabo, Z. *Manual of Microvascular Surgery.* Davis & Geck, Pearl River, New York, 1975.

B. Microsurgical Application in Resurfacing Large Plantar Defects of the Foot

Resurfacing of large ulcers on weight-bearing surfaces of the plantar aspect of the foot requires thick, glabrous, sensible skin to withstand the direct pressure and the shearing forces during weightbearing. Thin split thickness skin grafts alone have been used (1). Patients, however, exhibit a tendency to shift weight from the grafted areas to the other non-grafted portions of the foot (2). Flap skin with a subcutaneous pad reduces the shear forces and diffuses the weight over the contact surfaces.

NON-MICROSURGICAL APPROACH

Cross-leg cutaneous or myocutaneous flaps offer a relatively safe source of composite tissue for resurfacing of large plantar defects. The skin, detached after a substantial length of time to allow neovascularization from the recipient foot, is tailored to fit the plantar defect (Fig. 8B.1). The pedicle detached from its cutaneous nerve supply may develop minimal protective sensation by ingrowth of cutaneous nerves from the surrounding foot skin. In the neurotropic foot, reinnervation in the anatomic sensory nerve distribution is precluded.

Disadvantages of this technique include: a prolonged immobilization time, a two-stage operation, and randomization of the flap without discrete nerve supply.

MICROSURGICAL APPROACH

The neurovascular island flap, either as a transposition flap isolated on the neurovascular pedicle or as a free microvascular flap, can resurface the weightbearing plantar foot with skin of satisfactory texture and feeling (3). Return of a useful pressure sensation reduces neurotrophic ulceration thought to be due to inability to perceive friction during walking (4). Free neurovascular flaps from the foot have been used extensively in hand reconstruction (5–11). Donor two-point discrimination averages 32 mm on the dorsum of the foot, 11.3 mm

on the lateral surface of the great toe, and 16.4 mm on the medial surface of the second toe (5). The flap is supplied by the vascular territories of the underlying axial artery.

The "dorsalis pedis flap," extending from the extensor retinaculum proximally to near the web space distally, can supply as much as 14 × 12 cm of skin from the dorsum of the foot if the "random" areas are properly delayed (12), making it ideal for coverage of neurotrophic heel defects (Fig. 8B.2).

The first web space flap between the first and second toes is nourished by the dorsalis pedis artery and its terminal branches (first dorsal metatarsal artery, dorsal and plantar digital arteries) (13) (Fig. 8B.3).

Resurfacing of the entire plantar surface of the foot may combine the anatomical vascular territories of both described flaps. (Fig. 8B.4).

Cortical reeducation in the free microvascular neurosensory flap is minimized by direct anastomosis of the donor nerve included in the free flap to the anatomically correct sensory nerve.

Mechanical limitations of the donor foot are minimal (14), although take of the split thickness skin graft over the tarsal bone and extensor hallucis longus may be slightly delayed (6).

CASE REPORT

A 22-year-old female sustained a degloving injury of all of the soft tissues of the left foot distal to the ankle when she caught it beneath a train. Initial treatment was by debridement and coverage with split thickness skin graft. The entire plantar surface of the foot was anesthetic and unstable. Three months later, she underwent a free neurovascular island pedicle flap from the dorsum of the contralateral foot. The flap measured 19.0 cm in length and 12.0 cm in width. The dorsalis pedis artery was anas-

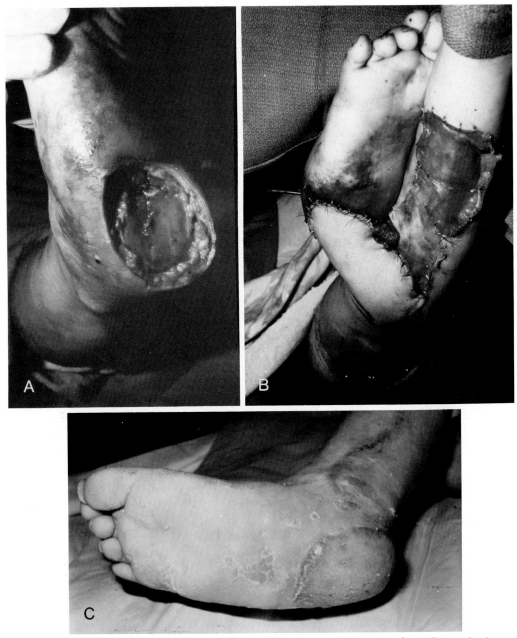

Figure 8B.1. Cross-leg myocutaneous flap. *A*, 8 × 6 cm neurotropic ulcer plantar heel post debridement *B*, cross-leg medial gastrocnemius flap attached to defect. *C*, at 4 weeks, flap was detached, tailored, inset. At 6 months, protective sensation is negligible.

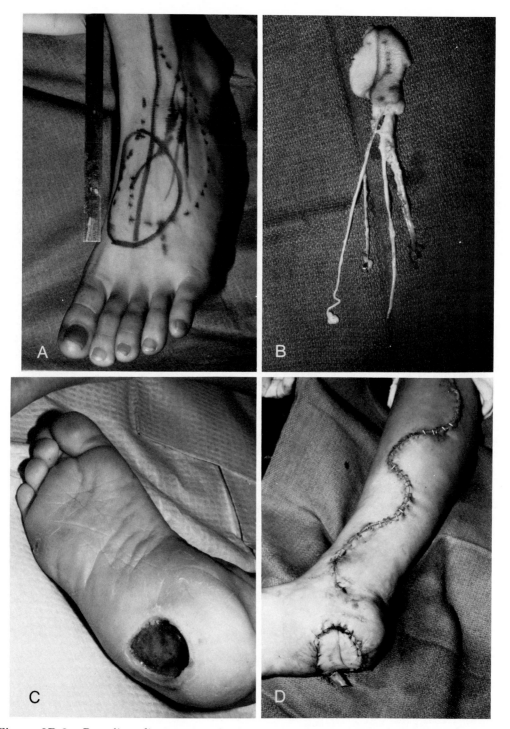

Figure 8B.2. Dorsalis pedis neurovascular flap. *A*, central axis of flap is dorsalis pedis artery. Cutaneous innervation is via superficial peroneal nerve terminal branches. *B*, flap detached with nerve and vascular pedicles. *C*, neurotropic heel defect. *D*, flap inset after anastomosis of dorsalis pedis artery to recipient posterior tibial artery and superficial peroneal nerves to posterior tibial nerve.

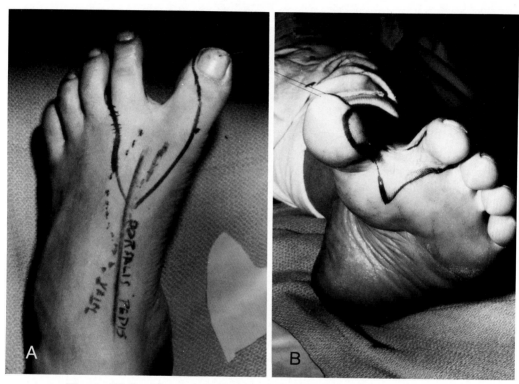

Figure 8B.3. First web space flap. *A*, dorsal view *B*, plantar extension.

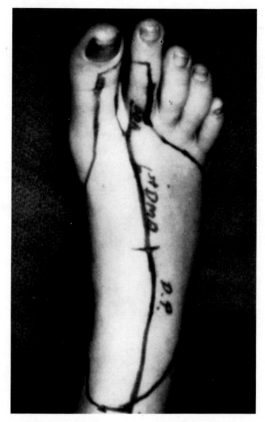

Figure 8B.4. Combination dorsalis pedis and 1st web space flap, useful for coverage of entire plantar surface.

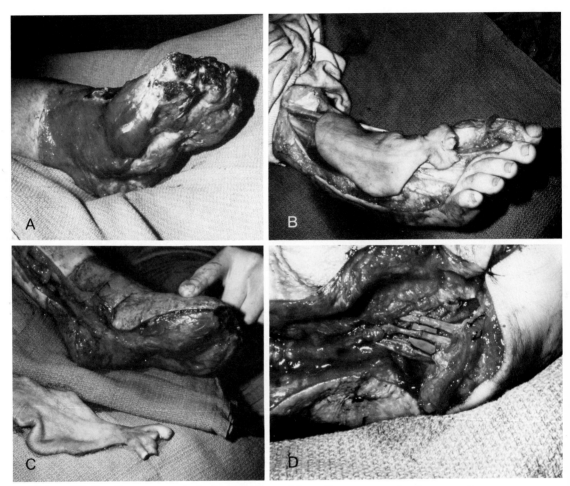

Figure 8B.5. Case report. *A*, degloving injury of foot. *B*, neurovascular flap from donor foot. *C*, flap detached and ready for inset onto plantar surface. *D*, microsurgical repair of arteries, veins, nerves (see text). *E*, flap inset. Note covering over metatarsal heads. *F*, weightbearing on flap.

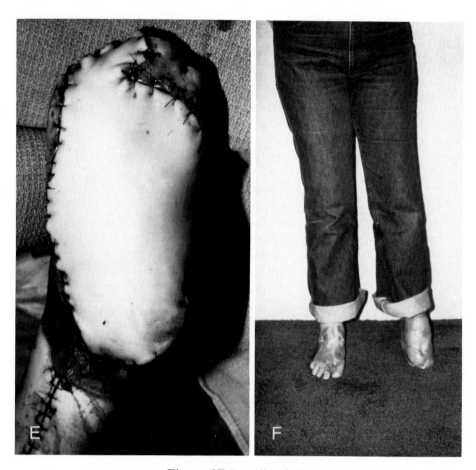

Figure 8B.5.   (*E* and *F*)

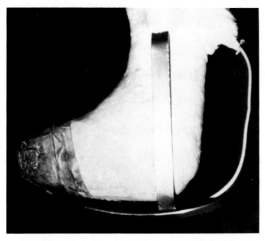

Figure 8B.6. Cast fixation with metallic cradle protects foot until reinnervation has recurred.

tomosed to the posterior tibial artery of the recipient foot. The superficial peroneal and deep peroneal nerve were repaired en bloc to the tibial nerve of the recipient foot. Both superficial and deep veins were anastomosed. The first web space extension on the flap was used to cover the first, second, and third exposed metatarsal heads (Fig. 8B.5).

Long term, the successful flap transfer provides thick soft tissue coverage and protective sensation for progressive weightbearing. Cast fixation with metallic cradle to preclude direct weightbearing on the foot is used for several months postsurgery until the reinnervation of the flap has occurred (Fig. 8B.6).

References

1. Wolfering E. A., Thorpe, W. P., Reed, J. K., and Rosenburg, S. A. Split thickness skin grafting of the plantar surface of the foot after wide excision of the neoplasms of the skin. Surg. Gynecol. Obstet. 149:229, 1979.
2. Sommerland, B. C., and McGrouther, D. A. Resurfacing of the sole: Long-term follow-up and comparison of techniques. Br. J. Plast. Surg. 31:107, 1978.
3. Kaplan, I. Neurovascular island flaps in treatment of trophic ulcerations of the heel. Br. J. Plast. Surg. 22:143, 1969.
4. Snyder, G. B., and Edgerton, M. T. The principle of the island neurovascular flap with management of ulcerated anesthetic weightbearing areas of the lower extremity. Plast. Reconstr. Surg. 36:518, 1965.
5. May, J. W., Chait, L. A., Cohen, B. E., and O'Brien, B. M. Free neurovascular flap from the first web space of the foot in hand reconstruction. J. Hand Surg. 2:387, 1977.
6. Ohmori, K., and Harii, K. Free dorsalis pedis sensory flap to the hand with microvascular anastomosis. Plast. Reconstr. Surg. 58:546, 1976.
7. Robinson D. W. Microsurgical transfer of the dorsalis pedis neurovascular island flap. Br. J. Plast. Surg. 29:209, 1976.
8. Daniel, R. K., Terzis, J., and Midgley, R. D. Restoration of sensation to an anesthetic hand by free neurovascular flap from the foot. Plast. Reconstr. Surg. 57:275, 1976.
9. Buncke, H. J., and Rose, E. H. Free toe-to-fingertip neurovascular flaps. Plast. Reconstr. Surg. 63:607, 1979.
10. Strauch, B., and Tsur, H. Restoration of sensation to the hand by a free neurovascular flap from the first web space of the foot. Plast. Reconstr. Surg. 62:361, 1978.
11. Morrison, W. A., O'Brien, B. M., Maclead, A. M., and Gilbert, A. Neurovascular free flaps from the foot for innervation of the hand. J. Hand Surg. 3:235, 1978.
12. McGraw, J. B., and Furlow, L. T. The dorsalis pedis arterialized flap: A clinical study. Plast. Reconstr. Surg. 55:177, 1975.
13. Gilbert, A. Composite tissue transfers from the foot—anatomcal basis and surgical technique. In Symposium on Microsurgery, edited by A. Daniller and B. Strauch. C. V. Mosby, St. Louis, 1976, pp. 230–242.
14. Joseph, J. Some aspects of functional anatomy of the foot. Ann. Phys. Med. 7:26, 1963.

CHAPTER 9

Soft Tissue Tumors

STEVEN J. BERLIN, D.P.M.

Tumors including soft tissue neoplasms, cystic lesions, and pseudo-tumors, represent a significant portion of the pathology of the foot. The purpose of this chapter is to discuss different types of tumors relating to specific tissues of the foot and to discuss certain problems with which podiatrists come in contact in regard to the location of benign or malignant neoplasms of the foot. It will not delve into the history or etiology or histologic differences of such tumors. ("Pure" inflammatory lesions are being excluded from consideration.)

Patients seeking care for a tumor or "growth" usually present themselves to the doctor with pain and/or swelling. It is well established that any expanding lesion may cause discomfort, particularly when in proximity to neural structures. "Swelling," on the other hand, is intrinsic in any space-occupying lesions; but it may be accentuated by inflammation, with edema and/or hemorrhage within or around a tumor. Primary cysts, of course, enlarge at a rate proportionate to their underlying nature, or "secretory" activity.

The patient may also seek consultation because of other signs or symptoms, such as the sudden appearance of a lesion, the rapid enlargement of an existing lesion, or other local changes which may occur over the course of months or years, such as change in coloration, bleeding, ulceration, appearance of satellite lesions, etc.

The history of the lesion is obviously an essential portion of the examination and may provide the leads which allow the doctor to make a more rapid or more precise diagnosis so that his treatment may be successful.

The physical examination places the lo-cation of the lesion; and this is crucial to making a clinical diagnosis, for various tumors have a propensity for different anatomic locations. For example, plantar fibromatosis involves the plantar fascia.

In addition to the history and physical examination, other diagnostic aids are available to augment the likelihood of accurate diagnosis and enhance the surgical evaluation of the lesion. These include radiological techniques, such as arteriography, CAT scan (i.e., computerized axial tomography), in addition to the "ordinary" x-rays. Another aid is among the least of all utilized: the punch biopsy. Biopsy techniques are among the most rewarding available, and frequently provide a precise anatomic diagnosis which may not be available otherwise. Remember that the only definitive diagnosis can be made by microscopic examination of the tissue excised. All other methods provide only inferential or circumstantial evidence. The biopsy, whether it is an excisional biopsy for a small lesion or a punch biopsy for a larger lesion, can help direct the successful surgical managment of many lesions.

SKIN TUMORS

Skin tumors represent the most frequently seen lesions requiring surgical treatment in podiatric practice. When the clinician excises any type of skin lesion, particularly when doing an excisional biopsy, the surgeon should follow the skin lines, to reduce the skin tension and the possibility of hypertrophic scarring. More importantly, the surgeon should allow adequate margins in all directions to enhance the likelihood of completeness of excision. Some skin lesions spread subdermally, which is rarely recognizable at the operating table. For this reason, the surgeon must be assured by the pathologist that there are adequate margins around the tumor; for the only hope of cure for most malignancies is complete surgical extirpation (Figs. 9.1 and 9.17).

VIRAL LESIONS OF THE SKIN

Viral lesions of the skin, particularly verrucae plantaris, can be very stubborn lesions to eradicate. Not only do they spread, but they often become more resistant after different types of therapy. When excisional procedures are used for removing warts, it is important to be sure of adequate margins; otherwise, the lesion may recur, and the post-operative recurrence may be resistant to chemotherapy or cryotherapy and require re-excision.

The curettement method, in the author's opinion, represents the easiest form of excision with the least likelihood of complications. However, the greatest "problem" with this procedure is the likelihood of recurrence due to inadequate or incomplete curetting. A curettement with a blunt-type dissection usually results in a cure; but cauterizing the base after blunt curettement increases the chance of success by reducing the potential of recurrence. The next most significant complication of blunt curettement procedures is curetting too deeply so that the basement membrane of the epidermis is disrupted. Generally, this results in prolonged healing, as well as increased discomfort and scarring. The author strongly cautions against the use of chemotherapy following blunt curettement where the basement membrane has been broached, since it frequently retards healing. Unfortunately, there is no single best method for the treatment of verruca plantaris; and whatever works best in the particular clinician's hands is generally the best form of treatment for him to use.

Other benign skin lesions may be encountered in the foot, such as fibromas, nevi, and keratocanthomas. Most have the potential to recur if not completely excised; and a few may undergo malignant transformation.

Preservation of the skin, particularly when dealing with the plantar surface of the foot, should be the goal of any surgeon. Yet one of the major surgical errors of omission occurs when the surgeon inadequately excises a lesion. An error of commission occurs when the lesion is excised more widely than necessary. The former results in recurrence; the latter may require

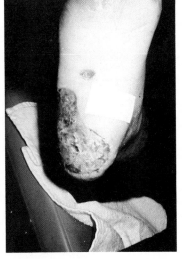
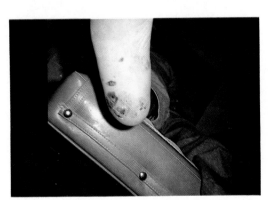

Figure 9.1. Melanoma. *Left,* multiple nodular melanomas are identified on the plantar aspect of the heel and arch. *Right,* the wide excision of the multiple lesions with split thickness skin graft. This patient died approximately 6 months later with severe metastasis. It is doubtful that amputation in this particular case would have meant the difference between survival and death (courtesy of Gerald Krieger, D.P.M.).

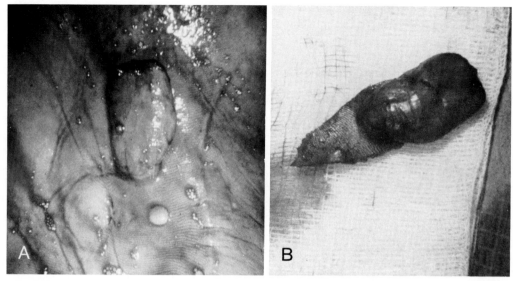

Figure 9.2. Dermatofibroma. *A*, this shows an extremely large plantar dermatofibroma and also small distal lesions. Wide surgical excision of this lesion was performed. *B*, represents the complete excision of the lesion and the adjacent lesion with wide skin margins. Complications developed due to lack of skin on closure and required skin grafting after excision of such a large lesion.

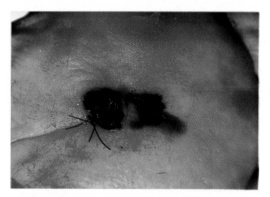

Figure 9.3. Nodular melanoma. Large ulcerating melanoma was a primary lesion. These highly metastatic lesions require aggressive surgery, and amputation of the foot is often the treatment recommended.

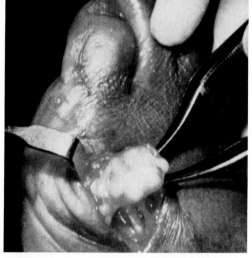

Figure 9.4. Lipoma. This lesion was located on the dorsal lateral aspect of the foot between the fourth and fifth metatarsal shaft, an uncommon location for a lipoma. Generally, complete excision results in a cure. However, the surgeon should be aware of the fatty offshoots which also must be excised to prevent recurrence.

skin grafting if of unusual size or if healing is complicated (Fig. 9.2).

Malignancies of the skin, particularly melanomas, especially need adequate excision. It is extremely important with melanomas to carefully evaluate the depth to which the tumor invades (Clark's level). Recent studies have shown that adequate excision of the more superficial melanomas may have a high rate of success. For example, melanomas less that 0.79 mm in thickness and not deeper than Clark's level I are almost always completely resectable and virtually curable. Even deeper lesions have a better prognosis if thoroughly excised, which, of course, is the most important requisite of any cancer surgery.

Any lesion which changes color, bleeds, or increases in size should be biopsied as early as possible to rule out the chance of a malignancy. Failure of surgeon to recognize the malignant potential of such lesions may result in medico-legal altercations or may even lead to the death of the patient. Any lesion excised from the foot, even if it is believed to be a wart or other viral lesion, should be excisionally biopsied if small or incisionally biopsied if larger, prior to definitive resection (Fig. 9.3).

TUMORS OF ADIPOSE OR FIBROUS TISSUE

Fibromas and lipomas usually cause minimal problems for excision unless they are very large. Some lipomas, however, have lateral extensions which must be incorporated in the resection to prevent the possibility of recurrence. In most instances, these tumors are easily managed surgically. Fortunately, the malignant counterpart, or liposarcoma, is extremely rare; and adequacy of excision of such malignancies often requires massive surgery or amputation (Fig. 9.4).

When these benign tumors are unusually large, there may be technical difficulties in surgical closure; or removal of the tumor may produce a large void, creating a post-operative hematoma or seroma, with the potential for infection or delayed healing following excision. A drain should be employed to reduce the possibility of a hematoma or seroma. This drain may be left in place for several days, or weeks, if necessary. Compression is also an important post-operative procedure to reduce the dead-space formation and resultant complications. It is thus very important for the surgeon to carefully evaluate post-surgical wounds after the excision of any large lesion (Fig. 9.5).

Of the benign fibrous lesions of the foot, the most difficult to treat is plantar fibro-matosis, which is more or less specific to the plantar fascia, although there are other fibromatoses elsewhere in the body. However, fibromatosis may occur within the fascia of the dorsal aspect of the foot as well. These fibromatoses have a high recurrence rate and need wide primary surgical excision, encompassing approximately 0.5–1 cm of normal plantar fascia around the margins. Plantar fibromatoses may suggest soft tissue malignancies because of their lateral extension and careful clinical evaluation is necessary to insure the likelihood of complete surgical excision. In rare cases, plantar fibromatosis may involve the entire plantar area of the foot so that a complete plantar fasciectomy must be performed to adequately excise the lesion; but even after "complete" excision of the plantar fascia, there is no guarantee that this fibrous tumor will not recur. When dealing with plantar fibromatosis and the overlying skin is not freely moveable, that non-moveable portion of the skin should be excised with the lesion, thus helping to reduce the possibility of recurrence. Seldom do any major structures become involved during the surgical excision of the plantar fascia; however, nerves may be entrapped in post-operative fibrosis, causing significant discomfort and subsequent paresthesias in the area of involvement (Fig. 9.6)

Fibromas are true neoplasms and usually create little or no problem and are easily excised, if not too large, since their borders are better defined than in plantar fibromatosis. Dermatofibromas are fairly common but are usually small and easily excised if reasonable borders are obtainable.

Periungual fibromas often create some surgical difficulty. There is a significant recurrence rate with fibromas involving the nail bed and nail fold region. One of the complications is a post-operatively deformed nail, resulting when the nail matrix is involved by the lesion or in the excision of it (Fig. 9.7).

Fibrosarcomas and dermatofibrosarcomas are rare lesions of the foot, but require meticulous, wide surgical excision, as do all

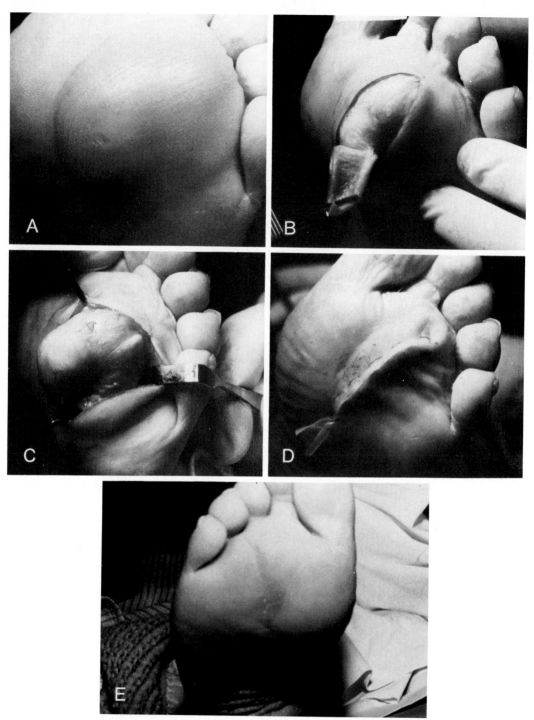

Figure 9.5. Epidermoid inclusion cyst. *A*, reveals a significantly enlarged mass along the plantar aspect of the second, third, and fourth metatarsals with the central aspect of the lesion pedunculated and the skin attached to the underlying neoplasm. *B*, reveals the surgical excision of the overlying skin, which is closely adherent to the cystic mass. *C*, represents the complete surgical exposure of this large cystic mass. This type of lesion leaves a large tumor void and soft tissue deficit. The closing of soft tissue with deep approximation is necessary to reduce the possibility of a hematoma. *D*, represents closure of the large defect with placement of surgical drain. *E*, represents the final healing of the cyst approximately 8 months post-operatively. The author recommends approximately 3 weeks of nonweightbearing on all plantar incisions to reduce the potential of complications, particularly with scarring.

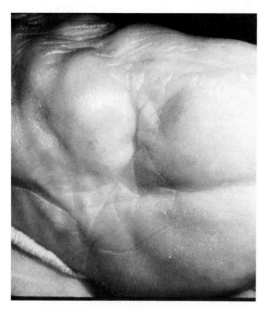

Figure 9.6. Plantar fibromatosis. This lesion was a recurrence from a previous lesion, about the size of a nickle. These lesions may appear as severe lesions on the plantar surface of the foot, act in some cases like a malignancy, and occasionally be confused histologically with fibrosarcoma.

malignancies. Depending on their degree of differentiation and their location and extent, amputation may be the treatment of choice (Fig. 9.8).

LESIONS OF MUSCLES, TENDONS, AND JOINTS
Ganglion Cysts

Synovial (or ganglion) cysts are the most frequent lesion involving the tendons and joints. They may arise from either tendon sheaths or parasynovial structures of the joints. They are generally freely moveable when involving tendinous structures and are generally nonmoveable when involving the joints. They may be of significant size, and if very large, can encompass nerves or major vascular structures, creating significant surgical management problems (Fig. 9.9).

The surgical excision of these lesions, especially when nerves or vascular structures are involved, requires meticulous dissection, in order to free these vital struc-

tures. In some instances, it becomes impossible to freely dissect nerves or vascular structures, which may preclude the possibility of complete resection and thus makes the probability of their recurrence very high. When these lesions are of such size, aspiration of the cyst during the surgical exposure often enhances the surgeon's ability to completely excise them. It should be pointed out that ganglion cysts are frequently located under the metatarsals and because of their mobility, these lesions often simulate Morton's neuromas. The surgeon should carefully evaluate lesions in the metatarsal regions to avoid missing a diagnosis of a ganglion or an adjacent intermetatarsal neuroma (Fig. 9.10).

Ganglion cysts have a fairly high recurrence rate. The author likes to avoid removing these cysts whenever possible and generally tries to aspirate them prior to any surgical intervention, since aspiration itself is potentially curable. At the least, it frequently eases the symptoms. After aspiration, a small amount of corticosteroid is instilled into and around the lesion to minimize the subsequent inflammation or fibrosis. Ganglion cysts which overlie bony surfaces apparently have a significant recurrence rate in the author's experience. We have found that removing the bony prominence underlying the ganglion cyst, whether it be a cyst of the tendon sheath or synovial structure, reduces the possibility of recurrence (see Fig. 9.18).

Digital mucous cysts, similar to ganglion cysts, have a high recurrence rate. It has been observed that excision of only the lesion and involved skin is inadequate, resection of the adjacent bony surface being required in most instances to reduce the potential for recurrence (Fig. 9.11).

Leiomyomas

Leiomyomas of the foot are uncommon and often pose very little surgical problem. They may occur in any area of the foot and usually arise from muscularis of the small blood vessels or from the erectopilorum muscles of the skin (Fig. 9.12).

Leiomyosarcomas, their malignant coun-

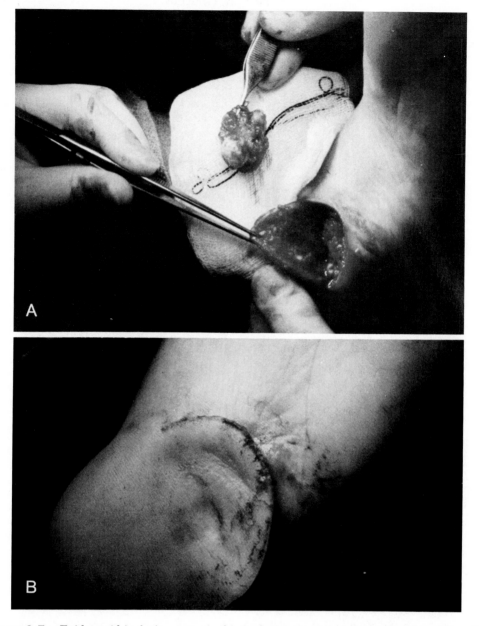

Figure 9.7.   Epidermoid inclusion cyst. *A*, this inclusion cyst created significant swelling. One can notice the close proximity to the underlying skin within the central portion of the incision during surgical exposure. *B*, represents the loss of vasculature of the underlying skin after the removal of the inclusion cyst. The surgical approach should have been a transverse incision through the central aspect of the lesion, excising out the skin involved. This may have prevented the wound breakdown and delayed healing in this region.

terpart, must be extremely rare in the foot, for the author has been unable to find a single reported case. But, as with all soft tissue malignancies, precise histological diagnosis is often relatively unimportant. What is important is wide surgical excision (or amputation) if there is to be any hope for surgical cure.

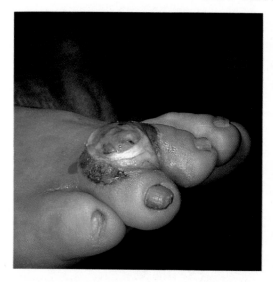

Figure 9.8. Dermatofibrosarcoma. These are rare lesions on the foot and have a high recurrence rate after surgery. Generally, radical surgical excision is necessary to completely eliminate the lesion and, in this particular case, partial amputation of the foot had to be performed.

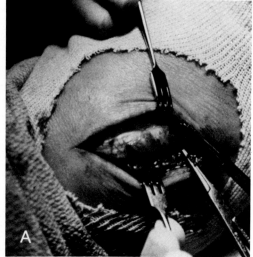

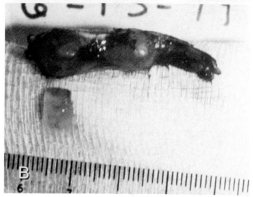

Figure 9.10. Ganglion cyst. *A*, large ganglion cyst extending from the calcaneus to the base of the fifth metatarsal. *B*, ganglion cysts may be multiloculated and, in some instances, dumbbell-shaped lesions. In this case, the ganglion cyst had closely infiltrated the muscular tissue, which had to be excised along with the cyst.

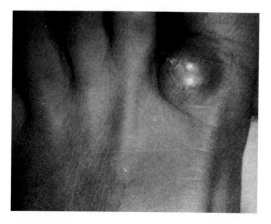

Figure 9.9. Synovial cyst. A large synovial cyst (ganglion cyst) located at the first metatarsophalangeal joint. Careful evaluation revealed the expansion of the lesion into the dermal structures of the skin, causing a significant stretching of the skin and loss of normal skin appearance. Surgical managment not only requires excision of the cyst, but also excision of a good section of normal skin overlying the cyst itself.

Rhabdomyomas

Rhabdomyomas, which are benign tumors of skeletal muscle, are extremely rare

anywhere; and again, the author has been unable to find a documented case occurring in the foot. On the other hand, rhabdomyosarcomas have been occasionally reported. These malignancies are generally of the embryonal type and are seen usually between the 1st and 3rd decades of life. As with any sarcoma, this lesion requires radical excision.

Giant cell tumors of the tendon sheath are seen in the foot with some frequency. These develop in and around joints or tendons. They may become very large and

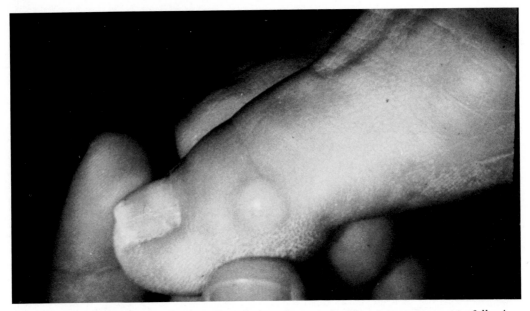

Figure 9.11. Digital mucous cyst. These lesions have a significant recurrence rate following surgery. Experience has shown that these lesions lie in close proximity to bony prominences of the joint. Excision of the bony prominences and, in some instances, partial joint resection in conjunction with complete excision of the cyst, is necessary to obtain a cure.

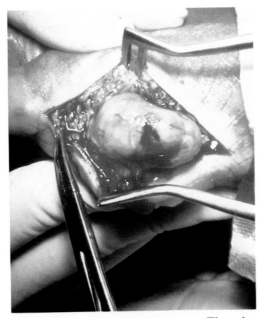

Figure 9.12. Vascular leiomyoma. These lesions are uncommon on the foot and are usually smaller than seen in this photograph (courtesy of Stuart A. Marcus, D.P.M.).

often appear as multilobulated, encapsulated lesions. Because of their close proximity to bony structures, the difficulty of surgical removal is increased. When clinical and radiological examination indicates that this tumor involves the bone, that portion of the bone involved should also be excised. Giant cell tumors also have a tendency to recur if inadequately excised. One cause of incomplete excision is due to their tendency to be multilobulated; and it must be remembered that all portions must be completely removed (Fig. 9.13).

Nodular Tendosynovitis

Nodular tendosynovitis is a variant of the giant cell tumor, but from a clinical standpoint, it is a more diffuse type of lesion, growing in several satellite regions from the main body of the lesion, making excision more difficult. Thus, because they are not as defined, meticulous dissection is necessary.

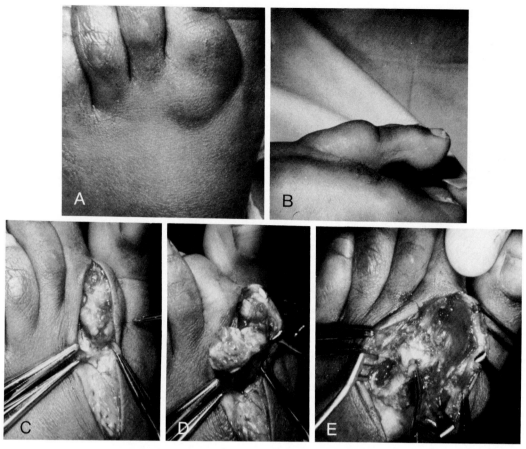

Figure 9.13. Giant cell Tumor. *A*, a large tumorous mass around the second metatarsophalangeal joint. *B*, represents the giant cell tumor and, because of its size, caused a dorsiflexion-type deformity at the second metatarsophalangeal joint. *C*, the surgical exposure of the brownish-yellowish mass. *D*, the mass as it is excised from the wound. *E*, the cavity in which the mass was isolated and the infiltration of the giant cell tumor into the head of the second metatarsal, which was later completely resected. It should be stressed that any benign lesion lying in close proximity to the bone can cause erosion or infiltration. Giant cell tumors and hemangiomas have a tendency to involve bone (courtesy of Mike Feinstein, D.P.M.).

Synovial Sarcomas

Synovial sarcomas are highly malignant lesions of the musculoskeletal system. Fortunately, they are relatively rare but, statistically, they are seen with some frequency on the foot and ankle. They are reddish to brown in color, nonencapsulated, and often blend into the surrounding tissue, making their margins difficult to discern. Because they may grow rapidly, the surgeon must be extremely aggressive in his endeavors to excise them. Usually, amputation is the treatment of choice (9.14).

VASCULAR TUMORS OF THE FOOT

The most frequently encountered vascular tumor of the foot is the hemangioma. Cavernous hemangiomas are probably the most frequently seen vascular lesions of the foot and vary in size depending on the vascular structure of involvement. From a clinical standpoint, they may become larger or smaller on activity, so that sometimes it is difficult to distinguish them from ganglion cysts. Cavernous hemangiomas often involve more than one vessel, posing a significant problem in excision. When they

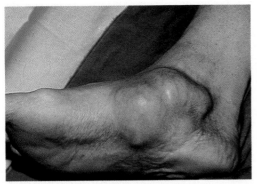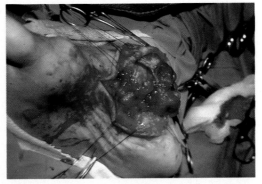

Figure 9.14. Synovial sarcoma. *Left*, these are aggressive and highly metastatic tumors. These lesions often require amputation when found on the foot. In some instances, depending on the histologic rate of synovial sarcomas, Mims salvage-type procedures may be performed. *Right*, the gross surgical appearance of the sarcoma which has no well-defined borders. Consequently, the complete surgical excision of this lesion is practically impossible on the foot (courtesy of Herb Rothfeld, D.P.M., and John Buchan, D.P.M.).

involve more than one vessel, posing a significant problem in excision. When they involve the major vessels of the foot, excision adequate to remove them may cause vascular insufficiency so severe that amputation is necessary. Arteriograms are often crucial in determining the extent of this type of vascular tumor prior to surgical intervention and to enhance the likelihood of a successful outcome. Because of the vascularity of these lesions, they may infiltrate bone and act in many instances like a malignancy. The possibility of heavy bleeding during their excision must also be a consideration.

Hemangiomas may involve nerves or tendinous structures of the foot, which also reduces the chance for surgically successful extirpation. The surgeon walks a fine line in the management of hemangiomas between being aggressive enough to excise the entire lesion, but not so aggressive as to compromise the blood or nerve supply. In some instances, the surgical excision should involve only the part of the lesion producing the discomfort, so as to decrease the patient's pain, but not jeopardize the involved limb. Following excision of large hemangiomas of the foot, it is imperative to adequately close the deep layers and insert a surgical drain. It is also important to carefully ligate any of the small vessels that enter the tumor, for a significant com-

plication in excising hemangiomas is the potential for great blood loss in or around the lesion. Fortunately, the blood loss may be less than with similar tumors in other areas of the body because of the smaller vascular structures in the foot. Edgerton has reported success in shrinking cavernous hemangiomas in juvenile patients with the use of corticosteroid injections (see Suggested Readings). The mechanism by which the steroids create a reduction in size of hemangiomas is unclear at this time, but it may be advantageous to use this as an adjunctive form of therapy following the incomplete surgical removal of large cavernous hemangiomas of the foot.

Kaposi's sarcomas are the most frequent vascular malignancies encountered in the foot. Often they are multiple and occur bilaterally. If adequately excised, a cure is a possibility; otherwise, they have a high rate of recurrence. These unusual tumors may also have a systemic involvement but the primary lesion may be first noticed on the foot. Following surgical excision, careful medical evaluation should be carried out and the appropriate medical specialist consulted (Fig. 9.15).

Hemangioendotheliomas are rare lesions of the foot and may be either benign or malignant. They are usually extensive and create significant difficulty during surgical management. The malignant lesion often

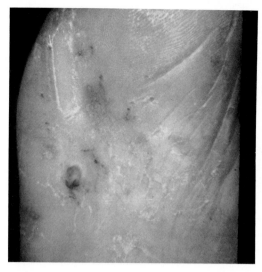

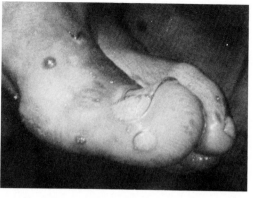

Figure 9.16. Exostosis. This clinical picture represents a small, fibrous, bulbous mass on the distal medial aspect of the great toe. Because of the irregularity of the soft tissue lesion, it can easily be confused with a dermatofibroma, verruca, or neurofibroma, as well as many different types of skin tumors. Histologically, this tissue is primarily fibrotic from an underlying exostosis of the great toe.

Figure 9.15. Pyogenic granuloma. This picture represents a small red granulomatous lesion on the plantar aspect of the foot. This lesion had been draining a serous-type fluid and was easily irritated on pressure. This is a benign form of capillary hemangioma, which can easily be confused with a melanoma, as well as other vascular and potentially malignant lesions. Surgical excision usually results in an adequate cure.

requires radical and/or block-type excision, or even amputation. Other vascular malignancies may be encountered on the foot, but they are, fortunately, extremely rare.

LESIONS OF NERVES

Neuromas are the most frequently found lesions of the foot, with the exception of skin lesions and, in most instances, they are the most painful. Morton's neuromas, found in the intermetatarsal spaces, have been the most publicized in the literature. Fortunately, these reactive tumors create no significant problem during surgery. However, two hazards the surgeon may encounter are inadequate excision or being too aggressive during surgical management and excising too much of the normal fibrofatty tissue in and around the neuroma. This latter type of aggressive approach often creates prolonged post-operative discomfort and healing. Post-operative fibro-

sis may develop within 2 or 3 weeks, and such patients complain of a painful lump on weightbearing following surgery. If this becomes a chronic problem, local corticosteroid injections in the surgical site, as well as aggressive physical therapy and protective padding around the region during weightbearing, often renders the patient asymptomatic. Traumatic and amputation neuromas occurring after surgical intervention in the foot clinically appear the same, and fortunately, cause fewer surgical problems than Morton's or intermetatarsal neuromas. This is not to say, however, that neuromas do not recur or that the operated area should not be protected with padding or necessary orthotics as a part of postoperative management. Failure to do so allows continued mechanical or other traumatic irritations and will often result in recurrence (Fig. 9.16).

Dermal neuromas are tiny neuromas in the deep dermis, which are being seen with more and more frequency microscopically, but are generally not clinically evident. They are often present overlying bone structures, particularly in close proximity to painful helomata. These neuromas may be the cause of severe pain underlying hyperkeratotic lesions. Often, the excision of a small wedge of overlying skin when resecting a bony prominence alleviates this particular problem. Neuromas may also occur in association with various scars and in puncture wounds. Meticulous physical examination is essential to even suspect the presence of such lesions.

Neurilemmomas (Schwannomas) are nerve tumors infrequently seen in the foot. They are usually well encapsulated; and when they involve small nerves, they present little problem during surgical excision. It is when they involve the major nerves, particularly the posterior tibial, that extreme care must be taken to prevent damage to the nerve trunk. Occasionally, such tumors may be shelled out of the nerve trunk, affording easy and successful nerve repair. The most significant danger occurs when a major nerve trunk is involved and neurolysis is necessary in order to adequately and totally excise the lesion. This may create paresthesias or permanent nerve damage.

Malignancies of nerve tissue are rare tumors in the foot but are similar to those occurring elsewhere. They are often slow growing and may or may not be painful and occasionally cause ulceration of the overlying skin, as with other types of sarcomas. Such tumors are highly malignant and when they involve the foot, amputation is the treatment of choice.

OTHER SOFT TISSUE MALIGNANCIES OF THE FOOT

Sarcomas of the foot are very rare, but when they occur, as has been mentioned throughout this chapter, aggressive surgical management is necessary in order to afford the best chance or any chance for cure. It is, of course, recognized how difficult it is for the surgeon to be both aggressive and conservative at the same time. Often, en bloc-type excision or even amputation is necessary to excise many of these tumors. When bone is involved by sarcomas, there

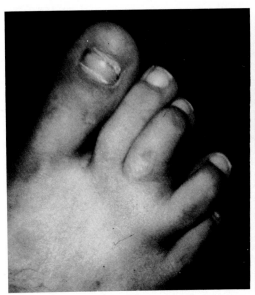 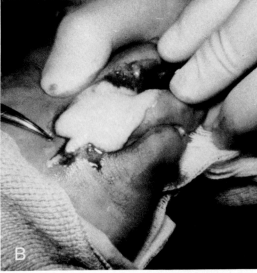

Figure 9.17. Epidermoid inclusion cyst. *A*, this photograph shows swelling of the dorsal aspect of the foot and significant spreading of the third and fourth toes. *B*, shows complications of exuding cellular material on the initial skin incision. The lesion was so close to the skin that the surgical blade pierced through the capsular structures, exuding this creamy white substance. It is important for the surgeon to evaluate the proximity of the lesion underlying the skin in order not to incise into the tumor or lesion involved.

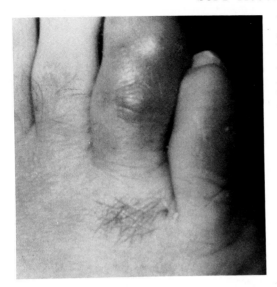

Figure 9.18. Calcified bursa. The figure represents an acute swelling and erythematous bulbous mass involving the fourth toe of the right foot. A similar clinical appearance is seen in acute cases of gout and rheumatoid arthritis. X-ray examination revealed a calcified mass, whereas histologically, it was a calcified bursa, appearing as an acute case of potential gout on clinical examination.

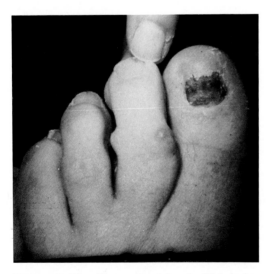

Figure 9.19. Tumoral calcinosis. This lesion represents irregular swelling within the digit of the second toe, seen on x-ray as a calcified mass.

is a much higher rate of metastasis, so that even more aggressive management is needed. It is not uncommon after an en

bloc excision is performed that radical amputation is necessary within a short time. One of the reasons for this is that amputation may become indicated after careful pathological evaluation of the tumor, in conjunction with other diagnostic aids, such as bone scans, arteriograms, and the presence of enlarged lymph nodes. Further, after surgical excision of sarcomas, it is often necessary to employ additional therapeutic modalities, such as radiation therapy and/or chemotherapy.

The greatest surgical errors include failure to use consultation with appropriate medical specialists, misjudgment of the histologic type of the tumor, and the overconfidence of the surgeon. The surgeon and the surgical pathologist must be a "team" and need to discuss difficult cases at length, and the surgeon needs to be assured by the pathologist of the adequacy of the resection margins before he can "rest easily."

Metastatic lesions to the foot are extremely rare and often present as inflammatory lesions. Such lesions can easily confuse the examining podiatrist and also pose significant problems for the surgeon and the pathologist as to the primary tumor site. Again, the desirability of a close working relationship between the podiatrist, the pathologist, the medical and surgical oncologist, and other medical specialists is emphasized.

SUMMARY

It has been the purpose of this chapter to describe various lesions of the foot and problems that podiatrists may find with them. It is extremely important for the podiatric surgeon to be aggressive, in particular, and conservative, in general, to prevent an overly aggressive approach to benign tumors or lesions. It is also extremely important to realize that lesions involving plantar skin, joints, nerves and vascular structures, and the skin, in general, all may cause complications (Fig. 9.19). The surgeon should have a good working relationship with his pathologist, for he will need to rely heavily on the biopsy interpretation.

Suggested Readings

Berlin, S. J. et al. *Skin Tumors of the Foot: Diagnosis and Treatment.* Podiatric Medicine & Surgery, Futura, 1974.

Berlin, S. J., et al *Soft Somatic Tumors of the Foot: Dx & Sur Mgmt,* Podiatric Medicine & Surgery, Futura Pub Co—1976.

Casara, M. D., et al. False-positive bone scan in bone tumors of the lower limb. Eur. J. Nucl. Med. 2:179–181, 1977.

Drzeweick, K. T., Ladefoged, C., and Christensen, H. E. Biopsy and prognosis for cutaneous malignant melanomas in clinical stage I. Scand. J. Plastic Reconstr. Surg. 14:141–144, 1980.

Edgerton, M. D. The Treatment of hemangiomas. Ann. Surg. 183:517–532, 1976.

Gall, Sim, Pritchard, MD Metatastic Tumors to the Bones of the Foot, Cancer, Mar 1976.

Gilbert, Kagan, Winkley, MD Soft Tissue Sarcomas of the Extremities: Their Natural History, Trt, & Radiation Sensitivity, J of Sur Oncology 7:703–317—1975.

Hara, B., and Lowe, B., Eds. *Complications of Foot Surgery,* Williams & Wilkins, Baltimore, 1976.

Ignoffo, R. J., and Friedman, M. A. Therapy of local toxicities caused by extravasation of cancer chemotherapeutic drugs. Cancer Treat. Rev. 7:17–27, 1980.

Morton, D., et al. Limb salvage from a multidisciplinary Treatment approach for skeletal and soft tissue sarcomas of the extremity. Ann. Surg. 184:268–278, 1976.

Ratz, J. L., and Barlin, P. L. Liquid-crystal thermography in determining the lateral extent of basal cell carcinomas. J. Dermatol. Surg. Oncol. 7:27–31, 1981.

Shiu, M., Castro, E., Hayden, S., et al. Surgical treatment of 297 soft tissue sarcomas of the lower extremity. Ann. Surg. 182:597–602, 1975.

Simon, M., and Enneking, W. The management of soft-tissue sarcomas of the extremities. J. Bone Jt. Surg. 58A:317–327, 1976.

Stephens, F. O., and Harker, J. S. The Use of intra-arterial chemotherapy for treatment of malignant skin neoplasms. Aust. J. Dermatol. 20:99–107, 1979.

Wu, K., and Guise, E. Metastatic tumors of the foot. South. Med. J. 71:807–808, 1978.

CHAPTER 10

Repair of Tendons and Soft Tissues

JAMES H. LAWTON, D.P.M.

Tendons are flexible fibrous tissues that offer great resistance to a pulling force. They consist of closely packed, parallel collagenous bundles. Fibroblasts are found between the parallel collagenous bundles. Tendons glide in the tissue by one of two mechanisms: 1) in a sheath and 2) in paratenon. The tendon and sheath pass across a joint or around curves and bend to produce a pulling mechanism with a defined vector direction and force. The sheaths and fascia prevent the tendon from bowstringing across the joint. The tendon and the sheath work essentially like a piston and cylinder, and the tendon glides on a thin film of synovial fluid. This mechanism consists of two layers of synovia: a visceral (epitenon) covering the tendon, and a parietal layer (sheath) lining the fascial tunnel through which the tendon glides. Two layers join to become the mesotenon. This mesotenon is loose, filmy and allows the tendon to glide. It is located on the convex side of the tendon away from the friction, and contains the vascular structures for the tendon.

The blood supply is distributed to the tendons in bundles of vessels from both ends and enters the tendon on the mesotenon side, runs longitudinally in the epitenon, and sends branches along the septa. The major neurovascular bundle is located at the proximal one-third of the muscle belly. The concave side bears friction and is relatively avascular. The fibrous septum runs from the epitenon and divides the tendon into bundles called endotenons. The paratenon is an elastic, pliable tissue that allows the tendon to glide. It fills the space between the tendon and the immovable fascial compartment through which the tendon moves, and is attached at its end to the fascia or some fixed structure. The tendon and paratenon pull in a straight line and act to keep a joint in proper alignment.

ANATOMY

Tendons are a type of dense connective tissue fashioned into fibers and arranged in an orderly parallel pattern. These longitudinally orientated collagen fibers are composed of a large number of fibrils and are surrounded by a loose areolar connective tissue called endotendineum. The endotenon is a relatively acellular tissue which carries the blood vessels which then reach the tendon through the mesotenon. The blood supply is longitudinally oriented and is fed segmentally through the mesotenon.

Fibroblasts are the only cell type present. The peritendineum surrounds a group of fibers. These bundles of fibers are called fascicles. The whole tendon, composed of a variable number of fascicles, is enclosed in a thick connective sheath, the epitendineum (22). The tendon sheath is lined with synovial tissue which is found whenever a tendon is forced to turn a corner.

Another major consideration is the overall architecture of tendons and the precision of movement required. Such function and degree of motion is determined by the number of neuromuscular end-plates. When gross motion is necessary, such as in the leg, only a single axon is required to fire many neuromuscular end-plates; when precise motion is required, then a single axon is required to fire fewer neuromuscular end-plates.

GLIDING MECHANISM

The tendon sheath is not responsible for the tendon's ability to glide because it lacks elasticity. Gliding mechanism of tendons is essential but depends exclusively on the paratenon, an elastic connective tissue covering which enables it to stretch several centimeters. The entire tendon is covered by the paratenon, which is firmly attached and doubled over at both ends of the tendon. Where the tendon sheath is absent, the tendon and overlying paratenon are enveloped in fatty areolar tissue. It is imperative to preserve this elastic structure to insure proper gliding of the tendon. If the paratenon is stripped or damaged during tendon surgery, the tendon will develop post-operative adhesions that seriously interfere with normal physiological gliding. Minimal trauma and instrumentation is the rule to be followed when performing tendon surgery. Drying should be avoided by covering exposed areas with saline-soaked sponges. Simple but essential surgical principles will help restore the normal function of muscular and tendinous structures, especially in light of the delicate structures necessary to produce this most important gliding mechanism.

Restoration of physiological function in a transferred tendon depends on two major factors: 1) blood supply, and 2) the degree of trauma. Tendons have been thought by many to be relatively avascular. However, the blood supply to tendons, as has been previously mentioned, is more adequate than generally appreciated. The mesotenon or vinculum, a delicate connective tissue membrane that connects the tendon with the floor of the sheath, transmits blood vessels to the tendon (6). These vessels do not penetrate the tendon fibers directly, but allow blood-borne cells that have the potential to synthesize fibrous tissue to migrate to tendon areas that require repair and/or nutrition. This concept of exogenous vascularization is significant, since intra-operative trauma by disrupting the mesotenon will not in itself result in adhesions. However, unless rigid hemostasis is practiced, hemorrhage can occur between tendon and paratenon or between paratenon and tendon sheath, which allows fibrous proliferation and resultant adhesions. Similarly, if a tendon is damaged along its longitudinal surface by rough handling or by partial laceration, and the interior of the tendon is exposed, then scar tissue often exerts a severe restricting influence (31, 32). No matter the method of disruption, whether it be direct trauma, spontaneous rupture, or ischemia, the reparative process is oriented toward the restoration of continuity. The traumatized tendon rarely, if ever, regains total pre-operative function. If the trauma is minimal, then the percentage of return of function will be greater. This must be kept in mind, especially in light of surgical repair which will further traumatize the tendon. If a tendon is completely transected, then the chance for return of full function is limited at best, and any further trauma in the intra-operative period will only further decrease the possibility of positive functional recovery. In the early stages following trauma, the tendon goes through a softening process during the first 5 days. It should be obvious that through this period the tensile strength of the tendon is extremely diminished. During tendon surgery, larger suture material will only serve to further traumatize the tendon, and thus reduce the potential functional recovery. Unless the traumatized tendon ends are in juxtapositional alignment, then healing cannot take place. Even when the tendon ends are in close proximity, there is a gap zone with accompanying fibroblastic proliferation. Within 48 hours after injury, the epitenon cells are proliferating vigorously to reduce the gap zone. When lacerated ends of a tendon are not in juxtaposition, or if there is any non-tendinous material between the ends, then cellular migration and fibroblastic proliferation to heal the tendon will be blocked, or at the very least, interfere with primary healing. While individual tissue systems have their own inherent healing tendency, all result and interact with each other in various phases of the healing process. Adhesions are formed from migrating fibroblasts and initially are not a complication of surgery but are an integral part of the healing response. Revascularization is initially from the surrounding tissue in a poorly organized pattern. Eventually, the revascularization pattern changes to a more normal longitudinal realignment, and within 8 weeks following the trauma and/or surgery, normal vascularity has been re-established. During the healing process, collagen deposition begins about the 4th day. The mucopolysaccharide concentration level is at its highest at about 4–8 days and then decreases. The amount of new collagen formation is in direct proportion to the degree of trauma. Initially, when new collagen is laid down, there is no specific pattern and its orientation is in a random fashion. At this point, it is nearly impossible to differentiate normal tendon tissue from fibroblastic adhesive tissue. When stress is placed across the healing area, these random fibers begin to assume a more longitudinal orientation. It has been discovered that a tendon is a piezoelectric substance and a material which is capable of converting mechanical stress into electrical potential.

Eventually, the amount of collagen in the healing area diminishes, and what remains completes its longitudinal orientation with multiple cross-linkages. The revascularization has been completed by this time in a longitudinal direction and the vascular supply to the surrounding adhesions decreases. When the adhesions become weakened, they no longer restrict motion and the gliding mechanism is restored. In other instances, the adhesions retain their restricted position and power, and thus are a complicating factor.

TENDON ANOMALIES

Anomalous insertions of tendons of the foot are quite common and produce functional changes. The normal foot changes from an excessively mobile adapter, functioning in a pronated attitude, to one requiring rigidity for leverage. Evolutionary development has brought about changes in bones, tendon insertions, and function of muscles. Most anomalous tendon insertions are traced to changes not keeping pace with the bony and/or functional changes. Usually, these evolutionary "arrests" tend to increase the pronatory attitude of the foot, and when the insertions appear earlier than the bony adaptation they tend to increase the supinatory and/or equinus attitude of the foot.

Peroneal Tendons

The peroneus longus tendon traverses the plantar aspect of the foot and sends slips to the base of the first metatarsal. In earlier forms of primate development, the peroneals were anterior muscles performing extensor functions. Insertions of the peroneal tendons lateral to the first metatarsal are considered regressive because they will interfere mechanically with effective stabilization of the first metatarsal. This is another consideration in the etiology of hallux abducto valgus. An anomalous insertion of the peroneus longus tendon more distal along the shaft of the first metatarsal causes excessive stabilization of the segment and is among a number of etiological factors resulting in plantar flexed first ray and subsequent medial sesamoiditis. Other peroneal anomalies involve the duplication or absence of one or both tendons. Tenoanastomosis (partial or complete) of the peroneus longus and brevis tendons has been reported. At times, a fourth peroneal muscle exists that enhances the action of the others. Insertions of the peroneus brevis have been seen as far distal as the fifth digit.

Posterior Tibial Tendon

This has many variations of insertions. Most hinder its power as an inverter.

Anterior Tibial Tendon

Sometimes this tendon sends an "ancestral" slip to the dorsal aspect of the first metatarsal, or even the first phalanx. This muscle in prehuman forms was a powerful digital dorsiflexor. It may still dorsiflex the hallux with its anomalous insertion or indirectly via branches with the extensor hallucis longus. A rarer anomaly is the absence of the extensor hallucis longus with a replacement from the anterior tibial. Insertion dorsally into the area of first metatarsophalangeal joint is detrimental to plantar flexion of the hallux segment, and a hypermobile first ray may develop. Tenectomy of this variant of the anterior tibial is indicated. Rarely, a slip of the anterior tibial has been found inserting into the talus, which may have a premature supinatory effect on the rearfoot.

Flexor Hallucis Longus Tendon

The role of this tendon may have been greatly understated as being primarily a flexor of the distal phalanx. It is the only tendon to lie directly under the sustentaculum tali, and it intimately hugs the posterior aspect of the talus and the lower tibia. It is unusually large in diameter and has a greater crural origin than any other leg muscle. Its position, size, power, and evolutionary implications suggest strongly that this is a key tendon for proper foot function. In cadaver experiments, it has been demonstrated that a significant increase in the range of ankle dorsiflexion is made possible by performing a tenotomy of the flexor hallucis longus behind the ankle joint. The function of this tendon is commonly influenced by the flexor digitorum longus, since there are frequently slips of one to the other. There may be slips of the flexor hallucis longus tendon into the calcaneus.

Smaller Digital Tendons

Smaller tendons, especially the intrinsics, are more commonly involved in anomalous insertions than are the major tendons, and deviations from textbook descriptions are almost the rule. Such deviation is a factor in dealing with digital mal-

alignments, since duplications or absences are frequently encountered.

TRAUMA

Rupture of a tendon affects the musculotendinous unit which activates joints which, in turn, is activated by other musculo-tendinous units, so that the full range of motion is solely controlled by a single unit. The muscle is most likely to tear in the midrange of contraction when it is overloaded and the tension is the greatest. The damage likely to occur includes: tendon avulsion from the bone, rupture at the musculo-tendinous junction, or muscle rupture. The younger the patient, the more likely that there will be muscle rather than tendon rupture. The reverse is true in older individuals. However, muscle ruptures are not a common clinical entity and have to be of an exaggerated nature to require surgical repair.

A tendon may rupture either during excessive stress, during normal activities, or when unusual strain is applied to the tendon unit. As a general rule, the best treatment following rupture of a tendon is accurate juxtapositional alignment of the ends with no tension until the healing is complete. Any evidence of contamination of the wound or necrosis of the tendon requires surgical debridement and excision. In some cases, the degree of trauma and necrosis and/or gapping may require the use of a tendon graft. If neglected, such cases usually require extensive surgical correction at a later date with a much poorer prognosis and long periods of rehabilitation.

Rupture of the peroneus longus tendon occurs as a result of a sharp inversion force to the foot and ankle when the muscle is contracted. Generally, pain, swelling, and tenderness are noted in the lateral ankle region. Immediate repair is recommended to prevent deformity.

Rupture of the tendo Achilles does not generally occur as a spontaneous act. Rupture occurs when forces exceed the tensile strength of one of the component parts of the unit. Tendo Achilles rupture may be the result of abrupt, excess, functional strain placed on a tendon that exceeds the range of motion of the triceps surae. A blow over the bone may cause fracture and the rupture of a taut tendon as well. Tuberculous tenosynovitis and rheumatoid tenosynovitis cause changes of attrition that result in spontaneous rupture of the tendo Achilles following a slight stretch.

Such ruptures cause a sudden onset of pain in the calf and the individual finds normal walking impossible (40). If the rupture is complete, there is inability to rise on one's toes while standing or plantarly flexing the foot in recumbance. One test is to plantarflex the foot against a given resistance. Thompson (36) developed a test whereby the calf muscles can be squeezed, and if the tendon is intact, then the foot will flex plantarly. However, if the tendon is ruptured, then there will be no motion in the foot. Ruptures of the tendo Achilles at the musculo-tendinous junction occur most often in the young, while ruptures near its insertion on the calcaneus are seen more in adulthood. If left untreated, the tendon may unite spontaneously, but in a lengthened position. If the rupture is at a lower level, it can be felt along the course of the tendo Achilles. If the rupture is at a higher level, only partial loss of active plantarflexion will be experienced. In this case, the rupture may be incomplete and there may be an intact tendon sheath with a ruptured tendon. It is difficult to detect any loss of continuity since there will be effusion of blood, and edema of the paratenon at this site. Ultrasonography may be useful as a diagnostic tool when dealing with ruptures of the tendo Achilles. Bruce et al. (40) reported on the use of diagnostic ultrasonography when confronted with cases when clinical examination left a question as to whether or not rupture was present. In active individuals, they felt that primary surgical repair was indicated, and thus this test aided these decision-making processes. For comparison, the untraumatized limb was also evaluated. Clinical examination in

the acute stage can be difficult and, thus, we should keep this method of diagnosis in mind for proper evaluation.

Although a ruptured tendo Achilles may be treated by immobilization, the healing will cause fibrosis and reduce the tensile strength of the normal tendon. Therefore, open repair of the tendo Achilles is recommended in many cases. In order to avoid adhesion of the scar to the underlying tendon, the incision is not made directly over the tendon. Instead, a posterior-medial incision is used. The surgery should be performed within 12 hours of the tendon rupture. Lynn (4) uses the plantaris as a free graft by fanning out the membrane, wrapping it around the anastomosed tendo Achilles, and suturing the structures. Should increased tension be necessary to rejoin the damaged tendon, Lindholm's technique may be useful (4, 55). The Bosworth technique has been found to be useful in repairing old tendon ruptures (4, 52). Post-operative cast application with the knee flexed and with moderate plantarflexion on the foot for approximately 14 days is indicated. The patient should obviously be kept off weightbearing during this time and after the 14-day period, a below knee cast may be applied with the foot held at a 90° angle for 1 week, followed by a gradual return to ambulation and weightbearing over the next 2–4 weeks, depending upon the degree of trauma. Another useful technique for untreated ruptures of the tendo Achilles has been advocated by Bugg and Boyd (60).

Certainly controversy will continue with regard to the proper clinical identification of an acute rupture of the tendo Achilles and the appropriate method of treatment. There still remains some uncertainty as to the absolute "best" approach for individual patients. Lea and Smith (3) are strong advocates of a nonsurgical approach to rupture of the tendo Achilles. They reported on eight cases and claimed a high degree of success and essentially abandoned surgical therapy. They did agree that the untreated Achilles rupture will heal with weakness and increased length but stated that there was limited loss to the patient if primary surgical repair was not performed. Total casting time is approximately 2 months with gradual ambulatory weightbearing, and graduated increases in dorsiflexion of the foot at the ankle with each cast changes. After completion of the casting, the patient is placed in a standard shoe with a one-inch heel elevation on the affected side. This lift is maintained for a period of one month and then discontinued. Lea and Smith reported that during the initial stages of healing, as in surgical cases, non-surgical patients were seen to have a considerable thickening at the site of trauma which decreased over a period of time, except in one case. This involved an open laceration of the tendo Achilles with an oblique transverse cut by a piece of glass. They stated that the time of follow-up was brief (approximately 1–3 years). There does seem to be some merit with this particular philosophy, especially with incomplete or partial tears or in contaminated wounds. However, in active collegiate or professional athletes or in complete ruptures with large gapping between the tendinous ends, primary closure appears to be indicated.

Teuffer (39) reported on 30 cases of traumatic rupture of the Achilles tendon involving athletes. At the outset, he stated that he did not use conservative therapy since he considered it "ineffective." His recommended surgical procedure was the use of the peroneus brevis tendon as a "sling" from lateral to medial through a transverse drill hole near the plantar aspect of the calcaneus. The rupture in the Achilles tendon is repaired initially and the peroneus brevis tendon is used as a medial and lateral reinforcement. He reported that, in 28 cases, there were excellent results, and in two cases good results. There was a delay in healing in two cases which eventually healed without further complications. There were no other complications in his series. All cases returned to athletic activities with guarded mobility in the two cases of good results, with intermittent pain

in the tendon or along the scar. Average follow-up was 5 years (2–7-year range) and the results are obviously impressive.

TENDON HEALING

Healing is different in the two types of tendons. In the sheathed type, there is very little reparative activity. When it is severed, the proximal end retracts and the tendon ends are sealed by epitenon. Granulation tissue forms so that with scarring, the tendon ends adhere to the sheath. Tendons severed in paratenon push out a proliferative material that arises from epitenon, endotenon, and paratenon tissue. The pseudopodia join, contract, and draw the tendon ends together. Any tendon that grows into fascia or a ligament will result in limited motion or end the gliding action of the tendon. The purpose of repair is to encourage progressive fibrosis and reconstitution. However, for this latter effect to occur, the tendon ends must be in "juxtaposition."

During the first 7 days of repair, the tendon ends are joined by a fibroblastic splint. Serous and granulation tissues then form a jelly-like union to bridge the tendons. During the 2nd week, the vascularity of the paratenon is increased and collagen proliferates. By the 8th day there is an ingrowth of tendon fibers and cells. From the 10th to the 14th day, the gap is bridged. By the 3rd week, the collagen fibers begin to mat and fibrose longitudinally. There is increased cell mitosis 1 cm back into each tendon end. During the 4th week, the resolution reduces swelling and decreases vascularity. The tendon is then capable of gliding to some degree.

Studies by Mason (44, 57) and Allen (58) show there is insufficient strength of union at the site of the tendon repair up to 15 days. From the 15th to the 21st days a fair degree of strength is present. After 3 weeks, guarded, minimal exercise is prescribed to improve strength. Maximal pull of the tendon is to be avoided for at least 1 month. Immobilization is recommended for 3 weeks to prevent rupture during healing. The mobilized tendon was found to be more edematous and adherent, while the immobilized tendon showed a better appearance and the least reaction to its surroundings.

REPAIR OF TENDONS

Mayer's rule (30) states that, when the origin and insertion of a muscle are approximated by repair of the tendons, ideally the tension should be zero. Slack should be taken out of the tendon before approximating the tendon ends. When a repair from an injury over 2 months old is made, the muscle has contracted. After tendon repair and healing, the muscle will achieve its proper length with exercise and activity. However, if the wound is more than 2 months old, there will be a wider gap between the tendon ends and a graft will be necessary. The tension on the muscle tendon unit must be adjusted to achieve the functional range of motion, and there should be some allowance for elongation of a muscle following rehabilitation.

If a muscle is placed under excessive tension, it loses strength; if placed under too little tension, varying degrees of muscle power are lost. The strength of a muscle is in proportion to its cross-sectional area, but its range of motion is in proportion to the length of the fibers. The objective is normal physiological tension so that loss of muscle strength will be minimized.

Suture materials for tendon repair include silk, wire, nylon, or synthetic materials, and the choice depends upon experience and preference. The size and the strength of the tendon are important factors. Stainless steel sutures cause the least reaction, glide easily, and provide strength. Kinks in the wire interfere with tendon gliding. These sutures may be used as a pullout type or they may remain in the wound. Suture material must be nonabsorbable in order to hold the tendon ends for a minimal of 3 weeks. Tantalum is inert but its tensile strength is low and it does not tie smoothly. The number of sutures must be kept to a minimum to prevent foreign body reaction and subsequent fibrosis. Therefore, a few strands of strong suture are preferable to many strands of a weak material. The sutures should be braided or spliced to the length of the tendon to prevent rupture during healing. The tendon ends are joined so that the fibers bend slightly like an accordion at the repair sight. If the tendon ends do not touch, healing may be delayed (Fig. 10.1).

End-to-end union of tendon is the most common technique employed (Fig. 10.2). The suture is woven diagonally through the tendon with two straight needles (Kieth) and crossed, then taken across the tendon gap and woven into the opposing tendon. The sutures are then pulled to remove all slack and tied. If it is a pull out wire, the suture should be pulled back and forth through the tendon to make sure that it can be withdrawn easily. For the pullout, the suture ends are fastened outside the skin to a padded button or disc (Fig. 10.3).

For major tendons, the pull out suture eliminates mechanical irritation and holds the tendon in place to insure good union. At suture removal, the tension on the pullout wire is from the muscle side. The other end remains passive.

When tendons of unequal diameter are sutured end-to-end, the exposed end of the larger tendon will grow a pseudo-podium which attaches itself to the surrounding tissue and contracts. This results in loss of

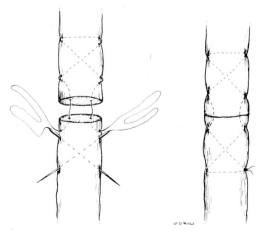

Figure 10.1. Bunnell stitch with tightening at the gap site to produce the accordion effect.

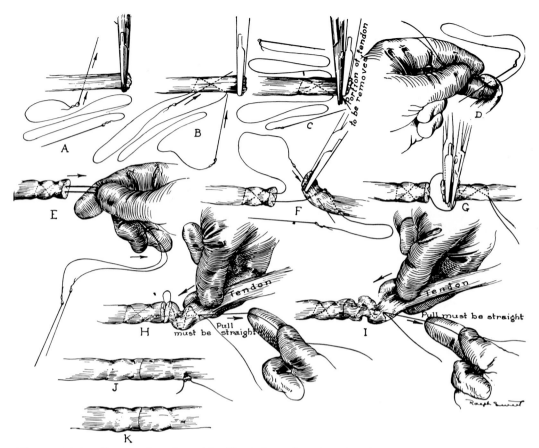

Figure 10.2. Suture of tendon with silk. *A–D*, with a thread and two needles, the sutures are laced traversing the tendon with each needle from 2–4 times and emerging through the end. *E*, all slack is drawn out. *F* and *G*, the suture is continued similarly up the other tendon. Both ends are brought out at the same spot. In placing the last strand in the second tendon end, the needle must not spear the other thread or they will not slip. By keeping the needles on separate sides of the tendon, this is avoided; or better, both needles may be thrust through the tendon simultaneously. *H* and *I*, to prevent the tendon ends from separating under strain, the slack is removed from the second tendon. To do this, one suture is pulled at a time as the tendon is shoved along it to be brought up snug against the other tendon end. *J* and *K*, there is only one knot; when tied, it sinks into the tendon at a place where it receives the least strain, since knots are the weakest parts of a tendon suture. (From *Bunnel's Surgery of the Hand*, 4th ed. Revised by J. H. Boyes, J. B. Lippincott, Philadelphia, 1964, with permission.)

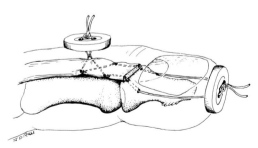

Figure 10.3. Tenodesis to bone with a proximal pull-out stitch, and proximal and distal external buttons.

gliding action. Therefore, the smaller tendon should be buried within the host tendon so that no free ends hang out following anastomoses. In the side-to-side union, the tendon ends are cut diagonally, overlapped, and sutured into position with buried or pullout sutures. In another technique, the tendon ends may be joined by overlapping. One tendon is passed back and forth through slits made in the host tendon, then the end of the running tendon is buried in

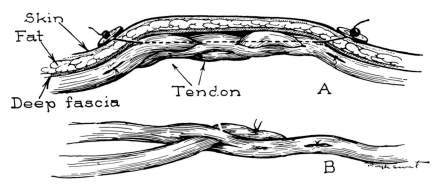

Figure 10.4. The tendon of an active muscle can be woven into one or more recipient tendons in tendon transfer operations. No free exposed tendon ends remain to become attached to surrounding tissues. (From *Bunnell's Surgery of the Hand*, 4th ed. Revised by J. H. Boyes. J. B. Lippincott, Philadelphia, 1964, with permission.)

the host and sutured into position (Fig. 10.4). With tendon grafts, the same technique is used as in suturing end to end (Fig. 10.5).

Immobilization is recommended so that the suture line of the tendon will be in a relaxed state for about 3 weeks. Sutures should not be relied upon to hold the repaired tendon ends together. After 3 weeks, guarded motion can be initiated. Maximal tensile strength of the tendon is not recovered for a period of 3–6 months.

An alternative to the standard Bunnell stitch, as was previously illustrated, was discussed by Ketchum et al. (1). They evaluated six methods of suturing as related to tendon repair, six types of suture material, evaluated the degree of return of tensile strength, and measured the degree of gapping that occurs with these various techniques. Their lateral trap suture demonstrated increased resistance to gapping and extreme resistance to rupture under stress. It has been shown that the lateral trap suture (Fig. 10.6) was 1.64 times as strong as Bunnell's stitch at the point of ultimate rupture and was 1.89 times as strong as the Bunnell stitch at the point of gapping. Of the suture materials tested, monofilament stainless steel produced the greatest resistance against both gapping and eventual rupture, having twice the strength of multistrand stainless steel and 1.7 times the strength of the strongest synthetic suture.

Tendon repair should be postponed if a

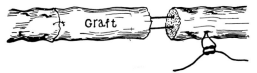

Figure 10.5. Method of interweaving tendons using withdrawable stainless steel wire. One tendon entwines through the other. Free tendon ends are buried. (From *Bunnell's Surgery of the Hand*, 4th ed. Revised by J. H. Boyes. J. B. Lippincott, Philadelphia, 1964, with permission.)

wound is contaminated and there is danger of infection because of increased scar formation. Tendons lining the infected tunnels of the pulling mechanism undergo ischemia and necrosis. This sloughing tendon tissue is replaced by a scar that adheres to the sheath and assures loss of the gliding action and contracture of the joint.

In multiple injuries affecting both bone and soft tissue, tendon repair has a low priority. Fracture reduction, vascular and nerve repair, and skin closure take precedence. Tendon repair is in order if it does not comprise fracture reduction. With a closed injury, crush, bruise, or partially severed tendon, the traumatized portion will swell and soften. In this state, a tendon can rupture upon exertion. Therefore, immobilization up to 3 weeks is recommended to avoid complications following trauma. As soon as healing allows, exercise is essential to prevent stiffness or loss of the gliding action of the tendon.

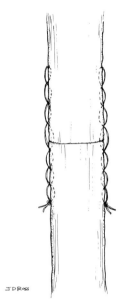

Figure 10.6. Lateral trap suture technique for tendon repair.

If the adhesion is light, the tendon may be free with minimal trauma and measures should be taken to prevent recurrence. If the tendon is bound down by a scar so that the gliding mechanism is not functioning, the following procedure is recommended. Attempts to free the tendon from its scar tissue are performed in the following manner. Begin sharp dissection in viable tissue. Identify the neurovascular structures and tendon while excising the scar back to normal tissue, fascia, or bone. Do not replace the tendon in the scar tissue since this will bring a return of the adhesion and immobilization of the tendon. If all of the scar tissue cannot be excised, interpose some paratenon or smooth deep fascia between the tendon and the scar tissue. This tissue is found in a large, thin, veil-like piece immediately overlying the fascia lata at the outer surface of the lower portion of the thigh. If the tendon is damaged within the scar and is not salvageable, excise that portion of the tendon and replace it with a tendon graft and its paratenon so that the gliding mechanism is restored. If the amount of scar tissue removed is excessive, the surrounding skin must also be free of any adhesion. A skin graft or a pedicle graft

may be required to furnish the soft bed of healthy tissue. Early exercise of the involved part is important because the paratenon may change to scar tissue.

TENDON LUXATION

An example of tendon luxation is the peroneus longus slipping out of its groove behind the lateral malleous as a result of trauma, a congenital absence of the malleolar groove, or a malunited lateral malleolar fracture. In chronic cases, the luxation occurs while walking, and there is acute pain and spasm of the peroneus longus. If the peroneal tendon luxation cannot be reduced manually, or if the reduction is unstable, surgery is required. Recommended is the creation of a periosteal flap to reinforce the sheath or an osteotomy to deepen the malleolar sulcus as described by Kelly et al. (45–47, 53, 54). Stover and Bryan reported traumatic displacement of the peroneal tendons in 19 patients, most of whom were involved in skiing accidents and were most probably caused by forceful dorsiflexion of the ankle followed by mild reflex contraction of the peroneal muscles. Post-operative care includes immobilization for 4–6 weeks, followed by progressive weightbearing and increased activities, physical therapy, and rehabilitation.

TENDON INFLAMMATION

Tenosynovitis, which is an inflammation of the thin synovial lining of the tendon sheath, should be treated promptly to avoid impaired function (33, 34).

Acute, infectious tenosynovitis is caused by a pyogenic organism. It may be the result of a puncture wound or a laceration that pierces and inflames the tendon sheath. The bacterial invasion and the resultant purulent exudate can involve the entire length of the tendon sheath, as well as adjacent joints. Most commonly involved are the long extensor tendons on the dorsum of the foot. Treatment with appropriate antibiosis must be prompt, followed by rest and elevation of the limb. Hot compresses should be applied until the purulent material organizes and the sheath can be incised and drained.

Chronic infectious tenosynovitis is a condition which is uncommon, and is caused by such diseases as syphilis and tuberculosis. The synovial wall becomes thickened and there is a fibrinous exudate which affects the extensor and peroneal tendons. The primary treatment is directed to the underlying systemic disease. The damage to the tendon or sheath may need to be repaired surgically if there is great impairment of tendon function.

Acute, uncomplicated tenosynovitis results from overactivity and most commonly affects the extensor hallucis longus, anterior tibial, and the Achilles tendon. There is swelling over the course of the tendon and occasional crepitation on range of motion within the sheath. The onset of pain is usually sudden. Treatment in the first 24 hours consists of alternating ice packs and heat applications. The part should be immobilized with adhesive straps or plaster casts. Avoid multiple repeated steroid injections at the trigger point since it may in time weaken the tendon and cause its rupture (29). In cases of chronic simple tenosynovitis, this condition can be caused by continuous shoe friction or undue pressure on the extensor tendons or the tendo Achilles. The result is an effusion of synovial fluid into the tendon sheath that causes swelling along the course of the tendon. Treatment consists of removal of the irritating factor. If there is underlying osseous hypertrophy, it must be resected.

Stenosing tenosynovitis occurs most commonly at the ankle where the tendons angulate about the bony structure and are enclosed in a fibrous sheath that acts as a pulley. The friction and pressure of activity inflames the fibrous sheath and constricts the tendon. Distal to the point of constriction, the tendon exhibits a bulbous swelling. The sheath may also undergo degenerative changes and fibrous elements may increase. Stenosing tenosynovitis affects the anterior and posterior tibial tendons, the extensor digitorum longus, and peroneal tendons below the lateral malleous.

The inferior retinaculum, which encloses the peroneal tendons, is also a possible location where stenosis occurs.

When there is inflammation in the common peroneal tendon sheath, there is a palpable thickening below the edge of the lateral malleous, and pain is aggrevated by subtalar motion. The inferior retinaculum is thickened and constricts the peroneal tendons. Conservative care requires immobilization. The surgical approach consists of excision of the peroneal sheath. If the anterior tibial tendon is involved, the transverse crural ligament is incised laterally and is allowed to heal in a lax position.

Hemorrhagic tenosynovitis is caused by trauma in which the epithelial lining of the sheath is ruptured, followed by hemorrhage and clot formation. There is severe pain and swelling along the course of the tendon and rest gives no relief. Evacuation of the hematoma and preservation of the involved tendon is recommended. Tendovaginitis is believed to be caused by repeated trauma that causes mild, chronic inflammation or thickening of the fibrous wall of the tendon sheath. The sheath becomes fibrous and thickens, constricting the tendon and causing swelling.

Paratendinitis results from excessive friction between the tendon and the surrounding paratenon caused by overuse. There is a mild inflammatory reaction in the tendons and in the surrounding tissue, with local edema. Crepitation is produced when the fibrin-covered tendon glides within the inflamed paratenon. Immobilization is indicated to reduce swelling and inflammation.

Acute tenosynovitis caused by rheumatoid arthritis is a granular reaction which infiltrates the synovial sheath and retards the gliding action of the tendon. Mucoid degeneration occurs and nodular masses form within the tendon.

More and more frequently we are observing and diagnosing an increased incidence of tendinitis and tenosynovitis as associated with increased physical and athletic activities by the American population.

Garth (2) had a case of flexor hallucis longus tendonitis in a ballet dancer with associated necrosis and spontaneous tearing of the tendon. If the fitness craze continues in this country, then such incidences will become commonplace.

Compartment Syndrome

The vigorous activity that overtaxes the muscles can cause pain in the anterior muscle compartments as a result of stress periostitis at the ligamentous attachment of the muscle, or myositis of the muscle group. With common shin splints, rest, physical therapy, and judicious strappings are indicated. Casts should be avoided because the increased pressure can aggrevate the pain. In a stress or fatigue fracture of the tibia, the anterior tibial compartment becomes tender, painful, and swollen. Muscle movement aggrevates the condition. Additionally, the severe form of anterior tibial compartment syndrome is accompanied by a low-grade fever, leukocytosis, paralysis of the extensor muscles, persistent extreme pain, anterior tibial sensory palsy, and marked muscle compartment tension. Swelling in the compartment causes venous obstruction so that muscle necrosis may ensue. The anterior tibial artery is not occluded. Fascial incision is imperative to relieve the pressure within the muscle compartment and to prevent complete necrosis and sloughing of the entire muscle.

BENIGN DEGENERATION

Tendons of the foot and leg rarely undergo ossification. Ossification of the tendo achilles can be seen near its insertion. Such ossification may limit ankle motion, depending upon the extent of the lesion. Sudden exertion may sometimes cause partial or complete rupture of the tendo Achilles, necessitating surgical repair. Ossified tendons elsewhere in the foot are often difficult to visualize radiographically because of the superimposed osseous structures.

A ganglion is a mucoid fibrous cyst originating adjacent to a joint lining or tendon sheath. This cyst increases in size and may be asymptomatic or symptomatic, depending upon whether or not it is subjected to irritation or pressure. It should be excised, including the fibrous tissue of origin at the base of the cyst.

Tumors of the tendon sheath are thought to originate from the synovial lining of the tendon sheath. They are benign in nature. Tumors of neighboring structures can involve the tendon, but tendons do not produce true neoplasms. Xanthomatous giant cell tumors are encapsulated masses that arise from the tendon sheath. These tumors may grow in size and exert pressure on adjacent structures and they should be excised.

As was mentioned previously, muscle rupture is a relatively uncommon condition. In the common "charley horse," the injury may consist of rupture of muscle fibers, a deep-seated hematoma, or a muscle spasm. In the case of muscle rupture, immediate surgical repair is recommended to prevent chronic pain or muscle weakness. In animal experimentation, the nuclei accumulate in the rounded-off end of the transsected muscle fiber and budding begins at about the 10th day. The muscle buds pursue in a regular course across the rupture and fuse with the opposing muscle fibers. Young connective tissue forms at the rupture site. In the repair of an old muscle rupture, adequate exposure must be made to determine the extent of the trauma and the degree of scarring. The intervening scar tissue is excised except for the rim, which is left on either side to act as a stay for sutures. Following repair of the ruptured muscle, the parts should be protected for approximately 3 weeks.

As an aftermath of untreated hematoma, calcium deposition and subsequent bone formation may appear in the musculature causing myositis ossificans. Once this develops, it must be allowed to complete the active phase of development. If there is surgical intervention during the active phase, the prognosis is poor since the recurrence rate will be high. Therefore, one should wait 18–24 months before surgically excising the lesion.

SURGICAL PROCEDURES

Tenotomy

Although tenotomy of the extensor tendon is generally performed through a stab incision for contracted tendons to the lesser toes, Z-plasty lengthening is the recommended procedure to minimize the recurrence of contraction. It may be performed along with capsulotomy of the involved contracted metatarsophalangeal joints (Fig. 10.7).

The extensor tenotomy of one or two lesser toes may cause increased contracture of the remaining lesser toes. Tenotomizing of three arborizations of the extensor digitorum longus can cause severe muscle imbalance and dorsal contraction of the remaining digital arborization, with subluxation in some cases. Sectioning all of the lesser digital arborization of the extensor digitorum longus can result in atrophy of the involved muscle. Following surgery, fibrosis within the tendon sheath or paratenon and in the joint capsule can cause greater deformity than was originally present. Therefore, Z-plasty tendon lengthening is preferred to tenotomy in order to maintain proper physiological tension and continuity of the tendon and to enhance function of the muscles and involved digits. The reader is referred to Figures 10.8 through 10.16 for review of the appropriate and recommended technique.

Tenotomizing of the flexor digitorum longus at the digital interphalangeal joint of the lesser toe through a medial or lateral stab incision to eradicate a symptomatic distal keratotic lesion in a contracted toe can be successful if post-operative splinting or an orthodigital device is used for approximately 1 month.

Tendon Balancing

Without adequate tendon balancing, iatrogenic deformities can occur. Transpositioning and shortening of the abductor hallucis tendon, excessive tightening of the medial capsule, and tenotomy of the conjoined adductor hallucis tendon create tendon imbalance that may result in hallux varus. Other surgical procedures that shun tendon balancing and biomechanical function will also result in various degrees of subluxation. Often, tenotomy of the conjoined adductor tendon is performed without sufficient regard to the intrinsic musculature. When the tendon is severed and the end left free, the muscle contracts and atrophies. In order to assure forefoot stabilization with tenotomy of the conjoined adductor tendon, it should be transposed to the neck of the first metatarsal, which will maintain some degree of intrinsic muscle activity.

Iatrogenic deformity will follow a medial sesamoidectomy if the flexor hallucis brevis tendon (medial slip) is not properly repaired. The forefoot plantar push-up test will show if the hallux is in proper alignment or if it is abducted and dorsiflexed. Failure to perform the required arthroplasty, tendon repair, and balancing may cause the hallux extensus to worsen until, ultimately, it may require a Jones tendon transfer with arthrodesis of the interphalangeal joint.

Tenotomy of the extensor hallucis longus tendon is quite common during bunionectomies. Tenotomy of the extensor hallucis longus without reattachment transfers the pull to the remaining lesser toes and can provoke contracture. Periodically, a tourniquet applied above the ankle may cause muscle spasm, resulting in the dorsiflexion of toes from contracture of the tendons. If this is suspected, then release the tourniquet before any tendon lengthening procedures are performed to prevent lax tendons. Mann (5) discusses a case of a 27-year-old female who had undergone subcutaneous extensor tenotomy for a dorsally contracted second digit. Following the procedure, she developed a flexion deformity of the digit which did not allow her to ambulate comfortably. Evaluation of this case and other cases should discourage the common use of "snap" tenotomy.

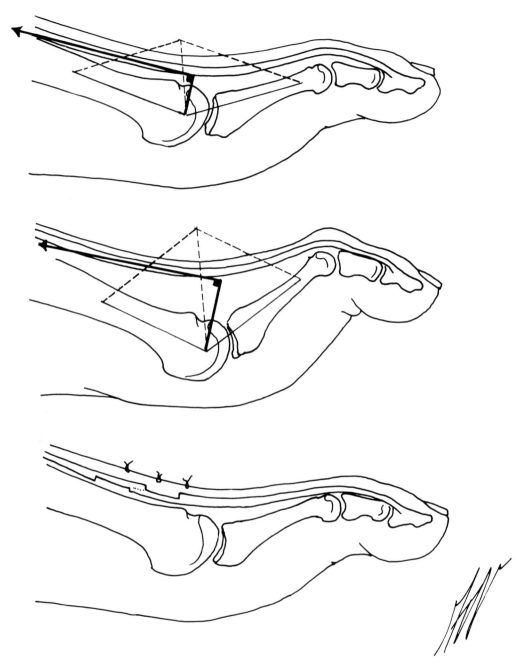

Figure 10.7. Sagittal plane relationship of the metatarsophalangeal joint. *Top*, normal sagittal plane, metatarsophalangeal joint angulation, and extensor moment of force. *Center*, retracted metatarsophalangeal joint: increased angulation and extensor moment of force. *Bottom*, post-operative restoration of normal metatarsophalangeal joint angulation and extensor moment of force.

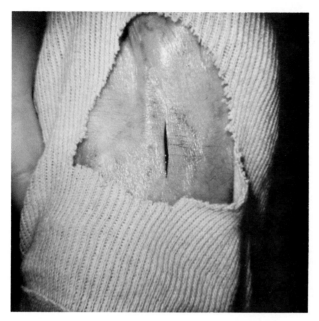

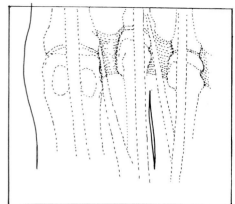

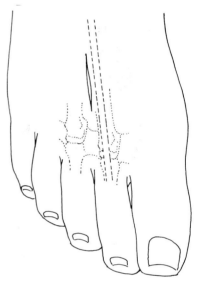

Figure 10.8. Placement of the incision between the second and third extensor digitorum longus tendons. Note the proximal placement and the length of the incision.

Free Tendon Graft

Two months after complete severence of a tendon, the involved muscle contracts and each end degenerates at least ½ inch. During surgical repair, it is necessary to excise the degenerated portion which shortens the tendon and creates a gap. If the tendon becomes short, a graft of normal tendon can be used. It should be slightly longer than needed since there will be normal contraction during the healing process. The source may be the plantaris tendon near the medial side of the ankle or a portion of the Achilles tendon. If a large graft is required, a flat piece of thick fascia lata may be taken through a small incision above the knee. *In vivo* autografts are superior to a chemically preserved homograft of fascia or tendon because the latter stimulates a foreign body reaction. The graft is initially nourished from adjacent tissues until vascularization occurs. Although the surface of the graft remains viable, patches of necrosis develop in the center of the tendon by the 7th day post-operatively. By the 11th day, growing cells appear in the graft, and necrotic tissue is replaced by regular tendon cells and fibers. During the 2nd and 3rd weeks, the graft is swollen and surrounded by newly formed vessels. Since the graft is fairly strong after 1 month, guarded exercise may be initiated. The danger of rupture is ended after 5 weeks if there has been no local trauma or infection at the surgical site.

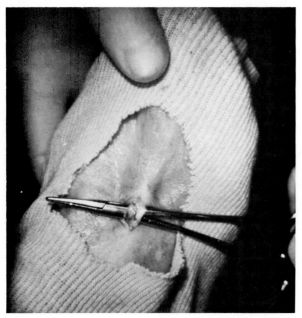
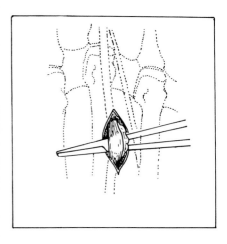

Figure 10.9. With a straight or curved hemostat, the tendon is fished out of the surgical site. Note that adjacent soft tissues are separated bluntly and automatically from the tendon.

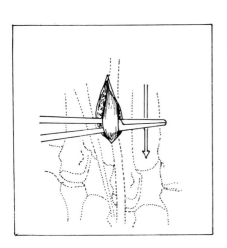
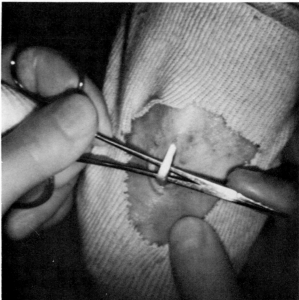

Figure 10.10. The tendon is pulled superiorly and anteriorly to free up the adjacent soft tissues which fall back into the surgical field.

Debate continues as to whether the grafted tendon becomes a part of the viable tissue or simply serves as a framework by which there can be migration of normal tendinous structures. Following tenotomy, there is complete replacement of lysed ten-

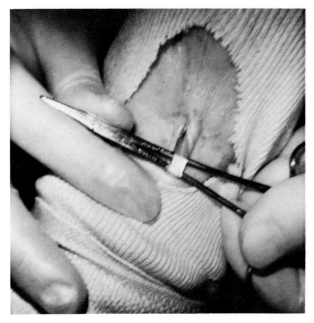

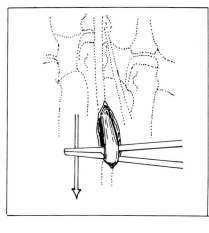

Figure 10.11.   The tendon is pushed proximally to free it in this direction.

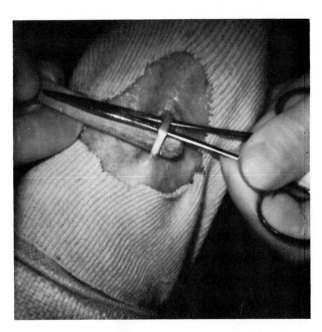

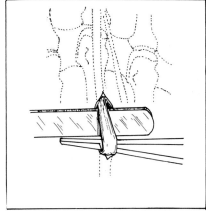

Figure 10.12.   A tendon board is placed under the tendon to separate it from the underlying soft tissue structures and to protect the latter.

don elements and this has been termed *regeneration.* Where there has been injury away from the site of surgery or trauma, there may develop new fibroblasts which

produce new bundles of collagen not in an overproductive manner, and this is referred to as *reconstitution.*

Various physiological studies have been

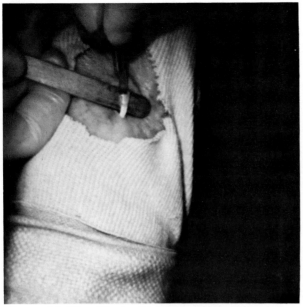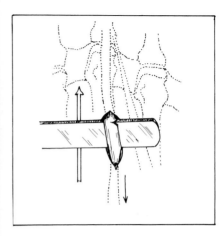

Figure 10.13. The tendon is cut distally from its center laterally. Note that cutting against the wood of the tendon board keeps the blade sharp and prevents shredding of the tendon. (Tissue shredding tends to produce mediocre post-operative results.)

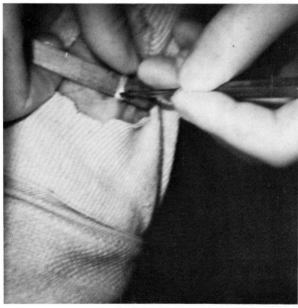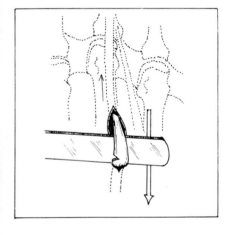

Figure 10.14. With the tendon board forced proximally and the toe slightly flexed to put the tendon on stretch, the proximal portion of the tendon is resected from its center to its lateral border.

done in attempts to understand the reaction to grafted tendon. Through various physiological and radiographic analyses, it has become more evident that an autograft acts more than as a basic framework for establishing new collagen material and re-

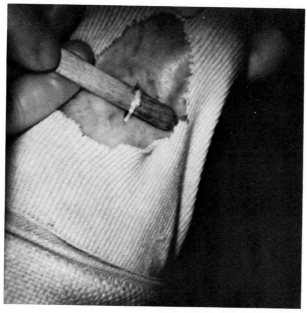

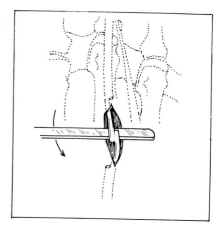

Figure 10.15.   The tendon board is turned on its side, the toe is flexed, and the tendon is slid into its lengthened position.

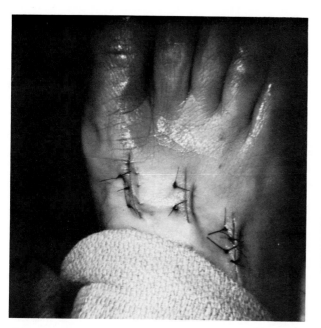

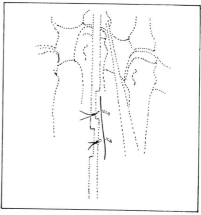

Figure 10.16.   The photo illustrates post-operative incisional margins after closure. Optimal areas are chosen by the surgeon, taking into consideration the patient's anatomy and the contractures involved.

placement of the graft. In contradistinction, an allograft does act as an inert scaffolding, and eventually all cellular elements are lost, and there is invasion and eventual replacement of this material by the host organism. A xenograft evokes a marked inflammatory response and, again, all tissue is replaced by host fibroblastic and collagenous material.

Basic surgical principles involving trauma to tendons must be followed. They should be familiar to most surgeons, but bear repeating since following these principles are of absolute necessity in attempts to yield more positive results.

1. Proper local wound care
2. Surgical repair as soon as possible
3. Aseptic technique
4. Appropriate debridement
5. Atraumatic tissue handling
6. Meticulous hemostasis

The slightest trauma in the intra-operative period may intensify the inflammatory reaction post-operatively and can be detrimental to repair. It is also essential that during the post-operative period guarded motion be maintained for an improved overall functional result.

The vast majority of previous work that has been done with regard to tendon grafts has been in relation to surgery of the hand, especially grafts involving the flexor complex. The function of the tendons of the foot are not quite as precise as the hand and therefore, our concern as foot surgeons is not always the same parallel concern as that of hand surgeons. Much can be learned, however, by review of the extensive work done by various hand surgeons over past decades. The most frequent complication following these tendon grafting procedures, and the most feared, is infection. This can lead to total failure of the grafting procedure and rather devastating consequences to function. Another concern is the formation of adhesions post-operatively. As long as the tissues are handled carefully, and whenever possible a tendon graft is surrounded by a fibrous sheath which can act as a barrier against adhesions, an improved functional result can be obtained. This was pointed out by Chacha (8) when he discussed autogenous grafts for replacement of lost flexor function in the digits of the hand. King et al. (9) discussed animal studies utilizing a Dacron polyester tendon

prosthesis. They reported a fair degree of success in these animal studies and showed that there was adequate connective tissue ingrowth within the fabric to allow for proper fixation and function, including when the prosthetic was attached to bone. Further studies in the human are needed, however, to see whether the prosthetic can withstand the load force, depending upon the demand made for the particular muscle or bony attachments, as well as stress when these prosthetics are sutured to myotendinous junctions.

Hunter and Schneider (7) discussed their ongoing work with damaged flexor tendons of the hand. They used silicone-Dacron reinforced prosthetics and the procedures were performed in two stages. The first stage being the implantation of a prosthetic device with attachment of the prosthesis at its distal end only. Three months post-operatively, the area was reoperated and the prosthesis removed with careful and meticulous respect for the newly formed sheath which now surrounded it. At the time of the second procedure, a free tendon graft replaced the prosthetic device within this newly formed sheath and allowed for better functional post-operative recovery and limitation of adhesions as was discussed previously. Furthermore, remarkable results using this particular technique is the ability to have a smooth, gliding motion of the part following free tendon grafting because of the newly formed sheath.

Hunter and Jaeger (10) further discussed the use of tendon implants and stressed that motion must be limited in the initial healing phase to allow for appropriate stability and increased tensile strength. The primary indication for using their two-stage prosthetic implants (silastic rods) was in cases following trauma where the gliding bed had been damaged. They stressed that this philosophy was based on tendon injuries and whether the patient was seen immediately or secondarily. Another advantage of their staged procedures is that since they are attempting to form a pseudo-sheath, and second-stage free tendon graft transplantation, that other types of reconstructive surgery following trauma (e.g., fracture fixation, capsulotomy, vascular repair, etc.) can be performed during the first stage of this procedure. The major contraindication when using this two-stage type procedure is when there is severe joint stiffness or poor vascular nutrition to the traumatized site which would jeopardize the success of the procedure. A major complication of this two-stage procedure is the development of synovitis around the transplantation site, or distal to it. Two major complications occurred after stage two and these were: adhesions along the tendon graft or at the proximal anastomosis, and rupture of the anastomosis of the tendon graft.

With regard to tendon repair in the foot, Holtz et al. (11) discussed a case following hallux abducto valgus surgery in which the extensor hallucis longus tendon had been lacerated and the hallux was in a plantarflexed position. In repairing the first metatarsophalangeal joint, they discovered the lacerated tendon, and after anastomosis, utilized silastic sheeting around the anastomosis in an attempt to allow for the proper post-operative gliding motion of the tendon, since without this elastic sheeting there would be the usual fibrosis and limitation of function of the tendon post-operatively. While their paper presented a 1-year follow-up on this particular procedure, it appears to have some merit since preoperatively there was no active dorsiflexion of the hallux and post-operatively there was active dorsiflexion of 25°. They further discussed the various conservative attempts and surgical attempts for prevention of adhesions to allow for the normal gliding motion. These included blocking agents which would attempt to isolate the tendon from the wound since one must understand that when dealing with tendon healing the "one wound-one scar" theory is applicable. Pharmacological agents have been used, such as cortisone, hormones, and enzymes, in an attempt to suppress the collagen synthesis of wound healing. For example, cortisone not only reduced the collagen synthesis, but decreased the tensile strength as well, which resulted in spontaneous rupture. The most promising potential success appears to lie with collagenase which will aid in decreasing adhesions. Production of a tendon sheath is another method that has met with some degree of success and has been previously discussed in relation to Hunter's research. Various types of pseudosheaths have been tried and the most promising results appear to be with silastic sheeting since it is apparently inert within the body substance. The most effective indication in the use of the silastic sheeting appears to be with secondary reconstructive surgery where the gliding mechanism of the tendon must be maintained. Where there has been loss of the tendon substance and further reconstruction is necessary, then the two-stage procedure utilizing a silicone rod appears to be more appropriate.

Finally, one of the most interesting new pieces of research was published by Gelberman et al. (12). Their animal study on dogs involved 20 adult specimens. They did a comparative study on tendon healing involving canine flexor tendons with one group being totally immobilized and the second group having controlled passive mobilization of the area. The significant portion of their study was that the immobilized tendons healed by ingrowth of connective tissue from the tendon sheath and cellular proliferation from the endotenon. The ingrowth of the tendon sheath, in the immobilized group, overwhelmed the epitenon response. There were definite signs of collagen reabsorbtion and protein synthesis was limited. By comparison, the passive, mobilized group healed by proliferation and migration of cells from the epitenon. There was limited ingrowth from the tendon sheath and greater activity in collagen production by using the controlled mobilization technique. Their controlled passive mobilization required daily exercises beginning on the first post-operative day, with 40–50 limited ranges of motion under a controlled situation. Their study did not suggest that total mobility was the appropriate post-operative therapy. It should be emphasized that their high degree of success in this study was based on a controlled passive range of motion and not an active unlimited type of motion. They further noted that Lindsay and Thomson (14) demonstrated cells in the epitenon and endotenon healed a traumatized tendon at the same rate, with the sheath removed, as tendons that had the tendon sheath intact. Gelberman's study (12) appears to show that early controlled motion in the healing process of flexor tendons demonstrate a change in the method of cell differentiation and invasion. One of their conclusions was that adhesion formation appears to be a primary inflammatory response which is stimulated by trauma to the tendon, tendon sheath, and surrounding tissue. Furthermore, this adhesion response is aided by total immobilization. The study produced evidence that the repair process of the controlled mobilized tendons is considerably different and improved from the totally immobilized group. These repeated controlled motions appear to disrupt the invasion of cells from the tendon sheath and inhibit their ingrowth which later reduced the degree of adhesions which had commonly been seen in the past. Furthermore, Duran (13) demonstrated that controlled motion of only 3–5 mm is sufficient to prevent strong bonding between the tendon and its associated sheath. Based on this information, it appears that ingrowth from the tendon sheath during the proliferative phase overwhelms the repair process from the epitenon and that this can be prevented by controlled mobility. This is certainly a new and yet exciting concept which should be applicable to the foot and the ankle and should be of great interest to podiatric surgeons. Follow-up work in the lower extremity, especially when dealing with major tendons which control function, needs to be carried out.

Tendo Achilles Lengthening

Prior to the performance of any tendo Achilles lengthening, the range of ankle range of motion should be evaluated to differentiate between ankle equinus, gastrocnemius equinus, or gastrosoleus shortening. The importance of this evaluation is made more clear in a discussion by Whitney and Green (16) when they discussed the syndrome of pseudoequinus in relation to anterior metatarsal equinus. They state that there was not a true lack of adequate dorsiflexion but was associated more with compensation due to the anterior metatarsal equinus. We should be careful, however, in discussing the use of tendo Achilles lengthenings in association with supinatory deformities of the foot. In dealing with a pes cavus deformity, where there is increased calcaneal inclination, lengthening of the tendo Achilles will obviously weaken the structure and thus not aid in the reduction of the elevated calcaneal angle. Reduction of the various structural deformities that occur with supination or pes cavus should be appropriately evaluated.

Lengthening of the tendo achilles has been a common surgical procedure during this century (21, 35). Many procedures have been proposed over this time and controversy continues in reference to the anatomy of the tendon (50). The standard Z-plasty lengthening procedure is made longitudinally, either in the frontal or sagittal plane. If there is varus deformity, the distal portion of the tendon is left attached to the lateral aspect of the calcaneus. In indicated cases, the capsule of the posterior ankle joint is divided to allow adequate dorsiflexion of the foot. Sufficient tendon length must be provided to allow adequate ankle joint motion in the sagittal plane. As mentioned previously, further evaluation of the flexor hallucis longus may be necessary, if after Z-plasty and posterior ankle capsulotomy inadequate ankle range of motion exists in the absence of osseous ankle blockage.

White (17) described a subcutaneous Achilles tendon lengthening using a transverse incision in the anterior half of the tendon above the insertion, with a second incision in the posterior half of the tendon, distal to the musculotendinous junction.

His surgical procedure was based on his theory that there was a rotational component to the tendo Achilles and that Z-plasty lengthening did not allow for the proper "sliding" of the tendon during surgery. He did, however, not report on any number of cases, the degree of success, or the extent of follow-up. Cummins et al. (18) discussed a number of cases with anatomical dissection of the adult tendo Achilles and once again proposed that there was a torsion effect in the tendo achilles complex. Jager and Moll (19) discussed the development of the human triceps surae but were primarily interested in the morphological development of the muscle mass of the gastrosoleus complex. Their schematic drawing, however, suggest that the gastrosoleus complex is fashioned with the soleus being anterior and the gastrocnemius posterior, but it is unclear whether this pattern follows through into the tendon complex. Dr. Leslie Arey, at Northwestern University Medical School, is one of the foremost international authorities on human embryology. On several occasions, when specifically asked about the potential torsion of the tendo Achilles, he denied that he had ever seen such a phenomenon in the human embryo. Furthermore, Clark (20) did an initial study of histological sections in five full-term, stillborn infants. His conclusion was that there was no torsion of the fibers that make up the tendo Achilles.

There still remain several questions on this entire matter. When indicated, there is definitely merit with the longitudinal Z-plasty technique. Those who advocate the subcutaneous method also state that they have had good clinical success, but there is insufficient published data in order to arrive at a strong conclusion. Over the past decade, we have observed a major complication following tendo Achilles lengthening, which is the enlargement of the tendon at the anastomosis at the posterior aspect of the ankle, which may be cosmetically unacceptable. Through our observations, it seems that two major factors in this procedure have been overlooked. First, extreme care must be taken during the sur-

gical procedure to avoid trauma to the body of the tendon and its associated sheath. Iatrogenic trauma cannot be overlooked as a factor. Secondly, we have observed several surgeons and have reviewed several cases where the tendon sheath was not properly dissected and retracted, and then properly sutured into place at the completion of the lengthening procedure. It should be obvious from our previous discussion on tendon healing that protection of the sheath and realignment of the sheath around the anastomosis is an essential component of this surgical procedure. Following these two concepts of atraumatic tissue handling and respect for and reapproximation of the tendon sheath, we have not encountered the complication of tendon enlargement post-operatively. Following the surgical procedure, the patient should be placed in an above the knee cast with 15°–20° flexion of the knee, and the foot held in a neutral position or in slight equinus. The patient is kept non-weight-bearing for 7–10 days post-operatively, after which time the cast is changed, sutures are removed, and a new, below knee cast applied. The patient is kept non-weightbearing through the 3rd or 4th postoperative week, after which time the patient is allowed to bear weight with crutch assistance for 7–10 days, and is instructed to begin controlled active exercises over the next several weeks since continued gradual increase in stress is needed to complete the healing process.

Gastrocnemius equinus is a component of the ankle equinus syndrome which clearly must be recognized and differentiated from the gastrosoleus equinus. Tenoplasty of the tendo Achilles is indicated when there is a gastrosoleus equinus. If the patient has an identifiable and measurable gastrocnemius equinus, then Z-plasty or subcutaneous tenoplasty is contraindicated. Where the patient has a clear gastrocnemius equinus, then the surgical procedure of choice, if conservative measures are unsuccessful, is the gastrocnemius recession procedure. These procedures are performed at the myotendinous junction to allow for the appropriate lengthening of the gastrocnemius component without weakening or compromising the soleus component.

The use of local corticosteroids should not be utilized on a routine basis. While the concept in trying to reduce collagen formation and maintain the gliding function of the tendon may be ideal, the decrease in tensile strength, which can occur with use of steroids, can have a devastating effect on the surgical outcome.

The debate will continue over the most appropriate technique for tendo Achilles lengthening. Further research is necessary to help clear up some of the potential confusion which surrounds this particular surgical procedure. Having specific criteria is essential in order to eliminate overutilization of this procedure.

Tendon Transfer

Most major tendon transfers are successful when the phasic activity of the tendon is preserved. A muscle that is active in the swing phase of gait will usually not contract actively in the stance phase, and vice versa. The peroneus longus, for example, when transferred to the dorsum of the foot to replace an inactive anterior tibial will continue to contract during the stance phase. By being put on stretch, it may passively resist some plantar flexion. When a choice between a phasic and nonphasic transfer is available, the phasic is recommended (15). Mixed transfers usually have a higher failure rate. In anticipating a nonphasic transfer, the ancestral function and position of the particular musculotendinous unit should be taken into account. Transferring the peroneal muscles into the dorsum can produce a successful swing phase muscle. The peroneal muscles were once anterior muscles serving as extensors.

Tendon transfers may affect the strength of a muscle, even if it is phasic. If muscular activity following the transfer is either too great or too little, the desired effect will not be achieved. The effect of a musculotendinous transfer to the donor site must also be taken into consideration. Since all articulations are serviced by a delicate balanced complement of tendon insertions, the removal or impairment of one tendon upsets the stabilizing balance. For example, transfer of the flexor hallucis longus to replace a deficient posterior tibial may be an effective transfer since both are power muscles and phasic at approximately the same time. But the hallux segment will become unstable during propulsion, and a new deformity may develop. An alteration must be made to minimize imbalance. Arthrodesis will weaken the antagonist and/or immobilize the part in a functional position.

During transfer, the tendon and the functioning muscle are mobilized, detached, or divided, and reinserted elsewhere in the bone or into another tendon. The purpose is to improve function, provide a substitute for weak or nonfunctioning muscles, stabilize the remaining muscle, and prevent the onset of deforming forces. Transfer is employed whenever damage to the major nerve trunks has weakened or paralyzed the muscle, so that its primary function is partially or totally lost. Along with transfers, adjunctive procedures such as arthrodeses, osteotomies, and repair of contractures from scarring, fibrosis and adaptive shortening must be considered to assure maximal stabilization and function. The transferred tendon and muscle must have the power to perform the intended function. When the transferred muscle is too strong, a new and opposite deformity can be created. The transferred muscle tendon unit needs sufficient amplitude to function efficiently, but whenever a unit is transferred, some amplitude is lost.

The proper rest length of striated muscle is determined by pulling of the tendon until there is an increase in passive resistance to further stretching. If the transplanted muscle is shorter or longer than its rest length, muscle power will be lost. The tendon should be implanted with minimal tension while the foot is in a good functional position. A straight line of pull is recommended for maximal efficiency and strength when the muscle tendon unit is transferred. Placing the tendon in a gliding tissue insures function without scarring or adhesions. The tendon should be kept away from bare bone, the raw surfaces of cut fascial planes, or a hole in the fascia.

Muscle tendon transfer is performed after all conservative treatments have proved inadequate, but it should be done before irreversible contractures occur or as soon as deformities and contractures can be safely corrected. If bone stabilizations and other associated procedures are contemplated, muscle tendon transfer can be delayed until maximal growth has been attained.

The sequelae of lower motor neuron lesions are more successfully treated than those of the upper motor neuron lesions. Those of nonprogressive diseases and chronic affliction are more successfully treated than those of progressive diseases.

Muscle tendon transfer evolved during efforts to rehabilitate patients with paralytic disease that caused impotence of a major muscle or muscle group in the lower extremities. These transfers involved the distal transposition of a normal and active tendon to a new position so that it may afford motor assistance to a partially paralyzed muscle, or motor substitution for a completely paralyzed muscle. Figure 10.17 indicates the cycle beginning with flaccid paralysis and continuing through progressive deformity and loss of function. The procedure of tendon transfer can reestab-

lish muscle balance and prevent long-term deformity and loss of function. By definition, the term transfer implies detachment of the normal muscle at its insertion, transposition to its new position, and then reattachment to its new insertion. Transfer, then, is not synonymous with transplantation, in which the muscle is detached at its proximal end (origin) and distal end (insertion) and moved to a new position. Translocation is the rerouted course of a normal muscle to aid the motor function of a less than optimal muscle, but without detachment.

Muscle tendon transfer has been involved in medical practice since 1882, when Nicolandoni transferred both peroneal tendons to the tendo achilles in a desperate attempt to overcome a calcaneus deformity in a patient with a paralyzed gastrosoleus muscle (Westin) (56). His operation, though theoretically sound, failed. A subsequent attempt at the "Nicolandoni operation" by his contemporaries also failed. With one poor result reinforcing another, muscle tendon transfers fell into disrepute until 1916, when Leo Mayer made a monumental contribution (30). He recognized that for a transferred muscle and tendon to function effectively, every detail of the procedure must be directed toward the preservation of normal physiologic and anatomic functions. At about the same time that Mayer's principles were being applied with some

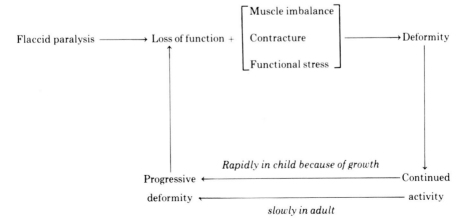

Figure 10.17.

success, Dunn and Hoke (27, 28) developed arthrodeses to treat the paralytic lower extremity.

Today, with few exceptions, tendon transfers in the lower leg and foot are combined with arthrodesis, because removing the tendon from the lateral aspect of the ankle joint and conveying it to another position increases the instability of the joint, and because stabilizing the joint permits the tendon to undergo its former function of stabilization and speeds up its conversion to its new function. With the evolution of electromyography, scrupulous selection of cases, improved techniques, preoccupation with the preservation of physiologic function, and sophisticated post-operative rehabilitation, tendon transfer alone is now a viable procedure.

Determining exactly how much tension the tendon should endure remains controversial. It is often recommended that the tendon should be reattached with "sufficient tension" to provide the transferred muscle with a maximal range of contraction. In an analysis of 125 muscle transfers, Reidy et al. (59) recommended that, generally, the joint should be brought into a position in which the muscle origin and its new insertion are approximated, with the tendon attachment made under slight to moderate tension. The interpretation of "slight to moderate" leaves much to the imagination. For each muscle there is a definite relationship between its "starting length and the amount of tension it can develop." When the muscle is passively shortened by approximating its origin and insertion, it develops very little contractile force. The greatest contractile force is developed when the muscle is at its "resting length." As the muscle is passively stretched beyond its resting length, the contractile force gradually diminishes, but the passive resistance of the connective tissue components gradually develop more tension so that the total muscle tension increases. This muscle length-tension relationship can be depicted rather graphically by the Blix curve as seen in Figure

10.18. Applying this relationship to the question of the tension under which a transferred muscle should be placed results in a conclusion that too much tension results in overstretching which causes fatigue and results in loss of power. If the tendon is not under any tension, then the slack will not be taken up by the muscle belly, and again, there is not enough power to function. The consensus of recent reports on muscle tendon transfer is that the tendon should be inserted under sufficient tension to hold the part in the position that it is expected to attain during its maximal contraction. The transfer should be protected by providing support in a position that allows maximal relaxation until healing is accomplished (56). Another important consideration is the strength of the muscles of the foot, particularly the antagonists. Westin believes that if the antagonist muscles are strong, there is little need for concern. If they are only fair, however, then less tension should be placed on the transferred muscle.

The introduction of electromyographic studies (EMG) was a most significant advancement in the field of muscle physiology (15). With the EMG, researchers were able to study the rhythmic, intermittent contractions of individual muscles as they functioned in normal walking. The concept of "phasic activity" emerged from these studies. In an EMG analysis of individual muscle groups of the lower leg and foot, Close and Todd (25, 48) determined that in normal subjects the anterior muscles of the leg were predominately swing phase muscles and the posterior or flexor muscles were stance phase muscles. Other authors have demonstrated that the pretibial muscle groups of the leg are active in both the stance and swing phases of gait (Rothbart).

An example of phasic transfer would be the shifting of the anterior tibial (a swing phase muscle) to the second metatarsal to replace a paralyzed peroneal muscle. Nonphasic transfers include the shifting of an active anterior tibial to the calcaneus to aid a weakened triceps surae muscle, or the

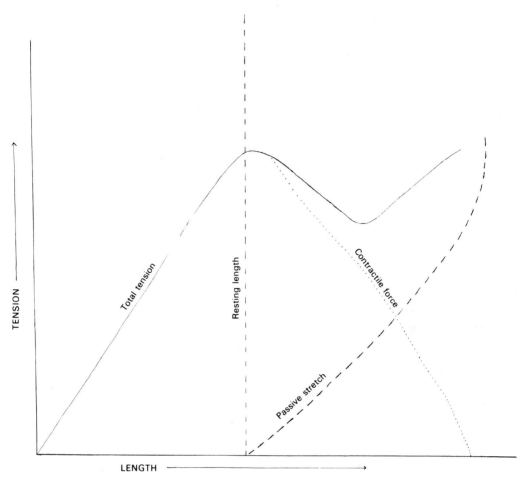

Figure 10.18. Blix curve. (From Salter, R. B. *Textbook of Disorders and Injuries of the Musculoskeletal System.* Williams & Wilkins, Baltimore, 1970.)

peroneus longus or brevis (stance phase) to the dorsum of the foot to replace paralyzed extensor muscles. The question of violating the patterns of phasic behavior and achieving a "functional transfer" is a most significant one. Furthermore, if transfers are done within the boundaries of phasic groupings, there is still a question as to whether these muscles can predictably retain their desirable activity. Close and Todd have shown that the patient can often make a voluntary effort to use an out-of-phase transfer, and the muscle makes a temporary phasic conversion. This change in the muscle's phasic activity is maintained as long as the patient concentrates on its use. As a general rule, however, non-phasic transfers should be avoided since the nonphasic muscle will not make this voluntary conversion. In addition, a nonphasic transfer can be detrimental. More important than avoiding nonphasic transfers is avoiding combined phasic-nonphasic transfers, since re-education of the transferred muscles becomes increasingly difficult and the likelihood of failure of both transfers is likely to occur.

In predicting the likelihood of a voluntary phasic conversion, transfer of the peroneus longus or brevis to the dorsum of the foot was most successful.

Muscle tendon transfer may be indicated in selected cases of neuromuscular disease in which certain isolated muscles or muscle groups are rendered ineffective by flaccid paralysis or are hyperinnervated by spastic paralysis. In addition to these cases, spastic deformities resulting from upper motor neuron lesions, such as cerebral palsy or corticospinal lesions, have traditionally been involved in muscle transfers. Muscle tendon transfer has also been advocated in the treatment of certain static deformities such as primary recurrent idiopathic clubfoot, as well as congenital convex pes valgus (vertical talus) and idiopathic pes cavus.

The inverter muscles of the foot—posterior tibial, flexor digitorum longus, and flexor hallucis longus—run medially to the oblique axis of rotation of the talocalcaneal navicular joint. The tibialis posterior inserts into the navicular, with fibrous expansions to the three cuneiform bones; and to the bases of the second, third, and fourth metatarsals; and into the toes. Both the subtalar and midtarsal joints are affected. The triceps surae is a very powerful supinator since the force of its contraction is exerted medially to the oblique axis of rotation of the talocalcaneal navicular joint. However, since it inserts into the calcaneus, it acts as a supinator of the subtalar joint only.

The evertor muscles of the foot are the peroneus longus, brevis and tertius, the extensor digitorum longus, and the extensor hallucis longus. The directional force developed by their contraction runs lateral to the oblique axis of the talocalcaneal navicular joints. The combined strength of these muscles is approximately balanced by the inverters of the foot, excluding the triceps surae.

The tendon of the anterior tibial passes anterior to the transverse axis of the ankle joint and medial to the longitudinal axes of the midtarsal and subtalar joints. It is a dorsiflexor and a supinator of the forefoot. In the normal foot, the anterior tibial passes through the axis of the talocalcaneal navicular joint and is a neutral muscle in so far as pure eversion and inversion are concerned.

A review of the literature reveals that practically every conceivable combination of muscle tendon transfer has been attempted. It is impractical to review every transfer or combination possible, but conditions amenable to transfer include the following:

PARALYSIS OF PERONEUS LONGUS AND/OR PERONEUS BREVIS MUSCLES

According to Duchenne (26), the action of the peroneal muscles produces eversion of the foot. Paralysis of the peroneus longus will cause overpowering by its antagonistic muscle, the anterior tibial, and result in a varus deformity. In addition to functioning as an evertor, the peroneus longus also exerts a plantarflexory influence of the first metatarsal. Therefore, an unopposed anterior tibial results in a metatarsus primus elevatus, dorsal bunion deformity, and eventual hallux rigidus. The peroneus brevis produces direct eversion with its antagonist being the posterior tibial. It is recommended that the deforming muscle force (anterior tibial) be transposed laterally to the base of the second metatarsal. In these cases, the active anterior tibial should never be transposed farther laterally than the third metatarsal because to do so risks inducing a valgus foot deformity. Transferring the anterior tibial to the dorsum is a phasic transfer and will function without the need for voluntary conversion.

PARALYSIS OF THE EXTENSOR DIGITORUM LONGUS AND EXTENSOR HALLUCIS LONGUS

The action of both of these swing phase muscles is dorsiflexion. Paralysis results in an equinus deformity because the action of the plantar flexors is unopposed. In order to re-establish muscle balance, the anterior tibial is transferred to the dorsum. Some authors have advocated the anterior transfer of the posterior tibial through the interosseous membrane to the dorsum (Turner and Cooper) (43). This particular transfer should be discouraged for two reasons: 1) it violates the pattern of phasic activity; and

2) transfers of any sort using the interosseous route should be avoided since it was observed that severe restriction of normal gliding was caused by invasion of the interosseous membrane and tendon by new bone formation.

PARALYSIS OF ANTERIOR TIBIAL

The action of the anterior tibial is that of dorsiflexion and inversion. It also opposes the plantarflexory effect of the peroneus longus on the first metatarsal. An unopposed peroneus longus causes an equinovalgus or cavovalgus deformity. A rational approach would be to transpose the peroneus longus anteriorly to the base of the second metatarsal, but the inherent problems of nonphasic transfer must be anticipated. As an alternative, Caldwell split the triceps surae and transferred the medial half around the medial side of the ankle to the second cuneiform.

PARALYSIS OF THE TRICEPS SURAE

The triceps surae produces plantar flexion, inversion, and also resists the pull of the intrinsic plantar flexor muscles, as well as the plantar fascia during the stance phase of gait. An ineffective triceps surae causes a calcaneus deformity of the rearfoot with the forefoot dropping into equinus. A muscle tendon transfer to a weakened or paralyzed triceps surae presents a unique situation in that two-thirds of the leg's musculature consists of the triceps complex. Selecting a muscle strong enough to substitute for the action of the triceps surae is the key problem. Therefore, transferring more than one muscle posteriorly to the calcaneous is advisable. Attempts should be made to keep transfers within the realm of phasic activity by using only flexor or stance phase muscles. The posterior tibial and peroneus longus tendons are particularly well suited for this purpose. Some authors have advocated translocation of the peroneus longus in the treatment of paralytic pes calcaneus. These reports, although limited in number and follow-up, claim that tendon translocations are more desirable than transfers in that: 1) in translocating a tendon, structures are displaced without disturbing the continuity; 2) suturing of the tendon is avoided; 3) the period of immobilization after translocation is shorter than after transfer; and 4) the muscle is immediately placed under tension, which prevents loss of strength. The primary disadvantages to peroneus longus translocation were dehiscence and necrosis of the skin incision. In fact, a study performed by Bickel and Moe (23) showed that in only three of the 13 cases in which that operation was performed did primary healing of the incision occur. Transfer in the form of an anterior advancement of the tendo Achilles for cerebrospastic equinus deformity has been reported. In this technique, the triceps is detached from its normal insertion and advanced to the posterior-superior portion of the calcanous. This weakens the muscle's resistance to dorsiflexion by reducing its mechanical advantage.

With regard to re-establishing the gliding motion, an excellent and simple method of restoring this mechanism, as recorded by Ober (30), involves carrying the transferred tendons through the compartment of the paralyzed tendon. The paralyzed tendon is withdrawn from the sheath and the transferred tendon is drawn through the sheath in its place.

Tenodesis

This technique, which entails suturing an end of a tendon to a bone, is accomplished by incising the periosteum to produce a small area of bone scar formation. The tendon is sutured flush against the scarified bone and fixed by passing sutures through a small drill hole and securing knots. Another method involves making a trap door in the bone to expose the medullary canal at the tenodesis. Just distal to the trap door, two drill holes are made through the cortex into the canal. The tendon, with the sutures placed at its end, is passed through the trap door and the sutures are pulled through the holes and secured. The trap door is then replaced. Several small drill holes in the trap door and the adjacent bone will assure that the sutures hold properly.

Post-operative Considerations

Proper post-operative care begins the moment the foot is immobilized. The joint should be splinted so that no strain is allowed on the tendon until firm healing is accomplished. Recommendations call for 4–6 weeks of immobilization in the corrected position. After an initial immobilization period, a bivalve cast or night splint is applied for approximately 6 months to assure rest and to maintain the optimal position for the tendon's new function. Gentle, actively assisted exercises are begun to give the patient a feel of the transfer and its new function. The patient must try to produce the motion that the transferred muscle formerly performed, while the foot is manually moved through the motion that the transfer is designed to provide. Exercises are continued as range and resistance are gradually increased, but the tendon is always returned to the resting length of its transferred position. Occasionally, the patient has difficulty in gaining control of this transfer, in which case it may be necessary to use electrical stimulation interspersed with exercise. Careful, functional re-education of the transposed muscle is essential, and undue fatigue and strain must be avoided until maximal function is attained. Transfers, when successful, tend to improve in motor power during the 6 months following immobilization. When stabilizing bone operations are combined with muscle tendon transfer, the tendon transfer should be avoided until the bony healing is completed.

An important aspect of successful muscle tendon transfer is the painstaking preservation of the physiologic function. It is important to perform a complete pre-operative survey with regard to the progressive nature of any underlying neuromuscular disease, the prognosis of future ambulation given appropriate transfers, the availability of muscle tendon for transfer, and the selection of possible surgical approaches.

When muscle tendon transfer is not sufficient to add necessary stability, concomitant arthrodesing procedures should be performed. Attention must always be focused on the paralyzed muscle's antagonist; the forces responsible for muscle imbalance. The goal of successful muscle tendon transfer is the re-establishment of muscle balance and the avoidance of long-term skeletal deformation and loss of function.

RESULTS

McGlamry (37) discussed the use of the anterior tibial tendon transfer as related to Charcot-Marie-Tooth disease, cerebellar ataxia, and dropfoot in which there is paralysis of all other anterior muscles. He accurately noted that the most essential decision to be made is exactly how far laterally the tendon needs to be transferred. If the muscle is transferred too far laterally, then it is possible to convert a severe talipes equinovarus foot pre-operatively into a rocker bottom flatfoot post-operatively.

Hoffer et al. (38) discussed in detail the use of the split anterior tendon transfer in the treatment of spastic varus hindfoot in children. Pre-operative evaluation included ambulatory electromyographs which demonstrated inappropriate anterior tibial hyperactivity. They also stated that this procedure can be performed in adults following cerebral vascular accidents. They reported on 21 feet involving 16 patients with varus deformity. The etiology of this deformity was cerebral palsy in nine patients, hydrocephalus in two patients, and acquired traumatic brain damage in five patients. In those patients where there was traumatic brain damage, it was recommended that reconstructive surgery be delayed for at least 2 years following the brain insult. Along with the split anterior tendon transfer, 12 patients had fixed deformities and required various adjunctive procedures including tendo Achilles lengthenings, posterior tibial and medial hindfoot releases, and one case of a calcaneal osteotomy. The soft tissue and tendon releases can be performed at the same time as the split anterior tendon transfer. However, as has been mentioned previously, a fixed bony deformity which requires a calcaneal osteotomy should be corrected initially, and tendon transfer delayed for at least 3–6 months or until there is satisfactory healing of the osteotomy site. In their study, all 16 patients pre-operatively required the use of braces and post-operatively only seven patients required the use of braces. There was residual fixed deformity in one patient, and in only one case of the 21 transferred tendons, did the procedure not work well. The key factor in their analysis was the ambulatory myographic studies which showed that the anterior tibial muscle was overactive and nonphasic. Post-operatively, there was no dramatic improvement in the gait electromyographic studies but, clinically, the vast majority of patients were improved. The importance of this analysis with ambulatory electromyography cannot be overemphasized. In their study, they noted that several other cases demonstrated spastic varus and that the ambulatory electromyographic study showed phase reversal of the posterior tibial muscle. Thus, in those cases, the posterior tibial tendon was transferred to the dorsal aspect of the foot where it performed as expected without training since it was already in reverse phase. Of their 21 transfers, deformity recurred in only two feet. During Dr. Sage's review of this study involving split anterior tibial tendon transfer (38), he noted that the use of the pulley suture with a split anterior tibial tendon transfer into the cuboid seemed to be more advantageous than the pullout tie-down suture technique, since there is danger for the tendon to be pulled from the tenodesis site, as well as the development of pressure sores on the bottom of the foot, especially when dealing with patients with neuromuscular disease.

Garceau (41) discussed his long-term follow-up with anterior tibial tendon transfer for recurrent clubfoot. He stated that the recurrence rate for unsuccessfully treated club foot was somewhere between 12–61%,

and in his series was approximately 50%. He emphasized that this operation was indicated only after prolonged and unrelenting conservative therapy had failed to prevent relapse of the deformity. The indications for this procedure are: 1) ineffective, conservative therapy, 2) flexibility of the foot joints, 3) patients under age 6 years; 4) peroneal weakness or total loss of function; 5) bowstringing of the anterior tibial on the anterior medial aspect of the ankle; 6) active abduction or eversion of the foot should not be possible, and 7) at least two recurrences of the deformity should have occurred before this surgical procedure is considered.

His report involved two sets of patients, the first group being 32 patients (with 38 operated feet) who were followed for 16 years. The second group involved 56 cases which had a follow-up period of 7 years or longer. His evaluation of the success of the procedure was broken down into several areas. In the first set, regarding appearance, 16 feet were rated excellent, 11 good, 6 fair, and 5 poor. With reference to gait, 14 feet were rated excellent, 10 good, 8 fair, and 6 poor. The degree of mobility was rated excellent in 18 feet, 10 good, 4 fair, and 6 poor. He also rated the degree of reduction of talipes equinus, varus, and adductus, with equinus reduction rated excellent in 15 feet, good in 12, fair in 4, and poor in 3 cases. The varus reduction was rated excellent in 23, good in 6, and poor in 2 cases. Finally, the degree of reduction of adductus was rated excellent in 22 cases, good in 5, and fair in 8 cases. Again, the major concern was exactly the degree of lateral transfer of the anterior tibial tendon. Of the 18 tendons which were transferred to the proximal end of the fifth metatarsal, 4 cases were rated excellent, 6 good, 4 fair, and 4 poor. Two of the cases with poor results were due to overcorrection. In two of the tendon transfer procedures, the anterior tibial tendon was anchored into the proximal end of the fourth metatarsal. Both of these procedures were rated excellent. Fourteen tendons were inserted into the cuboid bone and 4 were rated excellent, 7 good, 1 fair, and 2 poor. In 3 cases, the tendon was anchored in the lateral (third) cuneiform bone with 2 being rated as excellent and 1 poor. Finally, one tendon was anchored in the neck of the talus and it was rated as a poor result. Regarding the postoperative strength of the transferred muscle, 20 of the cases were rated excellent, 5 good, 4 fair, and poor results were reported in 5 feet. Following the transfer procedure, follow-up surgery was required in several cases with 3 feet requiring triple arthrodesis, 5 feet requiring open tendo Achilles lengthening, 1 foot requiring calcaneal osteotomy, 1 medial release, and 1 plantar denervation. In 1 case, the retransfer of the tendon to the original insertion was performed, but this did not achieve improvement. This retransfer involved one of the patients who had a poor result with overcorrection. Garceau (41) clearly states that the poor, overcorrective results were due to faulty pre-operative evaluation of the peroneal muscles and strongly encouraged the use of pre-operative electromyographic examinations. One of his final conclusions was that the transfer of the anterior tibial tendon for recurrent clubfoot should be just lateral to the midline of the dorsal aspect of the foot so as to avoid severe overcorrection.

Gartland and Surgent (42) reported a 7-year follow-up of posterior tibial transplant and surgical treatment of recurrent clubfoot. The primary indication for this procedure is recurrence of the deformity after prior correction has seemingly been obtained. Their theory was that the high percentage of potential recurrence of clubfoot deformity is secondary to muscle imbalance. Differentiation must be made, however, between a poorly treated clubfoot and a recurrent clubfoot. If treated by another practitioner, then detailed history from the parents should be made to determine whether the foot "looked normal" at any period during the conservative casting procedures or soft tissue surgical releases that may have been undertaken. If there had been inadequate reduction of the clubfoot

deformity, then tendon transfer is not indicated and should not be used to "shortcut" correct conservative soft tissue surgical procedures with this deformity. In their series, a recurrence rate was seen between an age range of 14 months to 8 years of age. They stressed the importance of flexibility of the foot and therefore recommended that even though the deformity had recurred, that the patient be maintained in maximum correction with plaster casts at least 1 month prior to surgery. The casts are then removed 2 days pre-operatively for proper work-up and skin cleansing. The transfer of the posterior tibial tendon from the posterior muscle group through the interosseous membrane is then sutured under tension and tenodesed to the third cuneiform. Their series involved 22 children (26 feet) with an average follow-up of 7 years. Several of these cases had had previous soft tissue releases, including two cases where an anterior tibial transfer had previously been attempted, and two other cases where there had been transfers of the tendoachilles. They suggested that adequate soft tissue and conservative measures be attempted, and that if recurrence continued to be obvious, then the posterior tibial transfer could be attempted after the child's second birthday.

The results of 14 feet (54%) were rated excellent, 8 feet (31%) with satisfactory results, and 4 feet (15%) without satisfactory results. Of the four failures, two of the feet had excessive adhesions because of strong adherence to the interosseous membrane not allowing the posterior tibial tendon to function.

In the two other feet that resulted in unsatisfactory results, the posterior tibial tendon was transferred incorrectly to the cuboid, thus resulting in severe pes valgo planus. When they further analyzed their results on the basis of age, they concluded that the best operative time was when the patient was 2–3 years of age, although they noted that recurrence can occur much later in life. They also noted that post-operatively there was an impressive degree of flexibility in those cases where the tendon transfer was successful. One final problem encountered was residual forefoot adductus following the tendon transfer procedure. Retrospective analysis showed that the metatarsus adductus had not been adequately reduced pre-operatively. If the child is older than 6 years of age, then base metatarsal osteotomies would be indicated. It has been emphasized before that any fixed deformities should be corrected prior to tendon transfer.

Acknowledgments—Thanks to Mary A. Doyle, D.P.M., for her valued assistance in the literature research for this chapter. Also, thanks to Jordon D. Ross, D.P.M., for his excellent illustrations which greatly added to the body of this chapter. A special thanks to Sherry Schulz, L.P.N., for her assistance and dedication in typing the manuscript for this chapter.

References

1. Ketchum, L. D., Martin, N. L., and Kappel, D. A. Experimental evaluation of factors affecting the strength of tendon repairs. Plastic Reconstr. Surg. 59:708–719, 1977.
2. Garth, W. P. Flexor hallucis tendinitis in a ballet dancer. J. Bone Jt. Surg. 63A:1489, 1981.
3. Lea, R. B., and Smith, L. Rupture of the achilles tendon nonsurgical treatment. *Clin. Orthop. Relat. Res.* 60:115–118, 1968.
4. Crenshaw, A. H., ed. *Campbell's Operative Orthopaedics*, 5th ed. C. V. Mosby, St. Louis, vol. 2, 1971, pp. 1464–1470, 1493–1495.
5. Mann, R. A. Complications in Surgery of the Foot. Orthop. Clin. North Am. 7:851–861, 1976.
6. Hurst, L. N. The healing of tendon, in *Biological Aspects of Reconstructive Surgery*. Kernahan, D. A., Vistnes, L. M., eds. Little, Brown & Co., New York, 1977, pp. 383–389.
7. Hunter, J. M., and Schneider, L. H. Staged tendon reconstruction, in *Instructional Course Lectures— AAOS*. C. V. Mosby, St. Louis, 1977, vol. 26, pp. 134–144.
8. Chacha, P. Free autologous composite tendon grafts for division of both flexor tendons within the digital theca of the hand. J. Bone Jt. Surg. 56A: 960–978, 1974.
9. King, R. N., Dunn, H. K., and Bolstad, K. E. A single unit digital flexor tendon prosthesis. Biomedical Material Research Symposium. No. 6, p. 157–165, 1975.
10. Hunter, J. M., and Jaeger, S. H. Tendon implants: Primary and secondary usage. Orthop. Clin. North Am. 8:473–489, 1977.
11. Holtz, M., Midenberg, M. L., and Kirschenbaum, S. E. Utilization of a silastic sheet in tendon repair of the foot. J. Foot Surg. 21:253–259, 1982.
12. Gelberman, R. H., Vande Berg, J. S., Lundborg, G. N., and Akeson, W. H. Flexor tendon healing and restoration of the gliding surface. J. Bone Jt. Surg. 65A:70–80, 1983.
13. Duran, R. E. Controlled passive motion following flexor tendon repair in zones two and three, in *AAOS: Symposium on Tendon Surgery in the Hand*. C. V. Mosby, St. Louis, 1975.
14. Lindsay, W. K., and Thomson, H. G. Digital flexor tendons: An experimental study. Part I. The significance of each component of the flexor mechanism in tendon healing. Br. J. Plastic Surg. 12: 289–316, 1960.
15. Mann, R. A. Tendon transfers and electromyography. AOFS surgery of the foot. Clin. Orthop. Relat. Res. 85:64–66, 1972.
16. Whitney, A. K., and Green, D. R. Pseudoequinus. JAPA 72:365–371, 1982.
17. White, J. W. Torsion of the Achilles tendon: Its surgical significance. Arch. Surg. 46:784–787, 1943.
18. Cummins, E. J., Anson, B. J., Carr, B. W., and Wright, R. R. The structure of the calcaneal tendon (of Achilles) in relation to orthopedic surgery. Surg. Gynecol. Obstet. 83:107–116, 1946.
19. Jager, J. W., and Moll, J. The development of the human triceps surae. Observations on the ontogenetic formation of muscle architecture and skeletal attachments. J. Anat. 85:338–349, 1951.
20. Clark, M. E. Morphology of the Achilles tendon in the newborn. JAPA 62:389–394, 1972.
21. Silverman, J. J. Device for stretching the triceps surae. JAPA 58:301–303, 1968.
22. Arey, L. B., ed. *Human Histology*, 2nd ed. W. B. Saunders, Philadelphia, 1963.
23. Bickel, W. H., and Moe, J. H. Translocation of the peroneus longus tendon for paralytic calcaneus deformity of the foot. Surg. Gynecol. Obstet. 78:627–630, 1944.
24. Boyes, J. H. *Bunnell's Surgery of the Hand*, 4th ed. J. B. Lippincott, Philadelphia, 1964.
25. Close, J. R. *Motor Function in the Lower Extremity: Analysis by Electronic Instrumentation.* Charles C. Thomas, Springfield, 1964.
26. Duchenne, G. B. *Physiology of Motion.* Translated by E. G. Kaplan. W. B. Saunders, Philadelphia, 1959.
27. Dunn, N. Stabilizing operations on paralytic feet. Proc. R. Soc. Med. 15:15–22, 1921.
28. Hoke, M. An operation for stabilizing paralytic feet. J. Orthop. Surg. 3:494–507, 1921.
29. Ketchum, L. D. Effects of triamcinolone on tendon healing and function. A laboratory study. Plastic Reconstr. Surg. 47:471–482, 1971.
30. Mayer, L. The physiological method of tendon transplantation. Surg. Gynecol. Obstet. 22:182–197, 1916.
31. Peacock, E. E. Fundamental aspects of wound healing related to the restoration of gliding function after tendon repair. Surg. Gynecol. Obstet. 119:241–250, 1964.
32. Peacock, E. E., and Van Winkle, W. *Surgery and Biology of Wound Repair.* W. B. Saunders, Philadelphia, 1970.
33. Salter, R. B. *Textbook of Disorders and Injuries to the Musculoskeletal System.* Williams & Wilkins, Baltimore, 1970.

34. Steindler, A. *Kinesiology of the Human Body.* Charles C. Thomas Springfield, 1955.
35. Tachdjian, M. O. *Pediatric Orthopedics.* W. B. Saunders, Philadelphia, 1972, vols. 1 and 2.
36. Thompson, T. C. Spontaneous rupture of tendon Achilles: A new clinical diagnostic test. J. Trauma 2:126–129, 1962.
37. McGlamry, E. D. Transfer of the tibialis anterior tendon. JAPA 63:609–617, 1973.
38. Hoffer, M. M., Reiswig, J. A., Garrett, A. M., and Perry, J. The split anterior tibial tendon transfer in the treatment of spastic varus hindfoot of childhood. Orthop. Clin. North Am. 5:31–37, 1974.
39. Teuffer, A. P. Traumatic rupture of the Achilles tendon: Reconstruction by transplant and graft using the lateral peroneus brevis. Orthop. Clin. North Am. 5:89–93, 1974.
40. Bruce, R. K., Hale, T. L., and Gilbert, S. K. Ultrasonography evaluation for ruptured Achilles tendon. JAPA 72:15–17, 1982.
41. Garceau, G. J. Anterior tibial tendon transfer for recurrent clubfoot. Clin. Orthop. Relat. Res. 84:61–65, 1972.
42. Gartland, J. J., and Surgent, R. E. Posterior tibial transplant in the surgical treatment of recurrent clubfoot. Clin. Orthop. Relat. Res. 84:66–70, 1972.
43. Turner, J. W., and Cooper, R. R. Anterior transfer of the tibialis posterior through the interosseous membrane. Clin. Orthop. 83:241, 1972.
44. Mason, M. L. Plastic surgery of the hands. Surg. Clin. North Am. 19:227, 1939.
45. Kelly, R. E. An operation for the chronic dislocation of the peroneal tendons. Br. J. Surg. 7:502, 1920.
46. Watson-Jones, R. Recurrent forward dislocation of the ankle. J. Bone Jt. Surg. 34B:519, 1952.
47. Watson-Jones, R., and Wilson, J. N., eds. *Fractures and Joint Injuries,* 5th ed. Churchill-Living-stone, London, 1976, vols. 1 and 2.
48. Close, J. R., and Todd, F. M. The phasic activity of the muscles of the lower extremity and the effect of tendon transfer. J. Bone Jt. Surg. 41A:189–208, 1959.
49. Bunnell, S. *Surgery of the Hand.* Lippincott, Philadelphia, 1956.
50. Arey, L. B. *Developmental Anatomy: A Textbook and Laboratory Manual of Embryology.* Saunders, Philadelphia, 1966.
51. Arey, L. B. Personal communication, 1975.
52. Bosworth, D. M. Repairs of defects in the tendo achilles. J. Bone Jt. Surg. 38A:111, 1956.
53. DuVries, H. L. *Surgery of the Foot.* Mosby, St. Louis, 1959.
54. Jones, E. Operative treatment of chronic dislocation of peroneal tendons. J. Bone Jt. Surg. 14:574, 1932.
55. Lindholm, A. A new method of operation in subcutaneous rupture of the achilles tendon. Acta Chir. Scand. 117:261, 1959.
56. Westin, W. G. Tendon transfers about the foot, ankle, and hip in the paralyzed lower extremity. J. Bone Jt. Surg. 47A:1430, 1965.
57. Mason, M. L. Rehabilitation of the hand. AAOS Instructional Course Lectures (Hand Injuries Symposium). 6:95, 1949.
58. Allen, H. S. Crushing injuries of the hand. AAOS Instructional Course Lectures (Hand Surgery Symposium). 9:195, 1952.
59. Reidy, J. A., Broderick, T. F., and Barr, J. S. Tendon transplantations in the lower extremity. A review of end results in poliomyelitis: I. Tendon transplantations about the foot and ankle. J. Bone Jt. Surg. 34A:900, 1952.
60. Bugg, E. I., and Boyd, B. M. Repair of neglected rupture or laceration of the Achilles tendon. Clin. Orthop. Relat. Res. 56:73–75, 1968.

CHAPTER 11

Forefoot Surgery

JAMES H. LAWTON, D.P.M.

Without a doubt, the overwhelming percentage of foot surgery is performed on the forefoot. Over the decades, the procedures performed literally number in the millions. A review of what has been performed in the past, as well as a continuing knowledge of updated information both biomechanically and surgically, is essential in the ongoing evolutionary understanding of this complicated area of podiatric surgery.

The primary assessment of the patient and the associated deformity cannot be taken lightly. While practitioners may have seen thousands of orthostatic and biomechanical deformities of the foot, the greatest pitfall is to begin to mentally classify these deformities into a small area of understanding and surgical approaches. Of primary importance is the patient's understanding of his deformity, his motivation in seeking medical and potential surgical care, and an evaluation of his expectations following attempts at surgical correction. The patients must understand that surgical therapy is a type of treatment among all the other types of treatment, and therefore not always curative. The patient may be seeking medical advice for relief of discomfort and some improvement of function. His expectations may not closely coincide with the goals of the attending surgeon. In this particular chapter, we will not attempt to discuss the most exotic or rarest of cases. Our intent is in the form of an update of the more common complications of forefoot surgery, as well as an attempt to discuss the ways to avoid them. While patient compliance cannot be totally controlled by the physician, we strongly urge the practitioner who is proposing a type of surgical treatment for a given deformity that he or she fully discuss with the patient the diagnosis, etiology, post-operative care, and the potential complications involved with the particular procedure. Surgical complications of the forefoot can be lessened by proper pre-operative evaluation, appropriate surgical approach and technique, and proper post-operative management. The proper compliance of the patient can also be maintained by open communication between the physician and the patient.

DIGITS

Hammertoes—Lesser Digits

As a single entity or associated with other biomechanical deformities, the patient presenting with a hammertoe digit syndrome of the lesser digits is seen daily by podiatric physicians and podiatric surgeons. An overlying keratotic lesion results from hypertrophy of the horny layer of the epidermis resulting in pain due to pressure from external sources. In studies done by Bonavilla (1), there was not only the expected cornification and hypertrophy of the stratified epithelium, but the reticular layer of the dermis beneath the stratified epithelium was heavily collagenized to a greater degree than one would normally expect. There was also a marked increase in the amount of capillary vessels and arterioles in the dermal layer. His conclusions were that there was a definite inflammatory response associated with these lesions, as well as a perineural scarring of the nerve filaments found on histopathological sectioning. In another study done by Freed (3), it was clearly shown that with this skin hyperplasia there was an associated cortical hyperplasia of the underlying bone which was demonstrated in 74% of his samples. His conclusion was that the type of cortical thickening associated with an overlying skin hyperplasia was the result of repeated and prolonged trauma to the periosteum. He further suggested that the cortical bone hyperplasia appears to develop earlier than the dermal thickening. Thus, periosteal inflammation would be followed by cortical hyperplasia which would eventually result in dermal inflammation and dermal hyperkeratinization. He clearly found that this type of cortical bone thickening is not similar to the situation in the development of exostosis. Beside these local effects, one would certainly be remiss if one did not also consider the overall biomechanical function of the foot as the primary etiological factor in developing these orthostatic digital deformities. However, such discussion is not within the realm of the goals of this text and has been adequately covered elsewhere.

Positive surgical results should be directly related to the surgeon's understanding of the healing process of the various tissues involved. Lewin (7) appropriately states that there is a definite relationship between the extent of injury, specifically to the periosteum, and the degree of osseous proliferation. Since the majority of surgical procedures performed on the lesser digits involves the resection of portions of the proximal and/or middle phalanx, a careful understanding of the bony healing in these areas is appropriate. Allbrook and Kirkaldy-Willis (8) demonstrated some rather interesting findings about bony resections and raw bony surfaces associated with joints. These studies were performed on monkeys and showed massive proliferation of fibroblasts from the cut ends of the periosteum and to a lesser degree from the medullary canal of the bone. In the first few weeks following surgery, there was obvious fibroblastic activity in order to form a "cap" over the raw, exposed bony surface. Eventually, these fibroblasts developed into prechondroblasts, chondroblasts and hypertrophic chondrocytes lying in a calcified matrix which were then invaded by capillaries and eventually by osteoblasts. If the degree of trauma has been limited, the practitioner will note, in follow-up x-rays of patients having undergone hammertoe

surgery, rounding of the peripheral edges, as well as the central portion of bone. Stern (6) appropriately analyzed the various factors in bone healing following hammer digit syndrome surgery and his conclusions were compatible with Lewin's statements that careful and limited trauma to the bone when resecting a portion of the phalanx will insure a limited inflammatory response. The following factors, with regard to bony resection, should always be kept in mind:

1. Make straight and even cuts of the bone;
2. Assure that the periosteum and bone are cut cleanly;
3. Avoid splitting and chipping of the bone;
4. Check that alignment and re-articulation are as accurate as possible.

If these factors are closely adhered to, then satisfactory results may be obtained since there will be an appropriate but limited inflammatory response following surgery. Stern pointed out that "regeneration" is an inappropriate term since osseous proliferation following hammertoe surgery is probably the result of the surgeon not closely adhering to the above factors. Again, the myth of "regeneration" was raised by Franklin (9), but if this single patient analysis "study" is scrutinized carefully, one will observe that the above stated factors were not closely adhered to and thus resulted in osseous proliferation which that author termed as "regeneration." We feel that this was an inappropriate conclusion. The standard rule of thumb should always be to remove as much bone as necessary to reduce the deformity. One can always further remove more bone if necessary. However, if there has been overresection of bone, inappropriate complications may result and are definitely iatrogenic in nature (2, 4, 5). Such an appropriate resection and realignment can be seen in Figures 11.1 and 11.2.

Post-operative Edema

The degree of trauma during surgery is not entirely associated with strictly the os-

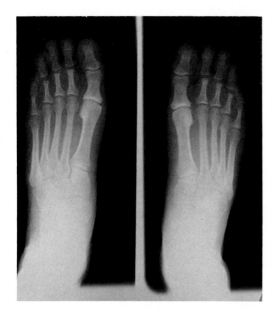

Figure 11.1. Post-operative A-P x-ray of both feet showing adequate excision of the heads of the proximal phalanges of the second, third, and fourth digits with proper alignment, rounding of the edges during healing, and proper rearticulation of the PIPJ.

seous tissues. Nor is the degree of trauma measured by the size of incisions. The surgeon must be constantly respectful to the soft tissues, i.e., skin, neurovascular bundles, capsule, and tendons. Following hammer digit surgery, when the patient complains of prolonged edema, or what has been euphemistically described in the profession as "sausage toe" (10), one should initially suspect that there has been over-traumatization of various tissue components. It becomes easy to blame the patient for excessive ambulation, or not following post-operative instructions, but the surgeon should also carefully re-evaluate his/her technique, especially when it has been observed that this is a rather common complaint of patients. Therefore, dissection and retraction of the associated soft tissues will help alleviate this unfortunate sequela. Such appropriate respect for unwarranted soft tissue injury will result in minimal fibrosis of the dermis, inappropriate hemorrhage and hematoma formation following

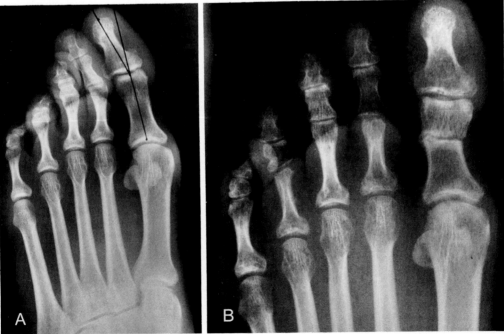

Figure 11.2. *A*, a patient with a symptomatic HAV deformity of the left foot and hammertoe deformities of the second and fourth digits of the same foot. *B*, shows proper post-operative alignment of the second PIPJ, adequate bone removed, and adequate reduction of the deformity. The head of the proximal phalanx on the fourth digit, however, has been excised at an angle which may lead to further stress and some periosteal proliferation in the future.

disruption of the vascular structures in the area, and limited fibrosis of the capsular tendon complex. The common rule of thumb is that if one carefully dissects and retracts the vascular structures and does not incise them, then they will not hemorrhage. If one does not interrupt or obliterate peripheral digital nerves, then patients will not complain of numbness or paresthesias following what should be a very basic type of surgical treatment. In avoiding excessive fibrosis of the skin, the patients will also be more pleased with the surgical result since their structural and functional digital deformity has been corrected, but also, the resultant scar will be more cosmetically acceptable. Beside analyzing the patient and the surgical technique, one should always take careful note of impending or current infection when one is dealing with excessive post-operative edema. However, when infection has been ruled out, then the above factors must be duly considered. In dealing with post-operative edema, there is certainly a normal amount of edema that occurs following hammer digit syndrome surgery. This may occur anywhere from 4–8 weeks post-operatively. Ways to eliminate or assist in control of this particular problem would include:

1. Digital splinting;
2. Physical therapy at home and in the office (massage, hydrotherapy, etc.);
3. Use of diuretics and/or oral enzymes when the edema is prolonged and symptomatic, although their use is questionable in such a localized area.

Flail Toes

It was mentioned earlier that only the appropriate amount of bone should be removed to correct a hammer digit syndrome of the lesser digits. Overexuberance in removing osseous tissue can lead to instability of the digit which, in many cases, results in symptomatic dissatisfaction with the procedure, as in Figures 11.3 and 11.4. In some cases there may be elongation of the second digit, which may be secondary to previous hallux abducto valgus surgery

which resulted in shortening of the first metatarsal and hallux. Thus, such a patient may desire further correction for cosmetic reasons, although there is not truly a hammer digit syndrome present. In dealing with such problems, a standard head resection of the proximal phalanx to the extent noted may lead to more flailness or instability of the digit rather than the patient's desired shortening effect for cosmetic purposes. A more appropriate procedure in such instances would be step-down diaphyseal osteotomy with wire fixation for appropriate stability during the bone healing process. Such a procedure would provide the patient with the appropriate cosmetic shortening of the digit and would also alleviate either the potential fibrotic ankylosis, which occurs at the destroyed proximal interphalangeal joint, or the flail instability of the digit following such a head resection. In Figure 11.5 there has been total head resections of the proximal phalanx of the fourth and fifth digits of the right foot. While this apparently satisfies the surgeon and the patient initially, the long-term results may not be as positive. The instability of these digits could lead to possible pain and edema in the future. Furthermore, atrophy of the fifth toe from excess removal of bone of the proximal interphalangeal joint may cause pain while wearing footgear and result in a "pinch" keratosis overlying the lateral aspect of the proximal interphalangeal joint due to the instability of the digit. It should be obvious through these examples and the previous discussion on bone healing that only the appropriate amount of bone should be removed to reduce the deformity. Stabilization of the digits in the first 21 days following surgery may be accomplished by applying an immobilizing dressing. Further stability may be obtained in such procedures with the insertion of a Kirschner wire through the middle and distal phalanx of the digit, and then reapproximating the proximal interphalangeal joint and retrograding the wire into the remaining portion of the proximal phalanx. This will provide further stability of the digit during the post-

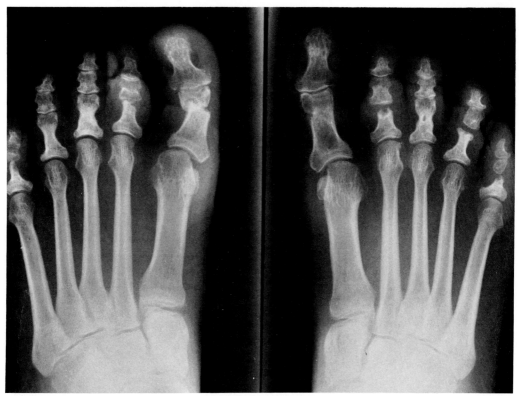

Figure 11.3. Post-operative x-rays following digital surgery bilaterally. There is abnormal angulation in removing the head of the proximal phalanx of the second digit left; excessive bone removed from the second and fourth digit of the right foot with resultant stress and excessive periosteal proliferation within the fourth digit of the right foot. Overreduction or removal of bone, especially in the fifth digit right foot, with resultant atrophy due to disruption of the circulation to the bone. Inadequate osteotomy of the left hallux with poor alignment and nonunion.

operative healing process and maintain the digit in its corrected position. These wires are generally removed approximately 3–4 weeks post-operatively unless the surgeon is attempting an arthrodesing procedure, at which time the wires may have to remain in for a longer period of time. As a general rule, the patients tolerate the insertion of the wires rather well. However, they should be informed pre-operatively that they will have metal wires protruding from the toes for approximately 21 days following surgery. When this surgical technique is performed, there are minimal complications with the use of the K-wires. During the retrograding of the wire through the remaining portion of the proximal phalanx, the wire should not pass through or across the metatarsophalangeal joint in hammer

digit syndrome surgery. If the wire does pass across the metatarsophalangeal joint, this may result in pain as well as post-traumatic arthritis of the metatarsophalangeal joint after removal of the wire, due to fibrosis following invasion and damage to the bone and cartilage of these joints (Fig. 11.6). An appropriate concern of surgeons who have not routinely used K-wires in the digits is the possibility of tract infection with the use of this technique. However, the literature does not support that concern. Following normal standards of care the percentage of tract infection following the use of K-wires is 1% or less. It should also be noted that, when using Kirschner wires, upon completion of the procedure, the wire is bent at a 90° angle to the long axis of the digit. This reduces accidental

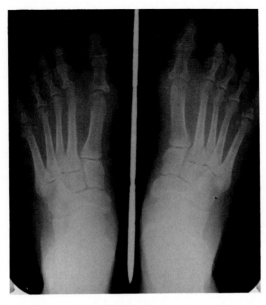

Figure 11.4. Excessive amount of the head and the shaft of the proximal phalanx has been removed from the fifth toes bilaterally, leaving a wide space at the PIPJ and potential for instability and hypermobility of the digit while not completely satisfying the cosmetic desires of the surgeon or patient.

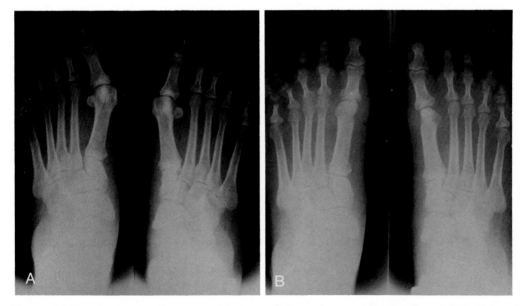

Figure 11.5. *A*, pre-operative x-ray of hammer digit syndrome of the fourth and fifth digits of both feet. *B*, post-operative x-ray with excision of the head of the proximal phalanx of the fourth and fifth digits being removed with malalignment left which possibly could result in hypermobility and instability of these digits resulting in pain and possible future surgery for reconstruction.

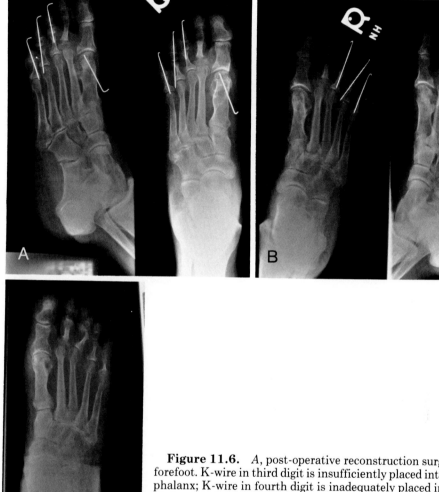

Figure 11.6. *A*, post-operative reconstruction surgery of left forefoot. K-wire in third digit is insufficiently placed into proximal phalanx; K-wire in fourth digit is inadequately placed in proximal phalanx and crosses into MPJ; K-wire in fifth digit crosses into metatarsal head which could result in post-traumatic arthritis. *B*, post-operative reconstruction surgery of the right forefoot. K-wire in fourth digit is inadequately placed for proper stabilization. *C*, post-operative x-ray of same foot seen in *B*. K-wire in third toe had been removed prematurely resulting in PIPJ subluxation and potential for future interdigital lesion.

trauma by the patient against a solid object which could possibly project the wire into the foot. Another potential complication could be that anywhere from several days to several weeks following the surgery, the patients may state that the wire has become loose with ambulation and is protruding farther out from the toe. These patients should be seen in the office immediately and evaluated as to the possibility of removal of the wire, depending upon the stage of the healing process at that particular time. The ends of the wires may be protected by adhesive tape or a small plastic cap which can be placed on the distal end of the wire.

Bony Atrophy

Another complication of overexuberant bone removal for hammer digit syndrome is the resultant potential for bony atrophy as seen in Figure 11.7. Beside the instability of the digit, excessive removal of the bone may disrupt the normal circulatory pattern into the proximal phalanx. The resultant effect is that the bone will be absorbed and atrophy back to its normal level of vascular penetration. At the same time, there will be soft tissue atrophy and the patient may be very unsatisfied with the result due to the "accordian" appearance of the digit. In these types of cases, the patients frequently complain of the inability to control the digit, especially when attempting to place their feet in footgear.

Conservative splinting of the digit can be uncomfortable and is generally not tolerated well by patients over a long period of time. Attempts at reconstruction of this avoidable complication in the past has included arthrodesis and/or syndactylization of the digit which may or may not result in patient satisfaction. Mladick (11) proposed a surgical procedure in such cases where a Z-plasty of the skin was performed to reduce the soft tissue contraction dorsally and insertion of a bone graft to provide stability to the digit, as well as some restoration of length to the digit which is cosmetically more acceptable to the pa-

tients. His recommendations certainly have some merit in terms of stability, restoration of function, and cosmesis.

A point must be made in this overall discussion of lesser digit hammertoe syndrome. It has been a common practice in some areas of podiatric surgery to invade either the proximal or distal interphalangeal joint for correction of a structural or positional deformity of the lesser toes and to invade or incise the capsular tendon complex in order to provide visualization for the bony surgery. Following the bony surgery, the capsular tendon complex is simply "laid" back into place. If these structures are not appropriately approximated with sutures, a resultant hypermobility or instability of the digit may occur. As stated earlier, with all types of surgery, one should have a comprehensive understanding of the healing of the various tissues involved. The surgeon can easily avoid this preventable complication of instability if he or she would take the time to approximate the capsular tendon complex in place, thus allowing the tissues to heal normally and provide greater stability to the digit. Although the resultant instability is not always a complaint of all patients, we have seen many patients over the years who do complain of unstable digits and hypermobility of the toe, and upon review of the operative record from the previous surgeon, it was noted that the capsular tendon complex was not approximated with suture material. Such routine re-approximation of these tissues certainly does not add an exorbitant amount of time to the surgical procedure.

In completing this discussion on basic hammertoe procedures, there are several interesting points that need further discussion. Too often with "routine" surgery, the surgeon does not make careful observations during the surgical procedure and, thus, important but minute details may be overlooked. An example would be the syndrome involving a hammertoe deformity of the fifth digit with an associated interdigital lesion between the fourth and fifth digits (15). A diagnosis is made where there is

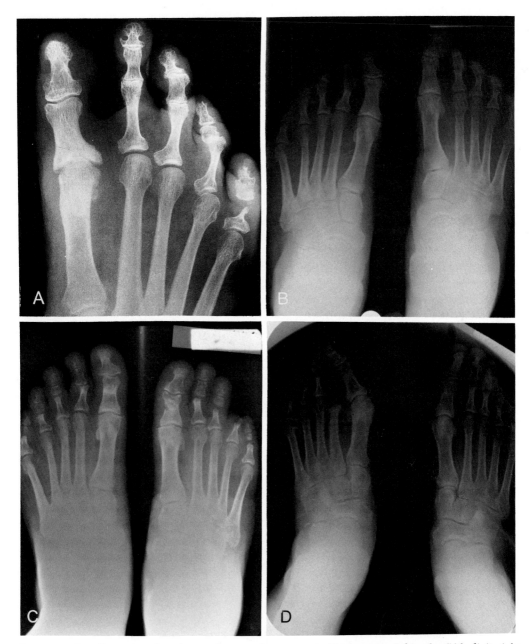

Figure 11.7. Bone atrophy. *A*, case 1: excessive amount of bone removed in the fifth digit right foot, disrupting the circulation and resulting in gross atrophy. *B*, case 2: pre-operative x-ray of hammer digit syndrome bilaterally. *C*, case 2: post-operative x-ray with malalignment of second digit bilaterally; too aggressive surgical technique when performing multiple lesser digital procedures resulting in gangrene of fourth digit right and resultant amputation. *D*, case 3: excessive trauma in attempting to correct hammer toe left foot which resulted in gangrene, amputation, and now an HAV deformity.

enlargement of the proximal phalanx at the head of the fifth digit, as well as enlargement of the lateral condyle of the base of the proximal phalanx of the fourth toe. The accepted surgical approach is excision of the head of the proximal phalanx of the fifth toe and lateral condyle of the base of the proximal phalanx of the fourth toe. It should be pointed out that we have observed erroneous diagnosis of this condition involving the head of the fourth metatarsal with inappropriate remodeling of the fourth metatarsal and further joint destruction. In the vast majority of cases, the base of the fourth digit is involved without involvement of the fourth metatarsal head and, thus, any further destruction of the fourth metatarsophalangeal joint is inappropriate. The lateral condyle on the base of the proximal phalanx is usually excised flush with the shaft of the bone. It is often necessary to resect the head of the proximal phalanx of the fifth toe because of bony hypertrophy on the medial side of the head.

The chief complication is subluxation of the fourth digit in the dorsal and medial direction. This subluxation may be caused by a lateral shredding of the capsule at the fourth metatarsophalangeal joint which precludes proper closure and creates muscle imbalance. A lateral longitudinal capsulotomy carried too plantarly will also section the intrinsic muscle leading to imbalance. A contracted extensor digitorum longus tendon to the fourth digit which is not properly lengthened will also create dorsal subluxation.

It is important, therefore, to properly perform the longitudinal capsulotomy so that the integrity of the capsule is maintained. A vertical capsulotomy on the medial aspect of the fourth metatarsophalangeal joint will also equalize tension at the joint. Forefoot push-up tests, and stance and gait analysis, should be performed to make certain the extensor digitorum longus tendon is not contracted. If it is contracted, Z-plasty tendon lengthening should be performed. The fourth metatarsophalangeal joint is then placed in proper alignment

and the capsule is closed. Proper subcutaneous closure should also add the needed strength to the lateral aspect. The skin is closed in the conventional manner. Following the surgery, the fourth toe should be splinted in a slightly abducted position.

The adductus type foot lends itself to dislocation because of the medial deflection of the digits at the metatarsal heads. Careful realignment of the proximal phalanx is essential.

If one carefully observes patients following surgery, the patient may continue to complain of pain in the fourth interdigital space. Galinski (13) pointed out the occurrence of a perineural fibrosis of the proper digital nerve in the fourth interdigital space which is the result of chronic fibrosis of the associated digital nerve following the juxtapositional irritation between the affected bones associated with compression and irritation from shoes. Surgical procedures involving the bony structures may be quite successful; however, the patient's pain persists and, therefore, true success of the surgical procedure is questionable. A few moments of extra time during the dissection phase, in both the fourth and fifth digital area, will occasionally reveal this associated reactive perineural fibrosis which should be excised. Too often in our desire for "speedy" surgery and the fact that we have seen "thousands" of these types of cases, we may not carefully observe these minute changes. Throughout one's surgical career, one should always re-evaluate one's techniques on a periodic basis and take the time and make the effort to observe and evaluate any pathological changes which may be noted at the time of surgery. As stated earlier, such astute observations will provide more positive surgical results and avoid a possible re-operation of the patient to alleviate their symptoms.

Another important point needs to be made involving hammertoe surgery, exclusively involving the fifth digit (12). Again, over a period of years, astute observation may be lost, and it has been well-documented that in a certain percentage of cases a recurrent keratotic lesion may be present over the dorsal-lateral aspect of the fifth toe following hammertoe surgery. In those cases where the initial keratotic lesion is only large enough to cover the dorsal-lateral aspect of the head of the proximal phalanx, a simple resection of the head of the proximal phalanx may be all that is necessary. However, either when the lesion covers both the head of the proximal phalanx and the middle phalanx, or when the lesion only covers the head of the proximal phalanx but routine radiographs show enlargement of the dorsal-lateral aspect of the base of the middle phalanx, then resection of that exostosis is indicated. This type of resection is not indicated in all cases. It is our feeling that careful clinical observation and radiographic analysis will lead the surgeon to the correct surgical procedure, perhaps including an exostectomy of the dorsal-lateral aspect of the base of the middle phalanx which, in the long run, may lead to a decrease in the recurrence rate.

Finally, we feel that a few comments are in order on the surgical procedure of excising the base of the proximal phalanx at the metatarsophalangeal joint for surgical correction of hammer digit syndrome (5). This particular surgical procedure has been used rather extensively. It has not proven to be of any significant benefit to patients, whether it is done as an independent procedure or in association with a syndactylization of the affected digit of the next largest toe. This is a joint destructive procedure which may lead to compensatory atrophy of the digit and thus an unfortunate cosmetic result, but also leads to instability of the metatarsophalangeal joint since there is loss of intrinsic muscle control by removal of the base of the proximal phalanx. In the past decade, we have examined numerous patients with prolonged complaints of pain, instability, stiffness, weakness and flaccidity of the affected digit or digits which then requires some attempts at reconstructive surgery and, in some cases, arthrodesis which is an unfortunate and preventable complication. The state of the

art in the last 40–50 years of hammer digit surgery has seen the use of multiple surgical approaches, most of which provide adequate reduction of the deformity, return to normal function without pain, resulting in stability to the lesser digit or digits. We do not recommend this particular procedure and feel that the surgeon can avoid this unless the patient's primary complaint in that area involves a bone tumor of the base of the proximal phalanx.

Post-operative Sagittal and Transverse Plane Deviations of Digits

Extensor contracture of the digits and lateral or medial migrations of the toes are common following surgery. The incidence is about 4 to 1 in favor of the second toe. The deformities include the following.

SAGITTAL PLANE

Simple dorsal contracture at the metatarsophalangeal joint is most common. It is characterized by an absence of bony changes. The entire digit is dorsiflexed on the metatarsal. The extensor digitorum longus tendon may bowstring and there may be extension contracture of the capsule. Subcutaneous metatarsophalangeal joint capsulotomy and tenotomy are frequent predisposing factors.

Simple dorsal contracture at the interphalangeal joints can occur following arthroplasties of the digits.

Complete or partial dorsal subluxation of the toe at the metatarsophalangeal joint frequently causes degenerative changes. This is most frequently seen following metatarsophalangeal joint arthroplasties, e.g., plantar condylectomy or other remodelings of the metatarsal head, or resection of the base of the proximal phalanx or all of the bone of the proximal phalanx.

FRONTAL PLANE

Rotational deformities of the lesser toes are uncommon. They are seen following arthrodeses with improper positioning.

TRANSVERSE PLAIN

Deviations of the digit at the metatarsophalangeal joints are frequent. Lateral deviation deformities are more common.

TRIPLANE

A combination of two or more of the above deformities, the most common involves extension contracture and lateral deviation of the digit at the metatarsal-phalangeal or proximal interphalangeal joints. Etiological factors include: healing defects or disorders; contracture of scar tissue in the skin, tendon, or capsule; delayed wound healing, and wound disruption with healing by secondary intention, infection, and hypertrophic scar or keloid formation.

Deficient techniques include: excessive removal of bone; improper remodeling of bony surfaces; failure to lengthen extensor tendons; improper splinting or immobilization; attempted reduction of an overriding second digit without repair of co-existing hallux valgus; and disturbance of the delicate intrinsic muscular balance in the extensor hood and flexor sling mechanisms.

Prevention of Post-operative Contracture Deformities

Traditional preventive measures include:
—Extra care for patients with a history of keloid or hypertrophic scar formations, e.g., the use of corticosteroids in wound;
—Sufficient mobilization of tissue during dissection;
—Closure in layers where indicated;
—Mandatory correction of an underlying hallux valgus deformity when repairing an overriding second toe;
—Immobilization of digits to allow for complete healing of soft tissues in corrected positions;
—Lengthening tendons farther than would seem necessary, because return of muscle tonus and physiologic shortening of the muscle will result in recurrence of the deformity.
Currently accepted preventive measures include:

—Using orthotic foot appliances to stabilize underlying functional or biomechanical pathologies that caused the deformities;
—Avoiding resection of the base of the proximal phalanges because joint stability is lost when the insertions of the lumbricales and interossei are removed;
—Careful placement and positioning of internal fixation devices, when used;
—Partial or complete surgical syndactylia to stabilize flail digits to adjacent stable digits;
—Revising the hammertoe repair procedure for the lesser toes that transfers the flexor digitorum longus tendon to the dorsum of the proximal phalangeal stump (after resection of the head of the phalanx) because of high incidence of resultant stiff toes and extension contractures.

Additional considerations include:

The subcutaneous "snap" tenotomy and capsulotomy at the metatarsophalangeal joint should be revised (16). If dorsal capsulotomy is required in an otherwise irreducible deformity, it should be performed with adequate exposure. This assumes that the extensor tendon is not severed at the level of the joint and that the incisions are confined to the dorsal aspect of the sling and not extended to the tendons, insertions, or expansions of the intrinsic muscles. The strong extensor sling originates from the tendon of the extensor digitorum longus proximal to the joint, so that severing the tendon and the extensor apparatus at the joint will not prevent extension of the proximal phalanx but will destroy the stabilizing influence of the intrinsic muscles. Lengthening of the extensor digitorum longus tendon is preferred to tenotomy. This should be done well proximal to the metatarsophalangeal joint, even to the level of the metatarsal bases, where several tendon lengthenings can be done with one incision. Sliding or Z-plasty techniques are helpful. When tenotomy of the extensor digitorum brevis is the choice, it must be remembered that this tendon exerts a stabilizing influence on the action of the extensor digitorum longus.

CORRECTION OF EXISTING DEFORMITIES

Early in the post-operative period, attention should be directed to signs of impending deformities. Measures that are effective during the first 60 days include the following:
—Splinting and immobilization by means of urethane molds or retainers;
—Use of other suitable splinting materials;
—Early injection of corticosteroids to minimize fibrosis and scar formation;
—Early tendon lengthenings.
Measures in longstanding deformities include:
—Tendon lengthenings;
—Skin plasties;
—Partial or complete surgical syndactylia of the involved digit to adjacent stable digits;
—Additional resection of bone;
—Arthrodesis.
Moldable Podiatric Compound was introduced in 1972. It is a silicone rubber compound that is mixed and cured in a plastic packet prior to application. It is molded to the foot or toes; the final product cures in 20 minutes to a semi-soft, durable, one-piece appliance that washes easily.

Clawed Hallux or Hallux Hammertoe Syndrome

The patient who has a symptomatic or asymptomatic dorsally contracted hallux at the metatarsophalangeal joint with flexion contraction at the interphalangeal joint may have any one of the following as an etiological factor:
—Post-traumatic arthritis;
—Post-operative arthroplastic joint destruction bunionectomies (Keller or Mayo);
—Bunionectomy procedure where both sesamoids have been removed;
—Neuromuscular disease resulting in a plantar-flexed first metatarsal with

contraction of the extensor hallucis longus tendon;
—Idiopathic clawing of the hallux with plantar-flexed first metatarsal and contraction of the extensor hallucis longus tendon;
—Untreated or improperly treated fracture or dislocation of the interphalangeal joint of the hallux.
Understanding the etiological factors causing this deformity will aid greatly in determining the appropriate surgical procedure. Without a doubt, it is commonly accepted that a fusion of the interphalangeal joint with either tendon lengthening or tendon transposition of the extensor hallucis longus provides the best long-term results. M'Bamali (14), in a report from England involving 26 patients and 36 feet operated on for this particular condition, recorded a total of 88.5% with good to fair results and only 11% of those patients with poor results. These cases involved a wide parameter of etiological factors, which were mentioned above, including neuromuscular disease. The Sir Robert Jones procedure involves the sectioning of the extensor hallucis longus tendon just proximal to its insertion at the distal phalanx of the hallux and transposing the tendon through a transverse drill hole in the first metatarsal and suturing it to itself for tension. M'Bamali initially did not provide any type of internal or external fixation for the interphalangeal fusion, but following his series, strongly recommended that some type of internal or external immobilization be provided and we would concur. An important factor involving this particular syndrome is the careful observation as to whether there is a rigid plantar-flexed deformity of the first metatarsal. If the first metatarsal is in a rigidly plantar-flexed position, then a dorsiflexory wedge osteotomy of the base of the first metatarsal would be appropriate. Otherwise, any soft tissue or osseous surgery involving just the first metatarsophalangeal joint and hallux would be unsuccessful. With any fusion procedure, careful denuding of the cartilage and subchondral bone and the articulating surfaces

of the interphalangeal joint of the hallux is essential. Next, appropriate positioning and fixation will insure proper fusion and adequate reduction of the deformity. Technical errors in the use of K-wires can be seen in Figure 11.8. Although there appears to be adequate denuding of the bony surfaces, the use of a single K-wire through the hallux provides inadequate compression, as well as the potential for axial rotation of the phalangeal segments in the frontal plane, and that type of motion may lead to statistically higher chance of nonunion, recurrence of the deformity, and pain. Another technical error is seen in Figure 11.9. Placement of cross K-wires will prevent any frontal plane rotation and will also aid in increasing compression over the fusion sight. One should also be sure that the K-wires do not cross at an osteotomy site so as to avoid an unwarranted, nonunion complication. Furthermore, K-wires should not pass through the first metatarsophalangeal joint unless one is also attempting a fusion of that joint. While the

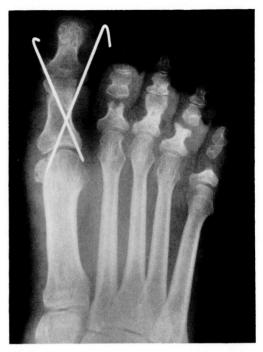

Figure 11.9. Post-operative x-ray at attempted fusion of right hallux IP with K-wires which cross the first MPJ and could result in first MPJ post-traumatic arthritis.

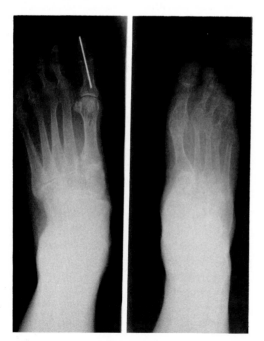

Figure 11.8. A-P x-ray showing attempted IP fusion of the left hallux with single K-wire which could result in some frontal plane axial rotation.

cross K-wires in Figure 11.9 may lead to a successful fusion of the interphalangeal joint, the size of the wires and the fact that they cross into and through the first metatarsal-phalangeal joint will more likely lead to limitation of motion of the joint, as well as traumatic arthritis, which could be rather debilitating to the patient. This complication can be avoided if, after the insertion of the K-wires, the first metatarsophalangeal joint is taken through a range of motion intra-operatively. If there is any restriction of the range of motion, or crepitation on range of motion, then the K-wires should be retrograded distally until the restriction and crepitation can no longer be seen or felt. If in doubt, do not hesitate to order intra-operative radiographs to insure proper wire position. Ideally, the K-wires are used in a cross fashion to avoid frontal plane motion, as well as sagittal plane motion. The wires do not cross at the osteotomy site but do cross two cortices in order to provide proper stability.

There will always remain the question as to whether this type of immobilization provides adequate compression for fusion. However, this type of fixation has apparently been proven over the test of time.

Finally, with regard to interphalangeal fusions of the hallux, there has been a great deal of discussion involving the "new" technique of utilizing screw fixation for improved stability as well as maximum compression which will statistically increase the chances of proper osseous fusion. This approach on the hallux involves a distal incision which, if over-traumatized, may result in excessive fibrosis and pain following the surgery. Also, it is recently been reported in a number of cases where screw fixation has been used for the hallux interphalangeal fusion that, within the first year post-operatively, there may be loosening of the screw and resultant pain which then involves removal of the surgical hardware. This can be seen in Figure 11.10. Adequate positioning and compression has been obtained with the use of a cancellous screw for fixation. While this might provide short-term, as well as long-term positive

surgical results, it could result in a rather difficult problem if the screw loosens over a period of time and requires removal. Since the shaft of the cancellous screw on its proximal portion is smooth, the bone will heal around it, making removal by simple stab incision and use of a screwdriver impossible because the bone along the smooth shaft of the screw has not healed in a threaded manner. Thus, we would like to recommend that if the surgeon chooses to use screw fixation for interphalangeal hallux fusion, then cortical screws should be used with a lag technique so that if loosening occurs and the screw requires removal, the removal procedure will be a minor one.

Arthrodesis of the Lesser Digits

Following the complications discussed earlier involving lesser digital hammertoe surgery or post-traumatic problems of the lesser digits, arthrodesis of one or more interphalangeal joints may be necessary. The same basic concepts and philosophies of arthrodesis in general, as well as digital

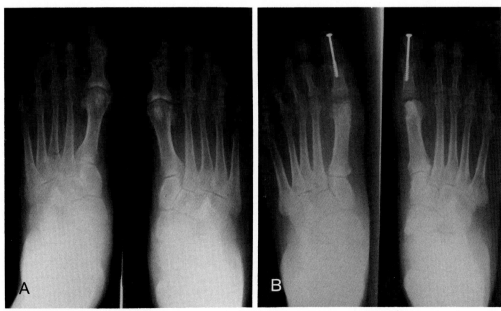

Figure 11.10. *A*, psoriatic arthritis of the IP of the hallux bilaterally. *B*, post-operative x-ray showing attempt at IP fusion using a cancellous bone screw. Threads of the screw in left hallux are within the fusion site, which is improper technique and could result in non-union and pain.

arthrodesis as was just discussed for the hallux, should be followed for the lesser interphalangeal joints. Adequate stability and function and structure will be obtained as can be seen in Figure 11.11.

Accessory Ossicle of the Hallux

A relatively common clinical deformity would be the patient who presents with an organized keratotic lesion of the plantar aspect of the interphalangeal joint of the hallux. In most adult patients, radiographs will reveal an organized, well-circumscribed, osseous accessory bone, and in some cases where bone has not been ossified, one may assume that the accessory tissue is of a cartilaginous nature. Various linear medial and transverse plantar incisions have been recommended for the excision of this accessory tissue. Hill (17) recommended a dorsal transverse approach which he felt was less traumatic than the previously mentioned approaches. It is our opinion that any one of these approaches has an inherent problem since we are dealing with a small area, but also, one must be cognizant of the important tendinous structures both dorsally and plantarly, especially since these accessory tissues, whether os-

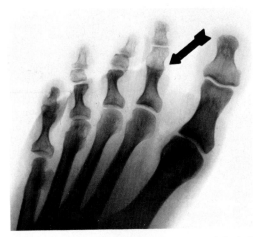

Figure 11.11. Post-operative x-ray of the left foot showing arthrodesis of the PIPJ of the second digit which was a reconstructive procedure following failure of previous standard arthroplasty procedure.

seous or cartilaginous, are imbedded in the flexor hallucis longus tendon beneath the interphalangeal joint of the hallux in the majority of cases. No matter what approach is undertaken by the surgeon, careful dissection is of the utmost importance. In removing accessory tissue, careful exposure is essential and extreme care must be taken during the excision of this abnormal tissue to avoid transection of the flexor hallucis longus tendon. If this tendon is either accidently or deliberately transected, then appropriate sutures of a horizontal or Bunnell type should be inserted with proper reapproximation of this tendon for normal position and function post-operatively.

Congenital Deformities

One of the most common pediatric congenital deformities seen in the podiatric office would that of underlapping or overlapping digits. For the most part, these conditions run a rather benign course and can be handled conservatively with appropriate orthopedic taping or splinting over a period of time. The neglected overriding contraction of the fifth toe is a frequent surgical problem. Multiple procedures have been proposed over the years, including skin plasties, tendon lengthening, tendon transpositions, and arthroplasty procedures. In describing the Butler procedure, Cockin (18) duly noted the high risk of this particular procedure through circumferential skin incisions. Care must be taken to preserve the neurovascular bundles; otherwise, catastrophic results in the form of gangrene and subsequent amputation will be an unfortuante consequence. He described good results in 91% of the patients in this study over a 10-year period. In 6% of the patients, elimination of the deformity went uncorrected and usually involved abnormal rotation. There was a 3% failure rate in his study, resulting in digital amputation. The most frequent complication of the "V-Y" plastic elongation of the skin would be an ugly scar formation and potential keloid formation with recurrence of the deformity. The proximal phalangectomy with plantar syndactylism, or excision of the base of the proximal phalanx with syndactylization of the fourth and fifth toes, generally provides good results, but has been criticized because it had resulted in complications or deformities.

In the adolescent and adult population, we have received positive results (unpublished) with the Lapidus procedure (5) of transpositioning the extensor digitorum longus tendon to the fifth digit after transection and rerouting it around the medial aspect of the proximal phalanx and suturing it to the lateral aspect of the fifth metatarsophalangeal joint capsule. This provides adequate reduction of the dorsal contraction as well as frontal plane derotation of the digit. In some cases where there has been either previous procedures performed or the deformity has been neglected, a capsulotomy may be necessary on the dorsal and dorsal-lateral aspect of the fifth metatarsal-phalangeal joint. In utilizing any of these procedures, meticulous dissection and surgical care must be of the utmost importance to the surgeon to avoid catastrophic complications.

POLYDACTYLY

A good example for the necessity of appropriate clinical examination and radiographic analysis for determination of the appropriate surgical approach would be those individuals who are born with a polydactyly and/or a polymetatarsia. A tremendous clinical pitfall is the snap clinical evaluation due to the obvious congenital deformity. Radiographs will certainly identify the accessory digit and/or metatarsal. However, a gross surgical error would be made if the practitioner does not appropriately examine the patient both neurovascularly, to determine his or her tolerance for the procedure, but also musculoskeletally. The rarely mentioned but extremely important aspect of pre-operative determination of which digit is to be excised is determining the normal musculotendonous insertions into the digits, since more often than not the accessory digit will have no

tendonous insertions or only weak, aberrant tendonous insertions. Thus, in polydactyly, it would be a mistake to always excise the most lateral digit since we have seen cases where the fifth digit (numbered from medial to lateral) is actually the accessory digit and the sixth digit is the normal fifth digit. This decision making process is made somewhat easier when there is an associated polymetatarsia since there is generally an accessory digit associated with this deformity which may or may not have any osseous structures within it. A gross and irreversible mistake would be made if the surgeon did not properly evaluate the muscle strength, tone, and function of the digits involved in order to determine the appropriate surgical approach. A good example was pointed out by Tozzi and Penny (19), who discussed the genetic inherited trait in an individual case. However, there was limited discussion involving the decision-making process as to which of the digits and metatarsals were to be excised and the rationale for the approach (see Figure 11.12).

The final congenital deformity to be dis-

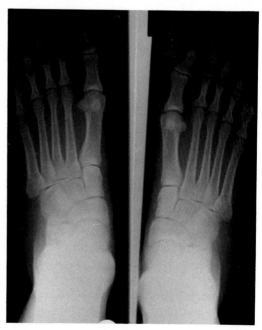

Figure 11.12. Pre-operative AP radiograph of patient with polydactyly accessory digit of the fifth digit of the right foot.

cussed involving the digits would be the rare condition known as macrodactyly. This is a rare deformity involving the fingers and toes with, to date, an unknown etiology but a suspicion of some form of neurofibrous disease. Tsuge (20) presented an excellent paper involving background, radiographic findings, genetic involvement, and some early surgical approaches to this deformity. His own surgical approach is described in detail. Extraordinary pre-operative planning is of the utmost importance in approaching children with this unfortunate type of deformity. Beside clinical and radiographic analysis, there must be detailed preplanning as to the surgical approach since most authors recommend a two-stage approach. We have found that both a two-stage and a one-stage approach yields satisfactory results. The surgical procedures must be performed with extreme care and with meticulous detail. The key component of success in performing surgery for such a congenital condition involves the preservation of the neuromuscular structures while excising profound amounts of adipose and fibrous tissue from the enlarged digit. There should be proper analysis of the radiographs pre-operatively to determine exactly the quantity of bone to be removed to help reduce the digital structure; however, in most of these cases, you will find that there is a normal size and shape to the developing phalangeal bones. The surgeon is cautioned that when involved with such cases, the two-stage approach is in the best interest of the patient, and that the second stage merely involves skin plasties to remove excessive amounts of skin which results from the shortening of the digit with the initial procedure. This secondary procedure to remove redundant skin may be performed within weeks to months after the initial procedure. The single-stage operation can produce positive results but runs a much higher risk of compromise to the neurovascular structures.

Neoplasms

A relatively uncommon problem presented to the practitioner involves the soft tissue and bony neoplasms of the digits. Most of the bony neoplasms would be in the form of chondromas, osteochondromas, and, on rare occasions, osteoid osteomas with even rarer sarcomas of bone. Soft-tissue tumors, beside verrucae, include ganglionic cysts, lipoma, leiomyoma, etc., as is seen in Figure 11.13 of an elderly patient with a benign lipoma on the dorsal aspect of the second digit of the left foot. Careful surgical approach, respect for neurovascular structures, and limited trauma to the skin, including proper nonconstricting suturing, can yield satisfactory cosmetic and clinical results. In dealing with areas of small and fragile neurovascular structures, one must take into account the patient's overall metabolic and medical status, vascular status, and the potential risk to the patient and survival of the digit (Fig. 11.14).

Neurovascular Complications

As with all forms of surgical trauma, especially of the extremities, there can result some unpredictable complications. Sudeck's atrophy or the classic post-traumatic sympathetic dystrophy is seen in a small percentage of patients. A condition known as mimocausalgia was described by Black (21) in a report on two cases. The standard course of treatment in these syndromes include physical therapy, local injections of anesthetics, exercise, oral vasodilators, and sympathetic spinal blocks. Finally, as with any of these situations or cases discussed in this chapter, when improper pre-operative clincal evaluation, inappropriate excessive trauma intra-operatively, or poor post-operative management and observation are not controlled by the surgeon, then neurovascular collapse and gangrene may result. There is no shame in informing a patient that his circulatory status could not sustain a given digital procedure. If the pre-operative evaluation shows poor vascular status, and the surgery is performed, then the results may be far more catastrophic than anticipated by both the patient and the surgeon alike. The same cannot be said when there is a catastrophic complication

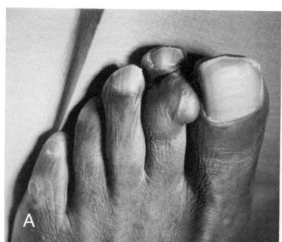
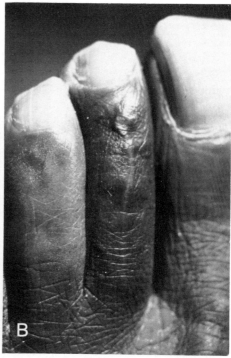

Figure 11.13. *A*, pre-operative AP photograph of the left foot showing a large, multilobular lipoma on the dorsal aspect of the second toe. *B*, post-operative photograph of the same patient following excision of lipoma utilizing to semiliptical incisions and careful dissection with plastic surgical closure of the skin and respect for the neurovascular structures.

with infection and/or amputation resulting. Unfortunately, when such complications occur and a retrospective analysis is made, in the majority of cases, there has been inappropriate evaluation of the patient pre-operatively or excessive trauma intra-operatively, both of which are iatrogenic problems and can be avoided.

On occasion, whether incisions are made dorsally on the digits or on the medial and lateral aspects, there can be associated adhesions, hypertrophic scar, and pain. Balkin (22–26) reported on the use of injectable silicone fluid for the relief of painful scars. The results are apparently quite gratifying and offer potential for the future. While his work in this area has been over a prolonged period of time, it is still to be proven what the long-term local and metabolic effects might be in patients where medical grade silicone fluid has been injected. Otherwise, when dealing with such

problems of surgical skin wounds, the standard procedures involve re-incision with excision of scar tissue with plastic closure, skin flaps, skin lengthening procedures when there is involved severe contracture, and local steroid injections to relieve pain.

LESSER METATARSAL SURGERY

Although in the past decade of podiatric surgery there has been an enormous discussion of various lesser metatarsal procedures, there has also been a limited amount of published material and data. A couple of texts and several articles have been published on the subject, in spite of the common use of various procedures to alleviate plantar keratotic lesions beneath the lesser metatarsal heads (50, 56). It seems apparent that much work is needed to determine the various indications and/or contraindications for the use of these procedures. In spite of the fact that Meisenbach (35) was the first to discuss the use of metatarsal osteotomies, for several decades the arthroplasty procedures, which in many cases destroyed the metatarsophalangeal joint, remained the most popular procedures. However, the past 10–15 years has produced various procedures with limited factual statistics which would enhance our overall knowledge of corrective surgery in this particular area (32, 51).

It is extremely important that the surgeon have a working knowledge of biomechanics of foot structure and function in order to make an accurate diagnosis of the patient's problem and complaints (54). Without a doubt, surgery is not the total answer when dealing with the intractable plantar keratosis beneath a lesser metatarsal head. Without a working knowledge of the biomechanics of foot structure and function, surgical errors and complications will continue to be made. The most glaring error is when the individual practitioner chooses only one particular procedure when patients present plantar keratotic lesions beneath one or more of the lesser metatarsal heads. Once an individual practitioner has "stereotyped" procedures without a knowledge of all available procedures, as well as a knowledge of the biomechanics of the foot, then the patient's best interests will not be served.

A few examples of variations which may result in lesions beneath one or more of the lesser metatarsal heads would be as follows:
—Pronation syndrome;
—Forefoot varus;
    —Lesion underneath the fifth metatarsal head;
    —Diffuse lesion beneath the second, third, and fourth metatarsal heads;
    —Hypermobility of the fifth metatarsal leading to a lesion beneath the fourth metatarsal head;
    —Hallux abducto valgus deformity with compensatory lesion beneath the second metatarsal head;
—Splayed forefoot associated with pronation syndrome with abnormal stress and friction beneath the lesser metatarsal heads with associated hallux abducto valgus.
—Pes cavus with lesions beneath either the first metatarsal head or first and fifth metatarsal heads;
—Abnormal length pattern of one or more of the lesser metatarsals;
—Idiopathic plantar-flexion of one or more of the lesser metatarsal heads;
—Exostosis or hyperostosis of one of the lesser metatarsal heads.

There must also be an accurate clinical analysis of the keratotic lesion itself in relation to size, location (whether directly beneath the metatarsal head or anterior to it), associated central enucleation, and degree of symptoms. Such discussion has been covered extensively in other texts and is not within the realm of this textbook.

We will not attempt to discuss all the various procedures that have been proposed within the last 60 to 70 years. Hatcher et al. (49) did discuss the historical background and the reader should also consult the textbook by Kelikian (68) for a more in-depth historical discussion. Hatcher did review, however, the various contemporary procedures, as well as their own success and failure rate with regard to lesser metatarsal surgery. This paper represents a fine piece of initial work since it is one of the few published articles in the area of research, and it makes one realize how much more important future published data will be.

Basic Principles

The following basic principles will be discussed briefly since they are an important adjunct to the overall discussion of lesser metatarsal surgery.

POWER EQUIPMENT

Power equipment permits more exact incisions and resection with a minimum of trauma to the surrounding tissues, and it provides smooth surfaces of incised bone to approximate and stabilize. The oscillating saw allows a perpendicular sectioning of a bone for osteotomies without trauma to the adjacent bones or tissues. The end of the blade of the reciprocating saw often damages tissues beyond the bone being excised. The rotary osteotome or Hall drill fails to cut a flat linear osteotomy and, if care is not taken, it burns the bone and prolongs union of the charred surfaces. The oscillating saw facilitates the correction of metatarsus adductus. Wedge osteotomies for all five metatarsals are likewise made easier. Contamination may occur, as bone dust and organic matter may be flung into contact with non-sterile surfaces (e.g., face mask) and may fall back into the sterile field. Therefore, the surgical site must be copiously flushed with suitable solution.

FIXATION

The stresses on and through a bone, as well as its shape, may directly determine the location of the osteotomy and the fixation required for stabilization. Internal fixation is required for biplane osteotomies as well as those in which the cortex is not intact. Stainless-steel fixation devices must be of acceptable metallurgical quality in order to avoid corrosive ionization. It has been observed that a profusion of callus appears when slight movement occurs, in contrast to the absence of callus after rigid immobilization during bone repair.

When one or two dorsiflectory osteotomies are done to the middle lesser metatarsals and the plantar cortex is preserved, fixation and plantar cast is a safer method of assuring good osseous alignment and repair. In a dorsiflectory osteotomy of the first ray, the forces acting on the first metatarsal make fixation and casting necessary. When either the medial or lateral cortex is preserved, internal fixation is necessary, in addition to external splinting with plaster casts. Weightbearing does not present a threat to good healing if adequate internal fixation and casting are assured. Apposition must be confirmed by immediate postoperative radiographs. Metatarsal osteotomy, whether singular or multiple, may be splinted by an ambulatory foot cast. The cast must meet the demand of immobilizing one joint proximal and distal to the osteotomized bone.

Immobilization, whether internal or external, or both, is crucial in preventing nonunion. Internal fixation is the attachment of two or more pieces of bone by a device usually made of metal or alloy. Tissue glues, such as methylmethacrylates, have been used.

There are six basic ways of attaching bone fragment: 1) by bone screws, which are usually made self-tapping so they cut their own threads; 2) by a long stem or rod that fits into the medullary cavity of the bone; 3) by tight, circumferential bands; 4) by onlay devices called plates, which are attached with screws or bolts; 5) by buried sutures; and 6) by staples.

Internal fixation should be considered only for temporary immobilization and not as a substitute for the stability of normal bones.

Wire Suture Fixation

Stainless-steel wire sutures are widely used, although their strength is limited. Sutures placed through holes drilled in bone secure good apposition, although absolute immobilization cannot be obtained. The effectiveness of wire sutures rests with the ability to drill holes so that passage of the wire permits tightening of the wire to close the osteotomy. Doubling the wire to form a loop and feeding it through the drill hole so that it can be pulled through with a crochet hook enhances the technique (Fig. 11.14). If the wire is too small, it may break or cut through the bone. If this occurs, a large gauge needle (18 or 20) may be cut and used as a sleeve in the drill hole. We have found that 2-0 (28 gauge) stainless-steel doubled is ideal in a 1.5-mm drill hole.

Arthroplasty Procedures

In this particular classification, metatarsal-phalangeal joint capsulotomies, ten-

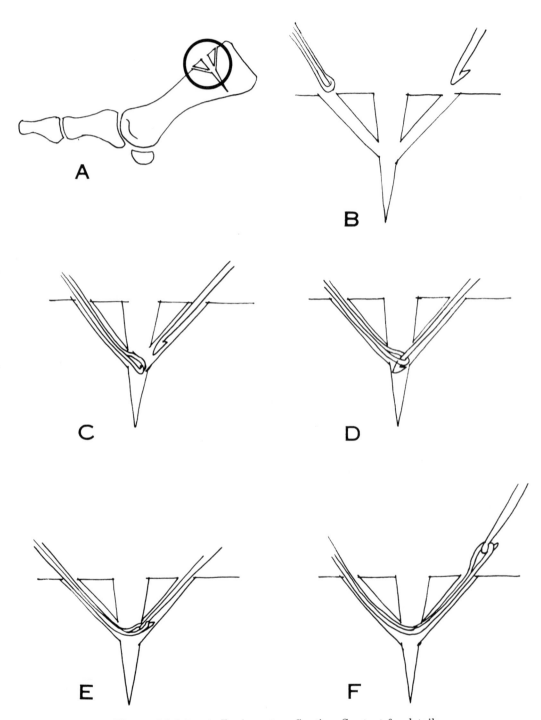

Figure 11.14.   *A–F*, wire suture fixation. See text for details.

oplasties, and other soft-tissue procedures would all be included but will not be discussed at length. Also included in this category are the partial metatarsal head resections, total metatarsal head resections (59), and plantar condylectomy. In these types of procedures, complications can be held to a minimum if there is limited injury to the capsule and associated tendons and collateral ligaments. Weinstock (31) accurately pointed out many of the post-surgical problems with these types of procedures. They were:

1. Metatarsophalangeal joint contraction;
2. Metatarsophalangeal joint subluxation;
3. Arthrodesis;
4. Pseudoarthrosis;
5. Transfer lesions.

As was stated earlier, proper evaluation and diagnosis are essential. McGlamry et al. (27) discussed the various clinical appearances of the lesser metatarsal-phalangeal joints when presented with a patient with a painful plantar keratotic lesion. Their paper included a proper discussion of the associated soft-tissue structures surrounding these joints and the biomechanics associated with the development of these deformities. The paper further discussed the objectives of surgical approach which would include:

—Establishment of proper length pattern without overshortening the bone;
—Proper alignment of the digit with the metatarsal shaft;
—Resection of any plantar hypertrophy of the metatarsal head(s);
—Meticulous preservation of the joint capsules and surrounding structures;
—Proper use of tenoplasties when indicated.

Complications of the partial or total metatarsal head resection have been discussed above, as well as in other articles or texts. It should be obvious that, whenever possible, one chooses a surgical procedure that does not result in joint destruction (Fig. 11.15).

We would like to briefly discuss the DuVries (2) procedure. Over the past decade, its use has been limited by the profession because of: 1) poor criteria and indi-

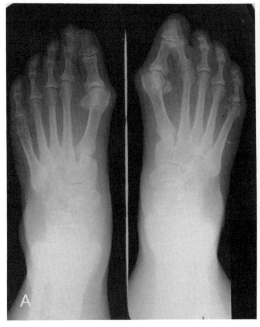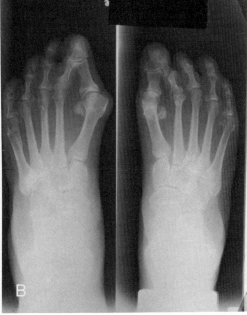

Figure 11.15. *A*, subluxation of the second MPJ right foot. *B*, post-operative partial metatarsal head resection of the second with resultant poor alignment, destruction of the joint, and instability.

cations for its use; 2) it is a less "dramatic" procedure than performing an osteotomy; and 3) poor results which may have been due to surgeon error rather than basic fault in the procedure. McGlamry et al. (28) pointed out that Giannestras had found satisfactory results in over 300 procedures performed in a 10-year period. They felt that the DuVries procedure was basically successful only when proper alignment of the toe was maintained post-operatively. Other authors, however, have reported varying complications with the DuVries procedure, including recurrence of the plantar keratotic lesion. Again, the above three factors cannot be discounted. McGlamry et al. (29) specifically discussed the use of DuVries plantar condylectomy procedure. They had used both an "H" and a "U" capsular incision in performing these procedures. They felt that the major complication or recurrence rate in utilizing this procedure fell in the areas of improper realignment of the toe at the metatarsophalangeal joint, as well as improper techniques in maintaining the digit in proper alignment for 6–8 weeks post-operatively. They recommended the use of a molded polyurethane retainer following healing of the surgical wound.

Two other factors must be discussed with regard to the plantar condylectomy procedure. It cannot be overemphasized that proper dissection is extremely essential in maintaining proper alignment of this joint post-operatively. This author has also seen numerous complications with this procedure which are iatrogenic in nature. Basically, if one properly evaluates the patient, clinically and radiographically, one sees that only a small portion of the plantar condyle needs to be removed parallel to the plantar surface (weightbearing surface) of the foot. However, in many cases, the surgeons become overexuberant and remove anywhere from one-third to one-half of the plantar aspect of the metatarsal head, leading to subluxations of the joint post-operatively, as well as a higher incidence of transfer lesions to other lesser metatarsals. In the Hatcher study (49), he showed a

success rate of partial metatarsal head resections of 64% which is greater than their overall average of 56.5% for all procedures performed in the lesser metatarsal area. Surgical procedures should not be abandoned or receive a "poor" reputation simply because of improper pre-operative evaluation or improper performance of the procedure itself.

Distal Metatarsal Osteotomy

OSTEOCLASIS

This is an intentional fracture to correct a deformity (51). Thomas (55) reported on a series of 39 pateints and 73 osteotomies. He osteotomized one or more metatarsal shafts of rheumatoid patients. Follow-ups ranged from 1 to 15 years and showed four failures, three of which were related to complicating circumstances, e.g., peripheral vascular disease.

Davidson (57, 58), like Thomas, recommended osteotomies of the shafts of the metatarsals. These procedures seem to fall into the classification of osteoclasis. Thomas accomplished his with an osteotome, while Davidson used a bone forceps. Davidson's goal was the relief of plantar keratosis. Thomas admitted "some incidence" of malunion but did not count it among post-operative complications. Davidson found that, of the more than 50 patients he osteotomized, pseudoarthrosis occurred in a "few" cases, but he expected that these would heal eventually (Fig. 11.16). Thomas stated that in four of his 73 osteotomies, a transfer of plantar pressure to the adjacent metatarsal head occurred, two of which were relieved by osteotomies. This technique has received some acceptance because of its simplicity and possible relief of the original lesion.

However, the lack of fixation brings about rapid and profuse callus formation. The less exposure used to incise the metatarsal shaft, the more it acts like a stress fracture. The adjacent tissues may support the position of the capital fragment and lessen the threat of pseudoarthrosis. How-

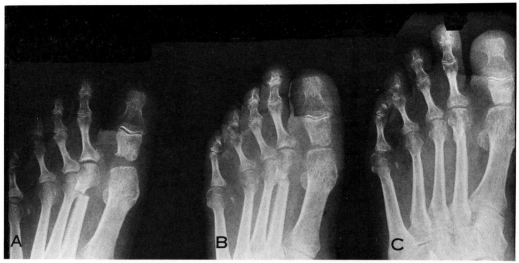

Figure 11.16. Osteoclasis of the second metatarsal. *A,* 3 weeks post-operative. *B,* 9 weeks post-operative. *C,* 14 weeks post-operative.

ever, the forces of contracted extensor tendons tend to displace the distal fragment.

The site of the osteoclasis dictates the degree of displacement. When the transection occurs proximal on the shaft in cortical bone, there is greater likelihood of displacement of the incised margin of the distal fragment, and the healing is slower (Fig. 11.17). In osteoclasis of cancellous bone precisely at the junction of the head and neck of the metatarsal, displacement will be limited by the intermetatarsal ligaments and capsule, and healing will be faster (Fig. 11.18).

Marked displacement often causes devitalization of the capital fragment. This may result in a prolonged recovery period, accompanied by tenderness on weightbearing, swelling, and delay in wearing conventional shoes. In some cases internal fixation with a K-wire can speed recovery.

Information is scant on the incidence of pseudoarthrosis following osteoclasis. Giannestras' study (71) of 776 patients who underwent a lineal osteotomy for shortening of a metatarsal for plantar keratomas showed that 18 (2.83%) resulted in nonunion; four were symptomatic and one required resection and bone grafting. Sgarlato (56) reports six non-unions in 400

metatarsal base-wedge osteotomies, a rate of 1.5%; all were asymptomatic.

The most frequent post-operative complications encountered with these distal procedures were pointed out by Weinstock (31). These are: 1) pseudoarthrosis; 2) rotation of the distal fragment; 3) non-union of the osteotomy site; 4) transfer lesions; and 5) excessive production of bony callus. Weinstock was discussing all forms of metatarsal osteotomies and their importance, in terms of location of osteotomies, i.e., distal, midshaft, or proximal. It should be pointed out that these complications deserve consideration when dealing with distal osteotomies.

COLLECTOMY

If nothing else, over the past decade, we should have learned not to be sold or convinced of the miracles and wonders of various procedures which have been developed with limited research and background. Whitney originated the prototype for the collectomy procedure in the 1960s. Levine (33) presented a paper which, once again, sold us on the belief of a simple procedure which brings almost "immediate relief" of symptoms and "long-term" comfort to the

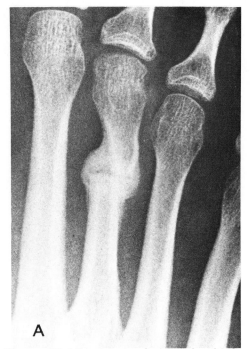
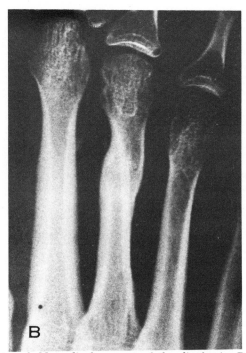

Figure 11.17. *A,* osteoclasis of the third metatarsal. Note displacement of the diaphysis. *B,* support of adjacent metatarsal promotes firm union.

patient. This particular procedure involved removal of a segment of cortical bone from a metatarsal shaft, deliberately not allowing for bony healing, and thus, allowing the distal metatarsal head to "float." The so-called long-term results of this study involved the presentation of three patients with a post-operative follow-up of 9–12 months. Certainly, this procedure did not result in positive results long-term, to the best of our knowledge. It is inadequate to assume that the "floating" of a metatarsal head to alleviate one problem somehow justifies either the pain that the patient may experience with a pseudoarthrosis, or the development of a transfer lesion to another metatarsal head, thus leading to further surgical intervention.

METAPHYSEAL OSTEOTOMIES

Literally, thousands of osteotomies of this nature, with varying shapes, have been attempted over the last several years, i.e., transverse, "V," arcuate (cresentic), etc. In

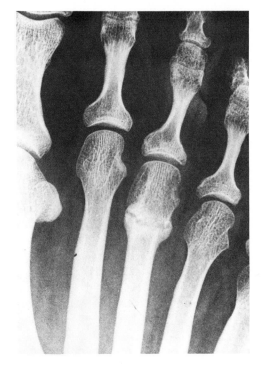

Figure 11.18. Osteoclasis of the third metatarsal at an ideal site.

the study by Hatcher et al., (49) two of the major complications were lack of toe purchase on the ground, which varied from approximately 45% in those cases of percutaneous metaphyseal osteotomy, 18–20% with distal metaphyseal osteotomies, and slightly over 50% with the distal "V" osteotomy; limitation of toe plantar flexion, which was slightly over 20% with the PMO, 15–16% in the DMO, and nearly 60% with the distal "V" osteotomy.

There are obvious basic deficiencies in a transverse metaphyseal osteotomy or realignment of the distal fragment to relieve the plantar keratotic lesion. By its very nature of being a straight, transverse, through-and-through cut, without proper immobilization and fixation, there can be the development of dislocation, pseudoarthrosis, and axial rotation of the distal fragment in the frontal plane. Depending upon the location of the osteotomy, aseptic necrosis is also a potential complication. This can be seen in Figure 11.19. The osteotomy may be performed too far distally, which would result in improper angulation as seen in the second metatarsophalangeal joint, as well as pseudoarthrosis in the third metatarsophalangeal joint bilaterally. The third metatarsal head in the right foot, because of the severe distal location of the osteotomy, may also result in aseptic necrosis of the distal fragment due to disruption of the metaphyseal vessel.

Unfortunately, the continued popular mode of treatment involves limited immobilization both internally and externally of the affected foot after performing a distal metaphyseal osteotomy. We have mentioned previously, on several occasions, the possibility of pseudoarthrosis which may be seen in Figure 11.20. It should also be noted that there can be the development of an excessive amount of bony callus which may complicate the post-operative symptomatology of the patient (Fig. 11.21). However, in this last case, there was a resection of the fibrous material with no further immobilization or fixation, resulting in a "free-floating" metatarsal head, increasing the chances of a transfer lesion. When performing reconstructive surgery for a non-union or pseudoarthrosis, the surgeon should keep in mind the various forms of fixation, as well as excision of the fibrotic material. Later in this chapter, we will discuss some various forms of fixating devices, but it would be important at this time to note that another form of fixation would be the use of an advancement cortical graft across the non-union area for stabilization and then the use of internal and external immobilization. One might also be able to use cortical freeze-dried bone for this purpose, in order to provide a scaffolding in an attempt to assure proper union. Perhaps such unfortuante consequences could be avoided if proper internal and external fixation were implemented, as can be seen in Figure 11.22. As pointed out by Weinstock (31), the osteotomy site can also be made proximal in the anatomical neck, thus leading to delayed or non-union with excessive bony callus formation, because the osteotomy site was performed in cortical bone. There may also be displacement, as shown in Figure 11.23. When such a serious complication occurs and is identified, the patient should be so informed and proper internal fixation with external immobilization applied, resulting in the avoidance of a potentially serious complication. This can be seen in Figure 11.24 of the same patient. Inner stability can be obtained when using an angulated type of distal osteotomy, such as the "V," since this can help prevent frontal plane rotation, as well as potential subluxation. However, it does not necessarily avoid the possibility of overabundant callus formation, delayed union, or non-union. Such complications can be seen in Figure 11.25 where there is not only displacement of the distal segment of the second metatarsal head left foot, but also, overexuberant callus formation of the second metatarsal osteotomy of the right foot; and in both areas, delayed union or non-union is possible, although it would be more probable in the left foot if this unfortunate subluxation was not corrected.

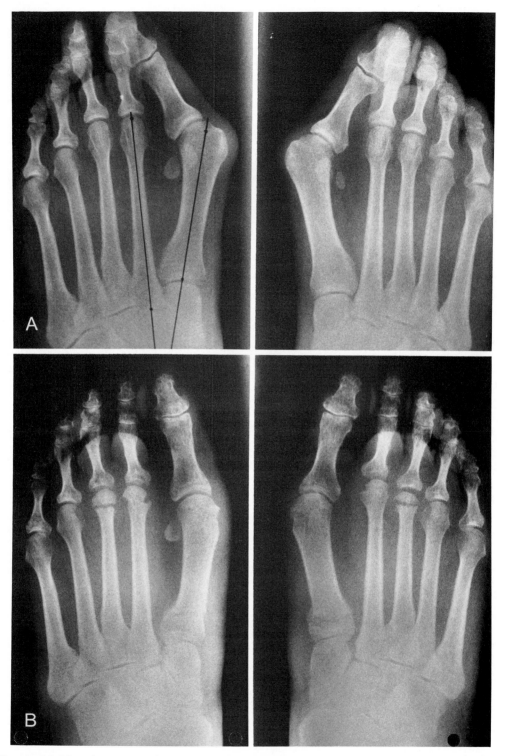

Figure 11.19. *A,* pre-operative x-ray. *B,* post-operative x-ray with angular displacement of the second metatarsal left; possible necrosis of the distal fragment of the third metatarsal right due to too far anterior placement of the osteotomy.

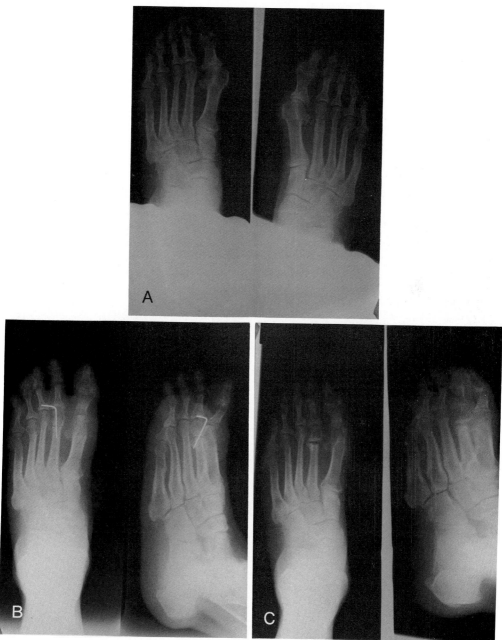

Figure 11.20. *A,* pre-operative x-ray with painful lesion beneath the second metatarsal-phalangeal joint of the left foot. *B,* immediate post-operative x-ray showing single K-wire and osteotomy at the anatomical neck. No plaster immobilization was used and the patient was allowed to ambulate. *C,* post-operative x-ray with delayed union due to inadequate fixation and immobilization.

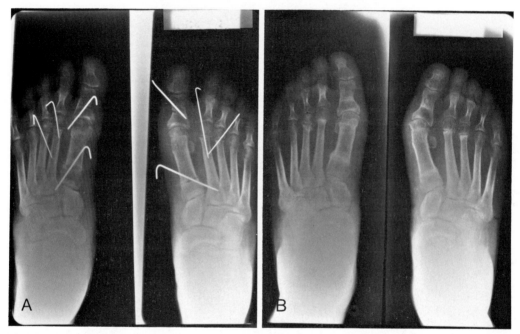

Figure 11.21. *A*, post-operative x-ray of multiple distal metaphyseal osteotomies bilaterally. *B*, 12 months post-operative nonunion with possible instability of the distal metatarsal fragment.

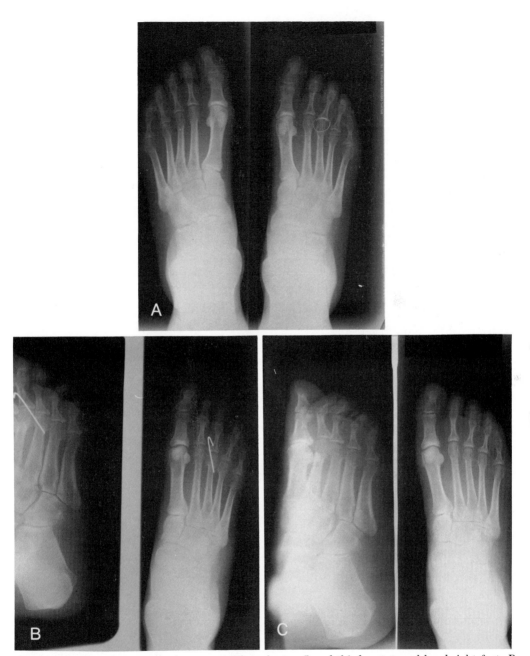

Figure 11.22. *A*, pre-operative x-ray with a plantar-flexed third metatarsal head right foot. *B*, one technique using K-wires with proper stabilization of the osteotomy sites. *C*, 12 months post-operative x-ray shows stable, healed osteotomy site.

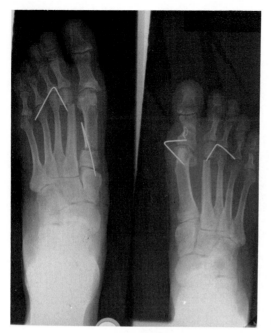

Figure 11.23. Post-operative x-ray showing displacement of the lesser metatarsal osteotomy.

Graver (34) presented a preliminary report on the reverse "V" osteotomy, but this was nothing more than a preliminary description of a procedure and does not lend itself to proper scientific analysis since there was limited follow-up. Hatcher et al. (49) reported a 66% acceptable result rate with the "V" osteotomy. An unfortunate consequence of this type of osteotomy appears to be the 50–55% occurrence of lack of toe purchase on stance, as well as an almost 60% incidence of limitation of plantar flexion of the digits post-operatively. The importance of this unfortunate and preventable type of surgical complication was stressed by Fenton and Butlin (36) in their article showing the necessity of reconstructive surgery following displacement of distal "V" osteotomies of the second and third metatarsals. They had to perform reconstructive surgery with proper fixation and immobilization.

Evaluation of Figure 11.26, including the pre- and post-operative and follow-up x-rays of this patient, could point out the inherent dangers of cortical osteotomy. Again, Weinstock (31) pointed out the in-

herent risks, prolonged healing, and high potential for delayed or non-union of this type of osteotomy. If it is the surgeon's choice to use such procedures, or angular or transpositional correction, then proper fixation devices should be applied and proper post-operative immobilization utilized (Figs. 11.27 and 11.28).

A more recent type of osteotomy has been the angulated osteotomy to correct lesions associated with the fifth metatarsal head or congenital varus angulation of the fifth metatarsal. Without the appropriate amount of intra-operative and post-operative treatment, dislocation of the distal fragment appears to be a common undesirable side effect. When such a complication is seen, immediate corrective measures are necessary, including attempts at closed reduction, but more than likely, open reduction with fixation will be necessary to obtain the desired clinical results. During the post-operative period, one should take note of serial x-ray examinations to be sure that

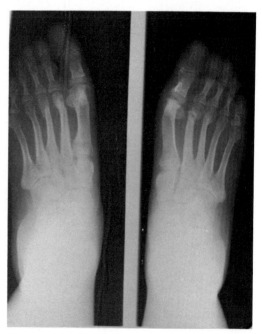

Figure 11.24. Patient seen in Figure 11.23 after a K-wire fixation and proper immobilization which resulted in proper healing and alignment (2 years post-op after further reconstructive surgery).

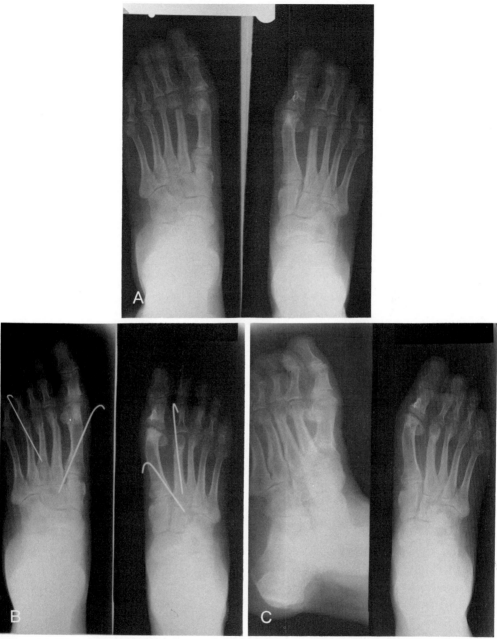

Figure 11.25. *A,* post-operative x-ray of an attempted distal metaphyseal "V" osteotomy second metatarsal head right. *B,* painful nonunion resulted and corrective reconstruction was undertaken with K-wire fixation and immobilization. *C,* post-operative distal "V" osteotomy of the second metatarsal right after reconstruction. However, excessive shortening can lead to lateral symptomotology. Note poor alignment of first metatarsal-phalangeal joint with prosthesis.

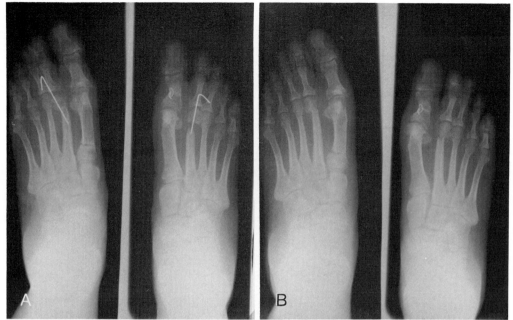

Figure 11.26. *A,* post-operative x-ray demonstrates poor alignment (*left*) and inadequate alignment (*right*). *B,* post-operative x-ray with malalignment left, and nonunion right.

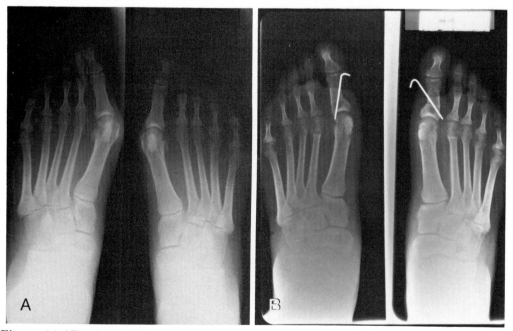

Figure 11.27. *A,* pre-operative x-ray. *B,* post-operative x-ray with apparent proper alignment of second metatarsal right but inadequate alignment of second metatarsal left which could lead to delayed union or nonunion. No form of fixation or immobilization was utilized.

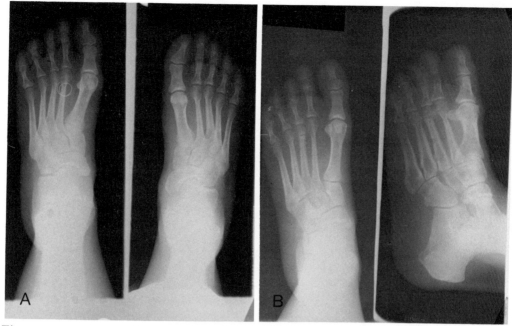

Figure 11.28. *A,* pre-operative x-ray. Accuracy of marker placement cannot be verified. *B,* post-operative x-ray showing delayed union of third metatarsal distal osteotomy (6 months post-op), and apparent discrepency with pre-operative x-ray which was under the second metatarsal.

the osseous structures are in their proper alignment and show proper osseous healing before the removal of any internal or external fixation, and the elimination of any external immobilization. Again, complications involving separation, displacement, or malalignment need to be treated as quickly as possible to avoid any unwarranted complications. Unfortunately, there has been recent discussion about the time frame for bone healing. In such cases, the practitioner did not inform the patient of the potential risks of future intervention. Such a delay in communication or not properly informing the patient of an unwarranted complication can lead to disruption of the doctor-patient relationship.

The same type of hazard can be seen with closing wedge osteotomy of the fifth metatarsal to reduce a varus alignment without the appropriate intra- and post-operative immobilization.

Buchbinder (52) reported on a 3-year series of 38 procedures with good to excellent results in 79% of the cases. His procedures involve the resurgent use of the DRATO procedure for Tailor's bunions. He utilized 25-gauge monofilament wire with a transverse through-and-through fixation and no form of external immobilization utilized other than that of a surgical shoe. In one case, where the patient traumatized the foot 3 weeks post-operatively, there was an apparent delayed union, but eventually went on to proper union after the patient was placed in cast immobilization. In the patients classified as poor results (8%), recurrence of lesion, transfer of lesion, delayed bony union, or painful union at the operative site occurred.

Proximal Metatarsal Osteotomy

Some practitioners have chosen to use proximal osteotomies of the metatarsals to alleviate a plantar keratotic lesion beneath one or more of the lesser metatarsals heads. These procedures include: 1) an extensor osteotomy (EO) which is a dorsiflexory base-wedge osteotomy; or 2) an extensor osteoarthrotomy (EOA) which involves the removal and destruction of the metatarsal cuneiform or cuboid articulation with subsequent dorsiflexion of the metatarsal and fusion. Again, Hatcher et al. (49) showed an acceptable result with the EO procedure of about 50%, and 33% acceptable result with the EOA.

A common complication of proximal metatarsal osteotomies is dorsal angulation (Fig. 11.29). Immediate post-operative radiographs should be taken to discover this, and repositioning and fixation should be affected. When poor position is discovered early enough (1 week), it is possible to pass a Kirschner wire through the metatarsal to achieve internal fixation.

If the cast is not used for a sufficient length of time in older patients, and the presence of external callus is not confirmed, dorsal angulation can occur even though the osteotomy seems to be clinically stable.

When adductory or abductory osteotomies are being done, it is vital that the cuts be made perpendicular to the long axis of the bone; otherwise, the wedge may be smaller at the inferior surface than the dorsum, so that when the osteotomy is closed, the bone becomes dorsally angulated as well as abducted or adducted.

Over the years, one of the major technical complications with the EOA is that the surgeons remove a wedge section of bone. Experience has shown us that by simply removing the articulating surfaces, which are in juxtaposition, provides adequate space, so that when distal plantar pressure is placed on the metatarsal head, that elevation can be obtained to allow for proper fixation and hopefully, that there will not be an overcorrection of the problem. Adequate fixation of an EO procedure can be obtained by the use of threaded or unthreaded K-wires, as can be seen in Figure 11.30. Care should be taken, however, to be sure that the osteotomy site is in the can-

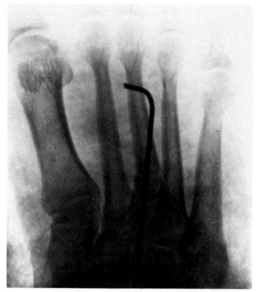

Figure 11.30. Post-operative x-ray of EO procedure in the third metatarsal with proper K-wire fixation. Osteotomy may be too far distal since it is in cortical bone and may result in delayed healing.

cellous bone of the base of the metatarsal and not in the cortical bone which possibly could delay healing. Another precaution was pointed out by Reinherz and Toren (37) with regard to the bone healing following adjacent metatarsal osteotomies. They reviewed the post-operative progress of 32 patients who had simultaneous adjacent metatarsal osteotomies, and their conclusion showed excessive post-operative swelling and excessive bony callus formation when osteotomies of the same type were performed on adjacent metatarsals. If, however, there were lesions beneath adjacent metatarsals and one osteotomy was performed at the base and the other one distally, the amount of post-operative edema and bony callus was reduced considerably. This is certainly an important consideration when dealing with multiple metatarsal osteotomies. When confronted with congenital deformities, such as an unresolved metatarsus adductus, in the adolescent or adult patient requiring multiple metatarsal osteotomies, it is essential that proper fixation and immobilization procedures be followed (Fig. 11.31). If the surgeon does not

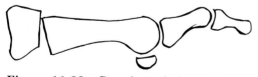

Figure 11.29. Dorsal angulation of the osteotomy site is a possible complication.

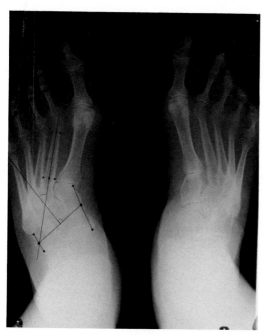

Figure 11.31. Pre-operative x-ray of an adult (untreated) metatarsus adductus requiring a Gartland-Berman procedure at a later date.

properly fixate the metatarsals, there may be subluxation at the osteotomy site which can lead to further complications, such as delayed union or nonunion, pain, or the development of further forefoot abnormalities in the future.

Finally, with regard to all types of metatarsal osteotomies, we would be remiss without a brief discussion or mention of the possibility or consideration of shortening following osteotomy procedures. Zlotoff (60), and then Schweitzer et al. (38), discussed the various angles and considerations, as well as the degree of metatarsal shortening following osteotomies. Let it be noted in their 1982 study that, with regard to distal osteotomy, there was an average shortening of 0.208 cm with "V" osteotomies, less shortening with distal and percutaneous metaphyseal osteotomies, but the least shortening occurred with the arcuate (cresentic), amounting to 0.15 cm. The greatest amount of shortening occurred with osteoclasis procedures, amounting to 0.33 cm. With regard to dorsiflexory wedge proximal osteotomies, there

was an average shortening of 0.20 cm. An important point in their discussion was the use of power equipment and the sharpness of the bars and blades which could result in bone burns and, thus, necrosis with additional shortening of the metatarsal. One should always take into account the pre-operative and biomechanical considerations to prevent excessive shortening, which lead to the development of further deformity in adjacent areas. The expertise of the surgeon performing the procedure cannot be discounted.

Pan-Metatarsal Head Resection

There are varying metabolic diseases which can result in the destructive process of the metatarsophalangeal joints of the feet. We shall now consider various aspects of these particular problems and hope to suggest ways of avoiding complications.

Healing of Incision

Wound dehiscence or slough may result from rough tissue handling. The use of Alis forceps for retraction is discouraged. Skin should not be reflected until the depth of the dorsal venous arch is reached. The skin flap should be hydrated with saline solution. Simple interrupted sutures are advised, as well as the elimination of traction resulting from plantar flexion. The choice of suture material has not been shown to be an important factor in the breakdown of wounds.

Vascular Impairment

Evidence of gross vascular impairment to the digits is not consistently seen in the rheumatoid patient. The actual grade of circulation in such patients always seems surprisingly good.

Persistent Post-operative Edema

This occurs irregularly and, in spite of occasional long-term persistence, it generally does not pose a problem to the patient. When it becomes a complication, the general disease state is apparently the cause.

ACTH, 80 units intramuscularly, helps to relieve the symptoms.

Digital Instability

Immediately following pan-metatarsal head resection, there is a definite flaccidity of the digits. This improves in 1–3 months, with most patients actively extending their toes within 3 months.

Contracture of Digits with Foreshortening of Foot

There is a definite fore-shortening of the distal segment on the remaining metatarsal stumps, depending on the amount of bony resection. If only the metatarsal heads are resected, this contracture is kept to a minimum.

Digital Deformities

Hammering usually does not recur. Transverse plane abnormalities improve with time.

Persistence of Deformity, Plantar Prominence, Keratosis, or Pain

Reduction of the deformity should be obvious at the time of surgery, with elimination of the plantar prominence accomplished immediately following resection of the corresponding metatarsal head and confirmed by digital palpatation of the plantar area. Keratotic formation and/or ulceration is rarely evident past the 3rd or 4th week. Persistence of pain has been seen on occasion, especially if moderate to marked edema has occurred. There is concurrent relief of pain with relief of the edema.

Recurrence of deformity, plantar prominence, callosity, or pain has not been observed past the first 3 months post-operatively.

Fitting and Use of Shoe Styles

The patient will usually return to the style and type of shoe that he or she favors. In severe cases of active rheumatoid arthritis in the midtarsal areas, the patient must be given advice as to the choice of proper footgear.

Management of Edema

Edema is present most often following surgery, within 7–30 days.

The three basic forms of treatment are physical therapy, bandaging and splinting, and medication.

PHYSICAL THERAPY TECHNIQUES

Topical Heat and Cold

It is accepted practice to prescribe the application of ice packs to the foot and ankle for periods ranging from 20–30 minutes during the day, to constant use. The application of ice packs for approximately 24 hours, followed by a switch to heat, is recommended. Hot packs or towels, a heat lamp, light cradle, and electric pads can be used.

Elevation

Elevating the extremity above the pelvic level is extremely important and should be done immediately. Repetition as often as possible during the rehabilitation period is imperative.

Hydrotherapy

Hot and cold hydrotherapy has been used extensively for 25 years, but its specific value is now questioned. Used two or three times daily, it may have some impact, but its indication at intervals of 2–5 days should be re-evaluated.

BANDAGING AND SPLINTING

Compression Bandages

Application of a compression bandage has great value. Elastoplast® is recommended.

Flexible Casting

Gauztex® stripping makes a useful and simple splinting device that is easily applied. It is particularly helpful after the initial union of the incision.

Rigid Casting

The wooden sole shoe is popular when immobilization is desired, but its use in the management of post-operative edema has not been fully substantiated.

Casting

Plaster bandages have innumerable applications and are quite acceptable. The restrictions on ambulation are often favorable to the inhibition of edema.

Urethane Molds

McGlamry and Kitting (30) have used polyurethane foam molds that are generally applied about 2–3 weeks after surgery. After the polyurethane is molded to the required shape and density, it is impregnated with a synthetic latex and sealed under shoe pressure for at least 6 hours.

Adhesive Splinting

A Band-Aid® or Elastoplast® applied to the digit, particularly the fifth toe, with mild to moderate pressure, helps to prevent the accumulation of fluids in the tissues. This can be pursued as needed.

INTERNAL MEDICATION

Enzymes

Enzymes are questionably recommended, particularly in those patients whose history indicates that edema will be a problem. The enzyme is most effective when it is prescribed at least 1 day pre-operatively and then for about 21 days post-operatively.

Diuretics

Patients with a history of edematous extremities are usually taking diuretics. If not, such therapy should be considered along with other methods of control.

In quite severe cases, when there is associated local inflammation, phenylbuta-

zone, although not specifically indicated for post-operative use, can be very effective.

The most commonly used procedures for multiple joint pains in the metatarsophalangeal joint areas involving metabolic disease, such as rheumatoid arthritis, osteoarthritis, or psoriatic arthritis, has involved the Hoffman or Clayton procedures (40, 41, 61). Brattström and Brattström (39) demonstrated the use of total head resections involving one or two metatarsals and then compared that with head resections involving the second through fourth and then the second through fifth. In their study involving 138 feet, there was a statistically higher percentage of excellent to good results when performing joint resections of the second through fifth metatarsals, including, in some cases, resections of the base of the digits (which I personally do not recommend). They also performed plantar incisional approaches in some of these cases, resulting in some skin necrosis or infection, but there was no delay in healing time. In their series of 138 feet, only one patient complained of scar pain when a plantar incision was used. Barton (42) did a retrospective analysis of forefoot reconstruction using varying techniques. He described a slightly less than 50% complication rate which included failure of primary wound healing, edema, hypesthesia of a digit or digits, plantar pain, and vein thrombosis. The failure of primary wound healing occurred in over 25% of those cases where a plantar incision was utilized, but a similar complication, when seen in dorsal incisions, was only viewed in approximately 20% of the cases. Due to the fact that the majority of these procedures are joint-destructive in nature, a review of several studies shows that the patient may actually have an increase in pain following the surgical procedure. This complication appears in a small percentage of cases and is due to the extent of trauma, and the manner in which the tissues were handled by the surgeon. In reviewing all of the results of Clayton (40), 63 out of 65 patients revealed that they were satisfied with the results. When the standard Clayton procedure is performed, without any adjunct procedure, instability of the digits is seen with subluxation or luxation at the remaining metatarsal-phalangeal joints, which can cause some future problems to the patient, as well as unsatisfactory cosmetic appearance of the foot. If only one foot is operated on, then the shortening that occurs in the operated foot may also present a problem in the future in the proper fitting of shoes.

Faithful and Savill (43) reported on 77 patients with forefoot reconstruction with a follow-up of from 2 months to 5 years (average, 2.2 years). Their complications included the development of hematoma in three feet, wound infection in seven, and delayed wound closure in seven. Overall, they reported a success rate of 80% where symptoms had been abolished and the patients were allowed to wear normal shoes without pain. In the discussion area of their paper, it was also noted that less positive results may be obtained in patients suffering from psoriatic arthritis.

Finally, MacClean and Silver (53) described the Dwyer procedure with forefoot reconstruction. His procedure resects the metatarsal heads of the lesser metatarsal-phalangeal joints and then uses a Kirschner wire fixation through the digit which is then retrograded into the metatarsal for proper realignment of the toe. He recorded a success rate of excellent to good results at 76%. The complications included two wound infections, four wound hematomas, one failed arthrodesis, one migration of the K-wire, one pin-tract drainage, one severance of a digital nerve, and one pulmonary embolism. There continues to be the debate in regard to surgical approach for these patients as to whether there should be a plantar approach, multiple linear incisions on the dorsum, or a transverse incisional approach. The latter can lead to several complications if the surgeon is not careful after his initial incision to preserve the linearly aligned neurovascular structures. Furthermore, if there is severe contraction and luxation at the metatarsal-phalangeal joints without considerable removal of bone, thus allowing a shortening, it may be

difficult to primarily close a transverse incision. Another consideration would be the use of one or two Z-plasty skin incisions on the dorsum of the foot to help alleviate the dermal contractions. Again, however, one must take careful note of the neurovascular structures, as well as careful underscoring of the skin flaps to avoid slough of these areas post-operatively.

Brachymetatarsia

On occasion, patients may present with a shortened, generally singular, lesser metatarsal. This may be due to congenital deformity or from iatrogenic complications from previous surgery. Due to abnormal weightbearing on the remaining metatarsals or a change in the biomechanics of the forefoot, reconstructive surgery may be necessary. McGlamry and Copper (44) reported on the surgical treatment for congenital brachymetatarsia. Kite previously theorized that this shortening was due to premature fusion at the epiphyseal line at the distal end of the metatarsal and occurred more often in the fourth metatarsal. It is important to note that when performing these procedures, intrinsic muscle resection may be necessary to allow for the proper lengthening. McGlamry and Cooper (44) utilized cortical bone graft with insertion of a Kirschner wire for fixation of the full length of the metatarsal. It may also be necessary to provide digital traction post-operatively to alleviate stress at the metatarsophalangeal joint following these lengthening procedures. The surgeon is cautioned in these cases to evaluate the patients properly to avoid necrosis and/or gangrene of the distal tissues, including the digit, since by lengthening, the neurovascular structures are stretched (Fig. 11.32). Such a complication was pointed out by Weisfeld and Kaplan (45) when reducing a zygodactylism brachymetatarsia. They also showed, however, that with careful observation and local treatment, a catastrophic complication can be avoided, and in the one case they presented, amputation of the affected digit was avoided. Again, through

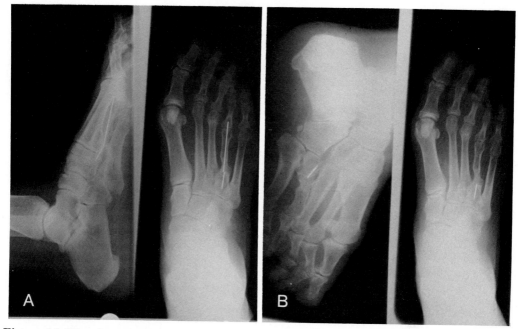

Figure 11.32. *A,* post-operative x-ray of attempted bone graft to reduce a congenital bradyme-tatarsia of fourth metatarsal right. The K-wire used was too small a diameter and placed at an improper angle resulting in breakage. *B,* bone graft appears to have healed well but broken wire is buried in proximal aspect of fourth metatarsal. As long as patient remains asymptomatic the wire need not be retrieved.

proper immobilization and fixation, autogenous bone grafts provide the most successful results in these types of cases, with delayed union and nonunion being the number one potential complicating factor along with neurovascular embarrassment.

Nonunions

Throughout this section we have constantly reminded the reader of the problems encountered with delayed unions and nonunions of metatarsal osteotomies. Proper fixation and immobilization cannot be overemphasized. Russell (46) discussed the use of compression bone plates and bone grafting following nonunion of metatarsal osteotomies. Walter and Pressman (47) further discussed this area of metatarsal nonunions and the use of an external fixation device for compression. Proper excision of the fibrous tissue in the distal and proximal segments of the metatarsal nonunion is of major importance. Depending upon the length pattern of the involved

metatarsal, bone grafting may be necessary, whether it is autogenous or homogenous. The use of internal or external fixation devices to obtain adequate compression and relief of the nonunion is dependant on the surgeon's expertise and experience. The use of internally placed electrodes to alleviate an identifiable nonunion has become a new mode of therapy over the past several years. This appears to have some positive ramifications for the future, but as yet the data is not complete.

Fractures

For the most part, fractures of the digits and the forefoot, including the metatarsal area, have not received the same type of long-term study and follow-up as have fractures in other areas of the body. It is not uncommon to see patients who have received insufficient treatment following forefoot fractures, since somehow the feeling is that forefoot fractures are not "important" or will not cause the patient permanent disability if treated at a limited level. An interesting closed reduction technique, suggested by Pritsch et al. (48) was formulated using K-wires for manipulation and external fixation of metacarpal fractures. While this has, to our knowledge, not been attempted to metatarsal fractures, it certainly is an interesting approach which could lead to less complications when dealing with noncomminuted fractures of the metatarsals. When one is presented with a comminuted fracture, as is seen in Figure 11.32, open reduction and proper fixation is recommended to avoid further complications, especially since we are dealing with the organ of the body that is the most important in locomotion and weightbearing. The usual complications following open reduction of fractures would include the careful observation and prevention of: 1) infection; 2) hematoma; 3) delayed union; 4) nonunion; and 5) thrombosis or embolism following prolonged nonweightbearing while the patient is in bed. One should be concerned about the possibility of thromboembolic disease following a comminuted fracture and an open reduction in an otherwise healthy patient or in one who has shown higher risk to the development of a complication. Then, use of subcutaneous heparin t.i.d. or q.i.d. in the hospital may be considered for prophylactic reasons.

Prosthetics

The entire subject of prosthetics has been covered very adequately in another chapter of this text. One would be remiss without a brief discussion or mention of this area in regard to lesser metatarsal surgery. It must always be remembered, that insertion of a prosthetic device at the metatarsal-phalangeal joint is a joint-destructive procedure and without proper analysis of the biochemical effects during the pre-operative period, as well as the potential hazards post-operatively, patients may be less than happy with their surgical results. Such an example is seen in Figure 11.33. Incomplete healing of the second metatarsophalangeal joint is seen, a radical resection has been performed, and insertion of a hinged im-

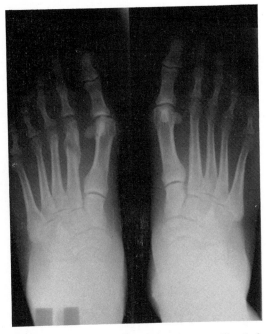

Figure 11.33. Pre-operative x-ray of healed oblique fracture second metatarsal left with incomplete reorganization.

plant has been improperly inserted (Fig. 11.34). Stability of this joint is extremely questionable and a dislocation of the implant is highly likely. Furthermore, there will be drastic changes in the biomechanical function of this forefoot resulting in transfer lesions, and perhaps, luxation of the adjacent metatarsophalangeal joints with the unfortunate consequence of further utilization of prosthetic implants.

In conclusion, it should be obvious through the review of this particular section that a great deal of scientific research continues to be needed when dealing with lesser metatarsal surgery. We need further quality studies and research over the long term to be able to clarify and present appropriate criteria for these various procedures. The success or failure rate should be based on reproducible, positive results that alleviate pain and symptoms.

HALLUX ABDUCTO VALGUS
Basic Principles

The amount of data available regarding hallux abducto valgus is voluminous.

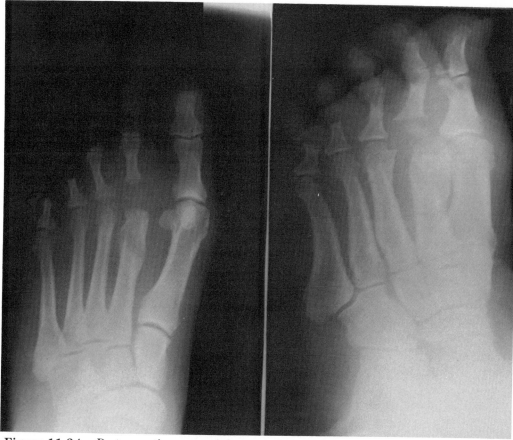

Figure 11.34. Post-operative x-ray of the same patient in Figure 11.33 showing inappropriate placement of prosthetic implant and overresection of bone.

Scores of articles have been written, both nationally and internationally. No single entity in foot surgery over the decades has had more opinions expressed, with variations on etiology and surgical procedural approaches. Discussion of the various contemporary procedures and their complications will hopefully alleviate some of the confusion regarding certain surgical approaches. It is not our intent in this section to discuss in detail the important criteria which must be utilized before attempting any one of the 75 to 100 various bunion procedures (68, 71). We will, however, interject a discussion of the important criteria when discussing the complications, for it is only then that we can hope to alleviate some of the continued misunderstandings of this deformity, and hopefully understand the approaches which will lead to higher rates and degrees of success (67).

While the orthopedic community continues to reject the concept, there is vast evidence which clearly proves that the primary etiological factor in the formation of the hallux abducto valgus deformity in human beings is directly related to the biomechanical malfunction of the foot, primarily associated with the pronation syndrome. The understanding of the normal and abnormal mechanics is not within the scope of this particular chapter, but has been covered very adequately by other authors, including Root et al. (62). In spite of their work, myths and inaccurate information abound in the literature. As late as 1981 (63), several noted authors continue to express the idea that shoe gear is the primary etiological factor in hallux abducto valgus deformity. It must be stressed that shoes are a contributing factor, but certainly not a primary one.

We would urge the formulation of sound criteria before any bunion procedure is contemplated and to avoid performance of individual or new procedures. Without criteria, the confusion will continue ad infinatum when dealing with this perplexing problem. The reason that the basic problem is so complex is because there are so many variables in terms of foot type, joint type, length patterns, degrees of deviation or subluxation, frontal plane axial rotation, angular variations, etc. Gerbert and Sokoloff (180) in their recent textbook adequately discussed the various pre-operative clinical and radiographic considerations which are essential in evaluating patients with a hallux abducto valgus deformity.

Frankel (70) emphasized the importance of determining whether the deformity was one of a structural or positional nature. Strong emphasis must be placed on his basic discussion since an error in judgement or evaluation as to whether a deformity is structural or positional will lead to failure of the procedure and an unsatisfactory clinical result.

Based on clinical observation over the past decade, as well as the study done by Schuberth et al. (73), in most cases it is unnecessary to do a lengthening of the extensor hallucis longus tendon. It appears that this does not have the bow string pathological effect on the hallux as has been described over the past several decades. Many surgeons do not properly evaluate their patients pre-operatively and, therefore, determine that an EHL tendon lengthening is necessary. During surgery with a tourniquet applied around a leg or ankle and the foot in an equinus position, an apparent "contraction" of the EHL tendon can occur. Since this study demonstrated that there is apparently no bow string effect, lengthening the tendon on a routine basis should now be called into question. During surgery, if one simply places the foot in a simulated weightbearing position, rarely does one observe a contraction of the EHL tendon. Also, if one is concerned about any lateral deviation of the EHL tendon during the time of closure, part of that closure should include sutures through the tendon sheath, but not through the tendon, so as to place the tendon in a more dorsal position post-operatively.

Another area of controversy involves the first metatarsal sesamoids. The current criteria utilizes the position of the medial sesamoid to help determine the degree of displacement. It has been noted by several authors that removal or excision of the medial seasamoid without proper coaptation of the medial head of the flexor hallucis brevis tendon can lead to a HAV deformity. However, Inge (74) reported on two cases examined in New York with congenital absence of a medial sesamoid with no apparent weakness or deformity. One can only assume that while the sesamoid was absent, the medial head of the flexor hallucis tendon was intact and functioning normally. The greatest area of controversy, of course, revolves around the lateral sesamoid and whether it should be excised during a bunionectomy procedure. McGlamry (75) gives us a detailed anatomical discussion and first MPJ function in relation to the sesamoid. He also discusses special surgical considerations and how one can avoid complications. We shall discuss the various complications that can occur with various procedures, whether the lateral sesamoid is excised or is allowed to remain intact. In this day and age, it needs to be only mentioned as a reminder that excision of both sesamoids should be avoided, unless dealing with some invasive tumorous mass, gross infection, or gangrene, in order to avoid the hallux flexus or hammertoe deformity of the hallux.

Lawton and Evans (76) described a capsular tendon balance bunionectomy, pointing out that only a limited resection of the first metatarsal head is necessary to help reduce the deformity. One can only hope that the time has finally passed when surgeons continue to use the so-called "sagittal groove" as a landmark for resection of the medial and dorsal medial aspect of the first metatarsal head. In many instances, if that landmark is utilized, anywhere from one-third to one-half of the first metatarsal head will be resected, then that does not provide an adequate surface for re-articulation with the base of the proximal phalanx, as is seen in Figure 11.35. This has been described as "stacking" of the first metatarsal head which leads to crepitation, pain, limitation of motion, and either the increased potential for recurrence of the initial deformity or the development of a hallux varus. Another example of excess bone resection of the first metatarsal head with limited reduction in hallux position can be seen in Figure 11.36. We present here in Figures 11.37, 11.38, and 11.39 the appropriate post-operative appearance of the first metatarsal phalangeal joint in relation to the articulating surfaces of the head of the first metatarsal and base of the proximal phalanx.

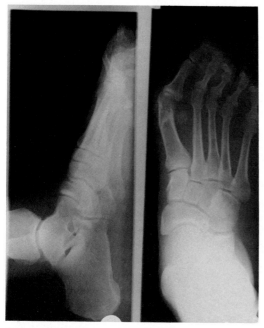

Figure 11.35. Post-operative x-rays demonstrating excessive removal of the medial aspect of the first metatarsal head which can lead to first metatarsal-phalangeal joint instability and a hallux adductus, or, as in this case, a recurrent HAV.

Joint Destructive Procedures (Arthroplasties)

Over 110 years ago, Hueter (149) described a procedure which excised the first metatarsal head in order to correct a hallux abducto valgus deformity. This procedure was later modified by Mayo and is commonly referred to now as the Mayo procedure (81, 112) (Fig. 11.40). Mayo (81) reported on 65 cases over an 8-year period with no discussion of any post-operative complications at that time. Rix (175) modified the Mayo procedure by using a capsular intra-articular flap which was based on the metatarsal rather than on the phalanx. He also transposed the abductor hallucis tendon, occasionally, more dorsally on the base of the proximal phalanx. He reported on 96 feet in 65 patients over a 15-year period (1951 to 1966). His post-operative follow-up involved 38 patients (59 feet) with an average follow-up of 6.5 years. Excellent results were seen in 17% of the patients. Good results were obtained in 61% with post-operative HAV less than 15°. In 22% there were fair results with slight recurrence which did not occur when the abductor hallucis was transposed (14 patients, 17 feet). In 6.8% of the patients occasional pain was experienced in the first MPJ. Average dorsiflexion post-operatively was 60° with no extension deformities. Post-operative lateral metatarsalgia occurred in 26% of the patients requiring further surgery or "arch supports."

Geldwert and Gibbons (80) reported a 7-year follow-up study on the Mayo procedure with their own personal modifications. They reported five major complications with this procedure, the first being the development of a plantar keratotic lesion beneath one or several of the lesser metatarsal heads. Secondly, they observed weak flexor power of the first MPJ. Thirdly, due to reactive fibrosis, there is a limitation of joint motion at the first MPJ. Fourthly, in some cases, patients developed a hallux elevatus. And lastly, other patients developed a hammertoe deformity of the hallux post-operatively. In their study, 45% of the pa-

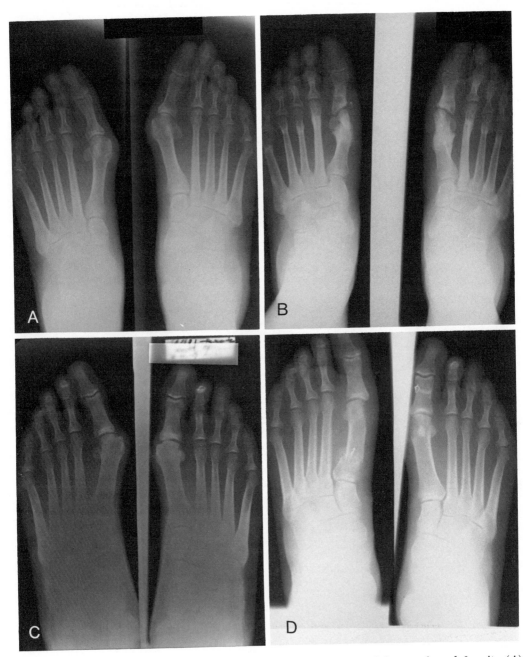

Figure 11.36. Case 1: Pre-operative x-ray demonstrating hallux abducto valgus deformity (A) and excessive removal of the medial eminence from the first metatarsal head with a Mitchell osteotomy, resulting in "stacking" with potential instability of first metatarsophalangeal joint (B). Case 2: Pre-operative x-ray with bilateral HAV (C). Using the "sagittal grove" is inappropriate and can result in "stacking" of the first metatarsal head which can lead to restricted motion at first metatarsophalangeal joint (D).

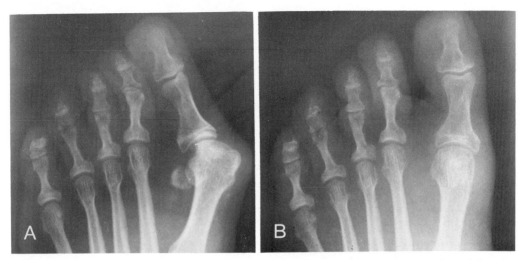

Figure 11.37. *A*, pre-operative x-ray demonstrating a severe hallux abducto valgus deformity. *B*, first MPJ correction with limited resection of the first metatarsal head and proper re-articulation with the base of the proximal phalanx.

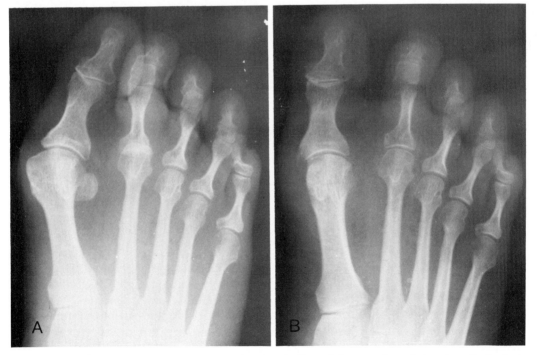

Figure 11.38. *A*, pre-operative x-ray showing hallux abducto valgus deformity. *B*, limited resection of the first metatarsal head allowing for proper re-articulation. If the medial aspect of the base of the proximal phalanx is prominent then it can be remodeled.

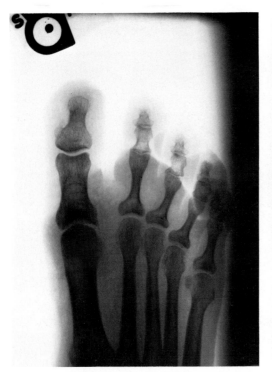

Figure 11.39. Post-operative x-ray demonstrating limited resection of the first metatarsal head with proper re-articulation of the base of the proximal phalanx.

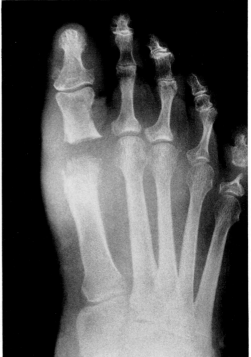

Figure 11.40. Post-operative x-ray showing a Mayo procedure of the first metatarsal head in conjunction with a Keller procedure.

tients revealed the occurrence of a lesion under one or more of the lesser metatarsal heads following surgery. Slightly less than 30% of the patients had significant limitation of range of motion or dorsiflexion at the first MPJ. Approximately 4% of the patients developed a hallux rigidus. In 47% of the patients where a hallux elevatus developed, which was generally attributed to the fact that there was a shortening of the hallux with weak flexion and contraction of the fibrotic tissue to hold the hallux in a dorsiflexed position. Finally, 10% of the patients developed a hammertoe deformity of the hallux which is attributable to the loss of the vector force of the flexor hallucis brevis tendons, reducing its power to below physiological levels.

Another interesting statistic was that 28% of the feet on which a Mayo procedure was performed had a recurrence of the HAV deformity. We would concur with their conclusions that the Mayo procedure should

be utilized as a salvage procedure when dealing with bone tumors, osteomyelitis, or as a palliative procedure in a geriatric patient who fulfills the medical requirements for surgery and who will not place the first metatarsophalangeal joint under great stress with excessive ambulation.

Bingham (146) discussed the use of the Stone procedure which Stone had been using for 50 years but had never published. Bingham reported on 54 patients (80 feet) over a 6.5-year period. Overall his complications included two patients with first MPJ stiffness; three patients questioned the cosmetic appearance of the hallux due to shortening; two patients with rheumatoid arthritis complained of post-operative metatarsalgia, but seven other patients with pre-operative metatarsalgia showed reduced symptoms. Collins (176) reported that a hammertoe deformity of the hallux (2–5%) may be anticipated following the Stone procedure. His modification of the

Mayo-Stone procedures involved limited remodeling of the first metatarsal head, unlike the original procedures, with "reshaping" of the sesamoidal grooves, and transposing the abductor hallucis tendon as advocated by Rix (175). Collins (176) reported on 43 cases involving 75 feet with a 2–5-year follow-up. Three cases developed arthrodesis of the first MPJ; limitation of the first MPJ motion occurred in 31 cases with three being painful; two patients complained of metatarsalgia; and six patients had a residual HAV deformity of greater than 20° (175, 176).

As is common in podiatric surgery, the pendulum is swinging again. Keller (84, 85) published his first paper in 1904 regarding a surgical correction for a bunion deformity. For many years it was a popular procedure and still is with certain individual practitioners. In the past two decades, however, this procedure has been performed less frequently on an individual basis, but has been combined with the use of prosthetic joint replacement procedures which were first developed by Swanson. Of late,

however, we are again experiencing a resurgence in the use of the Keller procedure as the primary surgical procedure for HAV deformity without the use of a prosthetic replacement as seen in Figure 11.41. Upon resection of the base of the proximal phalanx, one essentially removes the intrinsic power of the hallux to flex in a stance and propulsive position. Flexor power of the first MPJ is essential for normal gait and function. Various modifications of the Keller procedure had been proposed over the years. McCain and Nuzzo (82) advocated the deliberate suturing of the sesamoidal ligament into the capsule of the first MPJ in order to avoid the proximal retraction of the sesamoid following a Keller bunionectomy procedure. Though others have advocated the suturing of the flexor hallucis brevis tendons into the remaining portion of the proximal phalanx in order to stabilize the hallux in a flexed position, Stamm (95), performed a Keller procedure and transposed the adductor hallucis tendon through the first metatarsal head in conjunction with a proximal first metatarsal osteotomy

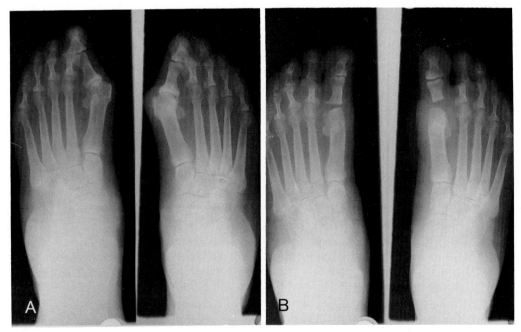

Figure 11.41. *A*, pre-operative x-ray of a hallux abducto valgus deformity. *B*, Post-operative x-ray demonstrating a Keller procedure which results in weakened instrinsic control and poor hallux toe purchase.

to reduce an elevated intermetatarsal angle. As with other modifications of the Keller procedure, a common complication of Stamm's procedure was the development of stress fractures of the lesser metatarsals post-operatively. In order to prevent further atrophy of the hallux, other authors have offered to "hourglass" the capsule at closure to prevent retraction and atrophy of the hallux post-operatively. Some have used a large K-wire or Steinman pin through the hallux and through the metatarsal head in order to stabilize and allow for fibrosis, which obviously will result in a hallux limitus or rigidus (95). McGlamry et al. (83) discussed their own appraisal of the Keller bunionectomy procedure for HAV correction. In a follow-up article in 1973 (86), they discussed two major modifications which included a medial "strap" of capsule with the base being proximal on the metatarsal head where there is significantly stronger tissue with resuturing distally to reduce the abductus deformity, as well as the use of drill holes on the plantar for re-attachment of the brevis tendons. They reported that in 2% of their cases, the resuturing techniques resulted in too great a pressure or tension which caused jamming or impaction of the phalangeal base onto the metatarsal head and produced a hallux limitus. Overall, however, these modifications appear to be worthwhile when in isolated instances a Keller procedure is indicated. In the patient's best interest, it is worthwhile to seek consultation when other, more technically involved procedures may be indicated, including the insertion of prosthetic devices (Fig. 11.42). At the same time, salvage or reconstructive procedures for previously performed Keller bunionectomies can be just as disasterous (Fig. 11.43). In this case, a hemi-angulated prosthetic has been placed into the proximal phalanx, but its position is poor, the functional result questionable, and depending upon the vascular status of the patient, it could result in some embarrassment to the digit due to traction on the toe with the placement of the spacing device into the first metatarsophalangeal joint.

Besides the other complications mentioned earlier, Ford and Gilula (87) reported on four patients who had sustained stress fractures of the second or third metatarsals following Keller bunionectomy. In their series, they had not seen similar complications with either the McBride (77), Joplin (150), Silver (94), or Peabody procedures (72). However, they also related that they had seen one case of stress fracture following a Mayo bunionectomy. Continued review from England on the Keller procedure performed by Wrighton (90) indicated that, post-operatively, 10% of the patients continued to complain of pain. He basically found the same statistical findings as were previously discussed by Geldwert and Gibbons 2 years later (80). Wrighton's study showed a 28% unsatisfactory result which divided into three basic categories: 1) anterior metatarsalgia deformity of the hallux (instability, excessive valgus; 2) dorsiflexion, dorsal subluxation, etc.); or 3) painful keratotic lesions on the lesser digits. Their conclusion was that the greater the amount of the base of the proximal phalanx that is removed (greater than one-third) the more potential complications occur. Another study done in 1972 by Soren (91) in New York, indicated poor results in 25 of 145 patients where an excessive amount of the first metatarsal head, as well as a Keller procedure, had been performed. He clearly stated that the "impairment of function and persistent pain were considered more important as the indication for operation of hallux valgus than the cosmetic demands of the patients." Markheim and Phillips (92) had similar complications following Keller procedures, but clearly stated that these procedures were probably contraindicated in the young or the athletic patient due to loss of push-off function of the hallux during gait. They did, however, recognize the importance of reducing an abnormal intermetatarsal angle which was also discussed in 1980 by Gora et al. (97). They combined their Keller bunionectomy procedures with an opening wedge osteotomy of the first metatarsal involving 68 procedures. A total of 35.6% of their pa-

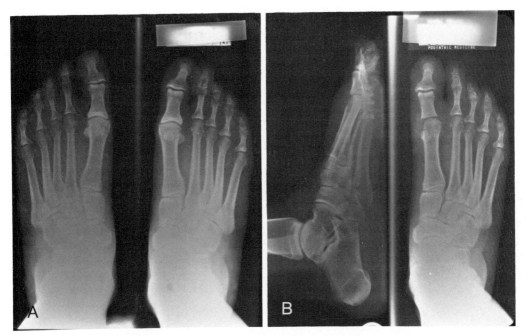

Figure 11.42. *A*, pre-operative x-ray of a hallux abducto valgus deformity bilateral. *B*, post-operative x-ray demonstrating the Keller procedure of the right foot. Note proximal position of medial sesamoid which indicates loss of intrinsic control.

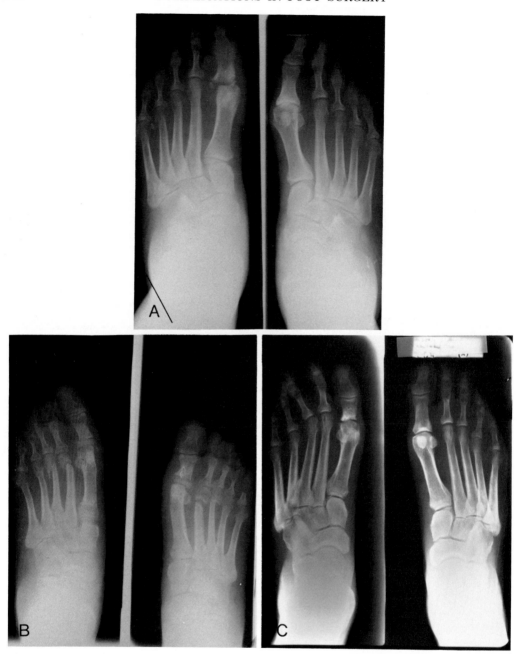

Figure 11.43.   Case 1: Post-operative x-ray following a Keller procedure with retraction of the digit and limitation of motion (*A*). Case 2: Post-operative x-ray showing insertion of hemiprosthetic after unsuccessful Keller with pain beneath second metatarsal and distal osteotomies, which resulted in stress fracture of left third metatarsal (*B*). Case 3: Post-operative Keller procedure (left foot) with atrophy of hallux and limited first MPJ motion (*C*). Case 4: Pre-operative x-ray with hallux limitus right foot (*D*). Case 4: Post-operative Keller procedure with irregularity and limited motion first MPJ; pain beneath second metatarsal head 4 months post-operatively and subsequent distal osteotomy (*E*).

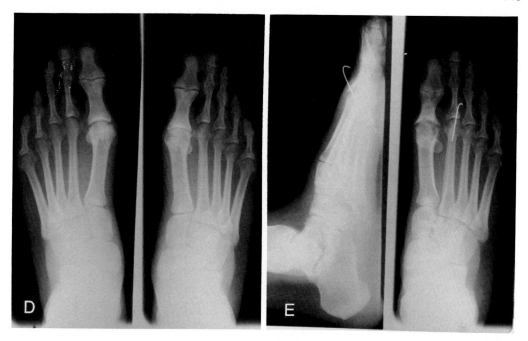

Figure 11.43. (*D* and *E*)

tients complained of residual pain post-operatively which most frequently involved the lesser metatarsophalangeal joints laterally. They also reported patient satisfaction in 59 cases with a percentage of improvement of 95%. One of the conclusions stated that by placing a graft and performing an opening wedge osteotomy, there appeared to be less pain in those patients where post-operatively the first metatarsal was longer than the second. In none of their cases was an implant prosthetic utilized; however, they did advocate its use for improved cosmetic and functional results. They also felt that it would allow for greater functional control and power of the hallux, thus eliminating lateral symptomatology.

An interesting side note to the analysis of all these cases is that nowhere is there a discussion involving the use of orthotics post-operatively as an aid to help control overall foot function and malalignment which we have discussed earlier as a primary etiological factor. We have emphasized before that surgical results are not necessarily based on surgical skills or limi-

tations of the individual, nor should the expectations of the patient be totally discounted. These are joint destructive procedures that have limited indications and criteria that can and should be used for salvage procedures when dealing with metabolic disease and their complications (176). Post-operative orthotic control has been, and will continue to be, emphasized throughout this section.

Capsulo-tendon Balance Procedures

In 1923, Silver (94) described the basic procedure for capsulo-tendon balance procedures, of which there have been various modifications. His work was followed by McBride (77–79), Hiss (120), and Stein (68). As a historical footnote, one should note that Fuld (147), in 1916, initially described an abductor hallucis transposition, as did Hiss, but was never given the same type of recognition. Initially, as was stated by McBride, an attempt was made to realign the hallux at the metatarsal-phalangeal joint and to reduce the retrograde force on the first metatarsal from the malalign-

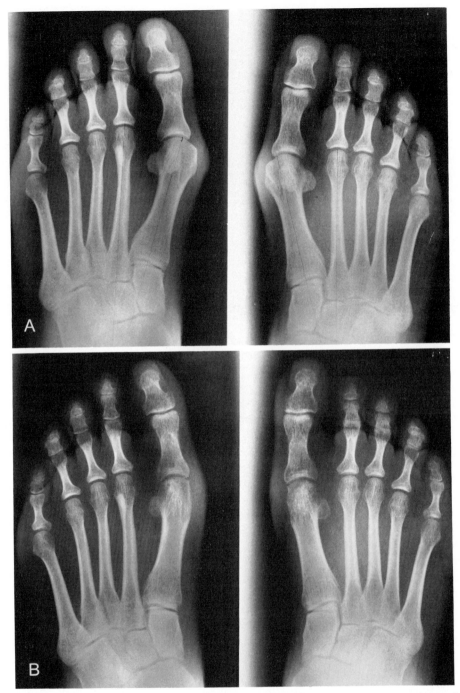

Figure 11.44.   Case 1: Pre-operative x-ray with bilateral hallux abducto valgus (*A*) and post-operative x-rays of Silver procedures (*B*). Case 2: Pre-operative mild HAV (*C*) and post-operative x-ray of bilateral Silver procedure (*D*).

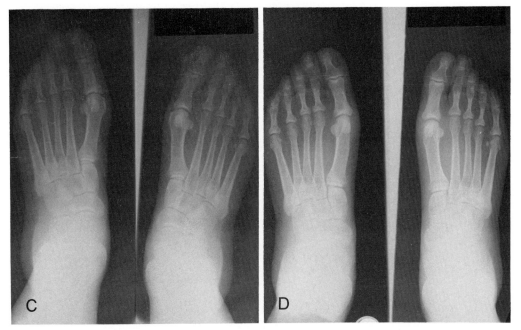

Figure 11.44.   (*C* and *D*)

ment of the hallux. McBride suggested that the lateral sesamoid be removed if it is "eroded, abnormal in shape, or displaced." In 1935 there ensued a professional debate between McBride and Lapidus as to the strength of the adductor muscle. McBride stated that there was a great advantage of the adductor forces over the abductor forces, including shoe pressure and contraction of the lateral head of the flexor brevis tendon. This is somewhat borne out by the electromyographic studies of Iida and Basmajian (69) who essentially demonstrated that, in the hallux abducto valgus deformity, the function of the abductor hallucis is essentially absent, and although the function of the adductor hallucis is considerably diminished, it still has a relatively overpowering effect on the abductor since, in their words, the function of the abductor hallucis is "nil."

An essential point in the entire discussion of capsulo-tendon balance procedure needs to be made here with reference to the positional versus structural deformities. In the continued debate between McBride and Lapidus (64), McBride stated that the metatarsus primus varus was of little significance. In 1953, he categorically stated that "the degree of varus of the first metatarsal is not of great importance." In this day and age, we would not concur with McBride's analysis and would emphasize that a capsulo-tendon balance procedure (Figs. 11.44 and 11.45) should only be performed when there is a positional deformity. Butlin (98) discussed some of the potential complications in the utilization of the McBride procedure, as well as his own modifications. He was one of the first to state that the most common reason for the development of hallux varus is the excessive resection of bone in the medial aspect of the first metatarsal. He also mentions hallux limitus and recurrence of the HAV deformity as potential complications. Excessive edema and/or hallux limitus following a McBride procedure is, generally, a cause and effect type of relationship between the extent of trauma during surgery. Considerable effort should be made by the surgeon to limit his exposure to the necessary tissues and to be able to visualize the neurovascular structures so as to avoid un-

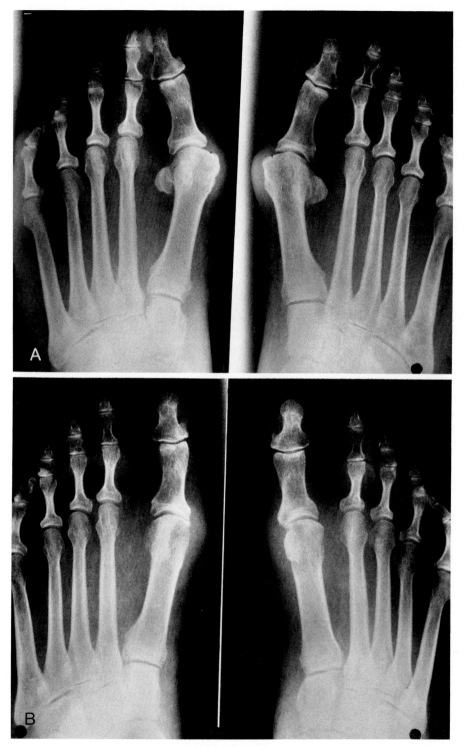

Figure 11.45. *A*, pre-operative x-ray of a hallux abducto valgus deformity. *B*, post-operative x-ray following a standard McBride procedure bilaterally.

necessary trauma and hemorrhage post-operatively. If one is having a high percentage of recurrences of the HAV deformity, then either the procedure is not being performed correctly or the pre-operative indications for the procedure were in error.

Hallux elevatus, of a minor nature, is also a potential complication, but little data has been published with regard to this particular problem. We are referring to the fact that in many cases the hallux does not engage the floor in a stance position following capsulo-tendon balance procedures. Either excessive trauma has been done, adhesions have formed dorsally with contractions of these tissues during the healing process, or the hallux is not bandaged correctly in a slightly flexed position immediately post-operatively and during the first few weeks post-operatively in order to avoid this particular side effect. Debate will continue, with regard to McBride's excision and transposition of the adductor tendon and its advantages or disadvantages, as well as resection of the lateral sesamoid. To state categorically that the lateral sesamoid should either never be removed or always be removed is inaccurate. As is typical, the truth lies somewhere between these two concepts. Patients should be analyzed individually.

Hansen (177) presents an interesting follow-up study of the McBride procedure involving 91 patients with an average follow-up of 6 years, 4 months. The problem of inability of toe purchase on stance is emphasized by Hansen for he had several patients with an inability to flex the hallux to the neutral position, and some as far as 10° above the neutral position (dorsally). Overall, he classified his results as good in 52% of the patients with an average post-operative valgus position of 0–25°. Fair results were seen in 35% of the patients where there was a (post-operative valgus position of 24–45°, or the development of a hallux varus deformity. Poor results (post-operative valgus of the hallux was greater than 45°, or a hallux varus) were seen in 13% of the patients. Another important point made by Hansen, which was common prac-

tice in the podiatric surgical community 10–20 years ago, was the foreshortening of the medial capsulotomy in order to avoid recurrence or relapse. Experience has shown that in a majority cases, shortening the capsule on the medial aspect of the first metatarsophalangeal joint is unnecessary.

Mann (99) discusses a few cases of hallux varus following the McBride procedure, but does not discuss in detail the etiological factors of the complication. He also states in one case when dealing with a rheumatoid foot that the McBride procedure is inadequate and that arthrodesis of the first metatarsophalangeal joint is primarily indicated. This appears to be a personal opinion based on a singular case, rather than an opinion supported by any statistical data. Complications of hallux varus will be discussed in more detail later, as well as other general post-operative complications that can occur with any form of bunionectomy procedure.

There continues to be debate surrounding the transposition of the adductor hallucis after excision from the base of the proximal phalanx. Many surgeons continue to "drop" the tendon into the first intermetatarsal space leading to atrophy of the tendon and its inclusion in surrounding fibrous tissue post-operatively. One never knows that at some future time it may be necessary to utilize that tendon, and we recommend that the tendon be sutured to the lateral capsule of the first metatarsal head. In reading McBride's work, one is never really satisfied with the explanations given, and unfortunately, this concept of transpositional suturing of the adductor will probably continue to be debated for years to come. A case to defend the transpositional technique, however, is presented in Figure 11.46. This particular patient underwent a McBride procedure, and approximately 2 years later fractured the base of the proximal phalanx on the operated foot. It was an intra-articular fracture which did not heal with immobilization and the patient subsequently underwent resection of the base of the proximal phalanx and insertion of a hemiprosthetic. However, since

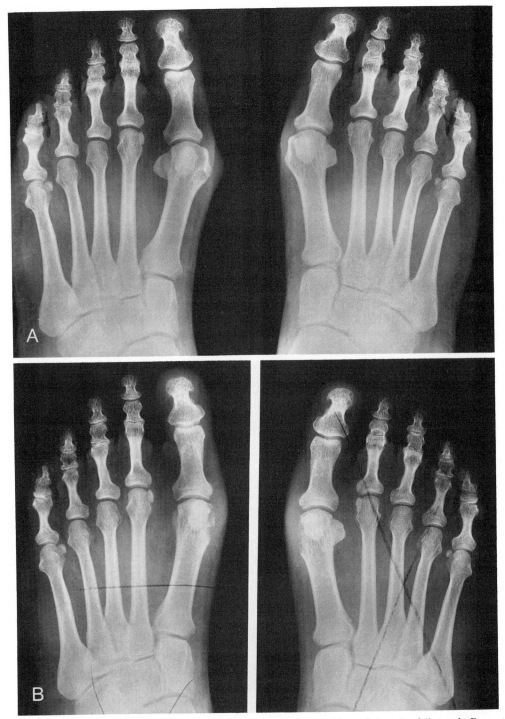

Figure 11.46. *A*, pre-operative x-ray of an hallux abducto valgus deformity bilateral. *B*, post-operative x-rays following a standard McBride procedure of the left foot and a Silver procedure of the right foot. *C*, patient subsequently fractured the base of the proximal phalanx intra-articularly and did not heal normally requiring the insertion of a hemiprosthetic device and the utilization of the transposed adductor hallucis tendon for lateral stability.

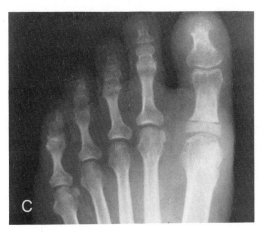

Figure 11.46. (C)

the adductor had been transposed, it was identified and utilized in the suturing technique to provide some lateral stability.

Splayfoot deformities were discussed by Joplin (150) with his soft tissue "sling" procedure. This procedure appears to be advantageous when there is flaccidity or hypermobility of the forefoot without structural deformity, but may be combined with structural correction procedures. Joplin reported that seven patients had recurrent plantar metatarsal keratosis with uncorrected hammertoes. Simple extensor tenoplasty was ineffective in correcting the problem and more aggressive correction of the hammertoes was suggested. A "few" of his patients complained of first MPJ stiffness post-operatively and he suggested early excercise would eliminate this problem.

Bishop et al. (178) advocated the Giannestras procedure for splay-foot which involved opening wedge osteotomies of the first and fifth metatarsals with bone grafting, and wire fixation across the metatarsal heads during healing. They reported 33% excellent results, 45% good, 14% fair, and 8% poor. Collapse of the bone graft accounted for many of the fair and poor results, and this complication will be discussed later.

Interphalangeal Osteotomies

In 1925, Akin (65) proposed an interphalangeal osteotomy to correct an inherent abnormal abduction of the hallux. The procedure was used relatively infrequently, but over the last decade, its use has increased. There continues to be some misunderstanding with regard to the pre-operative criteria, and perhaps the procedure is being overutilized, not only as a primary procedure, but also as a "cheater" procedure. There are basically three types of "Akin" osteotomies: distal, proximal and cylindrical. Distal osteotomies should be utilized when there is an abnormally high hallux abductus intra-phalangeal angle; the proximal procedure at the base of the proximal phalanx should be performed when there is an abnormally high distal articular set angle; the cylindrical osteotomy is indicated when there is an excessively long proximal phalanx, for shortening, as well as reduction of angulation. Various measuring techniques have been advocated over the years, including straight line drawings measuring the hallux abductus interphalangeous (HAIP) angle and the distal articular set angle (DASA). Other geometric measurements have been advocated, such as those developed by Gerbert and Melillo (181) and Gohil and Cavolo (100).

McGlamry et al. (101) discussed the cylindrical Akin osteotomy for excessively long proximal phalanges. They reported the potential for hyperextension of the interphalangeal joint of the hallux if the EHL tendon is not lengthened. They also noted that if there is an accessory ossicle on the plantar surface of the hallux IPJ, that this should be resected at time of surgery, since, in their opinion, the ossicle interferes with the function of the long flexor tendon. With the cylindrical osteotomy, there is also the increased potential for delayed or nonunion because of difficulties with fixation. In Figure 11.47, we see a case of a long hallucial proximal phalanx, but post-operatively, there is abnormal angulation of the distal portion at the site of the osteotomy. Care

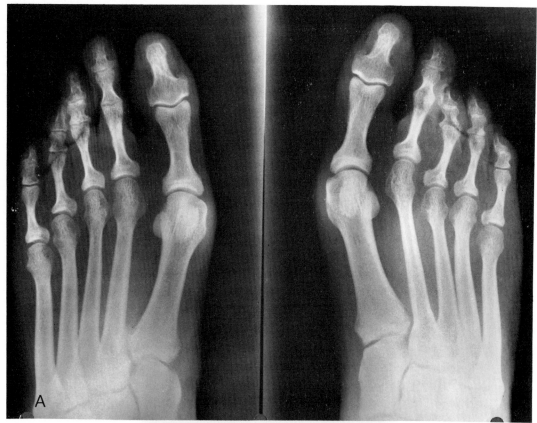

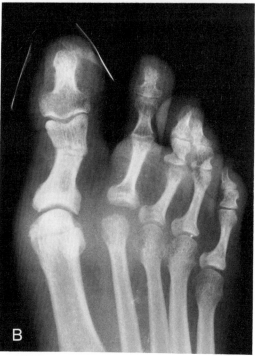

Figure 11.47. *A,* pre-operative x-ray of an hallux abducto valgus deformity bilaterally with elongation of the proximal phalanx. *B,* post-operative x-ray demonstrating a Reverdin procedure of the first metatarsal head and a distal Akin procedure of the right hallux, with no fixation and questionable angulation.

must be taken to avoid this particular potential complication. It should also be noted that the normal position of the hallux is not in a perfectly straight or rectus alignment, as is seen in this last case, and, therefore, the patient may have difficulty ambulating with shoes.

Of the three basic types of hallucial phalangeal osteotomies, the proximal osteotomy is probably the most frequently utilized (Fig. 11.48). Seelenfreund et al. (102) reported on their results with proximal osteotomies of the hallux involving 150 patients (253 feet). Three feet required reoperation and they performed a Keller procedure. Their complications included superficial infection, limited mobility at the first metatarsophalangeal joint, and pain at the first metatarsophalangeal joint. Complications occurred in 30% of the 50 feet reported. They also reported recurrence of the bunion deformity in 1% of the patients, and residual or recurrent valgus of the hallux in 2% of the cases. In their particular study, no screw, K-wire, or metal suture fixation was utilized, and they did not report any instances of delayed or nonunion of these osteotomies.

Various alternatives of the basic Akin procedure are described and discussed in detail by Gerbert et al. (103). They discuss various modes of fixation which do not include the current use of ASIF techniques and, the indications and use of the distal Akin procedure, criteria for which we have previously discussed (Fig. 11.49). Brahms (104) paper on the Akin procedure is nothing more than a description of the procedure with his own unique criteria. Like many other authors and contemporary surgeons, he does not offer any method of fixation other than soft tissue suturing. This, we feel, creates a paradox since, while we are trying to correct a malaligned digit, another goal of HAV surgery is proper range of motion and function of the first MPJ. Without proper fixation, one is forced to immobilize the hallux for an extended period of time to allow for proper bone healing which unfortunately may result in adhesions and splinting of the first

metatarsophalangeal joint. This is a poor surgical result from a functional standpoint (Fig. 11.50). Various techniques have been proposed, of late, to offset this paradoxical situation. Langford (105) discusses in detail the use of the ASIF technique for fixation of Akin osteotomies by use of cortical screws using a lag technique. He also points out some of the errors that need to be avoided, as well as some of the pitfalls in the use of K-wire fixation, which may lead to delayed or nonunion. If one is confronted with a hallux flexus deformity following an Akin procedure, Langford (108) further discusses the use of ASIF techniques for IP fusions of the hallux. However, in his latest study, cancellous screws were utilized, and although the author mentions that in one patient the screw needed to be removed 8 months post-operatively, he did not mention that the removal of a cancellous screw is far more difficult than if one uses a cortical screw and a lag technique.

Finally, Levitsky (109) discusses the use of a percutaneous osteoclasp for fixation of Akin osteotomies. While he discusses a single case, the presentation is incomplete in that he does not discuss success or failure rate or potential complications with the use of the clasp. While the osteoclasp system may have some merit, in our experience, it seems to be technically difficult to use; the degree of compression may vary from patient to patient and surgeon to surgeon and results are not always reproducible. In our opinion, this procedure should not be used as a "cheater" procedure to make the hallux "a little bit straighter" to satisfy the aesthetic needs of the surgeon.

Distal Metatarsal Osteotomies

The use of distal metatarsal osteotomies are primarily to correct an abnormally high proximal articular set angle (PASA); and/or for correction of an intermetatarsal angle, which is in the upper limits of normal where the first metatarsal segment is semirigid or rigid and, thus, less likely to reduce with a capsulo-tendon balance procedure. Another indication for a distal metatarsal

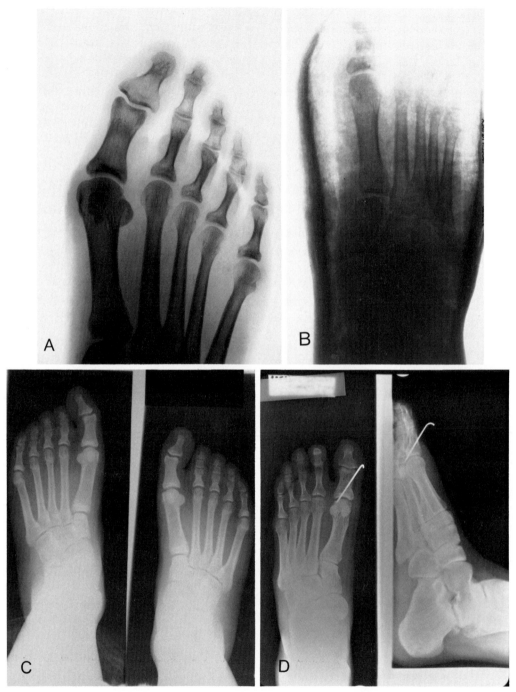

Figure 11.48. Case 1: Pre-operative x-ray demonstrating hallux abducto valgus deformity with abnormal distal articular set angle (DASA) (*A*) and post-operative x-ray showing a proximal Aikin of the right foot (*B*). Case 2: Pre-operative x-ray showing pronounced elevation of HAIP angle which would indicate a distal Akin procedure (*C*). Case 3: Post-operative x-rays of proximal Akin procedure but K-wire is into first MPJ which could result in irritation, synovitis, and restricted range of motion post-operatively (*D*). Case 4: Pre-operative x-ray with bilateral HAV and post-operative x-ray demonstrating Akin and Reverdin procedures (*F*); with Reverdin procedure performed at an inappropriate angle and K-wire fixation for Akin is inappropriately across the first MPJ.

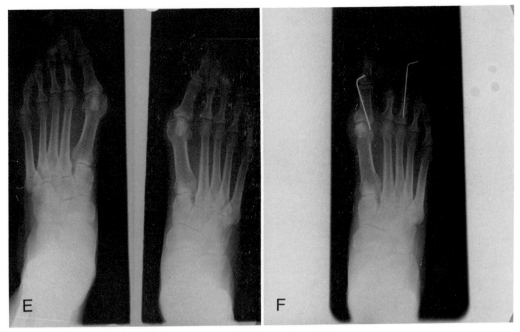

Figure 11.48.   (*E* and *F*)

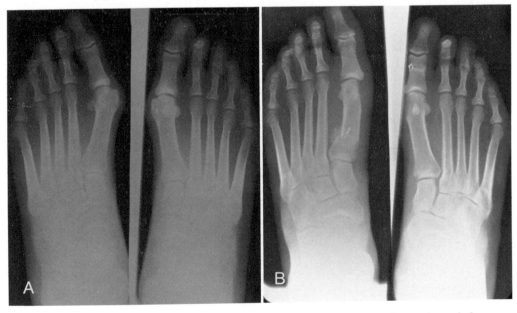

Figure 11.49.   *A*, pre-operative x-ray of an abnormally high hallux abductus interphalangeous angle. *B*, post-operative x-ray demonstrating a distal Akin osteotomy.

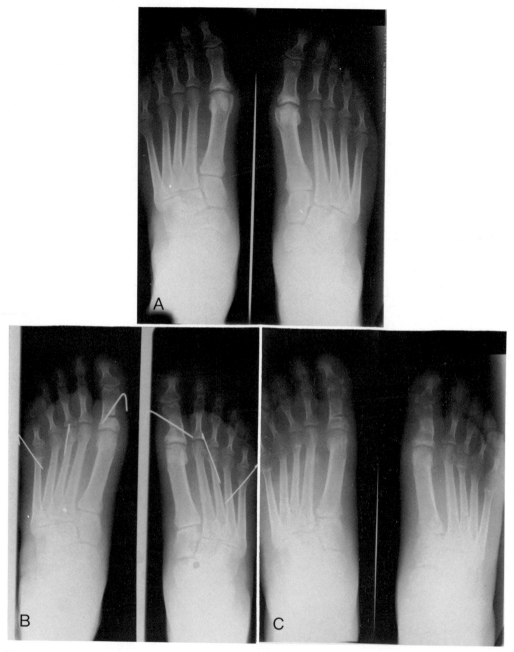

Figure 11.50. Case 1: Pre-operative x-ray demonstrating an abnormally high hallux abductus interphalangeal angle (*A*) and post-operative x-ray demonstrating a proximally placed Akin osteotomy with K-wire fixation. *C*, post-operative x-ray showing a nonunion of the Akin osteotomy left foot. Case 2: Pre-operative x-ray of HAV deformity with abnormal DASA (*D*) and post-operative x-ray left foot after Silver and Akin procedures with poor approximation of osteotomy site even with monofilament wire fixation (*E*).

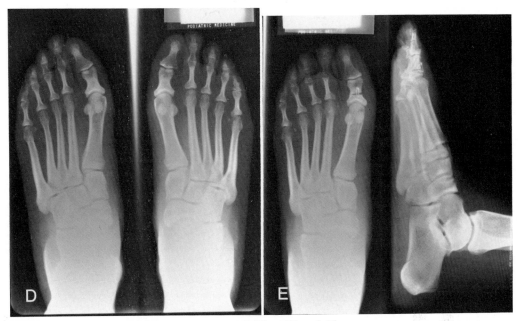

Figure 11.50. (*D* and *E*)

osteotomy is when there is a high hallux abductus angle with lesser metatarsal forefoot adduction, which would require placing the first metatarsal head, or its distal segment, in a more lateral position to compensate for the lesser metatarsal adductus and, thus, be able to reduce the abnormal position of the hallux. Several interesting techniques have been developed which we will discuss, both pro and con. However, a few basic principles must be noted before our involvement with specific procedures. First of all, recognition of the normal intermetatarsal angle is essential. Schoenhaus et al. (110) discussed the various intermetatarsal angles and their normal relationship to each other. However, their study did primarily deal with the lesser metatarsal angles. Gerbert et al. (180) discuss both the normal intermetatarsal angle, as well as normal versus abnormal proximal articular set angles. Another essential criteria is what is now referred to as the metatarsal protrusion measurement or metatarsal length pattern. Duke et al. (111) discussed the importance of metatarsal protrusion and how it can be correlated from radiographic analysis and how this can be pos-

sibly correlated with potential surgical procedures. While the surgeon may take special care in noting the intermetatarsal and proximal articular set angles, some may forget to analyze the length patterns, especially relating to the first and second metatarsals. Any procedure, such as a distal first metatarsal osteotomy, which has the potential to shorten an already anatomically short first metatarsal, will certainly lead to more lateral symptomatology postoperatively. Thus, if dealing with a negative metatarsal protrusion measurement, more proximal procedures are indicated. One should always be aware of the fact that, with distal first metatarsal osteotomies, the greatest risk is in relation to the vascular supply to the distal segment of the metatarsal. Because distal first metatarsal osteotomies have become more prevalent in the last few years, several authors have noticed the development of aseptic necrosis. Jaworek (113) has detailed the intrinsic vascular supply to the first metatarsal. For years, we have emphasized to students and residents the importance of adequate but limited dissection and underscoring the capsule of the first metatarsophalangeal joint on the medial proximal aspect, since under careful observation, one will notice the metaphyseal vessels as they course into the bone just proximal to the first metatarsal head. In an editorial, Jahss (116) duly notes the increased instance of distal asceptic necrosis by two methods. One, transection of the metatarsal head; two, stripping of its blood supply. Inadvertent damage was also noted by Jahss as being more common since the advent of "blind" outpatient foot surgery through tiny incisions. One is cautioned to duly note the primary indications for the use of a distal first metatarsal osteotomy, and then, when performing the procedure, to be mindful of the normal anatomy, including blood supply to the bone, so as to prevent undesirable complications. The preservation of cartilage of the first metatarsal head is a laudatory goal as expressed by Suppan (117). This procedure has its inherent risks. If the osteotomy site is placed too far proximal and interrupts vital circulation to the distal segment, then aseptic necrosis can result. Proximal placement of this osteotomy (Fig. 11.51) will have a higher incidence of aseptic necrosis, although it is not initially noted on the post-operative x-ray. Review of these patients 2, 3, and 4 years later is essential for post-operative evaluation.

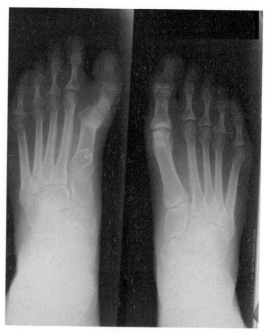

Figure 11.51. Post-operative x-ray with a transverse osteotomy of the Suppan type with shortening of the first metatarsal, and medial displacement with a hallux adductus.

REVERDIN PROCEDURE

A resurgence in the use of the Reverdin procedure, as was first described in 1881 (119), can be seen over the past decade. The primary criteria for the use of this procedure is the reduction of an abnormal proximal articular set angle (PASA) (Fig. 11.52). The major criticism of the procedure again has been aseptic necrosis of the distal segment, as well as reduction in dorsiflexion at the first MPJ due to trauma, adhesions, and fibrosis, as well as possible trauma to the sesamoidal complex. Funk and Wells (171) reported on their 10-year experience with the Reverdin procedure. They operated on 85 patients, involving 118 feet, and stated that their average bone wedge removed was 6 mm in thickness,

which seems rather large to us unless their patients had excessively high proximal articular set angles. There were no reported nonunions seen during follow-up questionnaire to 56 patients; results were as follows: nine patients had residual pain at the first MPJ with two patients having more pain than before the surgery, and seven patients with less pain than pre-operatively. There was one case of recurrence of the deformity, but 53 out of the 56 respondents stated that they were satisfied with the results. Their complications involved only some decrease in plantar flexion of the first MPJ which went unnoticed by patients. They also observed a reduction in the first intermetatarsal angle post-operatively of an average of 4.3° if the pre-operative angle measured greater than 11° (overall range from 7–20°). If the pre-operative first intermetatarsal angle was less than 11°, then there was a post-operative reduction of 1.5° on an average.

Several modifications of the basic Reverdin procedure have been offered over the

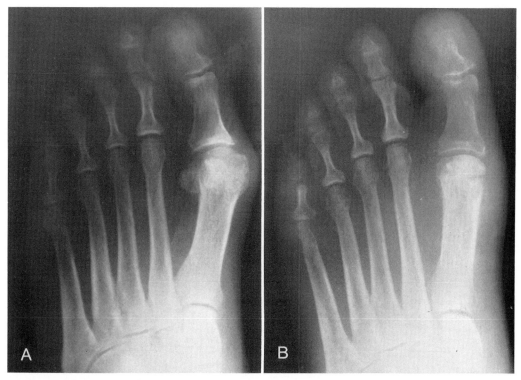

Figure 11.52. *A,* pre-operative x-ray showing a hallux abducto valgus deformity with abnormal proximal articular set angle (PASA). *B,* post-operative x-ray demonstrating a distal transverse osteotomy of the Reverdin type.

past 8–10 years. Beck (121) performed a Reverdin procedure, as well as angulated cuts dorsal-plantarly with a wedge section (base dorsally) much in the same manner as Watermann, to assist in post-operative dorsiflexion of the hallux. A similar modification has been advocated by Todd in a recent text. He pointed out certain potential complications, including incomplete correction of the PASA which resulted in recurrent HAV deformity, and overabundant removal of the wedge of bone which could result in a hallux varus deformity. There is also the possibility of a delayed or nonunion at the osteotomy site, but this appears to be a rare complication.

It is possible to have limited range of motion post-operatively with potential fusion of the sesamoids if the osteotomy site and sesamoids are not protected during performance of the procedure. Our experience has been in concurrence with Butlin and Beck, which showed an increase in exten-

sion of the first MPJ post-operatively when the Reverdin procedure was performed.

Another modification is the Laird procedure (180) which attempts to correct not only an abnormally high PASA, but also to reduce somewhat the metatarsus primus adductus angle, as is also seen in the Austin procedure (Fig. 11.53). Unlike the standard Reverdin procedure, which leaves the lateral cortex intact, the Laird modification reduces the PASA angle but also displaces the distal segment laterally and, if not fixated, can lead to displacement or inaccurate placement.

Another area for debate is the necessity for fixation with the Reverdin procedure. Over the past decade, recordings of several hundred Reverdin procedures which necessitated fixation in only two cases where the lateral cortex was disrupted have been reported in Illinois. If the osteotomy is well placed, and extreme care is taken to "thin out" the lateral cortex once the wedge has

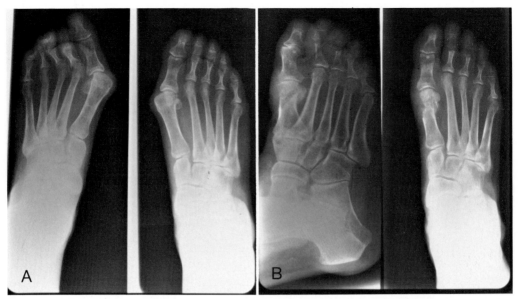

Figure 11.53. *A,* pre-operative x-ray demonstrating a hallux abducto valgus deformity with a slight elevation of the proximal articular set angle. *B,* post-operative x-ray demonstrating the Laird modification of the Reverdin procedure, with osteotomy too proximal.

been removed, then fixation is generally unnecessary (Fig. 11.54). If the lateral cortex has been broken, then various types of fixation are available, including monofilament wire, K-wires, and the use of absorbable and nonabsorbable sutures (Fig. 11.55). If there is any doubt at the time of surgery, then fixation should be utilized to prevent displacement. However, as in use of any technique, there can be technical errors. In Figure 11.56, the osteotomy was placed too far distal and may interfere with normal range of motion of the first MPJ post-operatively. At the same time, if some sort of fixation is utilized, one should be sure that the osteotomy site is closed as tightly as possible to eliminate any potential delayed or nonunion which may develop (Fig. 11.57) when a more proximal Barker procedure was performed (118).

We have previously stressed the importance of minimal resection of the first metatarsal head, but especially when performing a distal metatarsal osteotomy such as a Reverdin, the point needs to be made again. As can be seen in Fig. 11.58 of the left foot, there has been minimal resection and the joint easily re-articulates in proper

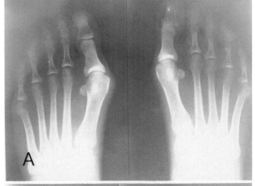

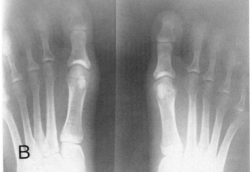

Figure 11.54. *A,* pre-operative bilateral x-rays with hallux abducto valgus deformity, and abnormal proximal articular set angle. *B,* post-operative x-ray demonstrating re-alignment with a distal Reverdin procedure of the first metatarsal bilateral.

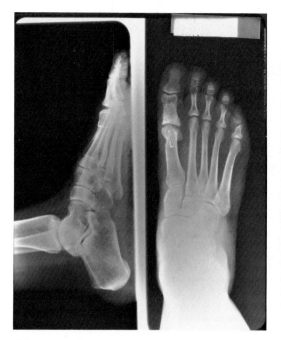

Figure 11.55. Post-operative x-ray demonstrating a distal Reverdin procedure with monofilament wire for fixation.

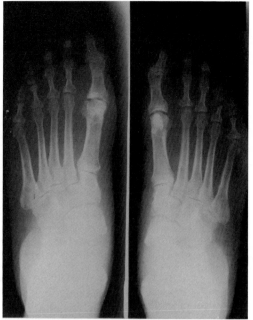

Figure 11.56. Post-operative x-ray of a Reverdin procedure with too distal placement of the osteotomy and distal irregularity from aseptic necrosis, which may interfere with the first MPJ function.

alignment. In the post-operative x-ray of the right foot, there has been too much bone taken off the medial aspect, and this may lead to the potential displacement of the medial sesamoid and a potential hallux varus post-operatively though the post-operative films show proper alignment.

Our only complications with the standard Reverdin procedure has been in six cases of acquired "dynamic" hallux varus involving 200 procedures. Post-operative review of these cases showed that the hallux varus deformity occurred only in cases where the adductor hallucis tendon had been transposed to the lateral capsule of the first metatarsal head, and the lateral sesamoid had also been resected. We now recommend that when performing the Reverdin procedure, the lateral sesamoid should not be removed if the adductor hallucis is released or transposed, or that the adductor hallucis tendon be resutured to its insertion after excision of the lateral sesamoid (Fig. 11.59).

In our opinion, the Reverdin procedure is a useful adjunct to capsulo-tendon bal-

ance procedures when dealing with structural deformity. The various modifications that have been mentioned may be useful in individual cases, but for the most part, the standard Reverdin procedure serves its purpose quite well without the necessity of primary or secondary modifications. Keep in mind, the more one makes a basic procedure more technically difficult, the more potential risks and complications can occur. Furthermore, the continued critique of the Reverdin procedure, that it causes either limitation of motion or trauma to the sesamoids due to the location of the osteotomy, has not been well documented. As with all types of bunion procedures, there may be a post-operative limitation of motion which may be attributable to the excessive trauma of the surgical procedure and inappropriate post-operative management. Trauma to the sesamoids can easily be avoided by placement of either Seeberger or Chandler retractors beneath the first metatarsal head on both the medial and

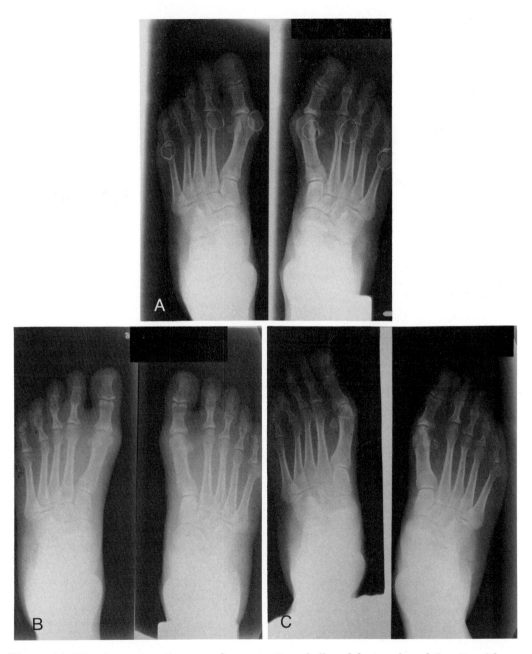

Figure 11.57. *A,* pre-operative x-ray demonstrating a hallux abducto valgus deformity with an abnormal proximal articular set angle. *B,* post-operative x-ray demonstrating a Barker procedure. *C,* post-operative instability of first MPJ secondary to distal asceptic necrosis resulting in recurrence of HAV.

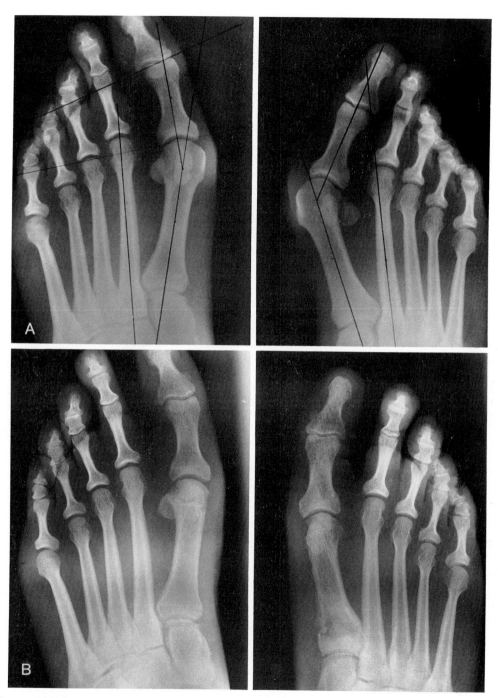

Figure 11.58. *A,* pre-operative x-ray of hallux abducto valgus deformity. *B,* post-operative x-ray of a distal Reverdin procedure with proper alignment of the left foot, but slightly more than an acceptable amount of bone removed from the medial eminence of the right foot which could potentially lead to medial sesamoid displacement.

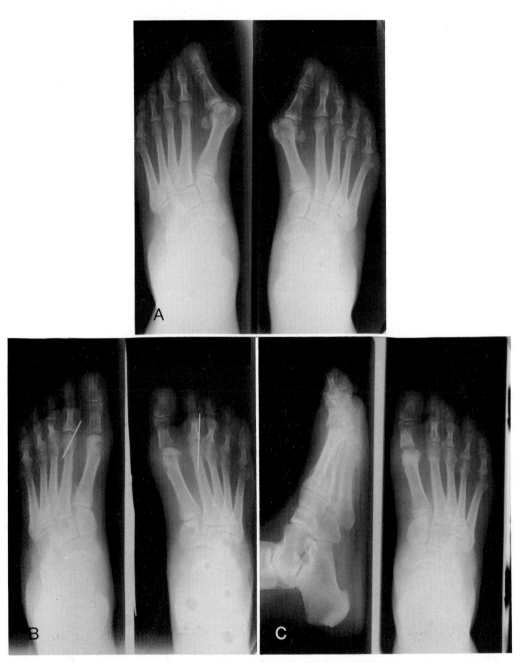

Figure 11.59. *A,* pre-operative x-ray demonstrating a bilateral HAV. *B,* post-operative x-ray with improper oblique angulation of Reverdin osteotomy right foot. Also note Keller procedures bilateral. *C,* post-operative x-ray following Reverdin-Keller procedure with apparently good clinical and radiographic alignment, but irregularity of distal first metatarsal head, limitation of joint motion, and questionable stability.

lateral aspects, thus protecting the sesamoids from trauma. Appropriate immobilization followed by aggressive physical therapy with active and passive exercises in an organized fashion can usually avoid most complications with any bunion procedure.

PEABODY PROCEDURE

The Peabody procedure (72) is designed for reduction of a high proximal articular set angle and a very slight elevated metatarsus primus adductus angle. The osteotomy is made more proximal in the area of the anatomical neck of the first metatarsal. Following Peabody's original description in 1931, a transverse osteotomy is made in the anatomical neck of the first metatarsal with a trapezoid segment being removed and the lateral cortex "fractured" to allow for proper realignment of the distal segment. If performed in this manner, then some form of internal or external fixation is necessary. Peabody recorded his results on 55 patients with 106 procedures. Of these, 16 patients reported complete satisfaction with the procedure. One patient reported weakness after long periods of walking. In another case, the patient continued to complain of "metatarsalgia," requiring a support in his shoe for relief. Of the 32 feet reexamined, the initial deformity was absent in 27 feet and a mild valgus deformity was seen in five feet. Mobility of the joint was good in 25 feet, fair in seven, poor in none, and absent in none. None of the patients reported any pain on range of motion. The average follow-up on these particular patients was 5–7 years after operation. Over the past 35–40 years, various distal osteotomies have been proposed for reduction of the intermetatarsal angle and/or reduction of an abnormally high proximal articular set angle. That does not mean that all of these authors recognized these criteria. They did seem to recognize, however, that there was a group of patients with structural deformity in which capsulo-tendon balance procedure was inappropriate. Again, without the use of proper criteria,

there are some obvious disadvantages to each one of these procedures.

HOHMANN PROCEDURE

In 1921, Hohmann described his transverse osteotomy of the anatomical neck of the first metatarsal (123). He also advocated its use on the fifth metatarsal in an attempt to reduce forefoot splay (Fig. 11.60). The most obvious problem with this procedure, and many other cases that we will exhibit later, is that while attempting to correct a moderately high intermetatarsal angle and/or an abnormally high proximal articular set angle, the surgeon does not take into account the metatarsal protrusion or relative length pattern between the first and second metatarsals. There is a certain amount of natural shortening with all osteotomies, and further shortening only leads to more lateral symptomatology post-operatively.

One of the keys to the Hohmann procedure, as originally described, is that the distal segment was not only displaced laterally, but then the distal segment was po-

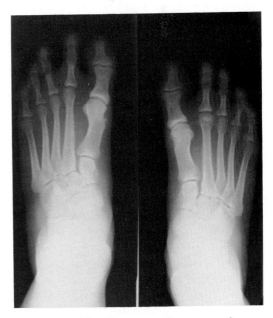

Figure 11.60. Post-operative x-ray after a transverse-oblique Hohmann procedure with K-wire fixation.

sitioned in a more plantar grade position (124–127). Several modifications of this original procedure have been proposed, including the more contemporary cresentic (arcuate) distal osteotomy. Again, the necessity for internal or external fixation should be obvious, although Hohmann, in his original procedure, did not advocate fixation of the distal fragment. This can lead to instances of displacement and failure of the procedure, as was pointed out by Winston and Wilson (122). They further pointed out that due to the location of the osteotomy, even with fixation, that pseudoarthrosis can occur. A further modification was advocated by Gibson and Piggott (169), in which a transverse osteotomy was made in the anatomical neck of the first metatarsal; then the dorsal half of the proximal portion of the first metatarsal shaft at its distal end was removed and then truncated into the metatarsal head which was now in a more plantar-grade position. They showed good to satisfactory results of 80.5% in 82 feet with poor results in 19.5%, where patients developed a nonunion which was then later treated with grafting and resulted in a hallux rigidus. Six other patients developed lateral metatarsalgia which resulted in more discomfort than their pre-operative symptoms. Of these cases, three patients stated that their original "bunion" pain had not resolved. In all of their cases, radiographs were taken within one week after the procedure, and in 11% of the cases, radiographs revealed unsatisfactory position with either incorrect angulation or displacement of the distal fragment. There also appeared to be several cases in which there was a loss of mobility of the first metatarsal-phalangeal joint. The most interesting comment of their study is that while they admitted that shortening of the first metatarsal is inevitable and averaged approximately 6 mm (as measured radiographically), they did not feel that excessive shortening was an important factor and, therefore, this should not deter the surgeon from fashioning a spike adequate for secure fixation. It is interesting to note that they did not relate

incidences of lateral metatarsalgia to this degree of shortening, which we feel should be obvious. As has been mentioned earlier, there was also no discussion with regard to post-operative follow-up and the use of orthotic devices.

An even more technically difficult modification of these basic procedures was advocated by Johnson and Smith (170) when they introduced the derotational, angulational, transpositional osteotomy (DRATO). While this particular procedure recognizes the structural deformities, it attempts to correct the deformities on all three planes, which obviously means that there must be a high degree of accuracy in the placement of the distal fragment. According to the authors, the major contraindications for this procedure are: 1) an extremely high intermetatarsal angle; 2) if bony adaptation has occurred at the articular surface of the base of the proximal phalanx; 3) if extreme valgus rotation of the hallux is adapted with the quantity of motion decreased; and 4) when arthritic changes have occurred. For the most part, this procedure has not met with acceptance due to these contraindications and due to the previously discussed technical difficulties. This is not to say that the procedure in itself does not have some basic merits in individual cases, as well as instances where the surgeon has a high degree of technical skill.

MITCHELL OSTEOTOMY

Since the original description of this procedure in 1945 by Hawkins et al. (128), this has become an extremely popular procedure in the correction of a bunion deformity. The basic procedure probably has also been overutilized since many surgeons have been looking for "the one procedure" to satisfy most, if not all, of the patients they evaluate with an HAV deformity. Mitchell (129) later modified the procedure by emphasizing the importance of also cutting the transverse osteotomy with a wider base plantarly so that the distal segment could be repositioned in a more plantar-grade position, as was emphasized by Hohmann. A primary indication for the procedure is in those patients with a semi-rigid or rigid first metatarsal segment and an intermetatarsal angle of approximately 14–16°. Another indication for the procedure is that it be performed on patients with a congruous or deviated joint. Finally, the metatarsal protrusion measurement will be +3 to 4 mm at a minimum since, by its very nature, the performance of this procedure will shorten the first metatarsal considerably. This last criterion seems to have been missed by most authors and, thus, there is a higher than normal incidence of lateral pain and/or the development of plantar keratotic lesions beneath the lesser metatarsal heads due to the shortening of the first metatarsal. Carr and Boyd (144) wrote of 36 feet with a follow-up of from 2–8 years. Less than 50% were rated as having an excellent result with approximately 40% having been rated as having a good result. Slightly more than 10% were rated with a fair result. Of those with good results, there was a lack of cosmetic correction in four cases; lack of relief of symptoms in three cases; inadequate correction of the deformity in five; and restriction of motion at the first MPJ in four. In three fair results, the primary complaint in two feet was a painful lateral metatarsalgia due to excessive shortening of the first metatarsal of approximately 7 mm. Another patient also demonstrated lateral metatarsalgia as well as excessive dorsal rotation of the distal fragment. Miller (168) modified the basic Mitchell bunionectomy procedure by advocating that the transverse cuts be made in relation to the long axis of the foot rather than the long axis of the first metatarsal. At the same time, a trapezoidal cut with the base medially was also made. The procedure could also correct a high proximal articular set angle, although this was not recognized as a factor by Mitchell or Miller. Certainly, the trapezoid type of excisional modification of the Mitchell procedure as advocated by Hammond, which has its base laterally, would grossly increase the normal or abnormal proximal articular set angle.

Miller reported that 91 of 101 procedures performed were satisfactory, or a 90% success rate. "Satisfaction" was determined by the patient and the surgeon. The primary criterion was the relief of symptoms and that the deformity had "improved." He stated that significant residual deformity was the leading cause of poor results which occurred in seven out of 101 procedures. As was mentioned earlier, the other common unsatisfactory results occurred in eight cases where patients complained of pain beneath the second metatarsal post-operatively. It was felt that if more attention had been made to tilt the distal fragment in a plantar-grade direction, that this complication may have been avoided. In his overall series, stress fractures occurred in three patients between 4 and 8 months postoperatively. These fractures occurred either in the second or third metatarsals and, again, there was no discussion of any orthotic devices post-operatively. Miller did state at the end of his paper that if the anterior articulating surface of the metatarsal head was pointing laterally, the trapezoid cut with the base medially was probably more appropriate along with the basic Mitchell procedure. Finally, Donovan (131) reported on 25 patients with 33 first metatarsal osteotomy bunion procedures of the Mitchell-Hawkins variety with an average decrease of the first intermetatarsal angle of 6.1° and an average decrease of the hallux abductus angle of 18.4°. The follow-up was from 9 months to 5 years and 3 months. The average healing time was 6–8 weeks. He did not report any cases of nonunions. There were some patients who did experience a reduction in range of motion at the first MPJ. No patients complained of pain when walking, even with high-heeled shoes. The most common post-operative complication, which occurred in 9% of the patients, was pain beneath the second metatarsal-phalangeal joint with increased symptoms in one patient who already had a plantar keratotic lesion in this area. In two of his patients, stress fractures were seen in the second metatarsal 3 months post-operatively, but they healed uneventfully. Donovan (131) further advocated the use of the previously mentioned trapezoid-type osteotomy with the base medially for patients presenting a high intermetatarsal angle, as well as an abnormally high proximal articular set angle. While we feel that the use of the Hawkins-Mitchell bunionectomy is certainly indicated in selected patients, we feel that the criteria previously mentioned needs to be followed more closely to insure a higher percentage of satisfactory results with a decrease in the type of complications which appear to be consistent from author to author.

Various other methods or modifications of distal osteotomies have been proposed, such as those by Pelet from Switzerland (132). His method was a modification of the Hohmann osteotomy with lateral transposition, as well as reduction in an abnormally high proximal articular set angle, but sets the distal segment back in a "niche" made in the proximal stump of the first metatarsal. He also utilizes cortical screws for fixation, using a lag technique. In his initial paper, he followed 20 feet for a minimum of 2 years post-operatively, and states that the technique is difficult and his initial poor results were probably due to failure to observe the proper indications, or failure in performing the operative technique properly. Some early complications were residual exostoses near the osteotomy site, as well as irritation from the head of the screw. Removal of the screw from 4–6 months post-operatively with simultaneous resection of the exostosis then revealed good results. To date, he did not report any secondary dislocation, delayed union, nonunion, or aseptic necrosis of the distal fragment. Pelet observed recurrence of the hallux abducto valgus deformity with pain and stiffness at the first metatarsal-phalangeal joint, as well as metatarsalgia beneath the second, third, and fourth metatarsal heads. He attributes the recurrence rate to those patients with a long hallux and suggests that an osteotomy of the proximal phalanx of hallux may also be indicated. Pelet also pointed out the danger in shortening of the first metatarsal.

Another modification of the Hohmann osteotomy has been the Wilson procedure, as was first described in 1936 (130). Wilson initially advocated the use of this procedure for hallux abducto valgus deformities which occurred, or were recognized in adolescence. Holstein and Lewis (133) further advocated the use of this procedure in all age groups in 1976. In Wilson's original paper from England involving 24 patients (130), he reported on one patient with a complete recurrence of deformity and on two patients with a moderate recurrence of deformity. He stated that there was no troublesome stiffness of the toe post-operatively, and at least 30° of dorsiflexion of the first MPJ was regained in all patients. In one patient, there was a persistent complaint of pain underneath the second and third metatarsal heads. In six patients, there was some keratotic lesions beneath the lesser metatarsal heads, but these had been present prior to surgery. In two patients, there was some complaint beneath the sesamoid bones, but the symptoms only lasted for a short period of time. He did advocate the use of post-operative plaster cast immobilization which was removed 8 weeks post-operatively, and bony union was identified 3 months post-operatively. Nonunion was not a complicating factor. Wilson did stress that the surgeon should avoid dorsal tilting of the distal fragment, which did occur in two of his procedures. While this has become a more popular osteotomy among certain practitioners of late, Wilson emphasized the importance of the proper angle of the osteotomy, as well as the proper visualization of the osteotomy site for appropriate correction. He did not advocate the use of any form of fixation post-operatively, but did hold the hallux in an overcorrected position, while in the plaster cast, for a period of 2 weeks, followed by repositioning of the hallux to a neutral position and reapplication of plaster casts. By comparison, Holstein and Lewis (133) performed 98 procedures over a 9-year period. Marked recurrence of the deformity occurred on one patient with partial recurrence of more than half of the correction in three patients. Again, they did not advocate the use of any form of fixation but did utilize post-operative plaster immobilization. Union of the bones were seen on an average 8 weeks post-operatively, and there were no reported cases of nonunion, but two cases of malunion. They did have a total of 17 patients who reported considerable pain beneath the lesser metatarsal heads post-operatively. The basic criteria for this procedure appears to be in individuals who have a 14–16° intermetatarsal angle, and who also have a positive metatarsal protrusion measurement which will offset the obvious shortening of the first metatarsal which occurs with this procedure. The angle of the cut is from distal-medial to proximal-lateral with lateral shifting of the distal fragment.

AUSTIN PROCEDURE

The basic Austin procedure (182) (Fig. 11.61) is a distal transpositional V osteotomy or Chevron osteotomy, which is used primarily for the correction of a moderately elevated intermetatarsal angle (14–16°), especially in cases where there is an abnormally high lesser metatarsal adductus. In 1962 (180), Austin presented his original concept in a paper to the American College of Foot Surgeons. Gerbert (135) has done considerable work with the use of the unicorrectional Austin procedure, as well as the bicorrectional procedure, which also helps to reduce an abnormally high proximal articular set angle. It should be further emphasized at this point that another important criteria is that the patient has at least a positive metatarsal protrusion measurement. Gerbert has appropriately pointed out in the basic technique that the apex of the V osteotomy is distal and the angle formed between the two cuts, both dorsally and plantarly, should be approximately 60°. If the angle of these two cuts is made at 90°, then there is potential for dorsal displacement on weightbearing. If the angle is less than 60°, then on impaction of the distal segment there may be cortical bone absorption and delayed union, as well as overproduction of bone on the

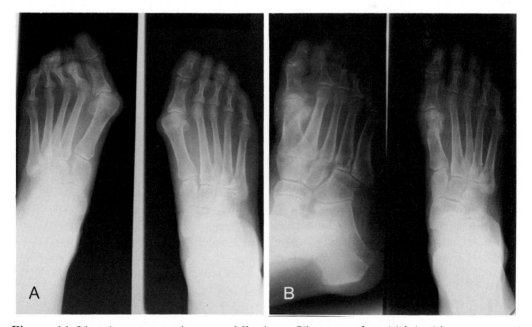

Figure 11.61. *A,* post-operative x-ray following a Silver procedure (right) with recurrence of the hallux abducto valgus deformity. *B,* post-operative x-ray following reconstruction with an arcuate osteotomy with too far lateral displacement of the distal segment, poor articulation at the MPJ, and hallux adductus.

plantar surface. In performing the procedure, staying at a right angle to the long axis of the first metatarsal going from medial to lateral is of extreme importance. Furthermore, one should preplan the distal portion of the "V" to be sure that the arms of the osteotomy do not meet too far distally, or even invade the metatarsophalangeal joint. Also, in shifting the distal segment laterally, the segment should not be displaced more than 50%, which can result in displacement or dislocation. Regarding the bicorrectional Austin to reduce an elevated proximal articular set angle, an overly abundant medial wedge can result in an overcorrection or a hallux varus, or too little a medial wedge can result in undercorrection with recurrence of the initial deformity. With common use of this procedure, simply impact the distal fragment once it has been shifted laterally, but care should be taken not to be overly aggressive with this impaction, which can lead to fracture of the distal segment. Cleary and Borovoy (136) reported on a case of traumatically displaced distal fragment following an Austin procedure without fixation, followed by open reduction with K-wire fixation, which resulted in proper alignment of the first metatarsophalangeal joint.

Johnson et al. (174) from the Mayo Clinic reported on the Chevron distal osteotomy which is essentially the Austin procedure. They reported on 18 patients (26 feet) and their basic procedure included a distal V osteotomy and the use of a short leg walking cast for an average of 32 days post-operatively. Their initial reason for using this procedure was that they found poor results with the Mitchell procedure due to considerable shortening of the first metatarsal and lateral metatarsalgia, which has been mentioned previously. Eighteen patients were contacted post-operatively with an average followup of 10 months after operation. They reported no complications with regard to infection, osteotomy displacement, nonunion, or aseptic necrosis of the first metatarsal head. Their primary indication was an elevated intermetatarsal

angle, which was approximately 15° in their study.

Miller and Croce (172), who used the same basic indications for the Austin procedure, did not mention the metatarsal protrusion measurement. They did mention the fact that this is a joint-preserving procedure, but must be carried out with accuracy. In utilizing the Austin procedure, Leventen (183) reported that in approximately 300 cases over a 10-year period, there had been no significant complications or recurrences. Lewis and Feffer (137) discussed a modification of the Chevron osteotomy of the first metatarsal which has a longer dorsal arm. They reported on 29 procedures performed on 17 patients and seemed primarily concerned with reduction of the intermetatarsal angle. Two of their patients had mild, occasional discomfort, but expressed satisfaction with the result. One patient had a gradual recurrence of the deformity over a 6-month period, which they attributed to "soft-tissue insufficiency." Another patient had gross undercorrection at the time of surgery. They also reported seven minor complications which they related chiefly to technical performance. They also reported that one patient suffered a post-operative fracture of the distal segment due to excessive distal extension of the osteotomy. In order to increase stability of the osteotomy and reduce post-operative pain, they did not advocate the use of post-operative plaster immobilization, and required 4 weeks of immobilization in a surgical shoe before returning to normal foot wear. An average reduction in the metatarsal angle was 4°, and reduction of the hallux abductus angle 13°.

There are definite similarities between the indications of the Austin and Mitchell procedures. As has just been pointed out by various recent studies, the Austin procedure appears to be far more stable with less shortening of the first metatarsal, as compared with the Mitchell procedure. Also, the Mitchell procedure requires precise fixation, as well as rigid immobilization to avoid nonunion, delayed union, or dorsal displacement of the distal segment. Both the Austin and Mitchell procedures have lent themselves to modifications which can also reduce the proximal articular set angle. The overall advantage seems to lean toward the Austin procedure with its modifications due to its overall post-operative stability. While the reader may feel that we have overemphasized the discussion of the metatarsal protrusion measurement, this is an area that has been incompletely discussed in the literature and needs further evaluation in the future.

Proximal First Metatarsal Osteotomies

When presented with structural deformity involving an excessively high first intermetatarsal angle, a proximal first metatarsal osteotomy may be indicated. When we previously discussed the distal osteotomy, the majority of those procedures involved an intermetatarsal angle of 14–16° with semi-rigidity or rigidity of the first metatarsal segment, as well as other possible structural deformities. However, when you are dealing with an intermetatarsal angle greater than 16°, whether the first metatarsal segment is rigid or hypermobile, a more proximal osteotomy is indicated. This theory was first proposed by Loisin in 1901, although he never actually performed any of the procedures. In 1903, Balacescu was the first to perform the technique as described by Loisin, which was a closing abductory wedge osteotomy near the base of the first metatarsal (114). Later, Lapidus, in 1934 (64, 173), stressed the importance of an elevated intermetatarsal angle or first metatarsal varus and its reduction in the overall surgical care of the hallux abducto valgus deformity. His contemporaries could not all agree with his proposals and a debate ensued.

CLOSING WEDGE OSTEOTOMY OF THE FIRST METATARSAL BASE

Youngswick, in a recent text (180), discusses the various pre-operative indications and contraindications for the use of this procedure. As a general rule, this procedure is combined with a capsulo-tendon balance procedure performed at the first metatarsal-phalangeal joint, as well as any other form of distal osteotomy which may be necessary to correct a distal structural deformity (107). The primary indications for the use of a closing wedge osteotomy of the first metatarsal base should be 1) abnormally high (greater than 15–16°) intermetatarsal angle or metatarsus primus adductus angle, and 2) a zero or positive metatarsal protrusion measurement. This latter indication, again, is essential since there is inherent shortening with this procedure.

Youngswick further discusses the possibility of a biplane-type closing wedge osteotomy when there is a rigid plantar-flexed first metatarsal, and a concurrent wedge can be removed with the base dorsal to elevate the first metatarsal segment. Another important point, is the use of templates for proper pre-operative measuring as to the exact degree and width of the appropriate wedge of bone to be removed. A key point is that the procedure should be performed 1–1.5 cm distal to the metatarsal-cuneiform articulation which will place the osteotomy site in cancellous bone, and will allow for more stable and more rapid healing, as compared to cortical osteotomies. Another important point made by Youngswick is that due to the location of the osteotomy, the epiphyseal plate should be closed prior to the performance of the procedure.

Various forms of fixation have been utilized over the years to maintain the bone in its corrected position. Monofilament wire is commonly used (Fig. 11.62). Overall, this provides adequate reduction but has limited ability in terms of compression. If the medial cortex is "thinned out" too much, it may result in fracture and displacement post-operatively, at which time the monofilament wire, generally placed only through the dorsal cortex, will be unable to prevent any dorsal displacement. K-wire fixation is also frequently utilized (Fig.

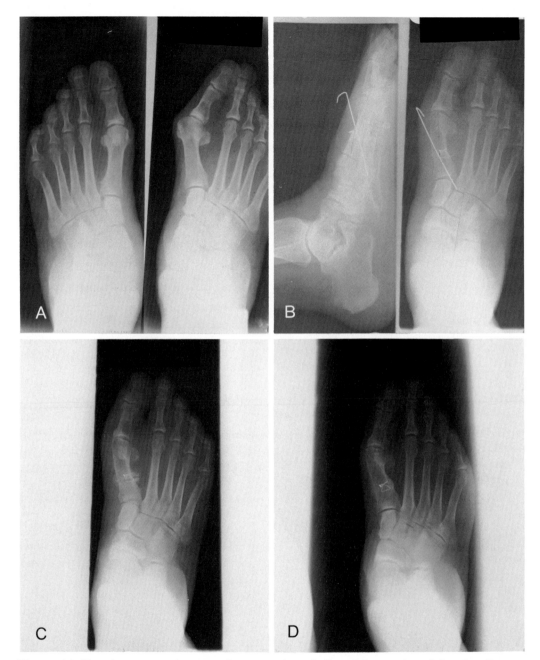

Figure 11.62. *A,* pre-operative x-ray demonstrating a hallux abducto valgus deformity. *B,* post-operative x-ray showing closing wedge osteotomy at the base of the first metatarsal with monofilament wire and K-wire fixation. *C,* post-operative x-ray showing exogenous callus formation due to too far distal placement of the osteotomy (cortical bone), inadequate fixation, and inadequate immobilization. *D,* post-operative x-ray with healed osteotomy but limited first MPJ motion and mild recurrence of HAV.

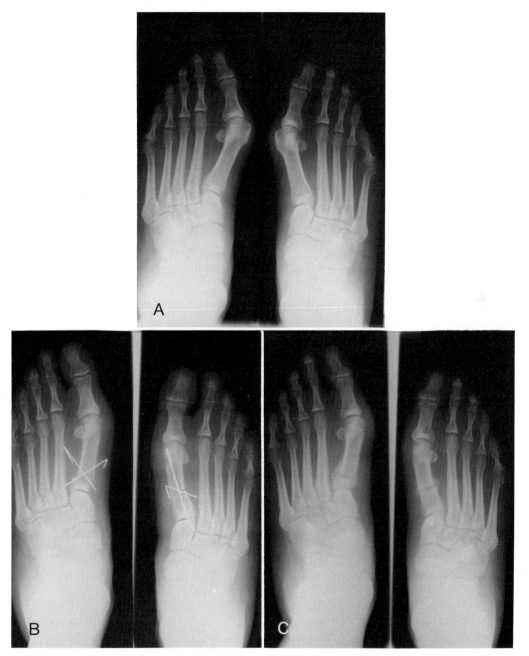

Figure 11.63. *A,* pre-operative x-ray with abnormally elevated first intermetatarsal angle. *B,* post-operative x-ray of a closing wedge osteotomy with K-wire fixation. *C,* post-operative x-ray showing exogenous callus formation bilateral; too far distal placement of right osteotomy; inadequate fixation and immobilization.

11.63). Again, care must be taken not to disrupt the medial cortex, as can be seen in the post-operative films, which may lead to potential displacement, and, if seen, the K-wire fixation should be maintained for a longer than average period of time until there is evidence of radiographic union (Fig. 11.64). Also, if the osteotomy is made too far distal in the cortical bone, then delayed union and long-term fixation and immobilization will be required. While the use of K-wire fixation can provide increased stability, the degree of compression at the osteotomy site is questionable, especially with the use of unthreaded wires.

Another device used for fixation is the Zlotof osteoclasp. There have been reports where the clasp has become loose and has required removal at a later date. The insertion of this fixation device is technically difficult and must be accurate to comply with the requirements for compression, which are designed into the device. This lends itself to technical error and varying degrees of compression, depending upon the technical skills of the surgeon, as well as the quality of the bone of the patient, which may lead to inconsistent results from patient to patient. Of more recent vintage, has been the use of AO screw fixation and the necessity to increase the obliquity of the wedge section to be removed so as to properly accommodate the insertion of the screw (Fig. 11.65) where a cortical screw was inserted. One should always be aware that it may be necessary to remove this screw and that the use of the lag technique is essential. Another common error is the counter sinking of the cortex of the metatarsal, which is essentially contraindicated because of the thinness of the cortex in the first metatarsal, and may result in poor compression and delayed or nonunion at the osteotomy site. Some surgeons have been using cancellous screws (Fig. 11.66). While the reduction of the osteotomy and the bony healing is evident, there may be some post-operative irritation from the head of the screw, and removal of this type of screw can be difficult, if not impossible, since the bone will heal around the smooth shaft of the screw, an area that is unthreaded. The most appropriate method seems to be the use of the cortical screw using a lag technique.

Unfortunately, while the use of the closing wedge osteotomy of the first metatarsal is used rather commonly, there is very little data that has been reported in the literature with regard to success rates and areas of complication. Youngswick (180) reported on a 10-year follow-up with the following complications:

—Overcorrection of the intermetatarsal angle;
—Undercorrection of the intermetatarsal angle;
—Inappropriate excision of a wedge piece of bone which can result in a "tear-drop" effect, and this defect on the medial aspect needs to be packed with bone;
—Fracture of the intact medial cortex which may result in dorsal displacement of the distal fragment;
—Delayed or nonunion of the osteotomy site;
—Osteoporosis due to prolonged immobilization;
—Dislodging or irritation from the internal fixation device which would require removal.

OPENING ABDUCTORY WEDGE OSTEOTOMY OF THE FIRST METATARSAL

In 1923, Trethowan (115) was the first to perform this procedure and he used the resected medial eminence from the first metatarsal head as the autogenous bone graft to be placed in the transverse osteotomy made at the base of the first metatarsal with the lateral cortex intact. The primary indication for this procedure is an elevated intermetatarsal angle between the first and second metatarsals. The procedure should also be utilized when there is a negative metatarsal protrusion measurement. Therefore, the major contraindication for this procedure would be when there is a positive metatarsal protrusion measure-

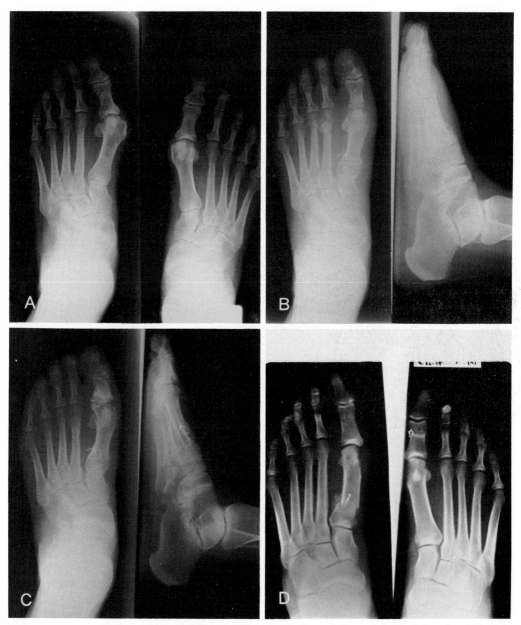

Figure 11.64. Case 1: Pre-operative x-ray of a hallux abducto valgus deformity (A); post-operative x-ray following closing wedge osteotomy at the base of the first metatarsal and the use of a monofilament wire, as well as the use of a hemiprosthetic at the first MPJ (B); post-operative x-ray showing healed proximal osteotomy but degenerative changes occurring at first MPJ (C). Case 2: Post-operative CWO with monofilament wire fixation, exuberent exogenous bony callus formation due to breakage of medical cortex, instability, and lack of immobilization (D).

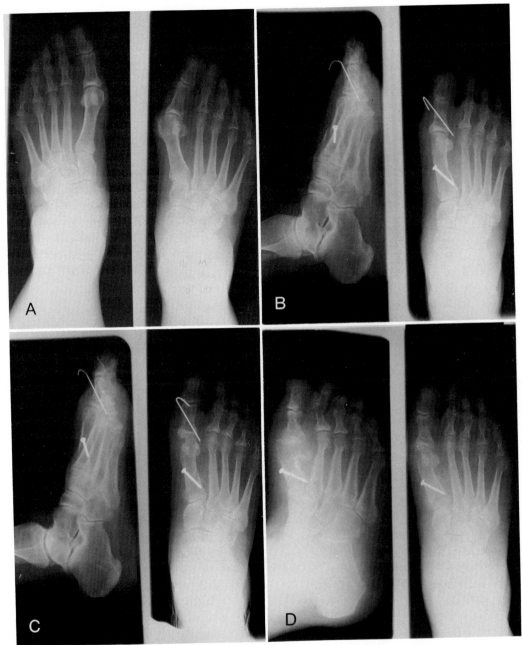

Figure 11.65. *A,* pre-operative x-ray with a hallux abducto valgus deformity. *B,* post-operative x-ray of a closing wedge osteotomy which is fixated with a cortical screw with inadequate alignment. *C,* post-operative x-ray shows inadequate osteotomy compression, exogenous callus formation, and instability. *D,* reconstructive surgery requiring debridement of delayed union and proper replacement of cortical screw using lag technique.

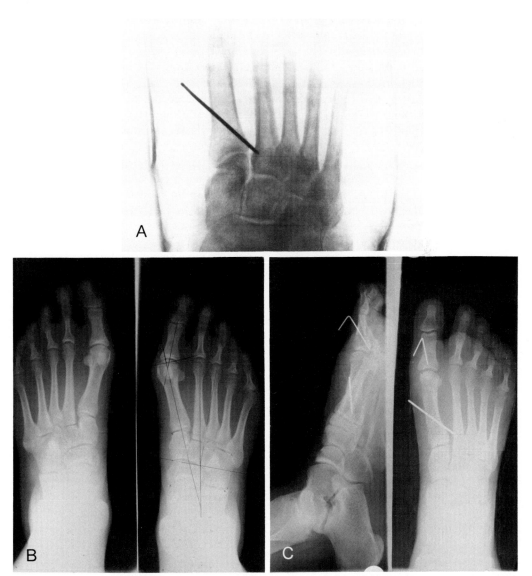

Figure 11.66. Case 1: Post-operative x-ray following an arcuate osteotomy of the base of the first metatarsal with K-wire fixation. The lack of visualization of osteotomy but improved structure is an indication of proper alignment and fixation. Cast immobilization was utilized (*A*). Case 2: Pre-operative x-ray with HAV deformity and elevated MPA (IM) angle (*B*); post-operative x-ray with a proximal arcuate osteotomy which shows good alignment and fixation, but was made too far distal in cortical bone, and most probably will result in prolonged healing time (*C*).

ment which could result in "jamming" of the first metatarsophalangeal joint and limited range of motion. Unlike many of the procedures previously discussed, the advantage of having a relative lengthening of the first metatarsal is an extremely important one. The major reason why this procedure is not used more frequently is that many surgeons have noticed that if they use the medial eminence of the first metatarsal head as the bone graft, there is compression of the graft during the post-operative healing period with loss of correction. Thus, an extremely important point to emphasize when performing an opening wedge osteotomy of the first metatarsal base is that cortical bone be used as a graft, whether it be autogenous or homogenous. We have found the use of cortical bone bank bone to be extremely advantageous, and the use of this freeze-dried cortical bone does not lead to compression. A major complication can occur if the cortical graft is placed too deeply in the osteotomy site or moves into the medullary substance, thus losing its dynamic effect. This results in undercorrection or recurrence of the elevated metatarsus primus adductus angle. Autogenous cortical bone can also be obtained with adjunct procedures such as Akin, Keller, or Keller with implant procedures.

Fixation is necessary along with immobilization post-operatively due to the inherent instability of this area after placement of the graft. There is limited data available regarding opening wedge osteotomies. Earlier this chapter, Youngswick provided us with some important areas of potential complications.

Haendel and Lindholm (141) pointed out in a 2-year follow-up study the various types of complications following first metatarsal wedge osteotomies. One of the key complications, which has been mentioned previously, is the development of a metatarsus primus elevatus, as was first described in 1938 by Lambrinudi (68). In Haendel and Lindholm's study (141), the normal declination of the first metatarsal

is approximately 10–15°. They accurately pointed out that the success of the procedure was dependent upon the type and location of the fixation device. It should be further pointed out that the correct angulation of the osteotomy cut is also essential to help reduce this type of complication. They also discussed how the use of monofilament wire does not adequately fixate the plantar cortex at the osteotomy site. Their study involved 53 patients with 59 closing wedge osteotomies having been performed. Overall, they showed that in 33% of their procedures, there was 5° or greater of first metatarsal distal segment elevation which is quite significant. Among the variants used in their study was the use of a type of thermoplastic immobilization (Hexolite®) versus plaster of Paris. The study showed that there was a decrease in the post-operative metatarsus primus elevatus in those cases where plaster of Paris had been used in comparison to the thermoplastic immobilization. Also, use of K-wires or AO screw fixation resulted in less elevation of the distal segment (106). Their conclusions include the use of cross K-wire or Steinmann pin fixation, as well as nonweightbearing casts for 4 weeks, and the use of ASIF screw fixation with a nonweight bearing period following surgery. Even with ASIF-type fixation and immediate weightbearing, they demonstrated that there can be displacement at the osteotomy site, excessive secondary bone formation, and loss of correction. Finally, use of internal monofilament wire can be utilized but should be passed through both the dorsal and plantar cortex on both sides of the osteotomy, which is technically more difficult than the procedure previously described, but should result in fewer complications of this type.

ARCUATE PROCEDURE

Several years ago, there was the development of a so-called cresentic osteotomy procedure to avoid the pitfalls in both the closing wedge osteotomy or opening wedge osteotomy of the first metatarsal base. Again, its use should be with those patients with a very high intermetatarsal angle between the first and second metatarsals. With the use of modern power equipment and properly shaped blades, the amount of bone removed at the osteotomy site is no more than 1–2 mm.

An important definitional change must be made at this time. As the reader has noted, we have used the term "arcuate" rather than "cresentic." Dr. John Comparetto has accurately noted that a crescent has two arcs and two radii. The procedure, as it has been performed over the last decade, has only one arc and one radius, and, thus, is truly an arcuate cut rather than a cresentic cut. We feel that this change in terminology is essential for accuracy.

A major advantage of this procedure is that it can reduce the first intermetatarsal angle without shortening the first metatarsal greatly, and therefore can be used in patients who have either a positive or slightly negative metatarsal protrusion measurement. If the metatarsal protrusion measurement is extremely negative, this procedure would be contraindicated. The major credit for developing this procedure must go to Dr. Robert Weinstock (31). If performed correctly, this procedure can quite adequately reduce a high abnormal intermetatarsal angle and, if fixated correctly, even on the initial radiographs, the osteotomy site is difficult, if not impossible, to visualize (Fig. 11.66).

The only available data with post-operative follow-up has been published by Clark in his chapter in the textbook by Gerbert and Sokoloff (180). This procedure also has the advantage of being able to either dorsiflex or plantarflex the distal segment, as was demonstrated by Clark. Our only variance with the basic procedure that he described is that in performing the arcuate osteotomy, the flange is left on the lateral side rather than on the medial side to allow for proper fixation with K-wires and allows for more lateral stability. In 1981, Clark reported that he had been performing the procedure since 1974 and had noted the following complications.

1. Overcorrection of the intermetatarsal angle;
2. Undercorrection of the intermetatarsal angle;
3. Delayed or nonunion of the osteotomy site;
4. Osteoporosis as a result of prolonged cast immobilization.

The reader should also take note that the osteotomy should be performed at right angles to the plantar surface of the foot to avoid elevation when moving the distal segment laterally. Due to the very nature of this type of osteotomy, it is inherently unstable and does not lend itself easily to the various types of internal or external fixation, as has been previously described with other procedures. Consistently good results may be obtained with the use of K-wires (0.045 or 0.062) or Steinmann pins (Fig. 11.67). The patient should be placed in plaster or thermoplastic immobilization with nonweightbearing for a period of 2–4 weeks, followed by weightbearing and continued use of cast immobilization, depending upon post-operative radiographs and evidence of osseous union.

MULTIPLE FIRST METATARSAL OSTEOTOMIES

The use of a double osteotomy of the first metatarsal to correct a structural deformity was first described by Logroscino in 1948 (152). He essentially utilized the techniques of Reverdin distally and Trethowan and Loison-Balacescu proximally. Further modification of this technique was proposed by Lidge (134) with his "3-in-1" technique (Fig. 11.68). In this particular type of procedure, there is correction of proximal structural deformity, distal structural deformity in the first metatarsal, and abnormal interphalangeal alignment of the hallux. He reported on 57 consecutive patients, 53 women and 4 men. There were a total of 92 feet operated on using this 3-in-1 technique. The age range was from 12 to 70

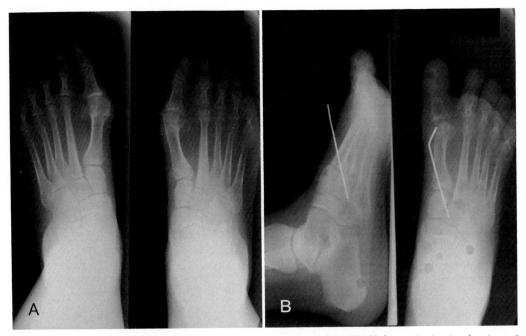

Figure 11.67. *A*, pre-operative x-ray of right foot of recurrent HAV due to lack of reduction of IM angle. *B*, post-operative x-ray of right foot after an arcuate proximal osteotomy with K-wire fixation. Overcorrection of IM angle can lead to a "static" hallux adductus.

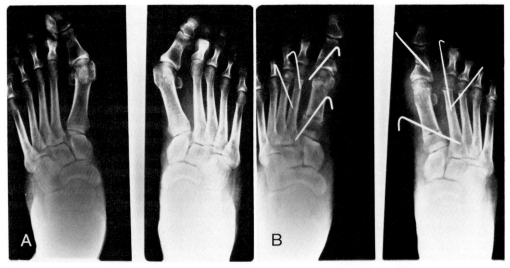

Figure 11.68. *a*, pre-operative x-ray of an hallux abducto valgus deformity. *B*, post-operative x-ray of "3 in 1" technique with a closing wedge osteotomy of the first metatarsal base, distal Reverdin procedure, and intraphalangeal osteotomy of the Akin type. Ostectomies bilaterally could be better approximated. Angle of some of the K-wires is questionable, and K-wire through left Akin crosses into MPJ which could lead to post-traumatic arthritis and limitation of motion.

years. In his overall study, 79% were satisfied with the results, while 13% felt that there was some improvement but were not entirely satisfied, and 8% were dissatisfied with the results.

In his complications, he listed that 20% of the patients showed mild swelling 3 months after surgery, in 5% of the patients pin migration occurred, and in 2% of the patients fracture of the pin occurred. In approximately 8% of the patients, joint stiffness was greater post-operatively than pre-operatively. As has been mentioned previously, dorsal displacement of the distal fragment is a possibility and certainly, statistically, is increased with these multiple osteotomies (Fig. 11.69).

The primary indications must be taken into consideration when performing multiple osteotomies of the first metatarsal and are as follows: 1) the reduction of an abnormally high first intermetatarsal angle; 2) an abnormally high proximal articular set angle; 3) paying close attention to the metatarsal protrusion measurement and choosing the individual procedures, both distally and proximally, to limit shortening

or to allow for lengthening; and 4) intraphalangeal osteotomy when indicated. Gerbert (180) in his text simply states that the overall complications with multiple osteotomies are inherent with the individual procedures themselves, and we have discussed those common complications previously. He stresses, however, the important use of pre-operative templates for accuracy and thus reducing, if not eliminating, the chance of overcorrection or undercorrection. Certainly, we would be remiss if we did not also emphasize the proper use of weightbearing and non-weightbearing casts for an appropriate amount of time due to the performance of these multiple osteotomies in a single osseous segment (Fig. 11.70).

The Lapidus Procedure

As has been previously discussed, Lapidus strongly believed in recognition of the "metatarsus varus primus deformity" as associated with or as a primary etiology of hallux abducto valgus. He correctly pointed out that "bunion" deformity is not so much a lateral deviation of the big toe as a medial

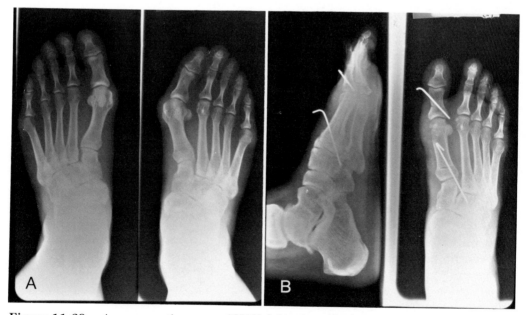

Figure 11.69. *A*, pre-operative x-ray of HAV deformity with abnormal MPA (IM), PASA, and DASA angles. *B*, post-operative x-ray tight of a "3-in-1" technique with proper alignment on A-P and lateral radiographs.

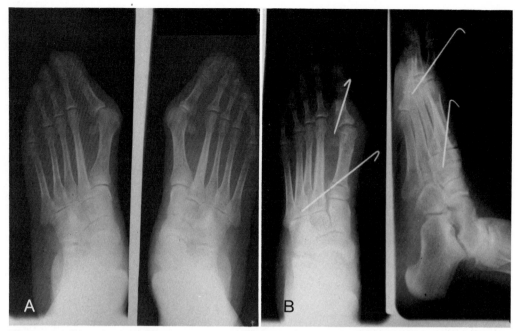

Figure 11.70. *A*, pre-operative x-ray with bilateral HAV with elevated MPA (IM) and PASA angles. *B*, post-operative x-ray of a Logroscino procedure with an Akin procedure ("3-in-1" technique) and K-wire fixation, but dorsal displacement of the distal osteotomy, either due to poor positioning, improper immobilization, or early weightbearing. Poor oblique angulation of distal Reverdin osteotomy, and K-wire in Akin osteotomy enters first MPJ.

protrusion of the first metatarsal head forming a bony proliferation because of constant trauma. He also emphasized the atavistic tendencies of certain foot types which allow for an increase in the metatarsus primus adductus angle and that soft tissue procedures are doomed to failure without correction of this high angle. He also made two other essential points: 1) shortening of the first metatarsal must be emphatically condemned as unphysiological and will result in biomechanical stress problems, and 2) he strongly advocated that each patient must be evaluated for structural and functional abnormalities, and that appropriate procedures be chosen based on those criteria. He did advocate that joint destruction of the first metatarsal base cuneiform articulation with fusion of this area will provide medial column stability, as well as reduce the abnormally high intermetatarsal angle. We feel that the primary indications for this procedure are:

1. Abnormally high first intermetatarsal angle greater than 15–16°;

2. Hypermobility of the first metatarsal with the subtalar joint held in a neutral position;

3. A positive metatarsal protrusion measurement.

We feel that the reason that this particular procedure has fallen into disfavor is that these criteria have neither been recognized or followed (Fig. 11.71).

Several technical points must be emphasized. First, while many authors have illustrated large wedge sections taken out to reduce excessively high intermetatarsal angle, in our experience, it is unnecessary to remove anything more than the articulating cartilage from the first metatarsal base and associated first cuneiform. Upon removal of the articulating surfaces, one will note that there is plenty of available space for reduction of the first intermetatarsal angle and that removal of a wedge would not only make reduction more difficult, but can lead to abnormal positioning. If extreme obliquity exists, then just the articulating cartilage can be removed and an

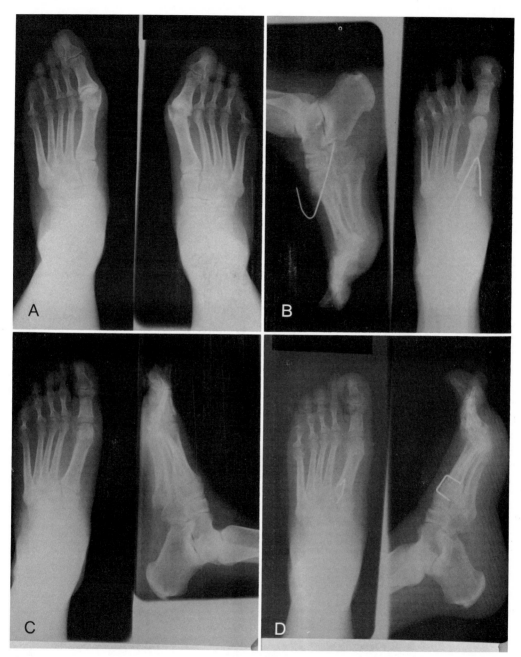

Figure 11.71. *A*, pre-operative x-ray of an hallux abducto valgus deformity. *B*, post-operative x-ray of Lapidus procedure with single K-wire fixation and a hemiprosthesis procedure at first MPJ. *C*, post-operative x-ray shows non-union of lapidus fusion. *D*, post-operative x-ray after reconstructive surgery to correct non-union with staple fixation.

opening osteotomy of the first cuneiform, with cortical bone graft, can be performed. Secondly, regarding positioning, one should take careful note to be sure to make vertical cuts and just remove the articulating cartilage. Unless one is trying to deliberately dorsiflex or plantarflex the first metatarsal segment, then wedge sections in the sagittal plane are unnecessary and can lead to untoward post-operative results (Fig. 11.72). Lapidus (173) reported again on his 28-year experience with his own procedure. While he quotes no statistics, he does state that his long-term experience with this procedure has been positive.

Gerbert and Sokoloff (180) properly emphasize the various complications, including shortening of the first metatarsal segment. In our own experience, we have found that this procedure provides excellent results when the previously mentioned criteria are followed. Without proper immobilization, fixation, and proper performance of the technique, then delayed or nonunion of the fusion site, as well as dorsal displacement of the first metatarsal, are potential undesirable side effects.

First Metatarsophalangeal Arthrodesis

As a result of complications of prior discussed procedures, undesirable side effects may necessitate the arthrodesis of the first metatarsophalangeal joint (153).

Acute pain may result at the first metatarsophalangeal joint following a Mayo-type procedure at the first metatarsal head. This may lead to some reduction in the stress pain that the patient experienced; however, it can also lead to more lateral symptomatology, as has been discussed previously with both the Keller and the Mayo procedures.

McKeever (93) was the first to discuss the deliberate arthrodesis of the first metatarsophalangeal joint. In 1941, he had a patient in which he performed a hallux abducto valgus correction and an infection ensued. After control of the infectious process, he noticed a rigid fibrotic ankylosis of the first metatarsophalangeal joint. He also noticed a reduction in the "metatarsus primus varus deformity," and that the "subjective" and "objective" evaluation appeared to be satisfactory. He then per-

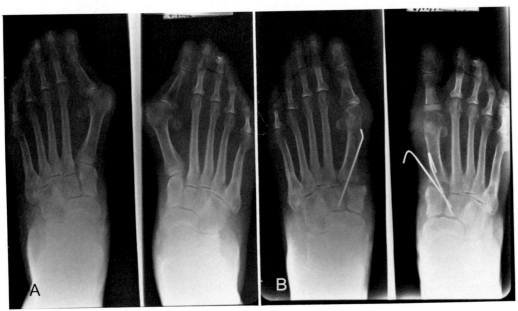

Figure 11.72. Case 1: Pre-operative x-ray with severe bilateral HAV (*A*); post-operative x-ray of attempted bilateral Lapidus arthrodesis procedure with excessive trauma, poor alignment, subluxation, and inadequate fixation (*B*).

formed several procedures in 1943 and 1944 on military personnel, but follow-up was impossible and the end results were unknown. In 1945, he began performing this type of procedure in private practice. He primarily used a fusion technique in which the cartilage at the first metatarsal-phalangeal joint was removed and the head was truncated into the base of the proximal phalanx and fixated with a cortical screw and washer. He stressed, however, that the position of the hallux is important, not the method by which the fixation is produced. An important point to be made by Mc-Keever's original article is that in men, the hallux should be fixated at approximately 15–20° of extension, and in women, who habitually wear shoes with medium heels, that the fixation be 15–25° of extension of the hallux. However, in women who wear high-heeled shoes at all times, that the hallux be fixated as high as 35° of extension. This obviously would create problems in any patient who cannot wear high-heeled shoes at all times. He stated that about 50% of the patients required no alteration in their shoe gear and that the other 50% required some temporary or permanent alteration with metatarsal padding. As originally described, McKeever advocated the use of this procedure for the relief of hallux valgus, metatarsus primus varus, and hallux rigidus. While the use of arthrodesis of the first metatarsophalangeal joint as described by Thompson and McElvenny (68) in cases of tuberculosis of bone appears to be indicated, the routine use of arthrodesis of the first metatarsophalangeal joint for hallux abducto valgus deformity or metatarsus primus varus, as advocated by McKeever, must be called into question.

Marin (138) further stressed that arthrodesis of the first metatarsophalangeal joint is not necessarily a salvage procedure, but when used as a primary measure, "gives a high percentage of excellent results." His primary indications were in cases of moderate to severe hallux valgus in middle-aged and elderly patients. Also, he used it in cases of hallux rigidus for the relief of pain. The primary contraindications were; 1) os-

teoporosis, as is seen in rheumatoid feet, and 2) where osteoarthritic changes of the interphalangeal joint has resulted in less than 45° flexion of this joint which may result in pain post-operatively. He advocated the fusion of the first metatarsal-phalangeal joint with the hallux held in 10° dorsiflexion in the sagittal plane. Marin reported on 200 procedures (180 for hallux valgus and 20 for hallux rigidus) over a 10-year period with 2% having a fibrous ankylosis which was painless. In 25% of his cases there was no associated lateral metatarsalgia; however, he did report 70% of his cases did have a slight metatarsalgia laterally and in 5% of the cases there was severe lateral metatarsalgia. He also advocated the fusion of the hallux in 2–5° of valgus, otherwise a plantar keratotic lesion may develop beneath the interphalangeal joint which may become symptomatic. In spite of the high percentage of patients who had lateral symptomatology post-operatively, he rated the overall procedure as excellent with limited sequelae. Finally, Fitzgerald and Wilkinson (139), reported on two series with a success rate of 91% and 86%, respectively. They noted that in a long-term follow-up of from 10 to 17 years, deterioration of the arthrodesis occurred only in those patients in whom arthritic changes developed in the interphalangeal joint. While they stated that external compression devices may have an advantage in rigid fixation, their major disadvantage is that weightbearing must be delayed until the apparatus is removed. In their method, they used primarily periarticular interosseous wire internal fixation for stabilization of the arthrodesis. They also noted that in cases where screw fixation was utilized for arthrodesis, pain may ensue from the head of the screw necessitating removal at a future date. Complications occurred in primarily two areas: 1) malposition of the arthrodesis, and 2) hallux interphalangeal arthritis. In approximately 16% of the patients, there were symptoms of pain directly attributable to improper position of the hallux in relation to the first metatarsal. In 9% of the patients, abduction and valgus rotation of the hallux, leading to a painful plantar keratosis on the medial plantar aspect of the interphalangeal joint resulted. Moynihan in 1967 noted arthritic changes in the interphalangeal joint following arthrodesis of the first metaatarsophalangeal joint, and Fitzgerald found this to be a 10% occurrence in his study. Fitzgerald and Wilkinson (139) advocated that the hallux be fused with approximately 20–30° of valgus position to allow the hallux to be accommodated in a normal shoe. A greater valgus position would result in crowding of the lesser digits. While they did not seem overly concerned about the exact percentage of dorsiflexion of the hallux at the metatarsophalangeal joint, they nonetheless advocated that approximately 20–30° of dorsiflexion seemed to be optimal. They primarily advocated the use of this procedure in patients with symptomatic hallux rigidus and hallux valgus with associated lateral metatarsalgia.

It would still seem that the importance of the first metatarsophalangeal joint is being overlooked in relation to biomechanical function if arthrodesis is used as a standard form of treatment for hallux abducto valgus. With the various surgical approaches now available, it still seems likely that this should be used as a salvage procedure for failures following surgical procedures at the first metatarsophalangeal joint. One should take note of the above studies since if arthrodesis is undertaken, there does appear to be a high percentage of successful results in terms of alleviating the patient's symptomatology.

Adolescent (Juvenile) Hallux Abducto Valgus

One of the most perplexing areas when dealing with a hallux abducto valgus deformity is when it involves an adolescent. This does not account for a high percentage of cases, and there is inconclusive evidence over the past 70 years concerning the exact approach in these cases (66). Because of the inherent anticipation of performing surgery on a growing child with active epiphyses, the tendency has been to utilize the most conservative approaches. There is also the erroneous conclusion that may be drawn from the patient's age that, for the most part, we are dealing with a positional deformity. On more careful analysis, the surgeon will be able to observe that there is a high degree of structural deformity involved in these cases. Thus, a more aggressive approach is indicated, but care must be taken not to interfere with the epiphyseal plates unless epiphysiodesis is being attempted. The same basic etiological criteria, as well as pre-operative criteria, must be maintained in the adolescent patient with a hallux abducto valgus deformity. On occasion, one can successfully perform a capsulo-tendon balance procedure which will adequately reduce the deformity and, if proper biomechanical maintainance is followed post-operatively, then recurrence can be reduced to a minimum (Fig. 11.73). The arthroplasty or joint destructive procedures should be avoided at all costs. Bonney and MacNab (143) from England pointed out that the results of the Keller operation performed on adolescent patients had been "uniformly bad." They also observed that the performance of metatarsal osteotomies showed distinctly poor results. However, it should be noted that many of their osteotomies were performed at midshaft to avoid injury to the epiphysis, and that the alignment and fixation were certainly inadequate. In their study, 34 out of 54 feet that had been operated on with a metatarsus primus varus deformity showed recurrence of the hallux abducto valgus deformity to the original state or to a larger angle than before surgery after intervals varying from 1 day to 3 months post-operatively. From their high percentage of failure, several conclusions were drawn which do have some validity, the first being that one must be able to control the first metatarsal segment and be sure that it is properly aligned in relation to the second metatarsal to prevent recurrence. Secondly, one must not obtain a "false" correction by soft tissue compres-

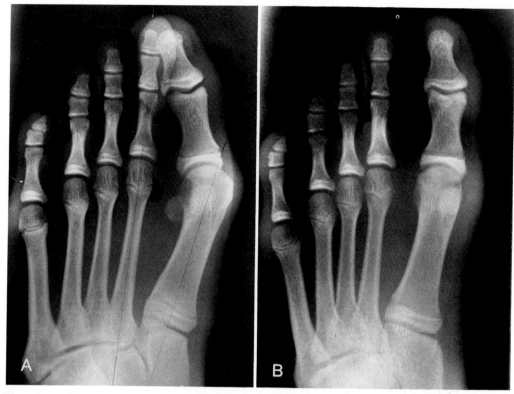

Figure 11.73. *A*, pre-operative AP x-ray of an adolescent hallux abducto valgus. *B*, post-operative x-ray following a McBride capsulo-tendon balance bunionectomy.

sion between the first and second metatarsals since, if the structural deformity has not been corrected, then recurrence is inevitable. Finally, with a first metatarsal osteotomy, the long axis of the entire first metatarsal must be controlled rather than just the distal segment. Furthermore, they pointed out that recurrence can develop from early weightbearing, inadequate immobilization, or more distal osteotomy while the proximal portion continues to develop in a "varus" alignment. Some general conclusions were drawn about potential complications which can also occur in the adolescent but have been previously discussed with reference to the adult population, such as 1) post-operative elevation of the first metatarsal following osteotomy; 2) limitation of motion at the first MPJ; 3) inappropriate removal of bone at the first metatarsal head; 4) recurrence of the deformity from soft tissue contractions (Fig. 11.74); or 5) overcorrection of the metatar-

sus primus varus deformity with excessive removal of the first metatarsal head, resulting in hallux varus. In order to avoid these potential problems, Bonney and MacNab felt that the most appropriate surgical therapy was an opening wedge proximal osteotomy of the first metatarsal with bone grafting from the medial eminence, as well as insertion of a screw through the first and second metatarsal heads in the transverse plane to secure the correction. They did state that the screw may be removed at a future date to prevent any bone stress or complications from its insertion, although their paper in 1952 did not draw any specific conclusions since they had just begun to use this particular procedure. Their overall conclusions were that one should avoid surgery until closure of the epiphysis since, in their particular study, 10 of 14 feet operated on before epiphyseal closure showed recurrence. However, there was a recurrence rate of nine feet out of 20

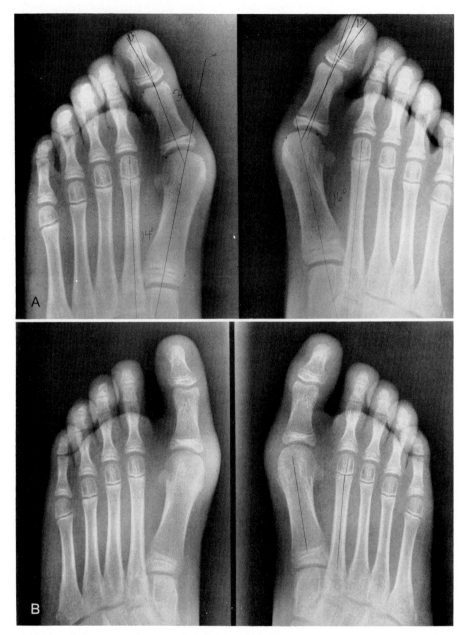

Figure 11.74. *A*, pre-operative x-ray bilateral of an adolescent hallux abducto valgus deformity with structural abnormalities. *B*, post-operative x-ray following a Silver capsulo-tendon balance bunionectomy with potential recurrence with first MPJ instability due to failure to correct the structural deformity.

operated on in which the procedure was performed after epiphyseal closure. One of their final interesting points was the possibility of a stapling or epiphyseal arrest procedure on the lateral side of the first metatarsal epiphysis, but they clearly noted that there were some technical difficulties with this "theory" and potential problems in growth which would have to be studied in more detail. There is currently no data available to support such a procedure, but it certainly lends itself to some potential research in the future.

Carr and Boyd (144) discussed the use of the Mitchell distal osteotomy for correction of a hallux abducto valgus deformity in 28 patients (five males and 23 females). The average first intermetatarsal angle was 13.5% pre-operatively with a range of 10–18°. The average follow-up following this procedure was 4 years with a range of 2–8 years. Of the 54 feet operated on, 41 were rated as excellent, with 10 rated as good, and three rated as fair. Of those patients rated as having a good result, they could not be classified as having an excellent result because of a lack of cosmetic correction in four, inadequate correction of the deformity in five, and restriction of motion at the first metatarsophalangeal joint in one. They concluded that the primary reason for all of these less than excellent results were due to excessive shortening of the first metatarsal or rotation of the distal fragment of the first metatarsal. In one patient with a fair result in a bilateral procedure, there was adequate correction of the intermetatarsal angle but excessive shortening of the first metatarsal (9 mm on the left foot and 7 mm on the right foot) and post-operative metatarsalgia bilaterally in the area of the second metatarsal head. In another patient with a unilateral procedure with a fair result, the pre-operative first intermetatarsal was corrected from 18° to 11°, but there was a residual hallux abducto valgus deformity. Carr and Boyd stated that the reduction of the first intermetatarsal angle must be to 9° or less in order to obtain proper post-operative results. In their conclusions, they empha-

sized that the first metatarsal should not be shortened more than 3–4 mm, which has been emphasized previously.

By far, the most detailed post-operative analysis of adolescent hallux abducto valgus surgery was performed by Helal (145). From 1966 to 1981, he polled 450 British orthopedic surgeons analyzing 842 patient records, but only 378 operations provided adequate pre-operative data. Several interesting patterns began to emerge with the help of this study and, hopefully, future data will allow the overall picture to become more clear. It is apparent that soft-tissue procedures or capsulo-tendon balance procedures have a much lower percentage of success. There may be inadequate reduction at the first metatarsophalangeal joint, poor correction of structural deformities can lead to stiffness and limitation of motion at the first metatarsophalangeal joint, as well as recurrence of the deformity up to 6 years post-operatively. In Helal's study, the Joplin procedure showed excellent results in 11%, good results in 49%, and poor results in 40%. The McBride procedure showed 14% excellent results, 32% good results, and 54% poor results. Improvement in these statistics was seen with the Peabody procedure where there was 34% excellent results, 32% good results, and 34% poor results. More drastic improvement in results is seen with the Mitchell procedure which showed 46% excellent results, 34% good results, and 20% poor results. Helal himself advocated the use of the Wilson lateral displacement osteotomy which showed 51% excellent results, 43% good results, and only 6% poor results. Of all of the cases analyzed, 92% of the patients were female and their ages ranged from 9–19 years. In 75% of these cases, the condition was seen bilaterally. To emphasize the hesitancy on the part of most surgeons, Helal showed that of 160 surgeons, only 2% operated on all adolescent hallux abducto valgus deformities, 5% avoid operating, and 65% operated on approximately 50% of their adolescent patients with hallux abducto valgus. He also took into account the fact that in many instances, the degree of morbidity following surgery was directly related to the experience and training of the involved surgeon, with a higher degree of morbidity in those cases involving younger surgeons.

Again, Helal primarily advocated the use of the Wilson displacement osteotomy. His most unfavorable results were found in those patients who developed a metatarsalgia laterally which followed a dorsal shift or tilt of the first metatarsal head. Helal emphasized the technical errors such as: 1) inadequate displacement of the osteotomies, and 2) an osteotomy that was too oblique or too transverse. In his series utilizing the Wilson osteotomy, none of the patients had relapsed into valgus. Further, he advocated that the age of the patient seemed to be an important factor and that the operation was best carried out in the early teens rather than at a later time. Whenever possible, he emphasized the avoidance of interfering with the metatarsophalangeal joint and categorically stated that to destroy the joint by fusion or arthroplasty procedures was not justified. He accounted for the failure of the capsulotendon balance procedures by stating that any attempt to realign the hallux at the first metatarsophalangeal joint alters the congruity of the joint and may cause degenerative changes of the articulating cartilage with subsequent pain and limitation of motion. He also mentions the feasibility of an epiphysiodesis as a rational approach to the problem of metatarsus primus varus. He further states, however, that too many of the patients present later in the growth curve and, thus, epiphysiodesis would not significantly influence the deformity since it goes unrecognized, either by the patient or physicians, for too long a time.

This most recent data appears to be clearing some of the cloud over the adolescent hallux abducto valgus deformity. When a structural deformity is identified and corrected, the radiographic appearance of the first metatarsophalangeal joint appears to be more stable with adequate correction, though it is not true that all adolescent patients with hallux abducto valgus deformity require structural correction since some of them will present with positional deformities. It is also clear that the majority of adolescent patients with hallux abducto valgus will have some underlying structural deformity which requires correction. Based on the available data, not to recognize this particular aspect of the deformity will only lead to a higher percentage of failure with undercorrection and the need for surgical intervention in the future.

Hallux Varus

Although there has been a limited amount of material published with regard to post-operative or acquired hallux varus deformity following hallux abducto valgus surgery, the overall incidence appears to be somewhere between 1–2%. In most cases, further surgery is necessary in the reduction of the hallux varus deformity and does not involve a simple approach, as one would assume on initial evaluation.

Janis and Donick (164) reviewed 1100 cases of McBride bunionectomies with hallux varus occurring in 18 cases or 1.6%. The following etiological factors of hallux varus were determined from that study:

1. Long first metatarsal or positive metatarsal protrusion measurement;
2. Round first metatarsal head;
3. Overcorrection of the first intermetatarsal angle;
4. Excessive resection of the medial aspect of the first metatarsal head;
5. Medial pull of the abductor hallucis;
6. Medial pull of the flexor hallucis brevis;
7. Medial pull of the EHL;
8. Inadequate capsular repair.

They observed that the varus deformity occurred in patients with an equal or long first metatarsal when compared with the second metatarsal, and did not occur in cases where there was a pre-operative negative metatarsal protrusion measurement. Clearly, when the patient presents a pre-operative first metatarsal head that is round, or when there is an excessive amount of bone resected from the medial aspect of the first metatarsal head, or when there has been overreduction of an elevated first intermetatarsal angle, then there will be a higher incidence of hallux varus (Fig. 11.75). Instability of the first metatarsophalangeal joint will occur upon poor capsular dissection. This was also pointed out much earlier by Seeburger and Bradlee (167) when they discussed various etiological factors involving hallux varus. The varus position of the hallux may not become evident immediately and can manifest itself anywhere from 6 months to 5 years postoperatively. They also pointed out the technical error of suturing the extensor hallucis longus tendon to the capsule, rather than suturing the tendon sheath, which may lead to inappropriate positioning and lack of motion of the tendon. Seeburger and Bradlee (167) advocated soft tissue releases to alleviate the varus deformity and advocated arthroplasty or joint destructive procedures only as a last resort.

Hawkins (166) discussed his concept of the acquired hallux varus and classified these cases into two categories, "static" and "dynamic." Static hallux varus was defined as having occurred following bunionectomies of the Mayo, Stone, Silver, Peabody, and Hohmann procedures. In his opinion, these procedures did not involve disturbance of the muscle balance even though the toe had been overcorrected. He anticipated that with time there would be gradual realignment. In the "dynamic" deformities, there was a disturbance of the muscle balance. Essentially, this occurs when the adductor hallucis tendon has been incised, the lateral sesamoid removed, and a lateral capsular release, which also includes the lateral head of the flexor hallucis brevis. This alleviates the lateral antagonistic opposition and allows for a medial overcorrection which has been seen in relation to the Reverdin procedure as mentioned earlier. Hawkins further pointed out that the great toe should not be corrected beyond the midpoint in its relation to the first metatarsal since there is a normal lateral deviation of the hallux of approximately 10–15°. Hawkins reported on 300 cases of the Stamm

procedure which involved adductor hallucis release and transposition, as well as an opening wedge osteotomy of the base of the first metatarsal. He reported on three cases of hallux varus in which either the lateral sesamoid had been excised or the lateral head of the flexor hallucis brevis had been released along with the adductor transposition. It was his conclusion that lateral displacement of the lateral sesamoid does not prevent correction of the hallux abducto valgus deformity and, thus, its removal is unnecessary. This particular concept has obtained some recent acceptability. Hawkins' method of correction of the hallux varus deformity included release of the abductor hallucis tendon from its insertion on the medial aspect and transposition to the lateral side of the base of the proximal phalanx where the adductor hallucis tendon had been removed. He also reported on the use of a fascial graft on the lateral aspect of the first metatarsal-phalangeal joint in one patient but did not feel that this was essential to the correction.

Feinstein and Brown (163) reported on 878 cases of post-operative bunionectomy, with a hallux varus (adductus) in eight cases following McBride procedures, one case following a Silver procedure, and one case following a modified Keller procedure, with an overall incidence of 1.13%. They emphasized that (following the work of Basmajian and Kerr) in only 19% of patients is the abductor hallucis tendon inserted into the base of the proximal phalanx. They stated that proper pre-operative evaluation must be undertaken along with the standard criteria since the occurrence of post-operative hallux varus appeared to be more prevalent in patients with joint hypermobility or subclinical Ehlers-Danlos syndrome. They also pointed out that excessive compression bandages and overcorrection of the hallux during the initial postoperative period can lead to the development of a hallux varus deformity. Further complications may occur with distal first metatarsal osteotomies of the Austin or Reverdin type where there is poor alignment of the distal fragment.

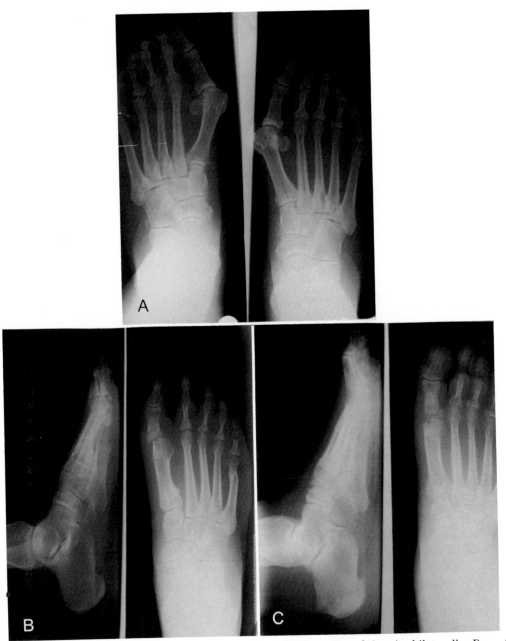

Figure 11.75. *A*, pre-operative x-ray of an hallux abducto valgus deformity bilaterally. *B*, post-operative x-ray of the right foot showing the hallux in rectus alignment and apparent stability of the first metatarsophalangeal joint, although the hallux should be in a more lateral position. *C*, post-operative x-ray of the left foot showing a hallux varus deformity of the "dynamic" type.

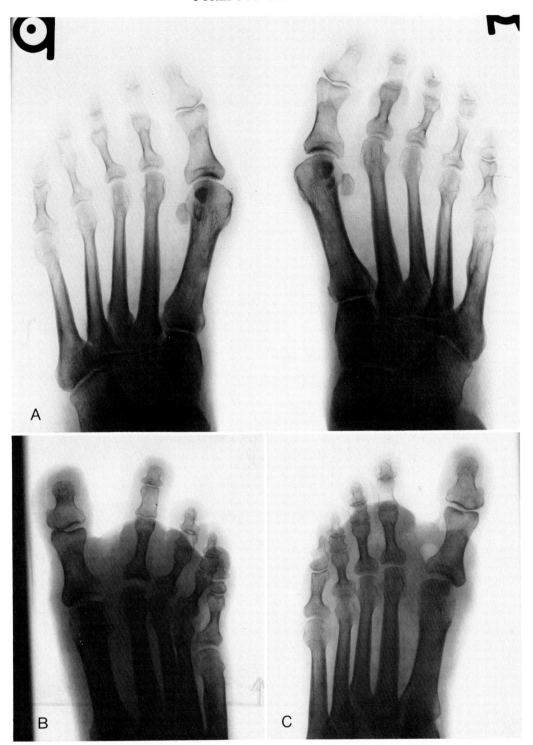

Figure 11.76. *A*, pre-operative x-ray of bilateral HAV. *B*, post-operative x-ray following a CWO and hemiprosthetic first MPJ procedure with a hallux varus deformity of the "static" type. *C*, post-operative x-ray showing a correction of static hallux varus (adductus) with use of a total hinge joint prosthesis first MPJ to provide stability.

Figure 11.76 demonstrates pre- and post-operative x-rays of a patient with a hallux abducto valgus deformity. The post-operative x-ray of the right foot shows a post-operative Silver procedure with the hallux in rectus alignment, whereas the position should be more lateral. In the post-operative x-ray of the left foot, there is a hallux varus deformity as a result of a lateral release and a wedge section removed from the capsule of the medial aspect of the first metatarsal-phalangeal joint. This dynamic type of deformity required further surgical intervention to correct this avoidable complication. It has been our experience that it is no longer necessary, as a routine matter, to shorten or remove a wedge section from the medial aspect of the first metatarsal-phalangeal joint capsule, especially in cases where there has been an excessive lateral release.

There have been various methods proposed for the reduction of the acquired hallux varus deformity. Midkiff (165) reported on soft tissue release with lateral capsulotomy and capsulorrhaphy on five patients with a more detailed description of one case of a severe, acquired hallux varus. After 1 year, he states that the results were satisfactory. Kimizuka and Miyanaga (162) reported on five cases of hallux varus following McBride procedures over a 20-year period. It should be noted that McBride had reported in 1935 on two cases of overcorrection following his procedure. Silver, in 1923, reported on two cases of static hallux varus after his procedure, but McBride's cases involved dynamic hallux varus. Kimizuka and Miyanaga reported overall satisfactory results with elongation of the extensor hallucis longus tendon and release of the abductor hallucis tendon. In one case, there was inadequate reduction and the patient complained of poor cosmesis. As a result, they now recommend a combination of the above procedures, as well as resection of the base of the proximal phalanx (Keller) with partial syndactylization between the first and second digits.

Wood (160) discussed the total joint

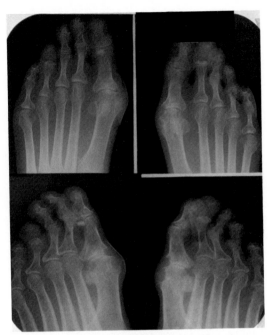

Figure 11.77. Pre-operative x-rays demonstrating gouty arthritis which must be recognized to avoid complications with whatever HAV procedure is being contemplated.

release (TJR) as performed at the University of Chicago and credited Gudas with its development. This appears to be a modification of previously mentioned procedures as advocated by Seeburger and Bradlee, and appears to be an adequate solution for the static type of varus deformity. The dynamic type of deformity is less likely to respond to this type of treatment. He reported on a single case, following a McBride bunionectomy. In his case presentation, there was apparent excessive removal of the medial aspect of the first metatarsal head which allowed for "stacking" and allowed the medial sesamoid to displace in a medial direction because of the lack of articulating surface.

Langford and Maxwell (161) further discussed the acquired type of hallux varus, involving a single case, but associated with a hammertoe deformity of the hallux bilaterally. It is not uncommon to see this type of interphalangeal deformity with a long-standing hallux varus. It should be emphasized at this point that when such a deformity occurs, that interphalangeal arthrodesis is indicated, as well as extensor hallucis longus tendon lengthening. Finally, they discussed the use of a total hinge joint prosthesis to provide stability at the first metatarsophalangeal joint. The use of arthroplasty or joint destructive procedures without prosthetics may reduce the varus deformity, but can result in other undesirable complications which have been discussed previously.

Once again, we emphasize the proper preoperative evaluation and appropriate criteria for the use of the various bunion procedures in order to avoid the post-operative hallux varus deformity. While the overall percentage of occurrence appears to be small, it can be a rather devastating complication to the patient. The recognition of the static versus dynamic type of development is an important one, especially when attempting to correct the deformity. Based on the various etiological factors of hallux varus, it is an avoidable type of complication, but one which will not be completely eliminated, even if strict criteria and preoperative evaluation are followed. There are always those cases where the patient may traumatize the operative site early in the healing phase, and, if recognized, aggressive conservative therapy would be indicated. Once recognition is made of the specific type of varus deformity, the best surgical approach is a step-by-step intraoperative regime from the most conservative total joint release progressing to osseous procedures, including the use of prosthetic devices.

GENERAL CONSIDERATIONS

Throughout this final section on hallux abducto valgus surgery, we have attempted to identify the various individual complications with the specific procedures involved. The surgical approach to hallux abducto valgus deformity is difficult and complex, and requires maximum effort on the part of the surgeon performing proper pre-operative evaluation, performance of the appropriate surgical technique, and controlled post-operative care. Dr. Earl

Kaplan has emphasized, in his many years of teaching, that each patient must be evaluated individually and the appropriate surgical approach must be undertaken only after careful history and physical examination. This particular point cannot be overemphasized. Various other complications can occur with any form of surgery on the foot and each area will be discussed here briefly.

Kirschner (179) discussed the various areas of overall complications that can occur, especially associated with hallux abducto valgus surgery. An allergic reaction to suture material can occur from time to time. A careful pre-operative history with regard to previous surgeries, or previous suture reactions, may assist in avoiding this type of complication. This complication may occur from 2 days to 3 years postoperatively. If a surgical knot on capsular suture is placed directly beneath the skin incision, it may then protrude, causing a localized tissue reaction. The same type of complication can occur if suture ends are not cut short enough and protrude through the incision line. At the same time, there may be a localized reaction to specific materials. When known, the materials should not be utilized. There are reports of patients who have come back 2–3 years postoperatively with a local small abcess along the incision line from deep, nonabsorbable sutures such as Tevdek®. Hematoma formation is a potential complication which is also preventable. As a general rule, when hematoma formation occurs, this is commonly due to poor surgical technique. When patients complain of severe localized pain beyond normal limits within 24–72 hours, and there is no evidence of infection, then hematoma formation must be suspected. This needs to be evacuated and hemostasis controlled to avoid further hemorrhage and potential infection. Poor surgical technique and mishandling of the tissue is a cause of wound dehiscence. Constant respect of the soft tissues and the neurovascular bundles must be of primary concern throughout the procedure. Dehiscence can also develop if there has been poor pre-operative evaluation of the patient with underlying arteriosclerotic disease or poor medical evaluation of metabolic disease. Morrison (158) emphasized several complications following forefoot surgery in rheumatoid arthritic patients. The results of this study involved basically forefoot reconstructive procedures with a plantar incisional approach. Several patients experienced pain along the incision line, although there was no delayed healing in any of the cases. In one case where there was a pre-operative diagnosis of psoriasis, the disease involved the suture line post-operatively, causing severe localized pain and tenderness and a poor functional result. Other patients in the series complained of pain along the incision line or on the plantar surface of the lesser metatarsals. It needs to be re-emphasized through this and other studies that plantar approaches should be avoided whenever possible since the complications that can occur are avoidable by dorsal incisions. Also, such approaches as advocated by Peterson for hallux abducto valgus surgery must be avoided since there is potential damage and stress to the neurovascular structures.

Post-operative osteoporosis may occasionally be seen and may be due to localized stress following surgery or as a subclinical form of Sudeck's atrophy. Appropriate physical therapy, therapeutic injections, and exercises should alleviate most symptoms. Post-operative anesthesia, paresthesia, or causalgia may occur following forefoot surgery. As a general rule, these too are avoidable since they generally occur when surgical technique is poor, and nerves are either lacerated partially or completely. The same symptoms may occur when sutures are inappropriately placed around nerves causing compression and disruption of the normal nerve pathway. Some patients may experience partial or complete anesthesia following surgery, even when normal techniques are followed. This is generally due to stretching of the nerves during retraction in performance of the surgical procedure, and normal sensation generally returns in 2–18 months.

Melillo emphasized in his chapter in the text by Gerbert and Sokoloff (180) the importance of appropriate capsulotomies and capsulorrhaphies. Mentioned earlier in this chapter was that shredding or inappropriate capsular dissection can lead to instability of the first metatarsophalangeal joint. Melillo emphasized that when this occurs, there are various procedures which can be performed to provide the necessary stability, and the reader is referred to that text for further discussion. He also discussed the unintentional laceration of the extensor tendon and appropriate methods for repair, including grafting, which may be necessary to allow for normal tendon function post-operatively, as well as continued stability of the first metatarsophalangeal joint.

Occasionally, one will see a mycotic infection post-operatively. The patients will complain of a "rash" which is pruritic and, as a general rule, does not lead to any serious complications if identified and treated appropriately. Localized bacterial infections should be seen no more frequently than in 1–2% of the cases. The vast majority of post-operative bacterial infections are directly related to inappropriate surgical technique and/or trauma by the surgeon during the operative phase. This is not directly related to the size of the wound. Excessive trauma to tissues can occur whether the incision is 1.0 cm or 10.0 cm in length. Johnson (155) pointed out the use of local antibiotic flushes intra-operatively, especially in cases involving multiple osteotomies, bone grafting procedures, and implant insertion. The use of kanamycin appears to be the most effective antibiotic flush. When dealing with bone grafting procedures, kanamycin should be diluted in Ringer's lactate solution, which is more physiologic to the grafted bone.

By definition, a delayed union of an osteotomy site occurs within the first 2–4 months. Careful support of the area and immobilization is indicated in order to prevent any further delay in healing or any unfavorable results. When an osteotomy has not healed by the 4–8-month period, diagnosis of nonunion can be made. Depending upon the location of the nonunion and the patient's symptoms, appropriate surgical therapy should be instituted to rectify the problem. While it is our desire to return these patients to normal ambulatory activities, one must have a clear understanding of normal bone physiology and the healing process.

When undercorrection, recurrence of the deformity, or overcorrection (hallux varus) occurs, then re-evaluation of the pre-operative analysis of the patient and/or the intra-operative surgical technique is indicated. Stiffness at the first metatarsal-phalangeal joint is generally due to an improper surgical technique or prolonged immobilization in bandages or splints which do not allow for normal rehabilitation.

Complications such as lateral metatarsalgia, stress fractures of the lateral metatarsals, flail hallux, hallux extensus, or hammer digit syndrome of the hallux are complications which are inherent with given surgical procedures which have been previously identified (Fig. 11.78). These complications may also occur when improper pre-operative evaluation or intra-operative performance of the procedure has lead to the performance of an incorrect procedure in a given patient.

Post-operative edema can be expected in the majority of cases by the very fact that surgery is being performed on a weight-bearing organ of the body. Wood (154) pointed out the appropriate use of compression dressings to equalize the intravenous pressure with the tissue pressure along with graded exercises to help reduce the stress on the venous and lymphatic systems. Prolonged periods of standing or ambulation should be avoided during the initial phases of healing. If the patient presents with a noninflammatory-type post-operative edema, then the application of ice and wrapping the lower extremity with a compression dressing or bandage is indicated. When there is inflammatory edema, then heat should be the treatment of choice. With excessive edema, the use of a salt-free diet and diuretics should also be considered and utilized when indicated. The use of

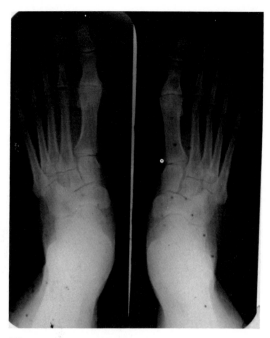

Figure 11.78. Pre-operative x-ray demonstrating enchondrom of proximal phalange right foot which could cause complications if a hemi or total prosthesis is contemplated due to poor bone stock for stability of prosthesis.

proteolytic enzymes has been used from time to time with some varying degree of success, although their mode of action and clinical efficiency have yet to be established.

Appropriate use of first MPJ capsulotomies needs to be understood in relation to whether there is any frontal plane valgus rotation of the hallux. The standard linear, inverted "L" or "Y" capsulotomies generally expose the first metatarsophalangeal joint adequately when there is no evidence of valgus rotation at the hallux. When there is valgus rotation at the hallux, then the various types of "V" or lenticular capsulotomies should be performed in order to not only realign the hallux in a more proper position at the first metatarsophalangeal joint, but also to eliminate the valgus rotation. The closing of the medial capsulotomy or suturing of the abductor hallucis tendon under extreme tension is not advised. During the initial post-operative pe-

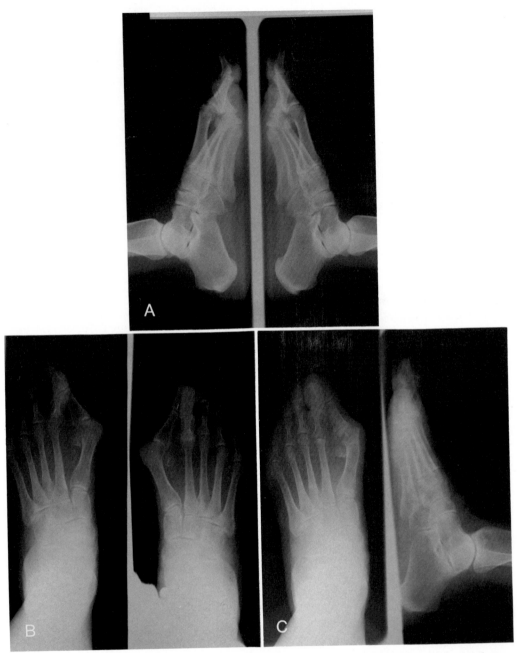

Figure 11.79. Case 1: Lateral weightbearing x-rays demonstrating metatarsus primus elevatus which must be recognized and treated with proximal osteotomy or arthrodesis along with appropriate first MPJ procedure (*A*). Case 2: Pre-operative x-rays of bilateral HAV (*B*) and postoperative x-ray, left foot, with recurrent HAV even with hemiprosthetic because structural deformity with elevated MPA (IM) angle went uncorrected (*C*).

riod, overcorrection of the deformity is ill-advised. If the appropriate surgical procedure has been performed to correct the positional or structural deformity, then simply bandaging the hallux in its normal alignment should be adequate. Do not rely on post-operative bandages to correct the deformity. Bandaging will not help and will not override either a positional or structural deformity if the appropriate surgical procedure has not been performed.

From a technical standpoint, one of the most difficult surgical procedures to perform on a human foot or ankle is the correction of the hallux abducto valgus deformity. The surgeon must perform a "balancing act" in order to appropriately correct this condition. While many of the rearfoot and ankle procedures appear to be technically more involved, as a general rule, the deformity is rather straightforward and the surgical approach is a direct one. During the past 100 years, much has been written about the surgical correction of hallux abducto valgus, and one can certainly expect considerably more data to be published. To avoid the complications which have already been identified, one must follow standard criteria, proper intra-operative techniques, and an organized post-operative regime in order to yield more positive results (Fig. 11.79). When there is an identifiable biomechanical abnormality as the primary etiological factor, then postoperative management and control of the biomechanical pathology must be implemented.

Acknowledgments—I wish to express my sincere thanks to my staff nurse, Sherry Schulz, L.P.N., for her dedicated time and effort in transcribing this manuscript. Furthermore, I wish to thank Mary A. Doyle, D.P.M., who was of enormous assistance in helping to gather the literature research material.

References

Digits

1. Bonavilla, E. J. Histopathology of the heloma durum: Some significant features and their implications. JAPA 58:423–427, 1968.

2. DuVries, H. L. *Surgery of the Foot*, 3rd ed. C. V. Mosby, St. Louis, 1973, pp. 379–467.
3. Freed, J. B. Histologic postmortem evaluation of bone hyperplasia accompanying digital clavus. JAPA 59:467–472, 1969.
4. Giannestras, N. J. *Foot Disorders.* Lea & Febiger, Philadelphia, 1967.
5. Kelikian, H. *Hallux Valgus, Allied Deformities of the Foot and Metatarsalgia.* W. B. Saunders, Philadelphia, 1965, pp. 282–336.
6. Stern, S. The repair of bone following hammertoe surgery. JAPA 59:473–478, 1969.
7. Lewin, P. *The Foot and Ankle.* Lea & Febiger, Philadelphia, 1959.
8. Allbrook, D., and Kirkaldy-Willis, W. H. The restoration of articular surfaces after joint excision. J. Bone Jt. Surg. 40B:742–764, 1958.
9. Franklin, L. Regeneration of resected phalangeal heads. JAPA 58:511–513, 1968.
10. Toth, S. P. Surgical fracture—"sausage toe." JAPA 60:364–365, 1970.
11. Mladick, R. A. Correction of hammertoe surgery deformity by Z-plasty and bone graft. Ann. Plast. Surg. 4:224–226, 1980.
12. Wiebe, E. L. Intermediate digital aphalangia. JAPA 63:522–524, 1973.
13. Galinski, A. W. Avoiding post-operative pain in digital surgery. JAPA 61:23–25, 1971.
14. M'Bamali, E. I. Results of modified Robert Jones operation for clawed hallux. Br. J. Surg. 62:647–650, 1975.
15. Van Pelt, W. L. A review of ten years of "hammertoe five" surgery. JAPA 59:385–389, 1969.
16. Bateman, J. E. Pitfalls in forefoot surgery. Orthop. Clin. North Am. 7:751–777, 1976.
17. Hill, J. H. Ostectomy of supernumerary sesamoid in flexor hallucis longus tendon. JAPA 60:237–238, 1970.
18. Cockin, J. Butler's operation for an overriding fifth toe. J. Bone Jt. Surg. 50B:78–81, 1968.
19. Tozzi, M. A., and Penny, H. L. Postaxial polydactyly with polymetatarsia. JAPA 71:374–379, 1981.
20. Tsuge, K. Treatment of macrodactyly. Plast. Reconstr. Surg. 39:590–599, 1967.
21. Black, J. R. Mimocausalgia. JAPA 70:430–432, 1980.
22. Balkin, S. W. Treatment of painful scars on soles and digits with injections of fluid silicone. J. Dermatol. Surg. Oncol. 3:612–614, 1977.
23. Balkin, S. W. Silicone injection for plantar keratoses. Preliminary report. JAPA 56:1–11, 1966.
24. Balkin, S. W. Plantar keratoses: Treatment by injectable liquid silicone. Report of an eight-year experience. Clin. Orthop. 87:235–247, 1972.
25. Balkin, S. W. Silicone augmentation for plantar calluses. JAPA 66:148–154, 1976.
26. Balkin, S. W. Treatment of corns by injectable silicone. Arch. Dermatol. 111:1143–1145, 1975.

Lesser Metatarsals

27. McGlamry, E. D., Kitting, R. W., Butlin, W. E. Prominent lesser metatarsal heads: Some surgical considerations. JAPA 59:303–307, 1969.
28. McGlamry, E. D., Butlin, W. E., and Kitting, R. W. Metatarsal shortening: Osteoplasty of head or osteotomy of shaft. JAPA 59:394–398, 1969.
29. McGlamry, E. D., Kitting, R. W., and Butlin, W.

E. Plantar condylectomy: Current modifications in technique. JAPA 59:345–348, 1969.

30. McGlamry, E. D., and Kitting, R. W. Post-operative urethane molds. JAPA 58:169, 1968.

31. Weinstock, R. E. Surgical judgment in metatarsal surgery for elimination of intractable plantar keratoses. JAPA 65:979–987, 1975.

32. Addante, J. B. Metatarsal osteotomy as a surgical approach for the elimination of plantar keratosis. J. Foot Surg. 8:36, 1969.

33. Levine, L. A. Collectomy: Lesser metatarsal neck resection. JAPA 62:447–458, 1972.

34. Graver, H. H. Angular metatarsal osteotomy. JAPA 63:96–98, 1973.

35. Meisenbach, R. O. Painful anterior arch of the foot: An operation for its relief by means of the raising of the arch. Am. J. Orthop. Surg. 14:206, 1916.

36. Fenton, C. F., and Butlin, W. E. Displaced V-osteotomies. JAPA 72:150–152, 1982.

37. Reinherz, R. P., and Toren, D. J. Bone healing after adjacent metatarsal osteotomies. J. Foot. Surg. 20:198–203, 1981.

38. Schweitzer, D. A., Lew, H., Shuken, J., and Morgan, J. Central metatarsal shortening following osteotomy and its clinical significance. JAPA 72:6–10, 1982.

39. Brattström, H., and Brattström, M. Resection of the metatarsophalangeal joints in rheumatoid arthritis. Acta Orthop. Scand. 41:213–224, 1970.

40. Clayton, M. L. Surgery of the forefoot in rheumatoid arthritis. Clin. Orthop. 16:136–140, 1960.

41. Hoffman, P. An operation for severe grades of contracted or clawed toes. Am. J. Surg. 9:441–449, 1911.

42. Barton, N. J. Arthroplasty of the forefoot in rheumatoid arthritis. J. Bone Jt. Surg. 55B:126–133, 1973.

43. Faithful, D. K., and Savill, D. L. Review of the results of excision of the metatarsal heads in patients with rheumatoid arthritis. Ann. Rheum. Dis. 30:201–202, 1971.

44. McGlamry, E. D., and Cooper, C. T. Brachymetatarsia: A surgical treatment. JAPA 59:259–264, 1969.

45. Weisfeld, M., and Kaplan, E. G. Surgical treatment of congenital zygodactylism and brachymetapody: A case history. J. Foot Surg. 16:24–34, 1977.

46. Russell, R. D. Use of compression bone plate after metatarsal nonunion. J. Foot Surg. 19:159–161, 1980.

47. Walter, J. H., and Pressman, M. M. External fixation in the treatment of metatarsal nonunions. JAPA 71:297–301, 1981.

48. Pritsch, M., Engel, J., and Farin, I. Manipulation and external fixation of metacarpal fractures. J. Bone Jt. Surg. 63A:1289–1291, 1981.

49. Hatcher, R. M., Goller, W. L., and Weil, L. S. Intractable plantar keratoses. JAPA 68:377–386, 1978.

50. Fielding, M. D., ed. *The Surgical Treatment of the Intractable Plantar Keratoma.* Futura, Mount Kisco, NY, 1974.

51. Wilner, R. J. Osteoclasis: A discussion. JAPA 63:1–7, 1973.

52. Buchbinder, I. J. DRATO procedure for Tailor's bunion. J. Foot Surg. 21:177–180, 1982.

53. MacClean, C. R., and Silver, W. A. Dwyer's operation for the rheumatoid forefoot. Foot Ankle 1:343–347, 1981.

54. Root, M., Orien, W., Weed, J., and Hughes, R. *Biomechanical Examination of the Foot.* Clinical Biomedronics, Los Angeles, 1971, vol. 1.

55. Thomas, W. H. Metatarsal osteotomy. Surg. Clin. North Am. 49:879, 1969.

56. Sgarlato, T. E. *A Compendium of Podiatric Biomechanics.* California College of Podiatric Medicine, San Francisco, 1971.

57. Davidson, M. R. A simple method for correcting second, third, and fourth plantar metatarsal head pathology, especially intractable keratomas. J. Foot Surg. 8:23, 1969.

58. Davidson, M. R. Non-stabilization metatarsal head osteotomies: A simple method for correcting second, third, fourth, and fifth metatarsal head pathology. J. Foot Surg. 10:121, 1971.

59. Davis, G. F. Cure for hallux valgus: The interdigital incision. Surg. Clin. North Am. 1:651, 1917.

60. Zlotoff, H. Shortening of the first metatarsal following osteotomy and its clinical significance. JAPA 67:412, 1977.

61. Marmor, L. *Surgery of Rheumatoid Arthritis.* Lea & Febiger, Philadelphia, 1967, pp. 221–235.

Hallux Abducto Valgus

62. Root, M. L., Orien, W. P., and Weed, J. H. *Normal and Abnormal Function of the Foot: Clinical Biomechanics.* Clinical Biomechanics, Los Angeles, 1977, vol. 2.

63. Wagner, F. W. Technique and rational: Bunion surgery. Contemp. Orthop. 3:1040–1072, 1981.

64. Lapidus, P. W. The operative correction of metatarsus primus varus in hallux valgus. Surg. Gynecol. Obstet. 58:183–191, 1934.

65. Aiken, O. F. The treatment of hallux valgus—a new operative procedure and its results. Med. Sentinel 33:678–679, 1925.

66. Piggot, H. The natural history of hallux valgus in adolescent and early adult life. J Bone Jt. Surg. 42:749, 1960.

67. Ebisui, J. M. The first ray axis and the first metatarsophalangeal joint. JAPA 58:160–167, 1968.

68. Kelikian, H. *Hallux Valgus, Allied Deformities of the Forefoot and Metatarsalgia.* W. B. Saunders, Philadelphia, 1965.

69. Iida, M., and Basmajian, J. V. Electromyography of hallux valgus. Clin. Orthop. 101:220–224, 1974.

70. Frankel, J. Structural or positional hallux abductus? JAPA 63:647–656, 1973.

71. Giannestras, M. J. *Foot Disorders: Medical and Surgical Management.* Lea & Febiger, Philadelphia, 1967.

72. Peabody, C. W. Surgical cure of hallux valgus. J Bone Jt. Surg. 13:273, 1931.

73. Schuberth, J. M., Cralley, J. C., and Wingfield, E. J. Extensor hallucis tendons of normal and hallux abducto valgus feet. JAPA 72:125–129, 1982.

74. Inge, G. A. L. Congenital abscence of the medial sesamoid bone of the great toe. J Bone Jt. Surg. 18:188–190, 1936.

75. McGlamry, E. D. Hallucial sesamoids. JAPA 55:693–699, 1965.

76. Lawton, J., and Evans, R. Modified McBride bunionectomy. JAPA 65:670–688, 1975.

77. McBride, E. A conservative operation for bunions. J Bone Jt. Surg. 10:735, 1928.

78. McBride, E. A conservative operation for bunions. JAMA 105:1164, 1935.

79. McBride, E. Hallux valgus bunion deformity—its treatment in mild, moderate, and severe stages. J. Int. Coll. Surg. 21:99, 1953.

80. Geldwert, J. J., and Gibbons, S. An end result study of the modified Mayo procedure. JAPA 64:976–982, 1974.

81. Mayo, C. H. The surgical treatment of bunions. Ann Surg. 48:300, 1908.

82. McCain, L. R., and Nuzzo, J. J. The "sesamoidal ligament" and its employ in the suturing of the Keller bunionectomy procedure. JAPA 59:479–480, 1969.

83. McGlamry, E. D., Kitting, R. W., and Butlin, W. E. Keller bunionectomy and hallux valgus correction. JAPA 60:161–167, 1970.

84. Keller, W. L. Surgical treatment of bunions and hallux valgus. N Y Med. J. 80:741, 1904.

85. Keller, W. L. Further observations on surgical treatment of hallux valgus and bunions. N Y Med. J. 95:696, 1912.

86. McGlamry, E. D., Kitting, R. W., and Butlin, W. E. Keller bunionectomy and hallux valgus correction. JAPA 63:237–246, 1973.

87. Ford, L. T., and Gilila, L. A. Stress fractures of the middle metatarsals following the Keller operation. J. Bone Jt. Surg. 49A:117–118, 1977.

88. Battey, M. A. The lesser metatarsal stress fracture as a complication of the Keller procedure. JAPA 70:182–186, 1980.

89. Zlotoff, H. Shortening of the first metatarsal following osteotomy and its clinical significance. JAPA 67:412, 1977.

90. Wrighton, J. D. A ten-year review of Keller's operation. Clin. Orthop. Relat. Res. 89:207–214, 1972.

91. Soren, A. Surgical correction of hallux valgus. Surgery 71:44–50, 1972.

92. Markheim, H. R., and Phillips, P. Surgical treatment of bunions. Surg. Clin. North Am. 49:1491–1498, 1969.

93. McKeever, D. C. Arthrodesis of the first metatarsophalangeal joint for hallux valgus, hallux rigidus, and metatarsus primus varus. J. Bone Jt. Surg. 34A:129, 1952.

94. Silver, D. The operative treatment of hallux valgus. J Bone Jt. Surg. 5:225, 1923.

95. Stamm, T. T. The surgical treatment of hallux valgus. Guy's Hosp. Rep. 106:273–279, 1957.

96. Hoffer, M. M., and Seaquist, J. L. Surgical correction of hallux valgus in cerebral palsy, in Bateman, J. E., Trott, A. W. (eds): *The Foot and Ankle.* Thieme-Stratton, New York, 1980, pp. 143–146.

97. Gore, D. R., Knavel, J., and Schaefer, W. W. Keller bunionectomy with opening wedge osteotomy of the first metatarsal, in Bateman, J. E., Trott, A. W. (eds): *The Foot and Ankle.* Thieme-Stratton, New York, 1980, pp. 147–154.

98. Butlin, W. E. Modifications of the McBride procedure for correction of hallux abducto valgus. JAPA 64:585–602, 1974.

99. Mann, R. A. Complications in surgery of the foot. Orthop. Clin. North Am. 7:851–861, 1976.

100. Gohil, P., and Cavolo, D. J. A simplified preoperative evaluation for Akin osteotomy, JAPA 72:44–45, 1982.

101. McGlamry, E. D., Kitting, R. W., and Butlin, W. E. Hallux valgus repair with correction of coexisting long hallux. JAPA 60:86–90, 1970.

102. Seelenfreund, M., and Fried, A. Correction of hallux valgus deformity by basal phalanx osteotomy of the big toe. J. Bone Jt. Surg. 55A:1411–1415, 1973.

103. Gerbert, J., Spector, E., and Clark, J. Osteotomy procedures on the proximal phalanx for correction of a hallux deformity. JAPA 64:617–629, 1974.

104. Brahms, M. A. Hallux valgus—the Akin procedure. Clin. Orthop. Relat. Res. 47–49, 1981.

105. Langford, J. H. ASIF Akin osteotomy. JAPA 71:390–396, 1981.

106. Muller, M. E., Allgower, M., Schneider, R., et al. *Manual of Internal Fixation Techniques Recommended by the AO Group.* 2nd ed. Springer-Verlag, New York, 1979.

107. Curda, G. A., and Sorto, L. A. The McBride bunionectomy with closing abductory wedge osteotomy. JAPA 71:349–355, 1981.

108. Langford, J. H., and Fenton, C. F. Hallux interphalangeal arthrodesis. JAPA 72:155–157, 1982.

109. Levitsky, D. R. Percutaneous osteoclasp fixation of Akin osteotomy: An alternative fixation technique. J. Foot Surg. 20:163–166, 1981.

110. Schoenhaus, H., Rotman, S., and Meshon, A. L. A review of normal intermetatarsal angles. JAPA 63:88–95, 1973.

111. Duke, H., Newman, L. M., Bruskoff, B. L., and Daniels, R. Relative metatarsal length patterns in hallux abducto valgus. JAPA 72:1–5, 1982.

112. Mayo, C. H. Surgical treatment of bunions. Minn. Med. 3:326, 1920.

113. Jaworek, T. E. The intrinsic vascular supply to the first metatarsal. JAPA 63:555–562, 1973.

114. Loison-Balacescu, J. Un caz de hallux valgus simetric. Rev. Chir. Orthop. 7:128–135, 1903.

115. Trethowan, J. *Hallux Valgus In a System of Surgery.* Hoeber, New York, 1923.

116. Jahss, M. H. Hallux valgus: Further considerations—The first metatarsal head (editorial). Foot Ankle 2:1–4, 1981.

117. Suppan, R. J. The cartilaginous articulation preservation principle and its surgical implementation for hallux abducto valgus. JAPA 64:635–656, 1974.

118. Barker, A. E. An operation for hallux valgus. Lancet 1:655, 1884.

119. Reverdin, J. Anatomie et operation de l'hallus valgus. Trans. Int. Med. Cong. 2:408, 1881.

120. Hiss, J. M. Hallux valgus—its causes and simplified treatment. Am. J. Surg. 2:50, 1931.

121. Beck, E. I. Modified Reverdin technique for hallux abducto valgus (with increased PASA of 1st MPJ). JAPA 64:657–666, 1974.

122. Winston, L., and Wilson, R. C. A modification of the Hohmann procedure for surgical correction of hallux abducto valgus. JAPA 72:11–14, 1982.

123. Hohmann, G. Symptomatische oder physiologische Behandlung des Hallux Valgus. Muench. Med. Wochenschr. 33:1042, 1921.

124. Hohmann, G. Uber ein Verfahren zur Behandlung des Spreizfuss. Zentralbl. Chir. 49:1933, 1922.

125. Hohmann, G. Uber hallux and Spreizfuss, ihre Entstehung und physiologische Behandlung. Arch. Arthop. Unfall-Chir. 21:525, 1923.

126. Hohmann, G. Sur Hallux Valgus Operation. Zentralbl. Chir. 51:230, 1924.

127. Hohmann, G. Der Hallux Valgus und die uebrigen Zehenverkruemmungen. Ergeb. Chir. Orthop. 18:308, 1925.

128. Hawkins, F. B., Mitchell, C. L., and Hedrick, D. W. Correction of hallux valgus by metatarsal osteotomy. J. Bone Jt. Surg. 27:387–394, 1945.

129. Mitchell, C. L., Fleming, J. L., Allen, R., Glenney, C., and Sanford, G. A. Osteotomy-bunionectomy for hallux valgus. J. Bone Jt. Surg. 40A:41–60, 1958.

130. Wilson, J. N. Oblique displacement osteotomy for hallux valgus. J. Bone Jt. Surg. 45B:552–556, 1963.

131. Donovan, J. C. Results of bunion correction using Mitchell osteotomy. J Ft. Surg. 21:181–185, 1982.

132. Pelet, D. Osteotomy and fixation for hallux valgus. Orthop. Clin. 157:42–46, 1981.

133. Holstein, A., and Lewis, G. B. Experience with Wilson's oblique displacement osteotomy for hallux valgus, in Bateman, J. E. (ed): *Foot Science*. W. B. Saunders, Philadelphia, 1976.

134. Lidge, R. T. Hallux valgus—surgical correction by three-in-one technique. in Bateman, J. E. (ed.): *Foot Science*, W. B. Saunders, Philadelphia, 1976.

135. Gerbert, J. Complications of the Austin-type bunionectomy. J. Foot Surg. 17:1–6, 1978.

136. Cleary, R. F., and Borovoy, M. A traumatically displaced Austin bunionectomy. JAPA 70:247–251, 1980.

137. Lewis, R. J., and Feffer, H. L. Modified chevron osteotomy of the first metatarsal. Clin. Orthop. Relat. Res. 157:105–109, 1981.

138. Marin, G. A. Arthrodesis of the metatarsophalangeal joint of the big toe for hallux valgus and hallux rigidus. Int. Surg. 50:175–179, 1968.

139. Fitzgerald, J. A. W., and Wilkinson, J. M. Arthrodesis of the metatarso-phalangeal joint of the great toe. Clin. Orthop. Relat. Res. 157:70–77, 1981.

140. Shaw, A. H., and Pack, L. G. Osteotomies of the first ray for hallux abducto valgus deformity. JAPA 64:567–580, 1974.

141. Haendel, C., and Lindholm, J. A. First metatarsal wedge osteotomies. JAPA 72:550–556, 1982.

142. Mann, R. *DuVries' Surgery of the Foot*, 4th ed. C. V. Mosby, St. Louis, 1978.

143. Bonney, G., and MacNab, I. Hallux valgus and hallux rigidus. J. Bone Jt. Surg. 34B:366–385, 1952.

144. Carr, C. R., and Boyd, B. M. Correctional osteotomy for metatarsus primus varus and hallux valgus. J. Bone Jt. Surg. 50A:1353–1367, 1968.

145. Helal, B. Surgery for adolescent hallux valgus. Clin. Orthop. Relat. Res. 157:50–63, 1981.

146. Bingham, R. The Stone operation for hallux valgus. Clin. Orthop. 17:366, 1960.

147. Fuld, J. E. Surgical treatment of hallux valgus and its complications. Am. Med. (Philadelphia) 14:536, 1917.

148. Hardy, R. H., and Clapham, J. C. R. Operations on hallux valgus. J. Bone Jt. Surg. 33B:376, 1951.

149. Hueter, C. *Klinik der Gelenkkrantheiten*, 1st ed. F. C. W. Vogel, Leipzig, 1871, p. 339.

150. Joplin, R. J. Sling procedure for correction of splay foot, metatarsus primus varus, and hallux valgus. J. Bone Jt. Surg. 32A:779, 1950.

151. Joplin, R. J. Some common foot disorders amenable to surgery. Am. Acad. Orthop. Surg. 15:144, 1958.

152. Logroscino, D. Il trattamento chirurgico dell'alluce valgus. Chir. Organi Mov. 32:81, 1948.

153. Lemperg, R. K., and Arnoldi, C. C. Intramedullary blood flow through arthrodesis-treated joints. Angiology 21:368–74, 1970.

154. Wood, W. A. Postoperative pedal edema. J. Foot Surg. 16:15–16, 1977.

155. Johnson, J. B. The prevention of wound infections with the use of local antibiotics. J. Foot Surg. 15:111–113, 1976.

156. Garner, R. W., Mowat, A. G., and Hazleman, B. L. Wound healing after operations on patients with rheumatoid arthritis. J. Bone Jt. Surg. 55B:134–144, 1973.

157. O'Duffy, J. D., Linscheid, R. L., and Peterson, L. F. A. Surgery in rheumatoid arthritis: Indications and complications. Arch. Phys. Med. Rehab. 53:70–77, 1972.

158. Morrison, P. Complications of forefoot operations in rheumatoid arthritis. Proc. R. Soc. Med. 67:110–111, 1974.

159. Mann, R. A. Surgical implications of biomechanics of the foot and ankle. Clin. Orthop. Relat. Res. 146:111–118, 1980.

160. Wood, W. A. Acquired hallux varus: A new corrective procedure. J. Foot Surg. 20:194–197, 1981.

161. Langford, J. H., and Maxwell, J. R. A treatment for postsurgical hallux varus. JAPA 72:142–144, 1982.

162. Kimizuka, M., and Miyanaga, Y. The treatment of acquired hallux varus after the McBride procedure. J. Foot Surg. 19:135–138, 1980.

163. Feinstein, M. H., and Brown, H. N. Hallux adductus as a surgical complication. J. Foot Surg. 19:207–211, 1980.

164. Janis, L. R., and Donick, I. I. The etiology of hallux varus: A review. JAPA 65:233–237, 1975.

165. Midkiff, L. C. Surgical hallux varus reduction. JAPA 64:160–162, 1974.

166. Hawkins, F. B. Acquired hallux varus: Cause, prevention, and correction. Clin. Orthop. Relat. Res. 76:169–176, 1971.

167. Seeburger, R. H., and Bradlee, N. Surgically induced hallux varus. JAPA 59:190–191, 1969.

168. Miller, J. W. Distal first metatarsal displacement osteotomy. J. Bone Jt. Surg. 56A:923–931, 1974.

169. Gibson, J., and Piggott, H. Osteotomy of the neck of the first metatarsal in the treatment of hallux valgus. J. Bone Jt. Surg. 44B:349–355, 1962.

170. Johnson, J. B., and Smith, S. Preliminary report on derotational, angulational, transpositional osteotomy: A new approach to hallux abducto valgus surgery. JAPA 64:667–674, 1974.

171. Funk, F. J., and Well, R. E. Bunionectomy with

distal osteotomy. Clin. Orthop. Relat. Res. 85:71–74, 1972.

172. Miller, S., and Croce, W. A. The Austin procedure for surgical correction of hallux abducto valgus deformity. JAPA 69:110–118, 1979.

173. Lapidus, P. W. The authors bunion operation from 1931 to 1959. Clin. Orthop. 16:119–135, 1960.

174. Johnson, K. A., Cofield, R. H., and Morrey, B. F. Chevron osteotomy for hallux valgus. Clin. Orthop. Relat. Res. 142:44–47, 1979.

175. Rix, R. R. Modified Mayo operation for hallux valgus and bunion—a comparison with the Keller procedure. J. Bone Jt. Surg. 50A:1368–1378, 1968.

176. Collins, W. R. A modified Mayo/Stone bunion operation. JAPA 64:630–634, 1974.

177. Hansen, C. E. Hallux valgus treated by the McBride operation. Acta Orthop. Scand. 45:778–792, 1974.

178. Bishop, J., Kahn, A., and Turba, J. F. Surgical correction of the splay-foot: The Giannestras procedure. Clin. Orthop. Relat. Res. 146:234–238, 1980.

179. Kirschner, C. Observations on complications after hallux valgus surgery. JAPA 64:216–236, 1974.

180. Gerbert, J., ed., and Sokoloff, T. H., assoc. ed. *Textbook of Bunion Surgery.* Futura, Mount Kisco, NY, 1981.

181. Gerbert, J., and Melillo, T. A modified Akin procedure for the correction of hallux valgus. JAPA 61:132, 1971.

182. Austin, D. W., and Leventen, E. O. A new osteotomy for hallux valgus: A horizontally directed "V" displacement osteotomy of the metatarsal head for hallux valgus and primus varus. Clin. Clin. Orthop. 157:25–30, 1981.

183. Leventen, E. O., and Austin, D. W. Film "Bunion Surgery, A New Approach." AAOS, San Francisco, 1975.

184. Comparetto, J. Personal communication.

CHAPTER 12

Implants

ALLEN M. JACOBS, D.P.M.
LAWRENCE M. OLOFF, D.P.M.

INTRODUCTION

Arthroplasty of the foot, or joint resection, has been an acceptable practice for many years. Standard joint resection arthroplasty remains a useful approach to selective arthritic, traumatized, or otherwise compromised joints of the foot, providing the surgeon recognizes the potentials for malalignment and loss of function. Synovectomy, adjunctive tendon balancing procedures, and arthrodesis also remain viable alternatives in the carefully selected patient. With advances in surgical techniques and biomaterials during the past two decades, reconstructive surgery has entered an era where restoration of extremity function has become a reality. Implant arthroplasty has an attractiveness over and above that of alternative procedures in that it most closely approximates what nature has intended us to have to facilitate daily activities. It allows for pain relief and stability, with the addition of mobility of affected joints. Unfortunately, limitations are expressed in terms of the biomaterials utilized, which can never fully serve as a substitute. Ushered in with this era are complications particular to these relatively new procedures.

Prosthetic materials vary greatly, but are so designed to possess certain common properties to make them suitable for implantation purposes (Table 12.1) (1). Various materials have fulfilled these requirements and because of biocompatibility have been utilized for implantation, including: metals, polyethylene-metal, polypropylene, and silicone rubbers. Recently, pyrolitic carbon is under investigative study for joint replacement (2). With the present state of the art, silicone rubber compositions seem to be more acceptable for use as prosthetic joints in the foot. The use of this material was first introduced by A. Swanson for use in the hand (3), and was later applied by him to the great toe joint (4). Present usage has expanded into many of the forefoot joints. Because of the widespread acceptance of these designed implants, emphasis will be directed to them.

It is not the intent of this chapter to single out implant arthroplasty as a hazardous procedure, but rather to serve notice to possible complications witnessed with their usage. As with most complications, iatrogenic contribution weighs heavily. Proper surgical technique and selective utilization will serve to minimize the potential hazards. All surgical procedures have inherent risks and complications, but early recognition is important to lessen morbidity. Emphasis will be directed to prevention, diagnosis, and alternative treatment regimens. Complications particular to all implants in arthroplasty of the foot (i.e., infection and biomaterial limitations) will be discussed first. Attention will then be directed to problems involving particular joint replacement procedures of the foot.

INFECTION

The risk of infection is a potential hazard with all surgical procedures, but is of particular concern in the area of implant surgery. Although the infection may be readily managed, it may necessitate removal of the implant, negating the initial intent of the surgical procedure.

Table 12.1.
Desirable Biomaterial Properties

Can withstand long contact with tissue enzymes without deterioration
Not induce sensitivity reactions
Not cause irritation or abnormal tissue reaction
Not become a focus for potential infection
Not have adverse effects on the hematologic components of blood
Not cause changes in the pH of tissue fluids
Not alter the electrical potential of the tissue cell

Prevention

Reports of the incidence of infection with silicone implants vary, but generally fall in between 1 and 2% (5, 6). Although this incidence falls within normal boundaries for the category of clean surgical procedures, the potential morbidity of an infected implant arthroplasty has prompted many to advocate the use of prophylactic antibiotics with this procedure (7, 8). A multitude of studies have been undertaken to assess the validity of this argument, but few have conclusively proven that the benefits outweigh the risks of side effects and colonization by resistant organisms (9). Strict adherence to good surgical technique remains the mainstay of prevention of infection, but prudent chemoprophylaxis is a seemingly good practice in this clinical setting.

With the multitude of antibiotics available today, one must sift through the available data to determine the best alternative drug for implant surgery. *Staphylococcus aureus* and *Staphylococcus epidermidis* are responsible for the majority of infections seen after implant arthroplasty (10), so one must choose an antibiotic whose spectrum of activities suppresses this particular indigenous population. While the semi-synthetic penicillins usually show good activity against *Staphylococcus aureus*, significant resistance to the penicillinase-resistant penicillins is found with *Staphylococcus epidermidis*. Because of this, cephalosporins appear to be the drugs of choice (11). Although individual choice holds precedence,

recent data suggests that cefamandole achieves the highest bone and joint concentrations.

In addition to choice of antibiotic, method of administration holds particular significance. It is most efficacious to administer antibiotics by means of intravenous infusion, generally just prior to the start of the surgical procedure (10, 12). In effect, what this does is allow for optimal drug levels during the time of potential contamination without the development of bacterial host resistance. In addition, tourniquet application 5 minutes after antibiotic administration does not appear to deleteriously affect antibiotic tissue concentrations (10, 13). The duration should not be continued beyond 24–72 hours because of the possibilities of super-infection or antibiotic side effects, with no decrease in the incidence of infection.

Early Infection

The key to the management of infection lies in its prevention, as was already discussed. But, despite strict adherence to basic precautions, infections will still occur. It seems that the presence of an implant or other foreign bodies interferes with the normal bodily defense mechanisms (11). When organisms reach the deeper tissues, the infection seems to propagate in the presence of an implant. Because of this, early discovery is of prime importance. More often than not, initiation of prompt treatment will salvage the surgical procedure and prevent the necessity for removal of the implant. Unfortunately, many surgeons elect to follow the "ostrich principle" and choose to ignore this complication until salvage procedures are no longer feasible (Fig. 12.1).

Infections early in the post-operative course are usually clinically easy to determine, while those that are delayed can be a diagnostic challenge. As with any other immediate wound infections, the cardinal signs of infection are usually present, although edema with implant surgery is somewhat more prominent than with other

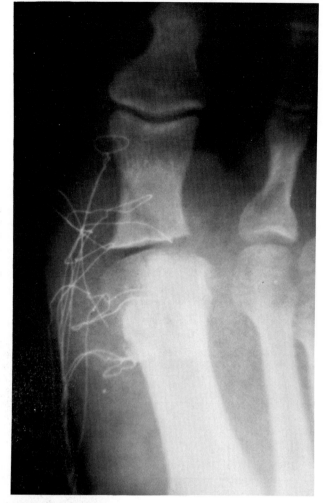

Figure 12.1. This patient had a deep infection at the site of a hemi-implant arthroplasty of the first metatarsophalangeal joint that was inappropriately treated. Implant removal was delayed until 6 weeks after discovery of the infection.

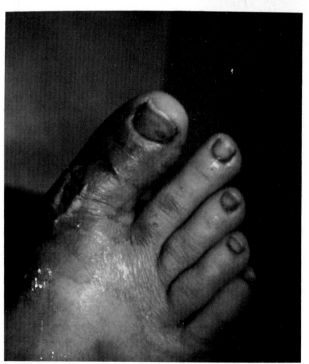

Figure 12.2. Infected first metatarsophalangeal joint implant site 1 week after surgery. Notice dehiscence, erythema, and edema. The patient had only minimal discomfort. Purulent drainage emanated from deeper tissues.

surgical procedures performed (Fig. 12.2). Increasing pain can often provide early subjective evidence of impending infection because patients undergoing implant surgery generally have minimal complaints of pain. This does not seem to be related to the ability of the surgeon, but rather that these patients have developed tolerance to pain from their arthritic joints over the years.

The presence of persistent fever following surgery is not always a reliable indicator of infection simply because of the multitude of factors which can contribute to temperature elevation post-operatively. When persistent fever occurs, and the impression is that of infection, the decision to continue the prophylactic antibiotic already administered is not warranted because the organisms responsible should be expected to be resistant to this particular antibiotic (10).

Many considerations are included in deciding the proper antibiotic before culture and sensitivities are available, including: gram stain results, the severity of infection, prevalence of infecting organisms in the particular hospital environment, status of host defenses, and complicating systemic diseases. When all these factors are taken into consideration, the surgeon has the added knowledge that without quick resolution the implant will be jeopardized. Even with resolution, prolonged infection may lead to excessive fibrosis which functionally limits the end results of the surgical procedure.

As stated before, diagnosis mostly rests upon clinical impression. If an error in judgement is to be made, it is best made on the side of safety. In other words, suspected infection is labeled so, until proven otherwise. Clinical determination can be assisted by the laboratory. White blood cell count elevations with a shift to the left and marked increases in the sedimentation rate will prove to be confirmatory. However, initiation of treatment is best left to clinical judgement, for accompanying laboratory deviations often change later. In addition, bacteriologic diagnosis is important to ensure antibiotic effectiveness. When a specimen is not readily obtainable, injection and aspiration of sterile saline might recover the offending organism for culture and sensitivity.

While the patient is undergoing antibiotic therapy, it is important to monitor drug concentrations for therapeutic purposes, as well as to guard against potential toxicity. Monitoring of drug serum concentrations are not routinely done, but are reserved for those patients receiving antibiotics that are potentially toxic or for those patients in whom infection is resistant to prescribed therapy (15). Determination of cephalosporin and penicillin levels is seldom necessary. On the contrary, determination of serum levels of gentamicin is usually performed because of potential toxicity. In this instance, peak and trough levels are obtained, where blood is drawn within 15 minutes of the last intravenous dose and within 1 hour prior to the next dose (15). This becomes important because peak levels of gentamicin should be above 4 mg to be therapeutically effective, and below 10 mg to avoid toxicity. In addition, trough levels above 2 mg are associated with an increased risk of nephrotoxicity (16). Antibiotic dosage is adjusted accordingly. In combination with serum concentration techniques, minimum inhibitory concentrations (MIC) are available. The antibiotic chosen is usually considered effective if the MIC is below the concentration of drug obtainable in the serum.

Local therapy is undertaken as to the preference of the individual physician and according to clinical findings. Often in mild infections, local care is as important to the overall treatment regimen as is antibiosis. Warm compresses, chemical and mechanical debridement, incision and drainage, wet to dry dressings, and elevations of the head of bed, will effect containment and assist in the cure of the infectious process.

The question of removal of an implant is a difficult one and dependent upon clinical findings. The answer becomes clear if the implant becomes exposed to the external environment, for certainly removal is necessary to facilitate healing. The presence of deep contamination of the wound also oftentimes dictates removal. When the infection stays confined to superficial tissues, trials of conservative care may be attempted.

If removal becomes necessary, options then exist as to whether to remain with a conventional arthroplasty or to proceed at a future date with reinsertion. This is best addressed on a individual basis. If stability and weight-bearing of the involved joints are severely compromised, reinsertion is preferred if feasible. If not feasible, an alternative method of obtaining stability is through arthrodesis. It has been suggested that a waiting period of 6 months to 1 year is preferred if reinsertion is planned (17). However, more important than time are the particular clinical circumstances. For example, if the infection progressed to osteomyelitis, the risks of exacerbation of the quiescent osteomyelitis by surgical intervention is high. This decision may be assisted by bone scanning techniques. Obviously, accurate diagnosis of the state of the osseous tissues is most important in making a decision. At the time of implant removal, numerous geographic cultures and bone biopsies will prove beneficial to future decisions. If the osseous tissues were not believed to be compromised, reinsertion is feasible. Scintigraphic examination may also prove useful to the surgeon when reinsertion is contemplated.

Delayed Infection

As stated earlier, the diagnosis of infection manifested weeks to months following implant surgery is a diagnostic challenge. When these patients present at this time with pain and signs of inflammation, a multitude of causes may be responsible (Table 12.2). Mechanical implant failure is one such cause to be considered. Mechanical failure may be a reflection of an infectious process, prosthetic breakage, or both. Also to be considered are cases of loosened implants, this applying to those prostheses which are luted or fixated to adjacent bone by either fibrous ingrowth or by polymethylmethacrylate. Reactive synovitis to implant particulate matter, or so called detritic synovitis, can also present weeks later with signs of inflammation and pain. A late manifestation of inflammation and pain is seen with ectopic bone formation, where regenerative bone irritates capsular and pericapsular soft tissue structures. With this myriad of potential disorders, extensive evalution is necessary to arrive at a diagnosis. Once again, the role is to assume infection until proven otherwise.

The dreaded offender of implant failure is osteomyelitis. Concern of existing osteomyelitis is most commonly initiated by two methods: either by suspicious findings on routine post-operative radiographs or by clinical presentation of pain and swelling. The former is not uncommon because the clinical manifestation of osteomyelitis is often subtle. Advanced destruction of osseous structures may be present without obvious clinical signs of infection after implant surgery (Fig. 12.3). The exhaustive work-up which follows is most dependent upon conclusive bacteriologic confirmation. Despite this, laboratory and radiographic studies will assist the surgeon in arriving at a conclusion.

The radiographic signs of osteomyelitis are well documented and adequately detailed in most standard textbooks of radiology (18). Findings of small radiolucent areas, cortical and medullary destruction, sclerosis, sequestrations, cloaca, involucrum, and subperiosteal calcification are demonstrated in varying degrees, depending on the extent and longevity of the infectious process. Conventional radiographs have their limitations in terms of time expression of the infectious process, for

Table 12.2.
Causes of Implant Failure

Soft tissue infection
Osteomyelitis
Prosthetic breakage
Detritic synovitis
Ectopic bone formation
Loosening of fixated implants

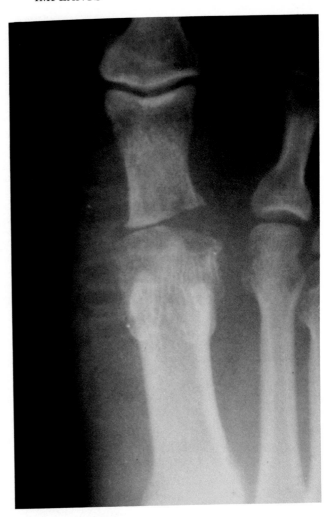

Figure 12.3. This is the same patient illustrated in Figure 12.1. This radiograph was taken 10 weeks after the original surgery. The attending physician withheld more aggressive therapy because the patient had only minimal symptoms. Notice the washed-out appearance of the metatarsal head and periosteal reaction on the proximal phalanx. The patient was later confirmed as having osteomyelitis.

positive findings are usually not present until 10–14 days after the onset of symptoms (19). In addition, some of these radiographic changes may be simulated by other entities which were previously discussed. For example, the radiographic changes seen with detritic synovitis may mimic some of those seen with osteomyelitis (Fig. 12.4). For these reasons, bone scintigraphy has been advocated as a useful adjunctive procedure in the early diagnosis and localization of osteomyelitis (19–27).

Bone scanning with technetium-99m phosphonates are obtained soon after the administration of the radiopharmaceutical, with delayed imaging performed a few hours later (25). Because of the additional time necessary for localization of the radiopharmaceutical to bone, certain pertinent clinical information is obtained. Immediate increase uptake, within the so called blood-pool images, is consistent with soft tissue infection. Delayed increased uptake may be consistent with osteomyelitis. Comparison of the two will help differentiate cellulitis from osteomyelitis (21, 25). As with most diagnostic tests, limitations are seen.

Although no radiopharmaceutical agents bind specifically to infected tissues, valuable information is obtained by sequential imaging, whereby technetium-99m phosphonate and gallium-67 citrate scans are used in combination. The method previously described for technetium scans is fol-

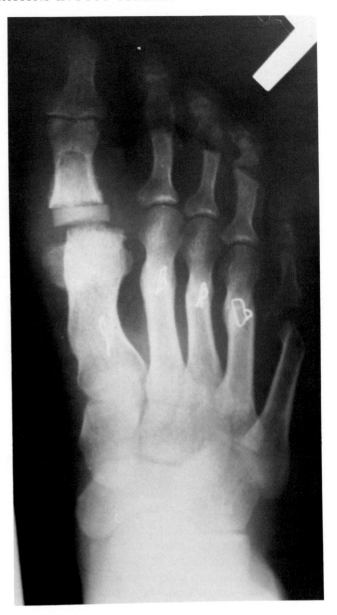

Figure 12.4. Notice the periosteal reaction and apparent destruction of the first metatarsal head. There were no clinical signs of infection. Intra-operative deep cultures and bone specimens were negative for infection. Synovial biopsy confirmed detritic synovitis.

lowed. Gallium-67 citrate is then administered, with imaging 2 days later. Osteomyelitis is suspected when localized uptake of both radiopharmaceuticals is witnessed at the same site (27). A positive technetium and negative gallium scan would rule out infection and suggest one of the previously mentioned entities discussed in the differential diagnosis. Why gallium localizes more accurately to infected areas is based upon three mechanisms: leukocyte localization, direct bacterial uptake, and lactoferrin binding (28).

The laboratory is also utilized for assistance in arriving at a diagnosis. Complete blood counts and erythrocyte sedimentation rates may prove useful. Expected laboratory findings are dependent upon whether the bone infection is acute or chronic. When acute, marked elevation of ESR, polymorphonuclear leukocytosis, and increases in the total white cell count may

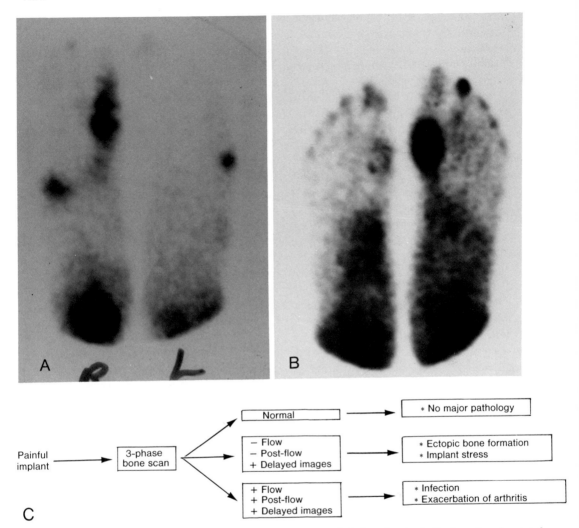

Figure 12.5. *A*, delayed imaging shows focal uptake and cleft at implant site 4 weeks after total implant arthroplasty. These findings are considered normal. *B*, delayed imaging shows diffuse uptake at site of total implant arthroplasty. ^{67}Ga citrate and aspirate of area confirmed deep infection. *C*, schematic.

be seen (29). In the case of chronic infection, white blood cell counts are usually normal, leukocytosis is unusual, but increases in the ESR may be seen. Exacerbation of a chronic osteomyelitis may also present with leukocytosis.

The laboratory proves to be of most benefit in terms of bacteriologic diagnosis. Isolation of the offending organism(s) is the ultimate test upon which the diagnosis is based. Previously discussed laboratory and radiographic methods are of valuable assistance, but isolation of the offending organism is the most conclusive evidence on which the diagnosis and treatment regimens should be decided. Pathogen isolation is obtained primarily by three methods: blood, surface, and deep cultures. Positive blood cultures are dependent on bacteremia, this being witnessed most commonly with acute hematogenous osteomyelitis. Even in this case, blood cultures are reported as being only 50% accurate (30). Surface cultures from dehiscence sites or sinus tracks are also unreliable for isolation of the offending pathogen (31). Deep cultures are obtained by either deep aspiration or surgical exploration. If open methods are performed, bone biopsy is obtained concurrently. Because of the lack of reliability with blood and surface cultures, deep cultures are obtained when infection is confirmed so that proper antibiotic therapy may be initiated.

Deep infection, with or without complicating osteomyelitis, is best treated with combined antibiotic and surgical therapy. Antibiosis is accomplished in the manner previously described as applied to superficial infections with the following exceptions. Generally speaking, prolonged parenteral antibiotic therapy for at least 4–6 weeks has been accepted clinical practice (32, 33). Unfortunately, long-term parenteral antibiotic administration is burdensome in terms of patient acceptance and medical costs. Because of this, alternative rationales of treatment have been suggested. One study showed promising results with short-term initial parenteral therapy followed by prolonged oral administration for treatment of acute hematogenous osteomyelitis (34). This might be applicable to selected cases of post-operative osteomyelitis, provided all the devitalized and necrotic tissue were removed. Other reports indicate success with long-term oral therapy (35). The method of antibiotic administration preferred by the practitioner should be dictated by the clinical presentation of each individual case. For instance, advanced destruction in infection will not be amenable to oral therapy initially, where variable serum concentrations and poor patient compliance may jeopardize the final outcome. In other words, patient convenience should not be a substitute for good clinical practice. It is also important to keep in mind that repetitive deep cultures are most important in long-term antibiotic therapy, so that varying sensitivity patterns may be detected quickly to allow for rapid antibiotic adjustment, so that therapy is not compromised.

As already mentioned, combined medical and surgical therapy is utilized for treatment of deep infections at implant surgical sites. The amount and type of surgical therapy is dictated by the clinical presentation and stage of development. In the case of early detected deep soft tissue infections or osteomyelitis, implant removal is usually necessary to facilitate healing. Some studies on early deep infected implants elsewhere in the body suggest a more conservative approach, whereby the implant is allowed to remain, all infected deep tissues are excised, the wound copiously irrigated, antibiotics employed, and primary closure obtained (36, 37). However, the success rate in these studies is rather low, and implant removal seems to be a safer approach to this problem. With early detection, followed by implant removal, medical management will usually allow for resolution of the infectious process without the need for more drastic measures (38). The exception to this rule is when abscess is present. In this case, decompression becomes necessary to prevent extension of bone necrosis (39, 40).

In established deep infections, more aggressive therapy is warranted. Implant removal is indicated, with no exceptions. Although medical management may prevent further spread into adjacent soft tissues and bone, therapeutic concentrations of antibiotics in the infected bone are not achieved because of compromised bone perfusion (41). Because of this, it becomes necessary to remove all grossly necrotic bone and soft tissues, sequestrum, and decompress the medullary cavity to facilitate healing. Because of the inability of the blood stream to deliver adequate concentrations of antibiotic, continuous closed suction irrigation can sometimes prove a useful adjunct in this clinical situation (42). The apparent advantage of this method, when combined with standard practices of debridement of necrotic tissue, is that the rehabilitation period is hastened by allowing for wound closure at the time of surgery (43). This method of management has drawbacks in that it requires close supervision in order to prevent the potential problems of clotting and secondary infection at the egress tube site (44).

Even while short-term goals are accomplished in the treatment of an infected implant, the surgeon should begin to consider the potential future problems. Surely, resolution of the infection is the primary responsibility, but decisions then exist as to management of the sequellae produced by the infection. The most disasterous sequellae would certainly be the necessity for amputation. When infection becomes impossible to control or is too extensive in terms of destruction, local ablation surgery may be necessary (41). Fortunately, this occurrence is unusual. More commonly, the patient is left with a standard resection arthroplasty. The functional and cosmetic results of a standard resection arthroplasty may be acceptable, but this has to be decided on an individual basis. Usually, excessive fibrosis is a consequence of the long-term infectious process, so that anticipated functional results are limited. When stability and function are necessitated, then alternatives that remain are arthrodesis or reinsertion of the prosthesis. Unfortunately, rigid criteria do not exist as to the safe timing for reinsertion. The same techniques are employed to make the diagnosis of osteomyelitis, and can also assist the surgeon as to the proper time for replacement of the prosthesis. Deep cultures, bone biopsy, and erythrocyte sedimentation rates may provide useful information as to whether the infection has resolved or progressed to a quiescent chronic state. Differential scanning also may provide answers as to the safety of reimplantation. As stated earlier, 6 months to 1 year has been suggested as the proper time period to confirm the clinical impression that the infection has resolved. Naturally, reimplantation mandates that sufficient bone architecture remain post-infection to receive and support the prosthesis.

BIOMATERIAL COMPLICATIONS

While infection is a complication en-countered with all implant surgical procedures, the use of biomaterials also carries the risk of certain universal complications that are related to the characteristics of the implantable material. These complications can be grouped into two broad categories: 1) those hazards related to the chemical and physical properties of the biomaterial, and 2) those related to improper application of the biomaterial. While these complications as a group are rather unusual, iatrogenic contribution accounts for the majority seen. To prevent such complications from occurring, the surgeon is obligated to have a basic understanding of the properties and limitations of the material which he is implanting in his patients. Although this knowledge is essential, it goes beyond the scope of this chapter. Certain properties will be discussed in a manner that is pertinent to the particular complication. Description will be limited to those biomaterials that are most commonly used in implantation procedures of the foot.

Improper Biomaterial Application

The most common causes for biomaterial failure are iatrogenic in origin. As previously mentioned, silicone elastomers have demonstrated many reasons for acceptability as implant materials (Table 12.3). Most importantly, medical grade silicones provoke minimal tissue reaction. Over the past several years, attention has been directed to isolated cases of reaction to silicone elastomer prostheses (47–53). This attention points to an important concept, that although silicone elastomers do not evoke tissue reaction en bloc, reaction to partic-

Table 12.3.
Advantages of Silicones

Heat-stable
Time-stable
Versatility
No adherence (excellent insulator)
Minimal tissue reaction
Not attacked or altered by body tissues
No toxicity
No carcinogenicity

ulate matter is possible. Detritic synovitis is the terminology used to describe the condition whereby a reactive synovitis forms secondary to particulate matter of silicone in the synovium around a joint in which an elastomer prosthesis was implanted. The origin of detritic synovitis has primarily three potential mechanisms: 1) as a result of a fractured implant, 2) improper usage of a prosthesis, and 3) inherent to the implantation of the elastomer itself.

The incidence of implant fracture is difficult to assess in the foot because of lack of detailed studies, but is reported in the hand as varying from 1–26.2% (54, 55). One would anticipate a higher incidence of fractured implants in the hand because of the greater torsional forces present in that portion of anatomy. It is readily apparent how particulate silicone is produced following breakage. The causes for breakage are mul-

tifactorial. It is impossible to predict what is the normal life expectancy of an implant, and this seemingly is best predicted by the years that a particular implant has been utilized without problems. However, ignorance as to the normal dynamics of implant function, as it relates to the physical properties of the elastomers, seems to be prevalent in contributing to early breakdown of prostheses (Fig. 12.6).

Silicone elastomers are so designed to produce an appropriate balance between hardness, elasticity, and toughness (54). This balance of properties allows for desired flexibility and longevity, with the ability to resist moderate deforming forces. Because implants undergo cyclical loading, the implant should confirm to Hooke's law. This implies that as the material is stretched during normal articular motion, the material should absorb this stress with

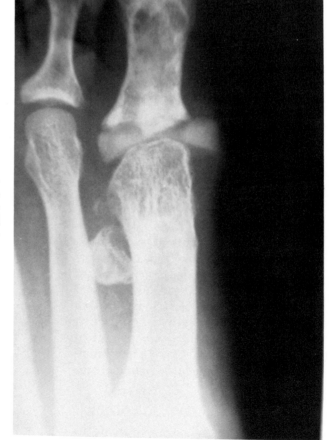

Figure 12.6.   Breakage of hemi-implant 3 years after surgery. Oversized hemi-implant and degenerative changes of first metatarsal head were felt to be contributory for failure of the implant.

no permanent structural change (Fig. 12.7). There is a point, beyond the functional demands, where permanent deformation occurs. The Swanson-designed silicone elastomer prostheses are designed to function within the "Hookian region" (54). This rule follows providing there are no flaws in the prosthesis itself. With an understanding of this concept, surgeons should gain an appreciation for not modifying the implant, because of the risks of creating flaws that will compromise the structural integrity of the implant. Inducing a flaw may lead to a laceration that will expand by a process known as "crack propagation" and eventually result in implant fracture (Fig. 12.8). The only modification that should

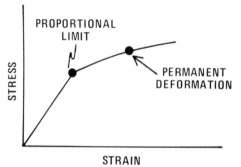

Figure 12.7. Plastic deformation.

ever be considered is trimming the stem in order to shorten it to adapt to a short phalanx, and even this should be limited to selected cases. The surgeon risks abrasion by the bone interface with formation of detric matter if he creates sharp points on the implant. This can result in fracture or intractable detric synovitis, either of which necessitates removal of the implant.

Flexible prostheses rely on the concept of minimal piston motion of the implant stems within the intramedullary canal. The ability of the stems to piston allows for prolongation of the implant life (56). Some surgeons feel uneasy about this concept because of the question of decreased stability. These fears seem unwarranted because the body reacts to the foreign body by enveloping the implant in a firm fibrous capsule. It is believed that this process takes approximately 3–4 weeks, and that the fibrous capsule takes on characteristics of the periarticular ligaments (56). This process of encapsulation results in good implant stability. To supplement encapsulation, the surgeon should take special care to preserve the capsular structures during surgical dissection. Preservation of the capsule is important because it serves as a latticework for the encapsulation process. The impor-

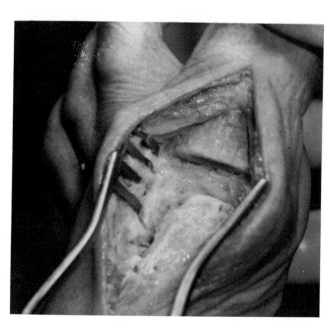

Figure 12.8. Breakage of implant at junction of stem and body of implant. Excessive trimming of the implant was responsible.

tance of this structure in stabilization of the implant becomes readily apparent when it is inadvertently damaged. For example, when a hemi-prosthesis becomes dislocated as a result of trauma in the early post-operative period, the capsular structures are oftentimes irreparably damaged. Simple reinsertion is not feasible because of the lack of stability and tendency toward redislocation (Fig. 12.9). External splinting or insertion of a double-stemmed hinged prosthesis then becomes necessary so that stability can be achieved.

A certain degree of motion is necessary for longevity of the prosthesis, and the encapsulation is not so firm as to limit motion entirely. The pistoning motion allows for greater dispersion of forces passing through the implant (56). This motion also allows for less resorption of the bone surrounding the implant. The greater incidence of fractures of those implants which become fixated to bone through fibrous ingrowth, as occurs in Dacron-impregnated prosthesis, bears testimony to the advantage of motion with flexible silicone elastomer protheses (55).

Another hazard related to improper implant usage is seen with hemi-implant arthroplasty. When a hemi-implant is contemplated, the condition of the opposing cartilage, against which the implant will function, must be accurately assessed. A hemi-implant that functions against abraded cartilage will result in the formation of particulate silicone from abrasive wear. The production of particulate silicone under these conditions, will initially cause detritic synovitis, and later will result in implant fatigue with eventual fracture. Before the advent of hinged joint prosthesis in the foot, single-stemmed prostheses were commonly utilized, regardless of the condition of the opposing joint surface. Today, degenerative changes on both sides of the joint mandate insertion of a total joint prosthesis in order to insure long-term function of the implant.

Biomaterial Failure

As discussed in the previous section, many of the cases labeled as so-called biomaterial failure are actually related to improper usage of the implant. However, there are isolated incidences of implant failure related to the chemical and physical properties of the implant itself. Included under these causes are: foreign body reactions, lipid absorption, and structural failure.

Foreign body reactions are a most unusual occurrence. Many of the cases indiscriminately labeled as implant rejection are in reality reactions to foreign materials that have become absorbed or adhered to the implant. The implant must be thoroughly cleansed prior to autoclaving because contamination by dust, lint, and fingerprints can occur (57). Synthetic detergents or oil-based soaps are not recommended because of chances of absorption (57). Silicones are gas-permeable, so cold sterilization methods should not be used. Attempts should be made to handle the implants with blunt instruments during surgery and avoid glove contact whenever possible. Strict adherence to these sterility rules, as well as company product recommendations, will help avoid these types of foreign body reactions. As previously mentioned, silicone elastomers produce little or no tissue reaction en bloc, but do evoke reaction when in particulate form. The production of particulate silicone by fracture and improper usage has already been discussed, but recent studies have shown that detritic synovitis can be produced from intact and normal functioning prostheses (49, 50). This may be a manifestation of normal wear properties of elastomer prostheses. The rough surface of the endosteum would be expected to create abrasive matter from the stem of the prosthesis (Fig. 12.10). The question as to when silicone particulate matter creates a problem remains unanswered. It has been suggested that detritic synovitis can mimic recurrence of an attack of inflammatory arthritis (49). Others report it is of no clinical significance (58). It has also been suggested that particulate silicone matter can migrate to a distant lymph node (47, 49, 51).

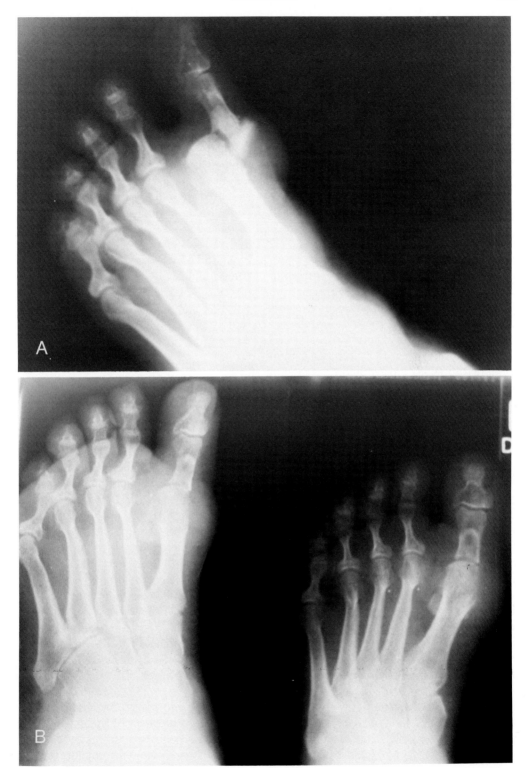

Figure 12.9. *A,* the patient tried to get out of bed the day of surgery, catching her toe on the bedrail with resultant dislocation. *B,* 4 weeks after external traction and removal of the implant in the same patient. The hallux was found to be stable and the functional result was acceptable.

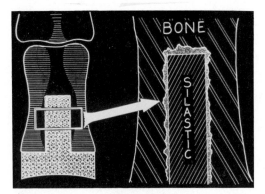

Figure 12.10. Endosteal surface felt to be contributory to abrasive wear of the stem of the prosthesis.

In our own experiences, the biggest problem clinically has been differentiating detritic synovitis from an infectious process. The clinical and radiographic findings are often similar, so that exhaustive evaluation is necessitated (Figs. 12.3 and 12.4). Synovial biopsy is the most reliable method of differentiation. Histologic sections of detritic synovitis show varying degrees of chronic inflammation, lymphocyte infiltration, and particles of refractile foreign bodies surrounded by or ingested by multinucleated, foreign body giant cells (48, 49, 52). While some cases of detritic synovitis appear self-limiting, most require implant removal and partial synovectomy to improve symptoms.

Structural failure is a subject that has not been adequately addressed in the past. As previously mentioned, silicone elastomer implants are designed to withstand the functional demands of the particular joints that they replace. Infinite flex life is expected when the implant functions within these boundaries (54). However, there are cases where functional demands may be exceeded, with resultant permanent deformation and eventual implant failure. For example, a professional athlete would produce more stress and strain on particular joints. Under these circumstances, an implant arthroplasty of the foot may prolong an athlete's productive years, but eventual replacement may be necessary (Fig. 12.11).

Patients expected to have increased functional demands should be forewarned of this possibility. The answers to these questions require additional research.

Some concern has been expressed in terms of the possibilities of implant failure being related to lipid absorption by the silicone rubber implants. This concern developed by the noticeable higher values of lipid found in silicone elastomer heart valves (57). This lipid absorption by prosthetic heart valves seems to show a time correlation. In addition, the synovial fluid of rheumatoid patients demonstrates a higher level of lipids. In an exhaustive *in vivo* study by Swanson et al. (54), it has been conclusively proven that there is no direct correlation between lipid content of joint implants and fracture rate (54). In that study no time correlation was demonstrated.

Polymethylmethacrylate

Although not used by itself, polymethylmethacrylate (PMM) is selectively used in implant surgery in the foot for those procedures that require its unique properties as a surgical cement, thereby fixating the implant to the bone. Commercially prepared, it comes in two packages, one containing a powder, the other a liquid. The powder contains previously polymerized polymer granules and necessary copolymer, while the liquid contains the monomer and a stabilizer (60). PMM is the finished product produced by the mixing of these two substances. The complications related to the use of PMM are both local and systemic.

The most common local complication of PMM use is bone necrosis, and this can occur by two mechanisms. The polymerization process produces an exothermic reaction that can cause osseous necrosis. In addition, the presence of the plastic cement against the marrow and endosteum can produce direct ischemia and prevent vascular regeneration (61). The development of ischemic necrosis creates the potential for gradual loosening of the prosthesis and

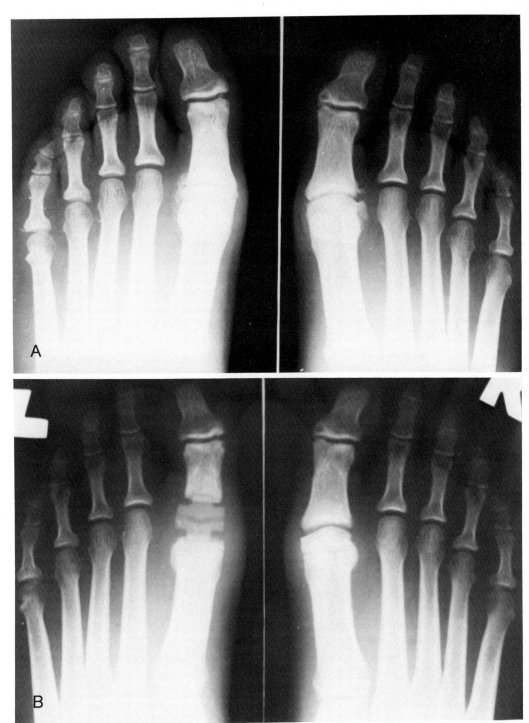

Figure 12.11. *A,* this 29-year-old male was unable to participate in basketball because of painful first metatarsophalangeal joint bilaterally. His goal in life was to play semi-professional basketball. *B,* same patient after total implant arthroplasty left foot and cheilectomy and Watermann osteotomy right foot. Implant was necessitated on the left foot because of severe degenerative changes. It was explained to the patient pre-operatively that an implant would make him pain-free but that the longevity of the implant would be questionable if he participated in sports. The patient has participated in his sport for 2 years without sequelae.

also increases the risk of sepsis. Beside ischemic necrosis, particulate PMM can produce local foreign body reactions (62). Either of these complications can necessitate removal of the implant, which results in the tedious task of removing the PMM from bone. Extreme care is taken not to leave any particulate PMM at the time of removal because of the possibilities of evoking the soft tissue reactions already mentioned.

Of greater concern are the different systemic reactions that can occur. Hypotension is most commonly seen and felt to be related to residual monomer absorbed into the bloodstream at the time of application (63). A more serious consequence is the possibility of fat emboli, which can be produced by the monomer effecting a breakdown of emulsified plasma lipids (63). Embolization to vital organs has been noted and related to the use of PMM and contributory to fatalities (64). The ingestion of PMM particles by macrophages can result in cell death with resultant tissue reaction (65).

SPECIFIC COMPLICATIONS OF IMPLANT SURGERY

General Considerations

The majority of complications in implant surgery of the foot are expressed by errors in pre-operative assessment, surgical judgement, technique, and post-operative rehabilitation. Before surgical intervention is undertaken, general considerations must be met to avoid standard surgical error.

The surgeon must first assess the patient as to suitability for implant arthroplasty. The patient's general medical status should be sufficient as with any elective surgical procedure. It is of particular importance in this case because implant arthroplasty mandates meticulous surgical technique and compromise is not acceptable. When the pedal complaints of a patient are so severe as to limit activity, and the patient's medical status is borderline for elective surgery, it may be more expedient to perform a conventional arthroplasty. Certainly of

prime importance is that the patient's neurovascular status be sufficient to undergo foot surgery. If doubt is expressed in this regard, vascular consultation should be obtained. Also of concern is the patient's mental status. The patient should be willing and capable to undergo the necessary rehabilitation program mandated with most of these procedures.

The surgeon should also consider those local factors that may compromise the surgical results. As with any implant procedure of the foot, the bone stock should be sufficient to accept and support a prosthesis. Although a functional musculotendinous unit is desirable, muscle imbalance is a relative contraindication. The problem that occurs in this situation is that abnormal joint mechanics will place undue stress upon the implant and may result in premature fatigue. Attempts should be made to selectively stabilize affected joints and to limit subluxatory forces by either releasing contractures or tendon-balancing techniques. It may be judicious to perform an arthrodesis in the presence of an upper motor neuron lesion that has resulted in pedal deformity and joint destruction. Also important is the status of the surrounding soft tissues. Skin coverage should be adequate so as not to limit joint motion.

With regard to the surgery itself, adherence to good surgical techniques will help to avoid many of the more common pitfalls particular to all surgical procedures. Careful attention and preservation of neurovascular structures is mandatory. Sharp dissection should be utilized wherever possible. Strict hemostasis is necessary to avoid hematoma, dehiscence, and infection. If a significant hematoma is discovered, it should be evacuated under aseptic conditions. Skin incisions should be so designed to allow for adequate exposure in order to minimize retraction and unnecessary undermining. This will prevent many of the dehiscences and skins sloughs encountered. The use of tourniquets will help expedite the surgical procedure, thus decreasing the chances of infection. On the other hand, tourniquet use is associated with greater post-operative edema. It is also advisable to irrigate the wound frequently and copiously to help limit contamination and remove debris.

The rehabilitation program is as important as the surgical procedure itself. Rehabilitation should be individually tailored to the intent of the surgery. In the case of a hallux abducto valgus deformity, corrective immobilization should be used for the period of encapsulation. This will help insure a stable prosthesis, as well as maintain the correction that was obtained. It is important to remember that bandaging is not a substitute for surgical realignment of deformities, but is supplementary to these corrections. When implant surgery is performed on the patient with hallux rigidus, the considerations differ significantly. In this case, early mobilization is preferred so that adquate increases in range of motion is obtained. In addition, it is sometimes necessary to stretch out any coexisting longstanding soft tissue contractures. Generally speaking, all flexible implant arthroplasty procedures in the foot are mobilized as quickly as possible to train the scar in order that collagen be realigned in the direction of tension (59). Mobilization of implanted joints is more often dictated by any additional procedures that were performed.

The following discussion will deal with specific complications of those procedures which are most commonly performed today. Mention will be made of some less commonly performed techniques, but will be limited in these areas because many of these procedures have been abandoned. Discussion will center around avoidance, recognition, and treatment of the more commonly encountered complications of implant surgery in the foot.

Hallux Limitus and Hallux Rigidus

There are a multitude of local and systemic causes of first metatarsophalangeal joint pathology that may necessitate implant arthroplasty (Table 12.4). Resultant deformities may be broadly classified into hallux valgus, hallux limitus, and hallux

Table 12.4.
Etiology of Hallux Limitus Rigidus

Inflammatory arthritis
RA
Gout
Psoriasis
Degenerative joint disease
Osteochondritis dissecans
Metatarsus primus elevatus
Neurotrophic joint disease
Previous first MPJ surgery
Sesamoid abnormality
Trauma

rigidus. Generally speaking, implant arthroplasty is considered when there is pain and/or deformity in association with loss of articular cartilage. The removal and replacement of a painful arthritic joint will in itself alleviate the patients' complaints most of the time, regardless of etiology. However, a universal approach to all patients, both medically and surgically, will lead to unnecessary complications. Surgical judgement, technique, and rehabilitation should be individually directed to each presenting etiology. Let us take the case of hallux limitus and rigidus first. Although many causes are responsible for the development of these deformities, the origins can be generally grouped into trauma, abnormal biomechanics, and inflammatory arthritis.

Trauma has been cited as the most common cause for hallux rigidus (66–79). Our own experiences suggest functional abnormalities as being far more common. Surgical reconstruction of the post-traumatic degenerative joint does not seem to pose nearly as many problems as the arthritic joint that is secondary to functional abnormalities. This holds true providing the patient's functional status was near normal prior to the traumatic episode. Although not always a reliable indicator, comparison with the opposite foot may yield useful information as to prior functional status. Certainly, secondary osseous alterations and soft tissue contractures must be evaluated and dealt with effectively at the time of surgical intervention. One type of trauma that seems fairly common is osteochondritis dissecans (70). Although implant arthroplasty is indicated for this problem, concern is often expressed in terms of implantation in the younger patient. Curettement of the fragment and defect down to subchondral bone may promote fibrocartilage that eliminates the patient's complaints and need for a prosthesis. Cartilage transplants may also be a viable alternative if the defect is larger in dimension. In long-standing cases, osteotomies that displace the useful range of motion in a more dorsal direction have proven to be a useful adjunct (68, 71, 72), providing secondary degenerative changes have not occurred. When secondary changes are present or the defect is large, implant arthroplasty is the preferred procedure.

As mentioned previously, there are the functional considerations that most com-

monly result in future complications. Hallux rigidus has been related to abnormal pronation (73–77) of the foot, especially in a rectus foot type (78). Because of this, one must first assess whether foot function can be controlled post-operatively. For example, a more vertical oblique midtarsal joint axis is not amenable to orthotic control (78). In this instance, abnormal foot function is going to exist post-operatively with resultant abnormal first metatarsophalangeal joint function. Although hemi-implant arthroplasty will initially alleviate the patient's complaints under these clinical circumstances, the surgeon will ultimately be disappointed with the functional results of the surgery (Fig. 12.12). Remembering that flexible prostheses are designed to accommodate the normal functional demands of the first metatarsophalangeal joint, this sit-

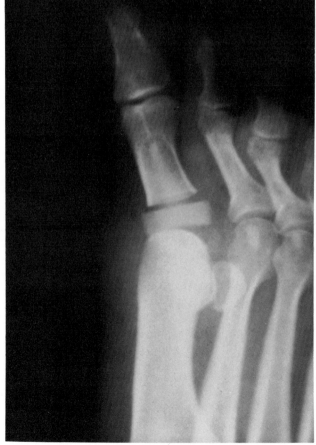

Figure 12.12. This is a stress view in a patient with a hemi-implant. Notice the abutting of the implant against the first metatarsal head and limited range of motion in this patient with metatarsus primus elevatus.

uation results in abnormal functional demands and inherent risks of future implant failure. Also to be considered is that metatarsus primus elevatus is a result of abnormal pronation in a rectus foot type and is a very frequent finding associated with hallux limitus (Fig. 12.13). The metatarsus primus elevatus deformity may be functional or structural in nature. The hallux has difficulty dorsiflexing on an elevated first metartarsal, whether it be functionally or structurally in this position. For these reasons, the surgeon should elect to perform a total joint implant procedure. The hinged prosthesis is not as directly effected by foot function or metatarsal position because the total joint prosthesis has its own built-in range of motion in the hinge (Fig. 12.14). In effect, this inherent range of motion compensates for a metatarsus primus elevatus deformity (Table 12.5). Because of these reasons, component prosthesis should be avoided under these clinical circumstances. Component prosthesis will be more adversely affected by first ray position (Fig. 12.15).

As previously mentioned, total hinge prostheses effectively compensates for abnormal functional or structural position of the first ray. Regardless of this, some may still feel more comfortable with the single-stemmed hemi-implant because of decreased morbidity when infection does occur. Recognizing the flaws in function that will normally occur with this approach, the surgeon should attempt to accommodate the smallest sized single-stemmed implant possible. The reasons for this are that smaller sized hemi-implants exhibit a better range of motion (Fig. 12.16). Unfortunately, the smaller prosthesis carries greater risks of bony overgrowth that can adversely effect the range of motion (Fig. 12.17). Total joint prostheses are applied in an opposite manner; larger sizes are preferred to lessen the chances of ectopic bone formation.

Beside altered osseous anatomy, soft tis-

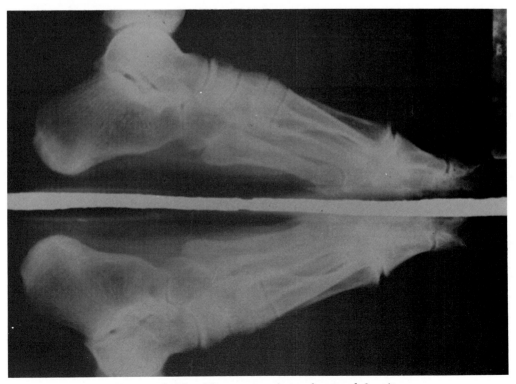

Figure 12.13. Metatarsus primus elevatus deformity.

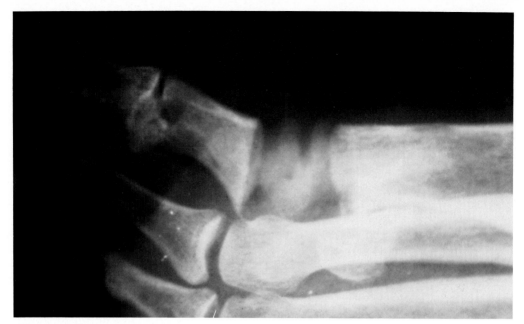

Figure 12.14. Range of motion of Swanson-designed total implant less affected by structural and functional deformities of the foot than the hemi-implant.

Table 12.5.
Comparison of Hemi and Total Joint Implants

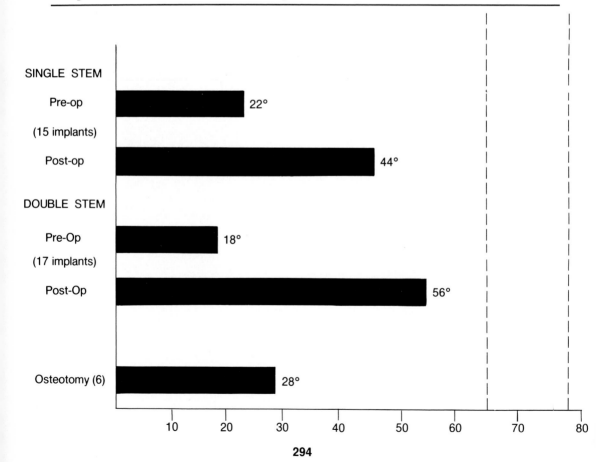

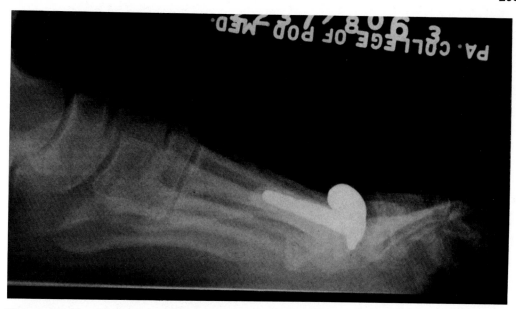

Figure 12.15. Limited motion of component prosthesis can occur if there is superimposed first ray deformities, as was seen in this patient.

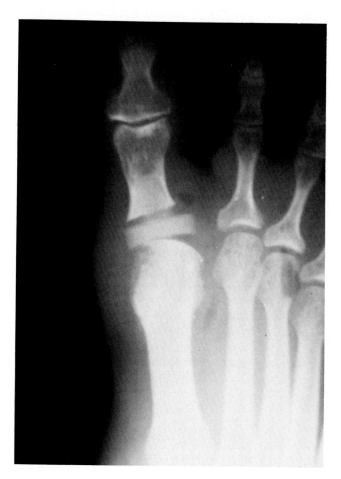

Figure 12.16. This oversized implant displayed a restricted range of motion. Eventual removal was necessitated because of fracture.

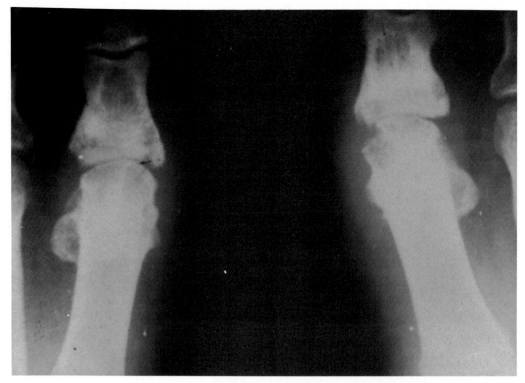

Figure 12.17.   This patient had bilateral hemi-implants 3 years previously. The smaller sized implant allowed for good range of motion but eventual bony overgrowth resulted in pain and limited motion. Revision was accomplished by total implant arthroplasty.

sue considerations also exist. One should expect a contracted flexor apparatus from longstanding hallux limitus deformity. Most often, resection of the joint creates enough shortening of the first ray to result in a relative lengthening of contracted flexor tendons. If severely contracted, it is best to avoid lengthening the flexor tendons for this will weaken the muscle and create problems with post-operative rehabilitation and risks of creating hallux extensus deformity. When contractures are felt to be significant, even after resection of articular surfaces, additional bone may be removed from the proximal phalanx if necessary. Extensive resection is not desired because it may remove the entire attachment of the flexor hallucis brevis and shortened stems are more prone to dislocate. Resection of the first metatarsal head should be kept at a minimum because it is not desirable to create the situation where the implant becomes weightbearing (Fig. 12.18).

As noted earlier, hallux rigidus surgery is designed to facilitate increases in range of motion. For this reason, passive and active range of motion therapy is encouraged early in the post-operative period. Sometimes, errors in technique create snags in the post-operative period by creating excessive fibrosis. Many of these errors are related to improper drilling, or reaming of the medullary canal. This is most commonly done on the phalangeal side. It is important to remember that the proximal phalanx is structured concave plantarly and convex dorsally. Improper orientation in this regard will result in perforation of the cortex with resultant adherent fibrosis to adjacent soft tissue structures (Fig. 12.19). In addition, ectopic bone formation is encouraged by this error which can result in irritation of pericapsular tissues with resultant pain on dorsiflexion. Similar problems, although not as common, can occur on the metatarsal side (Fig. 12.20). Also, it is important

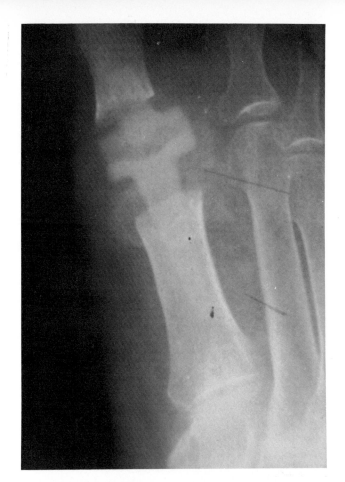

Figure 12.18. Too much bone was resected from the first metatarsal head. A transfer lesion developed under the second metatarsal head. Fatigue fracture of the implant is at risk in this patient.

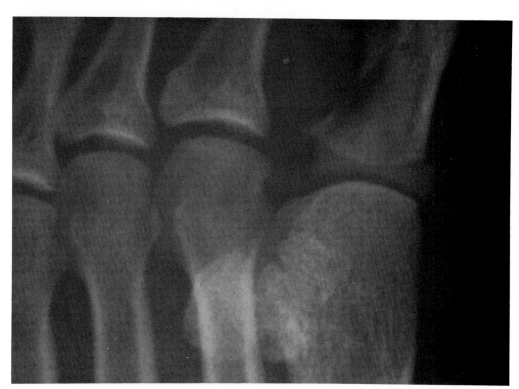

Figure 12.19. Notice the break in the plantar cortex of the proximal phalanx. Limited range of motion was seen. Ectopic bone formation caused pain on dorsiflexion.

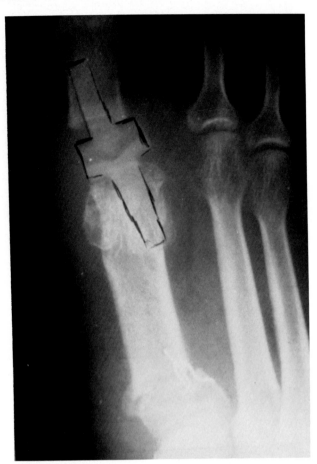

Figure 12.20. The cortex on the lateral aspect of the first metatarsal head was inadvertently drilled in this patient. Also, notice the improper seating of the implant.

that the medullary canal be drilled in a fashion that orientates the hinge of the total implant 90° to the long axis of the first metatarsal. This will allow for true sagittal plane motion to occur at the hinge. Failure to do so will result in increased torsional forces with greater risks of implant breakage.

Hallux Abducto Valgus

As with hallux limitus, implant surgery for hallux abducto valgus also requires special considerations. Naturally, implant surgery is not considered for all cases of hallux abducto valgus deformity, but is reserved for those cases that display articular degeneration from longstanding subluxation and improper function. Once again, the elimination of articular pain will be afforded by virtue of the implant itself. However, under

these clinical circumstances, the surgeon is most concerned with creation of a rectus hallux. This concern is based on several reasons for implant failure in the patient with hallux abducto valgus deformity. Of prime importance is the concern that residual deformity will allow the great toe joint to function improperly and result in undue stress upon the implant, these same forces having originally created articular degeneration. Secondly, there are often associated lesser toe deformities seen with hallux abducto valgus deformity, such as overlapping second and third toes, and correction of these digital deformities is doomed to fail unless the hallux is placed in a more rectus position. Third, but not of least importance, is that a rectus toe allows far more comfortable shoe wear and has better patient acceptance as far as cosmesis is concerned.

Similar to hallux limitus, hallux abducto valgus deformities are often associated with abnormal foot function. This deformity is seen with excessive foot pronation (79, 80) in association with an adductus foot type (78). Because of the implication that the deformity is often functional in etiology, the ability to control foot function post-operatively is necessary to insure long-term success of the surgery.

The creation of a rectus hallux requires careful evaluation of co-existing deformities of the first metarsal. In other words, proximal deformities must be concurrently realigned to insure adequate correction of the hallux abductus deformity. In this regard, it is important to assess for abnormalities of the metatarsus primus adductus and proximal articular set angles (81). The intermetatarsal angle, or relationship between the first and second metatarsals, is considered to be excessive when it exceeds 15° in the rectus foot and 12° in the adductus foot type (82). When excessive and not effectively reduced, correct alignment of the hallux becomes difficult. When the metatarsal is not realigned, it becomes necessary to perform an overzealous medial capsular correction which usually limits the range of motion post-operatively. This limited motion carries associated risks of bone resorption and/or fatigue fracture of the implant. It is best to reduce the intermetatarsal angle by either opening or closing wedge osteotomies at the base of the first metatarsal, depending upon the length of the metatarsal. With borderline cases of high intermetatarsal angles, a lateral release may afford effective reduction of the intermetatarsal angle.

Also of importance is the proximal articular set angle (PASA). This angle is formed by a line representing the bisection of the first metatarsal and a line representing the effective articular surface of the first metatarsal head, and is usually considered abnormal when in excess of 8° (82). Generally speaking, increases in the intermetatarsal angle parallel increases in the proximal articular set angle. The exception to this is found in adolescent hallux abducto valgus deformity where the lateral drift of the proximal phalanx is not accompanied by excessive deviation of the first metatarsal (80). Because degenerative changes of the first metatarsophalangeal joint in bunion deformity of functional etiology is more commonly seen in the older age group, one should expect abnormalities of both angles to be a relatively common finding. Failure to deal with the PASA will result in recurrence of deformity, undue stress on the implant, or limited functional results of the implant. Unfortunately, surgical correction of the PASA is not as easily accomplished as with the intermetatarsal angle. Osteotomies of the first metatarsal neck to reduce the lateral deviation of the articular surface carry potential problems when performed with a hemi-implant arthroplasty. For one thing, rehabilitation may be hampered by the longer recuperative time necessary for healing of the osteotomy site. Also, K-wire fixation is sometimes necessary to stabilize the osteotomy site, and this carries the risk of pin tract infection with obvious deleterious effects of the implant site. In addition, we have noticed an increased incidence of avascular necrosis of the first metatarsal head when these procedures are performed in combination. Reshaping of the metatarsal head to correct the PASA should never be done in concert with a hemi-implant because of resultant abrasive wear of the implant. We prefer alternative approaches to this problem. The least desirable alternative is to apply drill holes to the proximal phalanx medially in order that a capsular flap may be attached to retain the hallux in a more rectus position. Normally the hemi-implant should be wholly articular, but in this instance the implant is prevented from being wholly articular on its lateral aspect (Fig. 12.21). This may result in a medial impingement of the prosthesis with resultant abrasive wear. This problem has led to an alternative procedure, where a so-called Weil-designed angulated hemi-implant is used. This prosthesis in effect compensates for the lateral deviation of the articular cartilage by its design (Fig. 12.22).

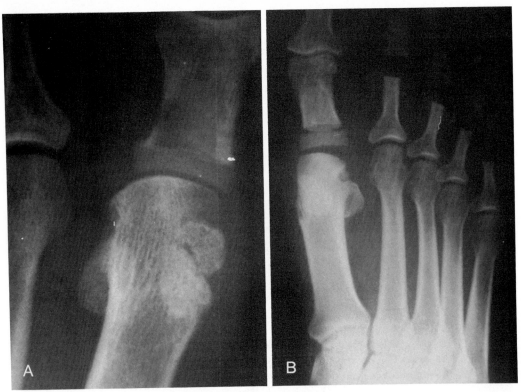

Figure 12.21. *A*, this hemi-implant is wholly articular with the metatarsal head and congruous. *B*, because of a high PASA, the implant does not articulate well on its lateral aspect. Medial impingement often occurs.

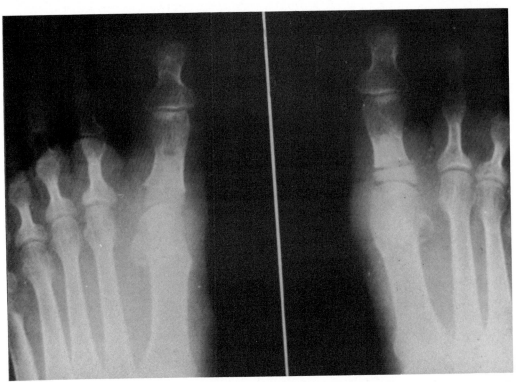

Figure 12.22. The Weil design angulated hemi-implant can sometimes be used to compensate for a high PASA.

Complications are seen with its usage as well. This design implant is seemingly more prone to displacement so that certain precautions should be used. Adequate lateral soft tissue release, reduction of the intermetatarsal angle if necessary, and the use of the previously described medial capsular attachment technique, will lessen the chances for recurrence of deformity or dislocation of the implant (Fig. 12.23). A third alternative is to eliminate the PASA by performing a total implant arthroplasty. By this method, the articular surface of the first metatarsal is removed perpendicular to the long axis of the metatarsal, thereby eliminating the PASA as a concern. This seems the best alternative in cases of abnormally high proximal articular set angles.

Technical errors previously discussed under the section on hallux limitus surgery are also of concern in regards to hallux valgus implant surgery. Of special concern with hallux valgus surgery is that resection of the base of the proximal phalanx be performed at right angles to the long axis of the bone. Failure to do so will result in probable recurrence of deformity, as well as stress upon the stem of the implant (Fig. 12.24). Also of special concern is the release of all soft tissue contractures. Adductor

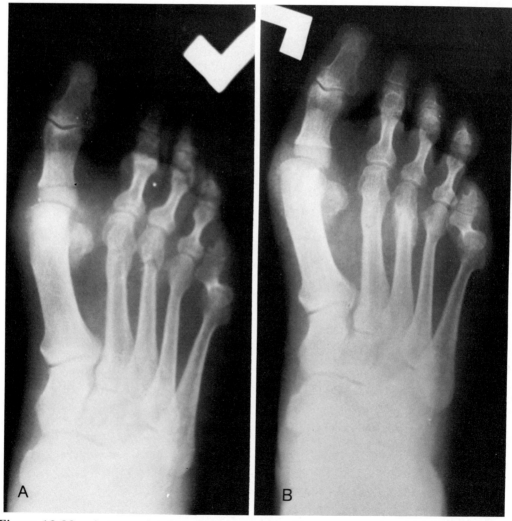

Figure 12.23. *A*, an angulated hemi-implant was used to compensate for a high PASA. Fibular sesamoidectomy, lateral release, and reduction of the intermetatarsal angle by osteotomy should have been performed. *b*, recurrence of deformity occurred 6 months later.

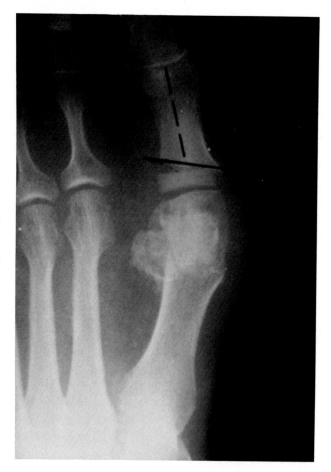

Figure 12.24. The base of the proximal phalanx must be resected at right angles to the bisection of the shaft, otherwise, recurrence of the deformity will be seen, as has occurred in this patient.

hallucis brevis, extensor hallucis brevis, and extensor hallucis longus are the more common soft tissue releases that should be performed. The fibular sesamoid is thought to be a contributory deforming force when the tibial sesamoid is in position four or greater (81). Under these circumstances, it should be released to allow for correct positioning of the hallux and to lessen the chances of recurrence. In addition, the articular surface of the fibular sesamoid may be eroded and contributory to the patients' complaints. In fact, the sesamoid bones are known to be affected by inflammatory arthritis (83). Sometimes removal will be difficult because the sesamoid bone may be ankylosed to the metatarsal head. Intracapsular approach, after resection of articular surfaces, will best facilitate removal when this occurs. Excision of the sesamoid will allow for improved tendon movement and

enhance chances for a better functional result. Freeing up of the tibial sesamoid may be necessary, but removal should be avoided because of resultant muscle imbalance.

Of particular concern with implant surgery in the patient with hallux abducto valgus are complications arising from associated inflammatory arthritis. Inflammatory arthritis often gives rise to subluxations, making hallux abducto valgus a frequently encountered associated deformity, especially with rheumatoid arthritis. In fact, the most severe hallux abducto valgus deformities are found with rheumatoid arthritis (78). When contemplating surgery in the patient with inflammatory arthritis, special considerations have to be afforded the patient. In the past, elective procedures were not performed during active stages of rheumatoid arthritis, but many feel this delay is no longer necessary, providing the disease can be suppressed by modern day therapy (84). Of greater concern are signs of vasculitis and neuropathy which signal a more severe disease process. Patients with psoriatic arthritis were thought to be at greater risk for infection, exacerbation of skin disease at surgical sites, osteolysis, and pronounced fibrosis which would jeopardize the surgical results. Newer thoughts feel that withholding surgery from the psoriatic patient is no longer justified (85). One must also be cognizant of the complications that accompany many of the anti-inflammatory drugs that these patients had been on for short- and long-term management (86, 87). X-rays of the cervical spine should be requested (flexion-extension and odontoid views) prior to contemplated general anesthesia, even in absence of symptoms, because of the possibilities of inducing cervical cord compression (88). One must remember that the cervical spine is frequently involved in rheumatoid arthritis. Because of these reasons, the best approach to the arthritic patient is one in which a close liason is maintained between the surgeon, rheumatologist, anesthesiologist, and physical therapist (89).

Lesser Metatarsophalangeal Joint

Implant arthroplasty of the lesser metatarsophalangeal joints has similar indications as the first metatarsophalangeal joint. In addition, use has been applied to short lesser metatarsals in order to restore length, for those patients that previously had isolated metatarsal head resections, for avascular necrosis, and as an adjunctive procedure to pan-metatarsal head resections for advanced forefoot destruction secondary to inflammatory arthritis. Despite the multitude of potential clinical applications, replacement of these joints has not gained widespread popularity because of inherent problems.

The most common problem has been adaptation at the phalangeal side of the joint. The smaller dimensions of the proximal phalanx has posed problems for inser-

tion of previously designed implants (90). This has resulted in necessary modifications of the implant by the surgeon with the resultant risks of early implant breakage. Recently, Swanson has introduced a flexible hinge prosthesis, similar in design to those used in the first metatarsophalangeal joint, with the exception that it is smaller in size. Although adequate followup is not presently available, this implant design seems promising for the future.

The previous difficulties with application of total implants have prompted replacement of just the metatarsal side of the joint; the ulnar head and Seeburger prosthesis (91) being two such examples. Replacement of the metatarsal head by these prostheses necessitated removal of large amounts of bone, and resultant stress fractures and transfer lesions under adjacent metatarsal head occurred. The undesirability of an implant being weightbearing in the foot is self-explanatory. Bone absorption at the implant-bone interface was fairly common. Despite these shortcomings, Swanson-designed condylar implants enjoy some popularity for use in the foot (Fig. 12.25). With less resection of bone, weightbearing does not seem to occur with these implants, so longevity would be expected. Unfortunately, the lack of retrograde stability often results in dislocation of these implants (Fig. 12.26). This necessitates fixating the implant to bone (Fig. 12.27) with resultant absorption of bone at the bone-implant interface. The newer hinged total prosthesis is seemingly the best prosthesis offered at this time.

As mentioned previously, bone resection should be kept at a minimum on the metatarsal side of the joint. Even when used to attempt restoration of length to a congenitally short metatarsal, bone resection should be limited to articular cartilage only on the metatarsal head. Overzealous resection will result in either fracture of the implant, dislocation, or transfer lesions.

Use of lesser metatarsophalangeal joint implants has been advocated for pan-metatarsal head resection procedures (92). Our

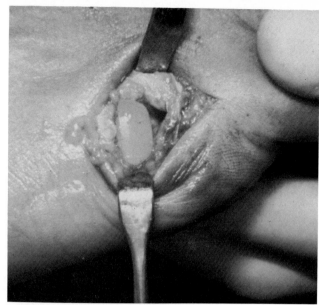

Figure 12.25. Application of a Swanson-designed condylar implant for replacement of the fifth metatarsal head. Dislocation is fairly common.

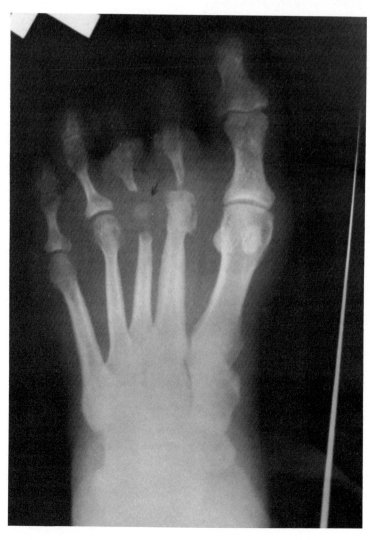

Figure 12.26. Condylar implant was utilized as a spacer in this patient who had previously underwent metatarsal head resection. Dislocation occurred 2 months after insertion.

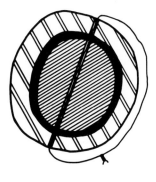

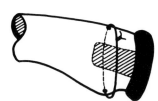

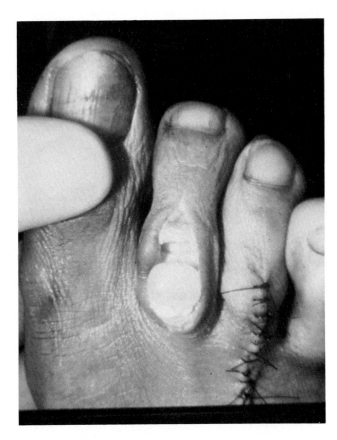

Figure 12.27. Method of tying in condylar implant in order to lessen the chances of dislocation.

Figure 12.28. Swanson-designed condylar implant being applied to retain length and function of the proximal interphalangeal joint of a second toe. One must be careful to insure adequate soft tissue covering.

own feeling is that this is usually not necessary. This procedure by itself usually has very uniform, acceptable results (93–96). The additional use of implants carries inherent risks that outweigh the potential benefits. This procedure is most commonly performed on patients with rheumatoid arthritis. Although comparable studies are not available in the foot, it is important to note the higher incidence of fractured implants in the hands in rheumatoid patients with severe disease (54). The good clinical results obtained with standard resection arthroplasty alone would suggest preference for implant abstention in this clinical situation.

Interphalangeal Joints

The use of implants in association with arthroplasty of the toes remains controversial. At present, condylar implants are utilized for this purpose (Fig. 12.28). In addition, development of a double-stemmed prosthesis has recently been introduced. Application remains limited and best suited for those patients requiring the need for additional length or in those patients who develop exuberant bone formation after conventional arthroplasty. The loss of retrograde stability by conventional arthroplasty usually does not create problems, provided the toe does not heal in a malaligned position. When this is a concern, the use of K-wires or interphalangeal joint fusion usually produces acceptable results. Because of their recent introduction, further research is necessary to determine the reliability and effectiveness of these prostheses.

References

1. Klasson, D. H., and Scheman, P. Purified carbon as a tissue replacement. Int. Surg. 62:179, 1977.
2. Hetherington, V. J., Kavros, S. J., Conway, F., Mandracchia, V. J., Martin, W., and Haubold, A. D. Pyrolytic carbon as a joint replacement in the foot: A preliminary report. J. Foot Surg. 21:160, 1982.
3. Swanson, A. B. A flexible implant for replacement of arthritic or destroyed joints in the hand. Interclin. Bull. 6:16, 1966.
4. Swanson, A. B. Implant arthroplasty for the great toe. Clin. Orthop. 85:75, 1972.
5. Millender, L. H., Nalebuff, E. A., Hawkins, R. B., and Ennis, R. Infection after silicone prosthetic arthroplasty in the hand. J. Bone Jt. Surg. 57A:825, 1975.
6. Sethu, A., D'Netto, D. C., and Ramakrishna, B. Swanson's silastic implants in great toes. J. Bone Jt. Surg. 62B:83, 1980.
7. Antimicrobial prophylaxis for surgery. The Medical Letter 21:73, 1979.
8. Veterans Administration Ad Hoc Interdisciplinary Advisory Committee on Antimicrobial Drug Usage. Prophylaxis in surgery. JAMA 237:1003, 1977.
9. Chodak, G. W., and Plaut, M. E. Use of systemic antibiotics for prophylaxis in surgery. Arch. Surg. 112:326, 1977.
10. Schurman, D. J., Hirshman, H. P., and Burton, D. S. Cephalothin and cefamandole penetration into bone, synovial fluid, and wound drainage fluid. J. Bone Jt. Surg. 62A:981, 1980.
11. Nichols, R. L. Use of prophylactic antibiotics in surgical practice. Am. J. Med. 70:686, 1981.
12. Mashford, M. L., Robertson, M. B., and Stewart, J. M. Use of prophylactic antibiotics in surgery. Med. J. Aust. 1:532, 1980.
13. Schurman, D. J., Burton, D. S., Kajiyama, G., Moser, K., and Nagel, D. A. Sodium cephapirin disposition and distribution into human bone. Curr. Ther. Res. 20:144, 1976.
14. Pollard, J. P., Hughes, S. P. F., Scott, J. E., Evan, M. J., and Benson, M. K. Prophylactic antibiotics following total hip replacement: A controlled trial. J. Bone Jt. Surg. 61B:118, 1979.
15. Hewitt, W. L., and McHenry, M. C. Blood level determination of antimicrobial drugs. Med. Clin. North Am. 62:1119, 1978.
16. Dahlgren, D. G., Anderson, E. T., and Hewitt, W. L. Gentamicin blood levels: A guide to nephrotoxicity. Antimicrob. Agents Chemother. 8:58, 1975.
17. Adams, J. P., and Neviaser, P. J. Complications of implant surgery in the hand, in Complications in Orthopaedic Surgery, 1st ed., edited by Epps, C. H., Jr. J. B. Lippincott, Philadelphia, 1978, vol. 2.
18. Shanks, S. C. A Textbook of X-ray Diagnosis. W. B. Saunders, Philadelphia, 1972, vol. 6.
19. Wald, E. R., Mirro, R., and Gartner, C. Pitfall in the diagnosis of acute osteomyelitis by bone scan. Clin. Pediatr. 19:597, 1980.
20. Duszynski, D. O., Kuhn, J. P., Afshani, E., and Riddlesberger, M. Early radionuclide diagnosis of acute osteomyelitis. Radiology 117:337, 1975.
21. Gilday, D. L., Paul, D. J., and Paterson, J. Diagnosis of osteomyelitis in children by combined blood pool and bone imaging. Radiology 117:331, 1975.
22. Handmaker, H., and Leonards, R. The bone scan in inflammatory osseous disease. Semin. Nucl. Med. 6:95, 1976.
23. Waldvogel, F. A., and Vasey, H. Osteomyelitis: The past decade. N. Engl. J. Med. 303:360, 1980.
24. Scoles, P. V., Hilty, M. D., and Seakinakis, G. N. Bone scan pattern in acute osteomyelitis. Clin. Orthop. North Am. 153:210, 1980.
25. Park, H. M., Wheat, L. J., Siddiqui, A. R., Burt, R. W., Robb, J. A., Ransburg, R. C., and Kernek, C. B. Scintigraphic evaluation of diabetic osteomyelitis: Concise communication. J. Nucl. Med. 23:569, 1982.
26. Berkowitz, I. D., and Wenzel, W. "Normal" technetium bone scans in patients with acute osteomyelitis. Am. J. Dis. Child. 134:828, 1980.
27. Ganel, A., Horozowski, H., Zaltman, S., and Farine, I. Sequential use of ^{99m}Tc-MDP and ^{67}Ga imaging in bone infection. Orthop. Rev. 9:73, 1981.
28. Hoffer, P. Gallium mechanisms. J. Nucl. Med. 21:282, 1980.
29. Roth, R., and Pressman, M. Clinical diagnosis of osteomyelitis. JAPA 67:709, 1977.
30. Mollan, R. A. B., and Piggot, J. Acute osteomyelitis in children. J. Bone Jt. Surg. 59B:2, 1977.
31. Mackowiak, P. A., Jones, S. R., and Smith, J. W. Diagnostic value of sinus-tract cultures in chronic osteomyelitis. JAMA 239:2772, 1978.
32. Norden, C. W. Experimental osteomyelitis: II. Therapeutic trials and measurement of antibiotic levels in bone. J. Infect. Dis. 124:565, 1971.
33. Norden, C. W., and Dickens, D. R. Experimental osteomyelitis: III. Treatment with cephaloridine. J. Infect. Dis. 127:525, 1973.

34. Cunka, B. A., Gossling, H. R., Pasternak, H. S., Nightingale, C. H., and Quintilian, R. The penetration characteristics of cefazolin, cephalothin, and cephradine into bone in patients undergoing total hip replacement. J. Bone Jt. Surg. 59A:356, 1977.

35. Bell, S. M. Further observations on the value of oral penicillins in chronic staphylococcal osteomyelitis. Med. J. Aust. 2:591, 1976.

36. Fitzgerald, R. H. Jr., Nolan, D. R., Ilstrup, D. M., Van Scoy, R. E., Washington, J. A., II, and Coventry, M. B. Deep wound sepsis following total hip arthroplasty. J. Bone Jt. Surg. 59A:847, 1977.

37. Amstutz, H. C., and Kass, V. Management of the septic total hip replacement, in The Hip: Proceedings of the Fourth Open Scientific Meeting of the Hip Society. C. V. Mosby, St. Louis, 1977.

38. Caldwell, G. A., and Wickstrom, J. The closed treatment of acute hematogenous osteomyelitis: Results in 67 cases. Ann. Surg. 131:734, 1950.

39. Curtiss, P. H. Jr. Bone and joint infection in childhood, in Instructional Course Lectures. C. V. Mosby, St. Louis, 1977, vol. 26, pp. 14–19.

40. Mollam, R. A. B., and Piggot, J. Acute osteomyelitis in children. J. Bone Jt. Surg. 58B:370, 1976.

41. Waldvogel, F. A., Medoff, G., and Swartz, H. Osteomyelitis: A review of clinical features, therapeutic considerations and unusual aspects. N. Engl. J. Med. 282:198–206, 260–226, 316–322, 1970.

42. Pressman, M. Continuous closed suction irrigation following postoperative infection of silastic implant. JAPA 67:746, 1977.

43. Dombrowski, E., and Dunn, A. Treatment of osteomyelitis by debridement and closed wound irrigation-suction. Clin. Orthop. 43:215, 1965.

44. Clawson, D. K., Davis, F. J., and Hansen, S. T., Jr. Treatment of chronic osteomyelitis with emphasis on closed suction-irrigation technic. Clin. Orthop. 96:88, 1973.

45. Reing, C. M., Richin, P. F., and Kenmore, P. I. Differential bone scanning in the evaluation of a painful total joint replacement. J. Bone Jt. Surg. 61A:933, 1979.

46. Braley, S. The silicones as tools in biological engineering. Med. Electron. Biol. Eng. 3:127, 1965.

47. Symmers, W. St. Silicone mastitis in "topless waitresses" and some other varieties of foreign-body mastitis. Br. Med. J. 3:19, 1968.

48. Aptekar, R. G., Davie, J. M., and Cattell, H. S. Foreign body reaction to silicone rubber: Complication of finger joint implant. Clin. Orthop. 98:231, 1974.

49. Christie, A. J., Weinberger, K. A., and Dietrich, M. Silicone lymphadenopathy and synovitis: Complications of silicone elastomer finger joint prostheses. JAMA 237:1463, 1977.

50. Bass, S. J., Gastwirth, C. M., Green, R., Knights, E. M., and Weinstock, R. E. Phagocytosis of silastic material following silastic great toe implant. J. Foot Surg. 17:70, 1978.

51. Christie, A. J., Weinberger, K. A., and Dietrich, M. Complications of silicone elastomer prostheses [letter]. JAMA 238:939, 1977.

52. Worsing, R. A., Engber, W. D., and Lange, T. A. Reactive synovitis from particulate silastic. J. Bone Jt. Surg. 64A:581, 1982.

53. Gordon, M., and Bullough, P. G. Synovial and osseous inflammation in failed silicone-rubber prostheses. J. Bone Jt. Surg. 64A:574, 1982.

54. Swanson, A. B., Meester, W. D., Swanson, G., Rangaswamy, L., and Schut, G. E. Durability of silicone implants: An in vivo study. Orthop. Clin. 4:1097, 1973.

55. Beckenbaugh, R. D., Dobyns, J. H., Linsheid, R. L., and Bryan, R. S. Review and analysis of silicone-rubber metacarpophalangeal implants. J. Bone Jt. Surg. 58A:483, 1976.

56. Swanson, A. B. Finger joint replacement by silicone rubber implants and the concept of implant fixation by encapsulation. Ann. Rheum. Dis. 28:47, 1969.

57. Roberts, A. C. Silicones and their application as implant materials. Biomed. Eng. 156, 1967.

58. Swanson, A. B. Complications of silicone elastomer prostheses [letter]. JAMA 238:939, 1977.

59. Carmen, R., and Kahn, P. In vitro testing of silicone rubber heart-valve poppets for lipid absorption. J. Biomed. Mater. Res. 2:157, 1968.

60. Binder, D. M. Hazards related to the use of acrylics, metals, and plastics in bone surgery. Arch. Podiatr. Med. Surg. 3:33, 1976.

61. Brooks, M., Murray, L., and Gallannaugh, S. C. Circulatory depression in bone after acrylic implantation. Clin. Orthop. Relat. Res. 107:274, 1975.

62. Willert, H. G., Judwig, J., and Semlitsch, M. Reactions of bone to methylmethacrylate after hip arthroplasty. J. Bone Jt. Surg. 56A:1363, 1974.

63. Breed, A. L. Experimental production of vascular hypotension, bone marrow, and fat embolization with methylmethacrylate cement. Cl. Orthop. Relat. Res. 102:227, 1974.

64. Cohen, L. A., and Smith, T. C. The intra-operative hazard of acrylic bone cement: Report of a case. Anesthesiology 35:547, 1971.

65. Pantusek, M. On the metabolic pathways of the methylmethacrylate. Fed. Eur. Biochem. Soc. 2:206, 1969.

66. Davies-Colley, M. R. Contraction of the metatarso-phalangeal joint of the great toe. Br. Med. J. 1:728, 1887.

67. McMaster, M. J. The pathogenesis of hallux rigidus. J. Bone Jt. Surg. 60B:82, 1978.

68. Watermann, H. Die arthritis deformans erossze, Lengrundgolentes. Z. Orthop. Chir. 48:346, 1927.

69. Mann, R. A., Coughlin, M. J., and DuVries, H. L. Hallux rigidus. A review of the literature and a method of treatment. Clin. Orthop. Relat. Res. 142:57, 1979.

70. Goodfellow, J. Aetiology of hallux rigidus. Proc. R. Soc. Med. 59:821, 1966.

71. Moberg, E. A simple operation for hallux rigidus. Clin. Orthop. 71:55, 1979.

72. Kessel, L., and Bonney, G. Hallux rigidus in the adolescent. J. Bone Jt. Surg. 40B:668, 1958.

73. Bonney, G., and McNab, I. Hallux valgus and hallux rigidus. J. Bone Jt. Surg. 34B:366, 1952.

74. Cotterill, J. M. Stiffness of the great toe in adolescents. Br. Med. J. 1:1158, 1888.

75. Giannestras, N. J. Foot Disorders: Medical and Surgical Management, 2nd ed. Lea & Febiger, Philadelphia, 1973, p. 400.

76. Jack, E. A. The aetiology of hallux rigidus. Br. J.

Surg. 27:492, 1940.

77. Nilsonne, H. Removal of the base of the proximal phalanx for hallux rigidus. Acta Orthop. Scand. 18:77, 1947.

78. Root, M. L., Orien, W. P., and Weed, J. H. *Normal and Abnormal Function of the Foot: Clinical Biomechanics*, Clinical Biomechanics Corporation, Los Angeles, 1977, vol. 2.

79. Hardy, R. H., and Clapham, J. C. R. Observations of hallux valgus. J. Bone Jt. Surg. 33B:376, 1951.

80. Piggot, H. The natural history of hallux valgus in adolescence and early adult life. J. Bone Jt. Surg. 42B:749, 1960.

81. LaPorta, G. A., Pilla, P., Jr., and Richter, K. P. Keller implant procedure using a silastic intramedullary stemmed implant. JAPA 66:126, 1976.

82. LaPorta, G. A., Melillo, T., and Olinsky, D. X-ray evaluation of hallux abducto valgus deformity. JAPA 64:545, 1974.

83. Resnick, D., Niwayama, G., and Feingold, M. L. The sesamoid bones of the hands and feet: Participators in arthritis. Radiology 123:57, 1977.

84. Libscomb, P. R. Surgery for rheumatoid arthritis-timing and techniques: Summary. J. Bone Jt. Surg. 50A: 614, 1968.

85. Lambert, J. R., and Wright, V. Surgery in patients with psoriasis and arthritis. Rheumatol. Rehabil. 18:35, 1979.

86. Kaye, R. L., and Pemberton, R. E. Treatment of rheumatoid arthritis: A review including newer and experimental anti-inflammatory agents. Arch. Intern. Med. 136:1023, 1976.

87. Ehrlich, G. E. Treatment of rheumatoid arthritis. JAMA 228: 94, 1974.

88. Cabot, A., and Becker, A. The cervical spine in rheumatoid arthritis. Clin. Orthop. 131:130, 1978.

89. Osmond-Clarke, H., and Mason, R. M. Combined medical and orthopedic management of rheumatic diseases, in *Textbook of the Rheumatic Diseases*, 4th ed., edited by Copeman, W. S. C. ECS Livingstone, London, 1969, p. 802.

90. McGlamry, E. D., and Ruch, J. A. Status of implant arthroplasty of the lesser metatarsophalangeal joints. JAPA 66:156, 1976.

91. Seeburger, R. H. Surgical implants of alloyed metal in joints of the feet. JAPA 54:391, 1964.

92. Aeby, C. H., and Leon, P. D. Utilization of Calnan-Nicolle implant. JAPA 68:167, 1978.

93. Clayton, M. L. Surgery of the lower extremity in rheumatoid arthritis. J. Bone Jt. Surg. 45A:1517, 1963.

94. Fowler, A. W. A method of forefoot reconstruction. J. Bone Jt. Surg. 45A:1517, 1963.

95. Hoffman, P. An operation for severe grades of contracted or clawed toes. Am. J. Orthop. Surg. 9:441, 1912.

96. Kates, A., Kessel, L., and Kay, A. Arthroplasty of the forefoot. J. Bone Jt. Surg. 49B:552, 1967.

CHAPTER 13

Diabetes

ALLEN M. JACOBS, D.P.M.
LAWRENCE M. OLOFF, D.P.M.

The pedal sequellae of diabetes mellitus are well known as evidenced by the large number of articles referencing such manifestations as ulceration (1–5), infection (6–10), vascular disease (11–15), neuropathy (16–20), and Charcot joint disease (21–24). It is now generally accepted that since the classic work of Banting and Best, in which the ability of insulin to control blood glucose was elucidated, the control of hyperglycemia, as well as the control of other chronic diseases, has permitted a large population of individuals to develop the long-term sequellae of diabetes mellitus. Formerly, such patients frequently expired from such phenomena as ketoacidosis or nephropathy rather early in the course of their disease, failing to thrive long enough to develop such problems as ulceration, gangrene, or Charcot joint disease. The common propensity of the patient with diabetes mellitus to develop major chronic lower extremity pathology is exemplified by entire textbooks which address the issue, and podiatric seminars which frequently allocate extensive periods of discussion to the subject. Podiatrists are frequently included in the team approach to the management of the diabetic patient, and have recently taken a more active role in the American Diabetes Association and its component societies.

One-half of all patients with diabetes mellitus will require surgery at some time in their life (25). As a result of improved methods of peri-operative control of serum glucose levels, as well as a greater understanding of the diabetic state, the operative mortality in patients with diabetes mellitus has decreased from 53% (26) in the 1930s to 3.6% (27) presently. No figures are specifically available regarding the mortality or morbidity associated with elective and non-elective foot surgery in patients with diabetes mellitus. 17.2% of diabetic patients undergoing surgery are reported to incur some type of post-operative complication, including wound infection (33%), genitourinary tract infection (33%), cardiovascular disease (8%), and delayed wound healing (4%) (27). With regard to general surgery, it appears that morbidity and mortality associated with surgery in the diabetic patient continue to remain higher than in control populations. Acute myocardial infarction and pulmonary embolic disease are the leading causes of post-operative death in the diabetic patient. A large number of abnormalities are frequently encountered in the diabetic patient admitted to the hospital for elective or emergency surgery, including obesity (58%), arteriosclerosis obliterans (31%), neuropathy (18%), and nephropathy (5%) (28). Significant lower extremity pathology is present in 8% of all patients admitted to a hospital and discovered to be diabetic on the occasion of their admission to surgery.

CLASSIFICATION OF SURGICAL PATHOLOGY IN THE DIABETIC FOOT

In recent years, the literature has reflected an attempt to classify the pedal lesions commonly encountered in the diabetic foot from a surgical or clinical perspective. Meade and Mueller (29) characterized infectious disease of the diabetic foot as belonging to one of three major categories (Table 13.1). The first of these, the dorsal phlegma, represents a cellulitic, non-localizing infectious process in which antibiotic therapy and control of serum glucose levels represents the mainstay of treatment. The deep plantar space abscess represents the second of the Meade-Mueller infectious processes, while the mal perforans, or pressure-induced neurotrophic ulcer, represents the third diabetic foot lesion not uncommonly encountered in clinical practice.

In a series of articles, Wagner (30–32) has presented a somewhat practical classification of commonly encountered diabetic foot lesions. In his proposed schema, a series of algorisms are presented which address the risk-benefit problem of therapeutic intervention for the surgical correction of pathology associated with the diabetic foot. Because the Wagner classification system is a surgical grading of diabetic foot lesions with diagnostic and therapeutic implications, and in view of the increasing popularity of this system, some discussion will be presented at this time.

Grade 0, diabetic foot lesions are pathologic but non-ulcerative lesions such as hammer toes, incurvated nails, bunions, or structurally plantarflexed metatarsals (Fig. 13.1). Although grade 0 lesions are found in the non-diabetic as well as the diabetic patient, they represent deformities which are well known to predispose patients to ulceration, infection, and gangrene in the presence of such factors as microangiopathy, sensory neuropathy, autonomic neuropathy, or large vessel disease. The grade 0 lesion presents the scenario of an area of increased pressure secondary to osseous deformity. When vascular and other factors permit, such lesions should be corrected, since they represent pre-ulcerative lesions, especially in non-compliant patients, patients with poorly controlled diabetes, or patients with significant autonomic or sensory polyneuropathy. The grade 0 lesion exemplifies the risk-benefit quandary faced by the surgeon confronting an obviously pre-ulcerative lesion in a diabetic patient. Certainly, removal of hyperostoses and correction of fixed bone and joint deformities should lessen the incidence of pressure-induced lower extremity pathology. What is worrisome to us is the reputedly high incidence of morbidity associated with foot surgery in the diabetic patient. Current literature suggests that diabetic patients may be evaluated for risk factors such as degree of vascular compromise, and that healing of foot surgery in patients with arteriosclerosis obliterans and diabetes mellitus may be predicted with a reasonable degree of success.

Because the grade 0 lesion (Table 13.2) represents a pre-ulcerative lesion, great care should be exerted to select those patients who are not at particularly high risk for poor wound healing. Anhidrosis is usually a manifestation of diabetic autonomic neuropathy and may impede wound healing. In general, the skin is affected in 30% of diabetic patients. Proper emollient therapy may be attempted prior to surgery in order to improve the condition of the skin in the area of an incision. In addition to anhidrosis, tinea pedis has been shown to affect up to 70% of diabetic patients in some studies.

When elective correction of a grade 0 lesion is contemplated, an examination of the foot and operative area should be made

Table 13.1.
Classification of Diabetic Pedal Lesions

Meade and Mueller (29)
    Dorsal phlegma
    Deep plantar space
    Mal perforans
Wagner (30–32)
    Grade 0: No ulceration (Fig. 13.1)
    Grade 1: Superficial ulceration (Fig. 13.2)
    Grade 2: Ulceration to tendon, bone, or joint capsule (Fig. 13.3)
    Grade 3: Ulceration to deep tissues with osteomyelities or deep abscess (Fig. 13.4)
    Grade 4: Gangrene localized to an area amenable to local radical amputation (Fig. 13.5)
    Grade 5: Extensive gangrene and necrosis

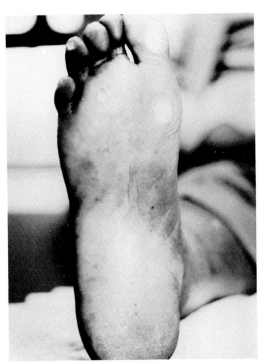

Figure 13.1. Wagner grade 0 dysvascular foot lesions. The grade 0 lesions are typified by pressure-induced keratomas, fixed digital deformities, and incurvated dystrophic nails. Such lesions frequently result in ulceration, complicated by secondary infection or gangrene.

Table 13.2.
Local Risk Factors in Grade 0 Lesions

Vascular
  Vasospasm
  Microvascular occlusive disease
  Medial calcific sclerosis
  Large vessel disease
Dermatologic
  Anhidrosis
  Tinea pedis, *Candida*
  Superficial infection
Hematologic
  Elevated hemoglobin A_{1C}
  Anemia
  Hyperglycemia
Osseous
  Undetected osteolysis, Charcot joint disease,
    or osteomyelitis

for evidence of tinea pedis. When suspected, a KOH study or confirmatory fungal culture may be performed, with the initiation of appropriate therapy. In addition to tinea pedis and anhidrosis associated with diabetic autonomic neuropathy, a variety of dermatologic lesions that may be found on the foot of the diabetic which may complicate wound healing are listed in Table 13.3.

Vascular evaluation of the patient with diabetes mellitus, as well as neurologic evaluation and control of the diabetic state, will be discussed later in this chapter.

Ulceration of the foot may be classified as grade 1, grade 2, or grade 3 (Figs. 13.2–13.4). As stated earlier, the grade 1 ulceration consists of a superficial soft tissue defect in which any infectious process is limited to the skin and superficial subcutaneous tissues. In a grade 1 lesion, no

osteomyelitis is present. The objective for management of a grade 1 lesion is to control and resolve any infectious process, secure healing of the ulceration, and prevention of recurrence by attention to correctable structural deformities or biomechanical abnormalities. The grade 2 ulcerative lesion is characterized by pathology of the skin, subcutaneous tissues, and fascial tissues. The presence of infectious disease must be established early and appropriate therapy instituted. When the infectious disease process extends to bone, joint, or deep spaces, a diabetic foot lesion is classified as grade 3. From a therapeutic standpoint, the differentiation of grades 1, 2, and 3 is essential and require a familiarity with a variety of radiologic, nuclear medicine, and often diagnostic modalities as they apply to the rheumatic consequences of diabetes mellitus. As a general rule, grade 2 and 3 ulcerative lesions require more aggressive non-operative intervention, as well as greater diagnostic acumen. The problems of early diagnosis and appropriate goal-oriented therapy are complicated by the fact that a tender, swollen, erythematous foot may characterize not only deep abscess, cellulitis, and osteomyelitis, but may be found in association with Charcot joint disease, diabetic osteolysis, and, in some cases, diabetic autonomic neuropathy. Soft tissue infection with ulceration may be

Table 13.3.
Lower Extremity Diabetic Dermatologic
Disorders

Anhidrosis
Tinea pedis
Carotenemia
Pruritis/pruritic excoriation
Rubeosis
Mal perforans
Diabetic bullae
Infarction
Tuberous xanthomata
Diabetic dermopathy
Eruptive xanthomata
Kyle's disease
Necrobiosis lipoidica diabeticorum
Erythrasma

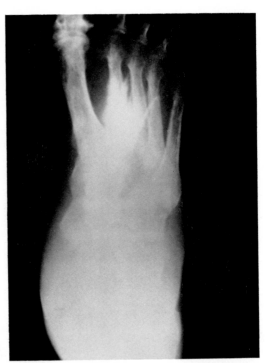

Figure 13.3. Sinogram of ulcerated heloma mollé showing extension into the central plantar space. Frequently, contrast media gently injected into an ulcerated digital lesion will reveal communication with the central plantar space. Spread of infectious organisms along the flexor tendon sheaths and plantar intrinsic musculature may explain pain, tenderness, and swelling in the arch area.

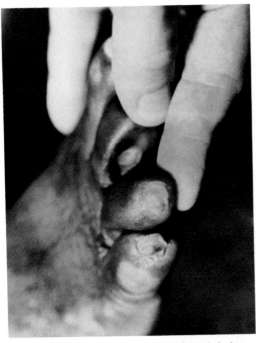

Figure 13.2. Ulcerated interdigital heloma mollé. Debridement of hyperatotic tissue in the diabetic patient frequently reveals the presence of undetected ulceration. In such cases, the presence of osteomyelitis must be considered by radiograph or bone scan.

present without osteomyelitis or deep abscess. Osteomyelitis may be present, but undetected due to a paucity of radiographic changes early in the course of the disease. Radiographic abnormalities such as diabetic osteolysis or Charcot joint disease may be mistakenly interpreted as osteomyelitic in nature, especially when such osseous abnormalities are found in proximity to soft tissue infectious disease. In the presence of deep ulcerations with infection, the presence of radiographic bone or articular abnormalities should be regarded as highly probable, but not diagnostic of osteomyelitis.

The grade 4 diabetic foot lesion is characterized by gangrene, extensive necrosis, or marked vascular or ulcerative and infectious disease clearly localized to one portion of the foot, and amenable to local radical amputation or debridement, when the patients' general medical status and lower extremity vascular status permit (Fig. 13.5). Grade 5 lesions are characterized by extensive areas of infection or vascular em-

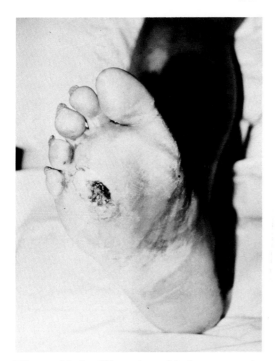

Figure 13.4. Ulceration with deep space abscess. Plantar ulceration with purulence, dorsal and plantar edema, erythema, pain, and tenderness are present.

barrassment, and generally represent disease requiring major vascular reconstruction or amputation.

SURGICAL ENDOCRINOLOGY OF THE DIABETIC PATIENT

Careful consideration must be given to the management of diabetes mellitus in the pre-operative, operative, and post-operative periods. Hormonal changes associated with the stress of anesthesia and surgery may result in an exacerbation of the glucose intolerance of a patient (27, 33). Careful monitoring of the fluid and food intake in the peri-operative period is often essential in order to avoid dehydration, electrolyte abnormalities, prerenal azotemia, ketoacidosis, or hyperglycemic, hyperosmolar, non-ketotic coma (27, 33).

The major objectives in the peri-operative period include:

1. Recognition and treatment of the diabetes, coexisting medical problems, and successful foot surgery;

2. Provision of an adequate amount of carbohydrate in order to inhibit catabolic proteolysis and lipolysis;

3. Provision of adequate insulin coverage in order to prevent hyperglycemia, hyperosmolality, ketoacidosis, and glycosuria while preventing hypoglycemia;

4. The avoidance of iatrogenic complications (27, 33).

As a general rule, minor surgical procedures and surgical procedures performed under local anesthesia do not require any alteration in the management of the diabetic patient (33). An attempt should be made to schedule diabetic patients for surgery early in the morning to minimize hypoglycemia which may complicate the NPO status. A late night snack on the evening prior to surgery is often recommended for this reason. It must be remembered that in order to maintain an adequate

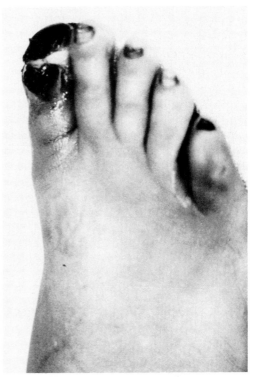

Figure 13.5. Wagner grade 4 lesion. Gangrene and infection are localized to a definable area. Where vascularity permits, such lesions are amenable to local radical amputation.

nutritional status of a patient, a minimum of 150–200 gm of carbohydrate must be available daily. Insulin, of course, must be available to promote utilization of these carbohydrate calories. When adequate amounts of carbohydrate calories are not available in the peri-operative period, hypoglycemia and ketoacidosis may result. The goal in the peri-operative period is to maintain blood glucose levels in the 150–250 mg/ml range. The balance between carbohydrate intake and insulin intake, fluid and foods, is considered together to achieve an appropriate serum glucose level.

As stated previously, in order to minimize the risk of hypoglycemia, surgical procedures on the diabetic patient should be scheduled early in the morning, and intravenous alimentation started at that time. Because the patient is NPO, necessary calories must be provided with intravenous solutions.

Anesthesia

Local anesthetics, as mentioned earlier, appear to exert little or no effect on blood glucose levels. Certainly, local anesthetics with vasoconstrictive properties due to epinephrine should not be used in the presence of marked peripheral vascular disease. Spinal anesthesia is safe in the diabetic patient, with minimal effect on serum glucose levels. The hypotensive effect of spinal anesthesia may be exaggerated in patients with diabetic autonomic neuropathy. Although some anesthetics may elevate blood glucose levels, 1% halothane or 5 mg phenoperidine and the thiopental/nitrous oxide-turbocurarine chloride techniques (25) appear to exert little effect on blood glucose levels.

Management of Diabetes in the Surgical Patient

Because the diabetic patient should be in the best possible nutritional balance at the time of surgery, hospitalization as much as 2–6 days prior to operation may be required. During this time, the diabetic state, nutritional status, state of hydration, and electrolyte status can be evaluated and abnormalities brought under control. Maintenance of blood glucose levels in the range of 150–250 mg/dl is considered ideal. Generally, mild to moderate hyperglycemia (200–250 mg/dl) is not hazardous, and is expected in the early post-operative period. Hypoglycemia is far more dangerous than mild or moderate hyperglycemia. When major foot infections are present, insulin requirements will fall abruptly following incision and drainage of abscesses. In the usual case, increasing insulin requirements 2–6 days following surgery reflect the presence of some complication, such as infection.

With regard to the control of diabetes in the peri-operative period, procedures should be classified as major or minor, and patients classified as being well controlled, poorly controlled without ketosis, or poorly controlled with ketosis or ketoacidosis. Opinion varies as to the best method of control, but in general most authors recommend the use of intermediate insulin (NPH or Lente) over that of regular insulin. As has been noted earlier, for minor surgical procedures, or brief procedures under local anesthesia, no alteration in diabetic management is required. If, for a surgical case under local anesthesia, the patient is NPO, then the usual carbohydrate content of that meal (50 grams or 1000 ml D5W) is given IV over a 4–6-hour period.

For major podiatric surgical procedures in patients whose diabetic state is well controlled, an intravenous infusion of 5% glucose in water or saline is started the morning of surgery. One half of the patient's usual dosage of NPH or Lente insulin is given subcutaneously. Intermediate acting insulins begin to affect glucose levels 3 to 4 hours following injection, peak at 8–12 hours, and exert a total effect over 18–24 hours. Regular insulin, with an onset of 30 minutes and peak activity in 2–4 hours, could result in hypoglycemia during the stress of anesthesia and surgery, and therefore is recommended as a supplement to NPH or Lente. When surgery is completed, the intravenous infusion with 5% glucose

½ DOSE NPH OR LENTE
+ D5W

is continued for a total of 2 liters D5W in 24 hours.

The second half of the patient's usual dose of NPH or Lente insulin is given in the recovery room. Other authors have recommended one-half the usual dosage of NPH or Lente on the morning of surgery, followed by a STAT blood glucose in the recovery room. Ten units of regular insulin is given for blood glucose levels of 250–350 ml/dl, while 15 units of regular insulin is given for glucose levels greater than 350 ml/dl. When surgical procedures exceed 4 hours, an intra-operative blood glucose level should be obtained. Because diabetic patients, especially those with autonomic neuropathy, are especially prone to silent myocardial infarction (painless MI), an EKG in the recovery room is recommended following procedures under general anesthesia. Moore and Fletcher (34, 35) have recommended that no insulin be given until the patient is brought to the recovery room, then use regular insulin based on serum glucose determinations.

In the days following surgery, a return to the patient's pre-operative insulin requirements should be noted. Failure to reduce insulin requirements, or increasing insulin requirements, may reflect post-operative wound infection, atelectasis, urinary tract infection, or other complication. Blood glucose levels are more reliable than urine testing, since the measurement of glycosuria is affected by diabetic renal disease with poor glomerular filtration, and poor bladder emptying in association with autonomic neuropathy. False positive testing with Clinitest® may result from such antibiotics as penicillin G, streptomycin, or cephalosporins, resulting in excessive insulin administration and hypoglycemia. Following surgery, the intermediate acting insulin is given in the usual dose. When urine testing is utilized, the intermediate insulin is supplemented with 3–6 units of regular insulin for each plus finding (1+; 2+; etc.).

For the first 24 hours following surgery, a blood glucose level is usually obtained every 6 hours. Two hundred grams of car-bohydrate should be given as 5 or 10% glucose in water or saline. Serum glucose levels are adjusted as necessary by regulating the dosage of regular insulin. If blood glucose levels fall below 150 mg/dl, the NPH or Lente insulin dosage should be decreased by 10–20%.

In the poorly controlled diabetic without ketoacidosis, 200–300 gm of carbohydrate should be provided daily. Patients not previously on insulin may be started on 10–15 units of NPH or Lente, with serum or urine monitoring one-half hour before meals, and regular insulin utilized to supplement the NPH or Lente.

Diabetic patients well controlled on oral hypoglycemic agents may be switched to insulin in the immediate peri-operative period, using 10 units of regular insulin for serum glucose levels greater than 200 mg/dl or urine glucose 3+ or greater. As stated earlier, it is important to remember that hypoglycemia due to overzealous control is more dangerous than mild or moderate hyperglycemia.

Pre-operative Hemoglobin

In recent years, a large number of publications have appeared regarding glycosylated hemoglobin, or hemoglobin A_{1C} (36–38). An association between hemoglobin A_{1C} levels and the healing of diabetic ulcerations has been noted. Hemoglobin A_{1C} is normally a minor hemoglobin fraction that results when hemoglobin A is glycosylated at the 2,3-diphosphoglycerate portion in a high glucose environment. Because erythrocytes survive in the peripheral circulation for an average of 120 days, and because the glycosylation process is largely irreversible, HgA_{1C} levels reflect the level of diabetic control for at least 4–6 weeks prior to testing. The normal serum level of glycosylated hemoglobin is 3–6%. The importance of the test in the pre-operative evaluation of the diabetic patient lies in the fact that elevated HgA_{1C} levels not only reflect poor diabetic control, but in addition, is associated with a variety of reversible hematologic abnormalities in leukocyte, lymphocyte, erythrocyte, and platelet structure and function. These abnormalities in cellular function reflect the first major, clearly demonstrable effects of hyperglycemia on hematologic function. Control of serum glucose levels in the immediate peri-operative period is often considered to eliminate the adverse effects of hyperglycemia with regard to such problems as impaired leukocyte function or poor wound healing in the diabetic patient. It now appears that such time-honored concepts are not entirely correct. As exemplified by hemoglobin A_{1C} levels, it is clear that even with the correction of serum glucose levels to acceptable surgical ranges, a period of time should be allowed in the case of elective surgical procedures for a reversal of the many hematologic alterations associated with poorly controlled diabetes mellitus. The delayed wound healing and increased morbidity associated with the diabetic surgical patient, even when surgical procedures are performed in the presence of normal range serum glucose levels, may be explained by the presence of these reversible abnormalities.

VASCULAR CONSIDERATIONS

Vascular disease represents the major cause of both morbidity and mortality in patients with diabetes mellitus (39). Four distinct types of vascular pathology appear to occur with increased frequency in the diabetic population: large vessel disease, microangiopathy, medial calcific sclerosis, and vasospasm. In patients with known diabetes mellitus, large vessel disease accounts for 75% of all deaths. Diabetic patients are five times more prone to gangrene and twice as prone to heart attacks when compared to nondiabetic patients (40).

The sequellae of diabetic peripheral vascular disease include such phenomena as rest pain, intermittent claudication, and ischemic ulceration. In the absence of overt signs and symptoms of peripheral vascular embarrassment, a complete vascular history, physical examination with attention to the peripheral vascular and noninvasive vascular trees, and noninvasive vascular testing should be performed on all diabetic patients undergoing foot surgery. Although some authors have presented evidence to the contrary, it appears that atherosclerotic vascular disease occurs more frequently, at an earlier age, and is more diffuse in the diabetic population (40). In insulin-dependent diabetes, histopathologic and clinical evidence of accelerated atherosclerosis can be documented after 10–15 years of diabetes when compared with age- and sex-matched controls (40). Clinically significant atherosclerotic lesions which may complicate surgery in the diabetic patient often have no relationship to the duration or severity of the diabetes. Microangiopathic disease characterizes diabetes mellitus, with basement membrane thickening present in 98% of overt diabetics, 53% of prediabetics, and 8% of nondiabetic controls (39). Thickening of the basement membrane is not related to severity or duration of diabetes.

With regard to vascular calcifications noted on radiographic evaluation of the foot and leg (diabetic medial arteriosclerosis), extensive vascular calcifications may be found in young and middle-aged patients, especially in poorly controlled diabetics. Medial calcific sclerosis represents an aging and mechanical stress effect, and although found with increased and earlier frequency among diabetic patients, represents a nonocclusive disorder. Diabetic medial arteriosclerosis does result in vessel nondistensibility which may interfere with the interpretation of noninvasive vascular studies (41).

Because significant peripheral vascular disease may complicate surgical wound healing, and because extensive vascular disease may be unrelated to the severity and duration of the diabetic state, the peripheral vascular status of all diabetic patients must be assessed prior to foot surgery. In addition to pre-operative vascular considerations, the podiatric surgeon must be prepared to evaluate and manage complications in the post-operative period.

Evaluation of the Vascular Status

Pre-operative vascular evaluation represents an attempt to detect the presence of vascular disease in asymptomatic patients, or to confirm the existence of vascular pathology in patients who demonstrate signs and symptoms associated with peripheral vascular disease. In either the former or the latter instance, an attempt is made through history, physical findings, noninvasive and, at times, invasive testing to "quantify" the peripheral vascular status of a particular patient. Ideally, those patients whose vascular status will permit a surgical wound (or an ulcerative lesion) to heal, can be differentiated with some degree of certainty from those surgical patients not likely to heal without sympathectomy, vascular surgery, or other major reconstructive vascular procedure. In practice, the evaluation of the peripheral vascular status of patients results in two major categories. Those patients who are likely to heal, and those patients who are not likely to heal.

In recent years, the ischemic index has gained popularity as a noninvasive method for determining the healing potential of a surgical wound or diabetic foot lesion (42). In order to calculate the ischemic index, a blood pressure cuff is placed just proximal to the ankle joint of the limb to be evaluated (Fig. 13.6). Either a Doppler ultrasound unit or plethysmograph is utilized to find and monitor the dorsalis pedis, posterior tibial, or perforating peroneal artery. Ideally, the cuff size should be 12% of the diameter of the ankle. Once the sounds or pulse volume recordings are obtained, the ankle cuff is slowly inflated until either the sounds are lost, or the pulsatile flow to the digits, as measured by a plethysmograph ceases. The pressure at which this stoppage occurs is noted. The ankle cuff is then deflated, and the pressure at which the sounds or pulsatile plethysmographic flow returns is again noted. This pressure, measured separately for each of the three major arteries supplying the foot, is the ankle pressure. Once found, the ankle pressure is

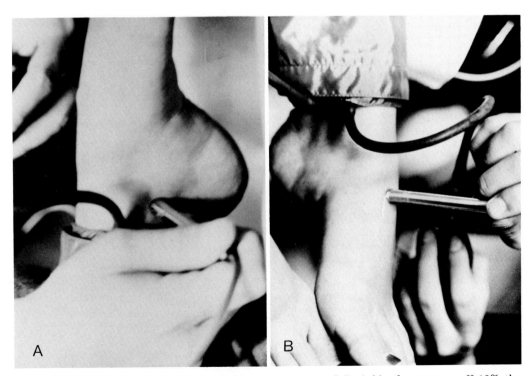

Figure 13.6. Method of obtaining ankle pressures. *A* and *B*; A blood pressure cuff 12% the diameter of the distal leg should be applied. The dorsalis pedis, posterior tibial, and perforating peroneal artery are individually studied with a Doppler unit, and the pneumatic cuff slowly inflated until audible sounds (or PVR tracings) are no longer heard. The pressure at which sounds or tracings are lost is the ankle pressure.

divided by the left brachial systolic blood pressure, as described by Windsor. The resulting number is the ischemic index, and has been cited by many authors as being of valuable predictive consistency. An ischemic index of greater than 0.45 (i.e., an ankle pressure greater than 45% of the left brachial systolic blood pressure) is predictive of surgical wound or pedal ulceration healing. In the nondiabetic patient, an ischemic index of 0.35 is considered adequate to obtain healing. Wagner, utilizing this criteria, obtained 90% healing of incision and drainage and local amputations in the feet of diabetic patients, and 97% healing in nondiabetic patients with arteriosclerotic lower extremity disease (41, 43).

Raines et al. (44) examined the relationship of the ankle pressure itself (rather than the ischemic index) to the healing of diabetic and nondiabetic foot lesions. They concluded that at ankle pressures of greater than 90 mm Hg, healing is likely. An ankle pressure of 80–90 mm Hg was associated with probable healing in diabetic foot lesions, and an ankle pressure of less than 80 mm Hg was associated with lesions unlikely to heal (44).

In addition to Raines, Strandness et al. (45), Yao (43), and others have demonstrated the predictive value of noninvasive evaluation of both the diabetic and nondiabetic patient with arteriosclerosis. In addition to their usefulness in the prediction of wound healing, ankle pressures appear to correlate well with a variety of clinical symptoms such as rest pain and intermittent claudication. It is generally accepted that rest pain and claudication represent severe degrees of ischemia which should contradict pedal surgical techniques. In the diabetic patient, it has been shown that rest pain is unlikely at ankle pressures greater than 80 mm Hg (at which pressure lesions are likely to heal), while it is likely to occur at ankle pressures below 55 mm Hg (at which pressure foot lesions are unlikely to heal).

Lieberman (48) has suggested that noninvasive procedures such as doppler blood pressure determinations and plethysmog-raphy suffer from the fact that they are subjective in interpretation, not sensitive for the detection of partially occluded vessels, and invalid when lower extremity venous pressures are increased. Similarly, Raines has shown that because of resistance to vessel closure, vascular calcification may artificially elevate ankle pressures by as much as 25 mm Hg.

With regard to the probability of healing, clinical impressions without some attempt at quantification are not good predictors of success. In an examination of factors which may predict the success or failure of amputations in the feet of 59 consecutive diabetic patients, Bailey et al. (46) showed that age, sex, method of diabetic control, smoking, presence of neuropathy or peripheral pulses, pre-operative BUN, and temperature all fail to correlate with success. This data is in agreement with other authors, suggesting that the presence of palpable foot pulses does not guarantee healing, while the absence of such pulses is not, of itself, a contraindication to surgery. In their study, Bailey et al. (46) demonstrated that pre-operative hemoglobin levels inversely correlated best with the prediction of healing for digital and metatarsal amputations in diabetic patients. One hundred per cent of patients with a pre-operative hemoglobin of less than 12.0 gm/dl (18 of 59 patients) healed, while 100% of patients with a hemoglobin of greater than 13 gm/dl (30 of 59) failed to heal. The authors suggested that in surgical procedures on the diabetic foot, artificial lowering of the pre-operative hemoglobin to less than 12 gm/dl might be beneficial. Kacy et al. (47), in a study of factors influencing the successful healing of below-the-knee amputations, reported that hemoglobin levels were inversely proportional to success rates only in patients with diabetes and concurrent cellulitis of the foot.

Nuclear Medicine Studies

Radiopharmaceuticals may be utilized to evaluate the healing potential of pedal lesions, to assess distal blood flow, and to evaluate the extent of arterial insufficiency.

The application of radiopharmaceuticals in the assessment of peripheral vascular perfusion may involve either clearance or delivery techniques. In the former, a radioactive material is injected intramuscularly (usually the gastrocnemius or tibialis anterior) or epicutaneously on the lower extremity (48, 49). The rate of clearance of the radiopharmaceutical usually bears some direct relationship to the rate of blood flow. Utilizing the latter methods, the radiopharmaceutical is injected intravenously and the accumulation of the radiopharmaceutical is dependent on the quantity of blood flow to the area. Failure of technetium methylene diphosphonate, a commonly used injectible radiopharmaceutical, to accumulate in areas of avascular necrosis infarction, and extensive frostbite, are cited as examples of the failure of intravenous radionuclides to accumulate in areas of absent vascular flow. Paradoxical negative bone scans (cold scans) have also been attributed to early septic vascular occlusion in osteomyelitis.

Researchers and numerous clinical studies advocated the use of the scintigraphy in the evaluation of peripheral vascular flow over plethysmography, oscillometry, doppler flow studies, ankle pressures, arteriography, and clinical signs and symptoms. Siegel et al. (51) has pointed to the inaccuracies of all vascular flow assessment techniques when compared to nuclear medicine studies. The use of scintigraphy for the evaluation of myocardial perfusion has become well established.

The utilization of thallium-201 for the evaluation of extremity vascular perfusion and the prediction of wound healing is well established (50). Originally, small amounts of the thallium-201 pharmaceutical were injected intravenously with the possibility of associated complications attendant to intravenous particulate matter. Modification of technique and improvement in the quality of the diagnostic materials injected have resulted in flow delivery studies which appear to be more accurate in the prediction of healing and the assessment of microvascular status than any presently available diagnostic technique. Siegal and Siemson (51) demonstrated that even in the absence of palpable pulses, or equivocal arteriographic findings, adequate peripheral vascular flow at the microvascular level may be present to obtain wound healing. Utilizing the diagnostic procedures advocated by these authors, the patient is given an intravenous injection of thallium-201. A photomultiplier tube gamma camera is placed over the selected areas of questioned wound healing. These sites, each 2.5 cm (from an ulcer, for example) are chosen. Five minutes following injection, counts for 1 minute are taken from the center of the ulcer and from each of the three selected areas which surrounded the ulcer. The average 1-minute count obtained from the selected periulcer areas are compared to the count from the ulcer itself. When the count surrounding the ulcer is greater than 1.5 times the ulcer count, or when an ulcer count of greater than 200,000 is obtained, healing should be expected.

The basis of this test, which prognosticates wound healing, appears to rely on the premise of reactive hyperemia. It has been suggested that thallium-201 accumulation represents a measurement of the body's ability to sustain an inflammatory response around the ulcer. The inflammatory response is necessary for wound healing to occur. In the absence of less than 1.5 times greater accumulations of thallium-201 in tissues surrounding the lesions, it is assumed that a patient is unable to mount an inflammatory response sufficient to obtain healing. A major advantage of this technique is the fact that as a test of microcirculation, thallium-201 scintigraphy is a reflection of ischemic pathophysiology. Arteriography may demonstrate anatomic narrowing, but does not demonstrate the actual physiologic significance of such narrowing. The concept of reactive or inflammatory hyperemia as a predictor of wound healing is not new. Bleeding from a surgical wound within 3 minutes of the release of a tourniquet has been said to be predictive of wound healing. In the histamine wheal test, the failure of a patient to mount a clinically observable inflammatory reaction to the intradermal injection of histamine phosphate is regarded as inconsistent with the expectation of wound healing. The observation of a poor or absent inflammatory response surrounding an ulceration or area of infectious disease is regarded as a poor prognostic sign, while the presence of marked inflammation is itself evident of microcirculatory patency.

The use of local clearance of radioisotopes in the evaluation of peripheral vascular flow is well-established. Kety (67) demonstrated the accuracy of the disappearance of intramuscularly injected radioactive sodium (24) as a measure of muscle blood flow. Thulesius (68) and Kappert (69) have demonstrated the usefulness of macroaggregated radioiodinated serum albumin in the evaluation of arterial insufficiency.

Local clearance methods with thallium-201 or xenon-133 are based on the utilization of radiopharmaceuticals that will diffuse freely from muscle or skin into capillary blood. The quantity of blood flow is the limiting factor in the clearance of these radiopharmaceuticals from an area under examination. Thus, the principle of measurement is that of evaluating the rate of clearing of the radiopharmaceutical from an area. The greater the quantity and the quicker a radiopharmaceutical is cleared from an area, the better the status of peripheral vascular perfusion.

Kostuik et al. (49) demonstrated the usefulness of epicutaneous xenon-133 clearance studies in the prediction of amputation healing. In their study, flow rates of greater than 1.5 mm/min/100 gm of tissue (skin) were associated with surgical wounds which could be expected to heal. They have advocated the use of epicutaneous xenon-133 clearance as a useful adjunct to clinical judgment in the determination of the level of amputation. Sejrsen (52) has demonstrated the usefulness of xenon-133 clearance in the evaluation of burns, while Moore (53) has also examined the use of xenon-133 clearance in the determination of wound healing.

Local clearance methods may also be performed by the injection of xenon-133 into the gastrocnemius or tibialis anterior muscles. Lassen and Holstein (48) have demonstrated the marked difference of xenon-133 clearance curves from the muscles of patients with peripheral vascular impairment, as opposed to normal subjects. Following intramuscular deposition of xenon-133, the patient in question exercises with a proximal tourniquet in place. On the completion of the exercise, the cuff is released and a scintillation detector coupled to a ratemeter is used to evaluate the clearance of the radiopharmaceutical from the muscle in the presence of reactive hyperemia.

The localization of thallium-201 and its quantification in the gastrocnemius muscle following intravenous injection and exercise has been evaluated by Seder et al. (50).

The evaluation of diabetic patients for evidence of vascular disease which may impair wound healing should include doppler auscultation of the posterior tibial, dorsalis pedis, and perforating peroneal artery. The Doppler unit, utilizing a signal frequency of between 10 and 20 MHz, reveals three distinct arterial sounds which may be recorded. The normal triphasic sound pattern, and more commonly, biphasic pattern, are consistent with arterial patency and adequate vessel distensibility. Monophasic sounds, especially when low-pitched, are suggestive of marked occlusive vascular disease. Extraordinary high-pitched sounds may be found in the region of stenotic vascular disease. The interpretation of doppler studies is necessarily subjective. The advantage of these studies lies in its ability to confirm the presence of patent arterial structures when palpation of pulses is difficult or equivocal. Additionally, the presence of abnormal doppler sounds is frequently associated with atherosclerotic or aneurysmal pathology. Dopplers may be utilized to detect the presence of pulsatile digital flow, and may likewise be used to evaluate arteriolar patency in the arch and in the web spaces. The major disadvantages inherent in doppler evaluation lie in the fact that, not only is it a subjective test, but like arteriography, it represents a nonphysiologic study. Despite the presence of doppler evidence of occlusive vascular disease, radioisotope studies have clearly demonstrated adequacy of the microcirculation distally to support wound healing. When used in combination with a cuff to determine the ischemic index, the Doppler ultrasonic evaluation of peripheral vascular status attains a greater predictive value.

As is the case with arteriography, doppler studies, palpation of pulses, and segmented blood pressure reflect directly the anatomic status of large vessels. Certainly, the increased incidence of macrovascular disease, and its earlier and more aggressive presentation in patients with diabetes mellitus, warrant careful scrutiny in the pre-operative patient for macrovascular disease. The unusual propensity of the diabetic for accelerated atherosclerosis may include other risk factors such as diet, obesity, stress, cigarette smoking, and noncompliance with regard to control of serum glucose. Hypertension represents another risk factor in the development of rapidly progressive atherosclerosis, particularly in black patients (63). Colwell et al. (39) have proposed a variety of mechanisms contributing to accelerated atherosclerosis in the diabetic, including endothelial injury from altered metabolism and immunologic endothelial damage from islet cell antibodies and insulin antibodies; direct hormonal damage has also been implicated. Mayne and others (54) have demonstrated increased platelet adhesiveness in diabetes mellitus. Odegaard et al. (55) have demonstrated increased "anti-Willebrand factor" in diabetic platelets. Breddin (56) has shown increased platelet aggregation to areas of damaged endothelium in diabetic patients. Bagdade (57) has shown defective clearance of very low density lipoproteins in some diabetics due to altered endothelial lipoproteins lipase activity.

Microvascular Evaluation

Functional and structural alteration in the microcirculation of the diabetic patient represents the most characteristic vascular change associated with diabetes mellitus. Because microvascular disease may exist despite the absence of clinically significant macrovascular disease, decreased peripheral tissue perfusion undetected prior to surgery may result in a relatively avascular surgical wound, with dehiscence and marked propensity to secondary infection. Conversely, as has been discussed previously, microvascular perfusion of tissue adequate to support wound healing may exist despite the presence of doppler or arteriographic evidence of significant large vessel disease, or the absence or peripheral pulses on palpation. The healing of surgical wounds for the correction of nail and digital pathology, or the healing of distal pedal infections or ulcerative disease, is highly dependent on microcirculatory adequacy. At the microcirculatory level, the sympathetic nervous system exhibits its greatest influence on vessel patency, so that the vasoconstrictive effects of this system become a major consideration. Vasospasm represents the clinical manifestation of microvascular functional disorders, in which symptoms and signs of diminished peripheral circulation appear, despite the absence of any demonstrable organic disease. At times, arterial spasm may be evident in the form of marked digital pallor, waxy color, decreased digital pedal skin temperature, a bluish or cyanotic-appearing hue, or Raynaud's phenomena. The effects of vasospasm appear to be accentuated by exposure to a cold environment or at times of emotional stress.

The deterioration of diabetic microcirculation has been detailed by McMillan (58). In addition to vasospasm, a variety of abnormalities appear to characterize diabetic microangiopathy. The most characteristic change appears to be capillary basement membrane thickening, as described by Siperstein (59). Kilo (60) has suggested that thickening of the capillary basement membrane, with resultant inability of oxygen to perfuse peripheral tissue, has a genetic basis and occurs early in the diabetic process. Colwell (61) and Spiro (62) have suggested that the basement membrane thickening occurring in diabetic capillaries may to some extent be reversed with good control of serum glucose levels. Microcirculatory problems may be accentuated by the increased plasma viscosity found to exist in patients with diabetes (58). The deformity of erythrocytes in passing through capillaries, as well as the tendency toward rouleaux formation, are reversibly altered in the presence of hyperglycemia. When erythrocytes lose the ability to deform, in order to pass through capillaries, and further demonstrate a tendency to aggregate, microcirculatory occlusion is the result. Of significant importance is the fact that plasma viscosity changes and erythrocyte functional alterations are reversible with time. When serum glucose levels are brought under control (e.g., 2–6 days prior to surgery) these alterations will remain for several weeks before reversal. Hemoglobin A_{1C} levels, when elevated, are usually indicative of poor chronic management of diabetes, and those hematologic changes responsible for functional alterations of capillary flow should be assumed to be present. The restoration of hemoglobin A_{1C} levels to normal values appears to be associated with a reversal of those changes in plasma viscosity, erythrocyte deformability, and erythrocyte aggregation tendencies which increase functional destruction of the microcirculation.

In addition to the signs and symptoms of functional disease of the microcirculation already discussed, digital plethysmography may be utilized to evaluate the effects of sympathetic activity on the microcirculation. Vasospasm, on digital pulse volume recording, is characteristically manifested by a normal or near normal wave morphology, but marked decrease in pulse amplitude. The effects of vasospasm may be inhibited by a variety of techniques. Prior to surgery, or during the post-operative period, the effects of "anti-vasospastic" therapeutics can be evaluated and a return to normal or acceptable pulse volume amplitude. Because a greater blood flow is required to heal a wound, as compared to

maintaining an already healed wound, the control of vasospasm in the peri-operative period is of the greatest importance. Because anxiety regarding hospital admission and possible serious complications with surgery may exacerbate vasospasm, firm psychological support must be given the patient. When necessary, tranquilizers or sedatives should be employed. Diazepam or florazepam are particularly useful. Posterior tibial nerve blocks with local anesthetics may be employed. Reduction of pain with analgesics or the use of a transcutaneous nerve stimulator is likewise helpful in the reduction of vasospasm from painful stimuli. A heating pad placed in the area of the abdominal aorta is frequently successful in the reflex dilitation it creates. The extremities should also be kept warm.

Medical therapy for the management of vasospasm remains promising, but increased incidence of side effects and uncertainty of success warrant drug therapy as a secondary choice for recalcitrant cases or surgical emergencies. The use of oral reserpine has been reported, while Willerson (64) has shown the successful use of intraarterial reserpine. The recent use of prostacyclin has been reported (70). Charles and Carmick (65) reported beneficial effects in the control of vasospasm for griseofulvin, while Varaai and Laurence (66) successfully reported on the use of methyldopa. Oral vasodilators such as tolazoline hydrochloride have been used with limited success. Surgical sympathectomy remains a controversial issue. The effects of sympathectomy are usually temporary, with results due to neural reanastomosis or endorgan hypersensitivity to norepinephrine. However, the maximum beneficial effects of the sympathectomy will occur during the period of wound healing, after which less tissue perfusion is required to maintain the healed wound.

Neuropathy

The neurologic sequellae of diabetes mellitus are well documented, particularly with reference to lower extremity signs and symptoms. Sensory and motor diffuse peripheral symmetrical polyneuropathy in the diabetic is a major etiologic factor in the evaluation of a variety of surgical lesions, including neurotrophic ulceration, tarsal tunnel syndrome, or interdigital neuroma. Localized neuropathic lesions, such as tarsal tunnel syndrome, may at times be difficult to distinguish from the early manifestation of diabetic mononeuritis simplex, mononeuritis multiplex, or polyneuropathy. Diabetic anhidrosis may result in wound dehiscence. Diabetic autonomic neuropathy can result in a variety of local and systemic disorders, increasing the morbidity and mortality associated with surgery on the diabetic foot.

Catterall (71) examined the results of foot surgery in patients with diabetes mellitus and found that local amputations in neuropathic feet consistently healed, as compared with ischemic feet, in which the long-term healing date (healed at 1 year) was only 35%. Other investigators, such as Cameron (72), noted in retrospective analysis that neuropathy was less common in patients with healed foot amputations than in those in whom it failed. The actual influence of neuropathy as an isolated factor in soft tissue healing following foot surgery is difficult to assess. In general, it appears that the sensory-motor polyneuropathy typically found in 45% of diabetic patients at any given time does not, in itself, alter soft tissue healing to a clinically significant degree. Autonomic neuropathy in the diabetic patient does appear to play a major role in soft tissue healing and will be discussed in detail later. Because the degree of

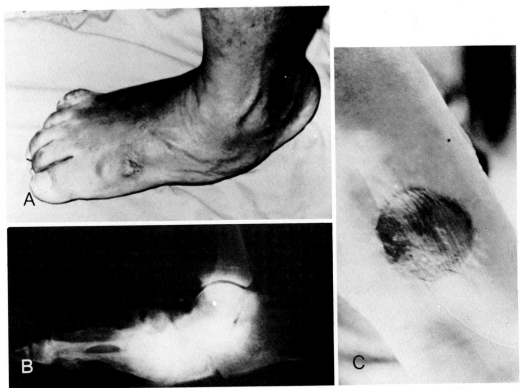

Figure 13.7. Cube foot deformity. *A,* collapse of the medial longitudinal arch with apparent widening of the foot secondary to abduction results in a foot with the typical cube foot appearance. *B,* demonstrates the typical hypertrophic type of neurotrophic joint changes seen in a cube foot deformity. *C,* ulceration below the midtarsal joint is not uncommon in a cube foot deformity. Resection of bone together with myofascial flap (flexor digitorum brevis) and split thickness were required to heal the defect. Despite the apparent "take," the skin graft eventually failed and required regrafting.

neuropathic disease present in a particular patient is not independent of vascular disease and metabolic status of the diabetes, the effects of diabetic neuropathy are difficult to define with reference to bone healing. Retief and Dreyer (73) were able to demonstrate delayed and defective bone repair in rats with experimentally denervated bone. Eloesser (74) was able to produce spontaneous lesions of bones and joints in cats by the surgical sectioning of the posterior nerve roots leading to an extremity. With reference to bone healing and the potential deleterious effects of diabetic neuropathy, a number of clinical entities found in the diabetic neuropathic foot, such as Charcot joint disease, osteolysis, spontaneous dislocation, and spontaneous fracture, might lead one to conclude that sensory-motor neuropathy plays a major role in the alteration of normal bone metabolism. While the mechanical stress placed upon the bones (and joints) are clearly altered by sensory neuropathy, or by deformities secondary to motor neuropathy, it appears that alterations in bone physiology, with regard to potential healing problems, are the result of autonomic nervous pathology, and its influence on the osseous vascular supply (88). Sensory and motor polyneuropathy do not appear to alter the healing of bone in the diabetic patient directly (75).

AUTONOMIC NEUROPATHY

Autonomic neuropathy is a complication of diabetes mellitus which may seriously alter soft tissue healing, bone healing, as well as the general peri-operative condition of patients undergoing foot surgery. A detailed description of the role of autonomic neuropathy has been presented by Schuster and Jacobs (76). The etiology of diabetic autonomic neuropathy remains obscure, and may relate to microvascular disease of the vasa nervorum, as described by Timperly (77), Olsson and Sourander (78), and Asbury and Johnson (79). Anderson (80), Clements (81), and Clark et al. (82) have suggested that diabetic autonomic neuro-

pathy occurs secondary to metabolic alterations in the nerve due to diabetes mellitus. The abnormalities may include depletion of neural myoinositol, glycosylation of neural proteins, sorbital accumulation within the nerves, or alterations in lipid structures and metabolic pathways.

Regardless of etiology, the onset of diabetic autonomic neuropathy is often insidious. The effects of dysfunction of the autonomic nervous system in diabetes mellitus may be catastrophic in patients undergoing foot surgery.

SUDOMOTOR AND VASOMOTOR DISTURBANCES

Sudomotor and vasomotor disturbances in diabetics affect the thermal regulatory processes of the body. The decreased ability of the body to sweat and to have reflex vasoconstriction in response to endogenous or environmental stimuli will lead to many problems, thus complicating post-operative wound healing. Vasomotor abnormalities were found to be more common than sudomotor abnormalities in diabetic neuropathy.

Sudomotor abnormalities will manifest as dyshidrosis or anhidrosis. The anhidrosis is present in 10% of patients with diabetic neuropathy. The sympathetic nervous system innervating the ecrine sweat glands is significantly damaged in this disorder. Injury to the post-ganglionic fibers appears to be responsible for the sudomotor dysfunction of the lower extremities observed in diabetic patients.

The often described disorder, anhidrosis, is a loss of sweating in the lower half of the body with excessive compensatory sweating in the upper half of the body. The distribution in the lower extremities is one of patchy loss of sweating, rather than a total lower extremity anhidrosis. Since the lower extremities cannot properly thermoregulate, the upper half of the body compensates by developing an observable hyperhidrosis (76, 78, 82).

Gustatory sweating, which may be defined as profuse facial sweating after eating, is linked with abnormal nerve regeneration between the autonomic nervous sweat regulators and salivary glands. The gustatory sweating, which may be observed in patients, must be differentiated from hypoglycemia and normal hyperhidrosis, seen after spicy food is eaten.

Clinically, the patient may complain of profuse facial sweating, intolerance to heat, or excessively dry skin of the lower extremities. In such cases, emollient creams and attempts to reduce the hypohidrosis are initiated several weeks before elective foot surgery. In semi-elective or nonelective cases, the problem of hypohidrosis may not be managed due to time limitations.

After truncal heating, disturbances in sudomotor function can be detected by faradic stimulation and testing for conductivity or by a variety of skin tests with compounds such as starch, quinizarin, or cobalt chloride. Recently, the galvanic skin response has been utilized for such purposes.

Galvanic skin response is a measure of dermal sweat gland activity by utilizing standard EKG apparatus. It is imperative that the podiatric surgeon check the feet of diabetic patients before elective or semi-elective surgery for evidence of anhidrotic manifestations. Anhidrosis appears to predispose the feet to fissures and secondarily to localized infectious processes, which have the ability to spread as a result of relative inability to localize the infection in diabetic patients. Lubricating skin creams, daily foot inspection for skin breakdown by the patient, and the prescription of proper shoegear play an obvious part in prophylaxis against the sequelae of anhidrosis in the lower extremities of diabetics (83).

Vasomotor dysfunction can be seen in up to 50% of diabetic patients with neuropathy. Vasomotor function can be closely linked to sudomotor changes because of their overlapping roles in thermoregulatory processes. A diabetic patient with vasomotor disturbances may complain of various sensations such as cold feet that require long periods of time to heat to the sensation of normal. Once the feet are warm and the stimuli removed, the feet may remain warm for periods of time lasting several hours.

Damage to the post-ganglionic autonomic nervous fibers is thought to be the site of dysfunction. Martin (84) has shown that the absence of reflex vasodilation is often of neuropathic origin. Tolazoline has the ability to act on smooth muscle directly and bypass that autonomic system. Using tolazoline on diabetics with vasomotor abnormalities, Martin found an increase in blood flow in previously constricted blood vessels, and his work has shown that vasomotor disturbances are of neuropathic and not vascular occlusive origin. The location of post-ganglion dysfunction was shown histologically by Barany and Cooper in 1956 (85).

Early denervation changes in the arterioles are speculated to be related to hypersensitivity to catecholamines and cold which cause increased vasoconstriction. The arterioles then go on to loss of vasoconstrictive properties with subsequent vasodilatation which will mimic the effects of a lumbar sympathectomy. The toes appear warmer than the hands. There is controversy remaining as to how responsive the feet are when there is cooling to the trunk portions of the body. Some authors have documented the loss of reflex vasoconstriction, whereas others have shown that the reflex usually remains intact. Under extreme conservation of body heat, the loss of vasoconstrictive properties in the lower half of the body will be compensated by vasoconstriction in the hands, which will mimic Raynaud's phenomenon.

Originally, lower extremity edema was thought by Rundles (86) to be secondary to increased vascular permeability from the vasomotor dysfunction. These observations have recently been disputed because of the high incidence of both renal and cardiac disease associated with diabetes that must be excluded as causes for edema.

Abnormalities in the lower extremities with regard to vasomotor function can be attributed to occlusive organic vessel disease; therefore, it is important to recognize that the vasomotor dysfunction may be occlusive or it may be in conjunction with autonomic disease. Peripheral nerves travel with the post-ganglionic sudomotor and vasomotor fibers. Abnormalities in sensorium, motor activity, sweat functioning, or vasomotor tone may all be seen to various degrees in the same patient. This complex, along with vascular disease, places the diabetic in a precarious position with regard to potential wound healing.

BONE HEALING

The role of the autonomic nervous system in bone and joint alteration in the diabetic patient has been examined by Bower and Allman (75), and termed a neurovascular reflex. A variety of bone changes may be found in the diabetic patient which can be explained, at least in part, by a neurally initiated vascular reflex which leads to increased bone vascular perfusion. Secondary to this increased blood flow, increased osteoblastic activity occurs, with osteopenia evident on radiographic examination. The resorptive changes of diabetic osteolysis, as well as atrophic changes seen in Charcot joint disease, could be explained on this basis. The spontaneous fractures and dislocations described by Bruckner (87), Feldman (89), and Normal et al. (90) often, with little or no history of trauma, could represent the effects of bone weakened by a vasomotor disturbance. Shim (91) demonstrated experimentally increased blood flow to the bones in dogs who had undergone lumbar sympathectomy.

In summary, it would appear that with regard to alterations in bone and joint physiology, the autonomic nervous system plays a vital role. The alterations in bone metabolism, and such clinical entities as spontaneous fracture or delayed bone healing, may be related to sudomotor disturbances in the presence of autonomic disease. Purely vascular and metabolic changes have been cited as other causes of the osseous abnormalities. The problem of establishing the exact nature of the bone changes encountered in diabetes mellitus remains to be resolved.

CARDIOVASCULAR MANIFESTATIONS

The recognition of the cardiovascular manifestations of autonomic neuropathy can lead to prevention of important sequellae in the peri-operative period. Resting tachycardia and postural hypotension are signs of autonomic neuropathy. Clinically, a resting heart rate of 90–110 beats per minute should alert the physician to the possibility of vagus nerve dysfunction. A patient with autonomic abnormalities in heart rate will not show response to carotid massage or administration of atropine or propanolol.

There is a normal cyclical variation heart rate which is dependent on vagal response. A good indicator of vagal dysfunction is a decrease of the R-R interval variation in the resting heart. Another test utilized is the Valsalva maneuver ratio, which is the ratio of the longest R-R interval to the shortest R-R interval during the maneuver.

Postural hypotension has been reported in 6–16% of patients with diabetic neuropathy. The fall in systolic blood pressure of 30 mm Hg or greater from supine to standing position is considered abnormal. Symptoms that usually occur on standing with systolic hypotension include dizziness, weakness, syncope, and visual disturbances. The pathophysiology of orthostatic hypotension is related to splanchnic pooling and a defect in plasma renin release from the kidneys. Another test of blood pressure is response of blood pressure after isometric exercise. This is accomplished with sustained hand grip test, wherein the diastolic blood pressure fails to rise greater than 10 mm Hg after isometric exercise, indicating a disturbance in the autonomic system (82). Clinically, one must be aware that a diabetic, once in the supine position, may be an increased risk for postural hypotension. Thus, in ambulating patients in the post-operative period, upon recognition of the signs and symptoms of autonomic neuropathy, it is advisable to insist upon assisted ambulations, elastic stockings, and Jobst therapy.

To prevent complications of orthostatic hypotension after prolonged bed rest, patients should follow a regimen of sitting up for short periods of time (with side rails up on the bed (92). α-Fluorohydrocortisone is currently the drug of choice in existing cases.

Page et al. (93) have demonstrated that insulin may increase the effects of orthostatic hypotension. Patients with postural hypotension may not respond with compensatory increase in heart rate. This hypotension may lead to a decrease in blood flow to the cerebral tissues. Patients with orthostatic hypotension may develop cerebral anoxia and syncope, which may progress to cerebral infarction or transient ischemic attacks.

Painless myocardial infarctions have been attributed to disease of the autonomic nervous system. In one study, 42% of all patients with painless myocardial infarctions were diabetic (94). This phenomenon has been related to abnormal cardiovascular and respiratory system physiology associated with autonomic neuropathy. It should be noted that patients with autonomic neuropathy show a higher incidence of cardiorespiratory arrest during lower respiratory infections or from general anesthesia during surgery (93). The use of cardiac monitoring is advised as a prophylactic measure for early recognition during surgery and under local anesthesia on diabetic patients who demonstrate the manifestations of autonomic neuropathy.

GASTROINTESTINAL MANIFESTATIONS

Gastrointestinal manifestations of autonomic neuropathy may complicate the peri-operative period of nonelective and elective foot surgery in the management of patients who are known diabetics. A wide range of gastrointestinal problems are associated with diabetics.

Originally, it was thought by Kassander (95) in 1958 that gastrointestinal changes could be directly attributed autonomically. In 1976, Campbell and his associates (96) showed that the gastric atony observed in diabetic autonomic neuropathy was not equivalent to that observed after surgical vagotomy. Debate and research continues to determine the exact extent of involvement of vagal neuropathy in gastrointestinal manifestations of diabetic neuropathy. Clinically, the most prevalent abnormal signs are reduced esophageal motility, gastric atony, diarrhea, constipation, and gallbladder enlargement. Radiographic, radioisotopic, and manometric changes of the gastrointestinal system that reflect the extent of autonomic disease may be noted.

The delay in the food reaching the small intestine will also contribute to poor diabetic control in the peri-operative period and the surgeon must be observant for signs of unexpected hypoglycemia. Gastric atony can also disturb the metabolism of oral hypoglycemic agents. Diabetic patients may develop heartburn-type symptoms because of decreased esophageal function and should be treated symptomatically (97). Constipation observed in such patients is probably the most common manifestation of gastrointestinal complaints, but diarrhea is most troublesome in terms of patient concerns.

The diarrhea is usually painless, profuse, and nocturnal in origin, and may be seen to affect patients up to 20 times daily, especially after ingestion of food. The etiology of the diarrhea is unclear at this time. Many treatments, consisting of antibiotics and antidiarrheal drugs, have been advocated by a variety of authors, all with limited success. Fortunately, both the surgeon and patient may be assured that the diarrhea is usually self-limiting.

The control of diabetic blood glucose levels may be hindered by gastric atony. Peri-operative constipation and diarrhea must be recognized. The judicial choice of anesthetic agents and peri-operative narcotics must be made in relationship to known diarrhea and constipation associated with diabetic autonomic neuropathy.

GENITOURINARY COMPLICATIONS

A variety of problems, including bladder dysfunction, impotence, retrograde ejaculation, failure to ejaculate, and loss of testicular pain sensation are encountered in genitourinary autonomic neuropathy. In patients with diabetes mellitus, some authors have indicated that up to 14% of patients studied were affected to some degree by symptomatology or signs of neurogenic bladder. This must be considered in the peri-operative period.

Bladder atony may be present with strain at micturition, slow urinary system, terminal dribbling, and frequency. This may develop into incomplete bladder emptying. A good discussion outlining this pathophysiology and autonomic involvement can be found in Clark et al. (82).

Once the bladder cannot be properly cleared of urine, the use of urine spot checks may become unreliable in monitoring the diabetic state and managing blood glucose levels in the peri-operative period. The surgeon should also bear in mind that incomplete emptying of the bladder is associated with higher incidence of bladder infection, which again may complicate both the peri-operative state and perhaps lead to a source of infection through the operative site by hematogenous spread. The surgeon must be aware of signs and symptoms, such as dysuria or increased urinary frequency. The associated urinary tract infection may complicate treatment of infections elsewhere in the body and lead to the observation of post-operative fever in the surgical patient. Pyelonephritis or kidney damage may result from longstanding urinary tract infections.

SENSORY NEUROPATHY

The usual presentation of diabetic sensory neuropathy is that of a bilateral, distal, symmetrical polyneuropathy. At any given time, Zimmerman (98) has stated that 45% of diabetic patients have signs and symptoms referable to polyneuropathy. A wide variety of clinical manifestations may be present as signs or symptoms of polyneuropathy, with loss of two-point discrimination, vibratory sense, and diminished or absent Achilles reflex among the earliest and most common findings. Typically, sensory loss is a "glove and stocking" type which typifies polyneuropathic disease. Less often, several individual nerves may be involved in causing sensory, motor, or combined motor neuropathy, in which case the term mononeuritis multiplex may be used. When an individual nerve is involved, the term mononeuritis simplex may be applied.

A complete discussion of the manifestations of sensory and motor neuropathy in diabetes is beyond the scope of this chapter, and the reader is referred to the suggested reading list for detailed information. The sequellae of sensory and motor neuropathy include neuropathic ulceration, usually ascribed as insensitivity to pain. The usual clinical scenario is that of a structural or functional abnormality of the foot, with hyperkeratoses (grade 0 lesion) progressing to ulceration because of a failure of the patient to avoid weightbearing on the compromised skin due to a lack of pain perception. The effects of motor neuropathy may complicate the clinical picture with contracted digits, and plantarflexed metatarsals resulting to further increase weightbearing abnormalities. Superficial or deep infection may occur, with deep plantar space abscess or osteomyelitis the potential result. Some authors, such as Deanfield (88), have attributed a larger role to autonomic neuropathy in the creation of mal perforans and other pressure-induced ulcerative lesions of the foot.

With regard to the usual lesions found in association with the neuropathic foot, attention is usually directed at resolution of infection, healing of the ulcerative lesion, and redistribution of abnormal weightbearing by nonoperative or operative means. As has been noted earlier, sensory neuropathy does not in itself appear to interfere with either bone or soft tissue healing.

Certain entrapment neuropathies, such as interdigital neuromas and tarsal tunnel syndrome, occur with increased frequency in the diabetic population. Tarsal tunnel syndrome, by definition, is a primary entrapment of the posterior tibial nerve under the laciniate ligament. Lam (99), Keck (100), and most recently Oloff et al. (101), have noted the high incidence of tarsal tunnel syndrome in patients with diabetes mellitus. Clinically, the signs and symptoms of sensory or motor neuropathy may simulate tarsal tunnel syndrome, and the reverse is also true. Thus, symptoms such as plantar parethesias, arch cramping or weakness, or numbness may be associated with tarsal tunnel syndrome, interdigital neuroma, diabetic polyneuropathy, or mononeuritis simplex or multiplex. When electrodiagnostic studies demonstrate isolated disease of either the medial or lateral plantar nerves, and when electrical abnormalities within tested muscles are restricted to the intrinsic muscles of the foot, the differentiation of typical early polyneuropathy from tarsal tunnel syndrome can be difficult. Because tarsal tunnel syndrome is characterized by normal conduction velocity of the posterior tibial nerve, and abnormal distal latencies of the medial and/or lateral plantar nerve, it is possible that many of the reported cases of tarsal tunnel syndrome in association with diabetes mellitus actually represent distal neuropathy. Roux (102) has studied the vascular anatomy of the posterior tibial nerve and noted that the particularly well developed segmental and longitudinal blood supplies probably reflect the high metabolic requirements for oxygen in this nerve. In his studies, Roux suggested that the posterior tibial nerve, by virtue of its extraordinary need for oxygen, was very susceptible to ischemic change from even minor degree of compression.

The possible microvascular ischemic changes which may be found in the posterior tibial nerve of patients with diabetes mellitus, together with the metabolic changes associated with diabetic peripheral nerves, may result in a posterior tibial nerve which is more susceptible to compression neuropathy. When the posterior tibial (or interdigital) nerves of patients with diabetes mellitus are viewed as "less than healthy" due to metabolic and vascular alterations, the concept of lesser degrees of compression creating an increased incidence of tarsal tunnel syndrome becomes plausible. Certainly, it would account for the increased incidence of tarsal tunnel syndrome described in the diabetic population. When the differentiation of diabetic polyneuropathy, mononeuritis multiplex, and tarsal tunnel syndrome become electrodiagnostically and clinically difficult, a sural nerve biopsy or sensory conduction of the sural as described by Behse et al. (103, 104) may be of value; similarly, sensory conduction studies of the superficial peroneal nerve as described by Lemont et al. (105) may be useful in the establishment of polyneuropathy, so that patients are spared a well-meaning but inappropriate surgical misadventure.

CLINICAL PRESENTATIONS OF DIABETIC AUTONOMIC NEUROPATHY

Cardiovascular
1. Resting tachycardia
2. Postural hypotension
3. Painless myocardial infarctions

Gastrointestinal
1. Decreased esophageal motility
2. Gastric atony
3. Diarrhea
4. Constipation
5. Gall bladder enlargement

Genitourinary
1. Bladder dysfunction
2. Impotence
3. Retrograde ejaculation
4. Failure to ejaculate
5. Loss of testicular sensation

Vasomotor
1. Altered skin temperature response
2. Hypersensitivity to cold
3. Neurotrophic joint disease
4. Osteopeonia
5. Spontaneous fracture
6. Spontaneous dislocation

7. Delayed osseous union

Sudomotor

1. Anhidrosis or dyshidrosis
2. Gustatory sweating

Other

1. Hypoglycemic unawareness
2. Pupillary abnormalities
3. Loss of sympathetic response to insulin

RADIOGRAPHIC AND NUCLEAR MEDICINE CONSIDERATIONS

In the presence of ulceration of the diabetic foot, pedal radiographs, nuclear medicine studies, sinograms, and other diagnostic modalities become essential in the assessment of the presence and extent of deep infection and osteomyelitis.

Soft Tissue Problems

The presence of soft tissue defects, sinus tracts, or abscess is not known in the diabetic foot. The presence of air density in soft tissues may be associated with soft tissue swelling secondary to a break in the skin, or may be evidence of clostridial or nonclostridial cellulitis or deep abscess. When the clinical signs of infection, bacteremia, or septicemia are present, gas-forming organisms must be suspected, and appropriate antibiotic therapy, as well as incision and drainage, initiated immediately. Diagnostic ultrasound may be utilized for the elucidation of deep space abscess, although at present, resolution with deep pedal abscess remains problematic. Subcutaneous crepitus in a febrile patient is an ominous sign with impeding bacteremia and septic shock a major concern. Although soft tissue swelling, air density, or other soft tissue manifestations of infection are present radiographically, the local clinical signs of soft tissue infection may be minimized by poor peripheral vascular status and decreased inflammatory response (106, 107).

With regard to soft tissue evaluation, vascular calcification representative of medial calcific sclerosis may be noted. Soft tissue calcification may be noted from the deposition of uric acid, particularly in poorly controlled diabetic patients in whom hyperuricemia due to urate excretion inhibition, dehydration, and increased protein catabolism is not an uncommon problem. Foreign bodies such as glass may be found in the plantar soft tissues of diabetic patients in whom the penetration of the object was undetected due to sensory polyneuropathy.

The definition of the extent of sinus tracts and abscesses is often difficult to determine on the basis of clinical and radiographic evaluation. Edema, erythema, warmth, tenderness and swelling of the arch and dorsum of the foot, and pain and frank ulceration with purulent drainage may suggest the need for incision and drainage. Because a traumatic technique and minimal disruption of noninfected tissue is essential in the management of soft tissue, attempts at localization of disease is of benefit.

Sinograms

With the use of sinograms, the depth, location, and extent of sinus tracts, soft tissue defects, and abscesses may be defined (Fig. 13.8). A sinogram is performed by the injection of a radiopaque contrast media into the soft tissue defect or sinus tract. In a simple abscess, a limited and generally well-defined area of contrast media is noted on examination of large amounts of contrast media, which produce less well-defined spacial presentation with the foot. When the contrast media is introduced, fluoroscopy, tomography, or multiple radiographic views may be utilized. With the use of the fluoroscope, the contrast media can be followed as it dissects fascial planes and joint spaces, or occupies defined areas of defect. With regard to conventional radiography, the anterior-posterior views allow determination of the location as well as the extent of a sinus tract or abscess uptake of contrast media. The lateral view provides information with regard to depth of involvement. Tomography and computerized axial tomography may be utilized with or without contrast media to localize and de-

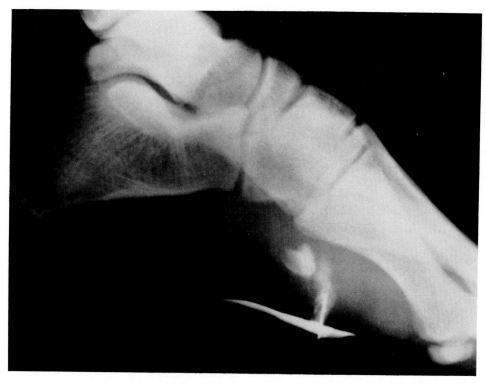

Figure 13.8. Sinogram showing the extent of sinus tract and possible communication with deep abscess within the foot which may be anatomically defined by the use of radiopaque contrast media.

fine the extent of soft tissue defects, and appear particularly useful in the evaluation of deep space pathology.

Once the exact location and extent of soft tissue pathology has been determined, the possible infectious nature of the disease process should be determined. The determination of the presence of soft tissue infection deep within the foot is initially a clinical diagnosis, with radiographic studies utilized to localize the area of major concern. Needle aspiration under fluoroscopic guidance may be used to obtain material for Gram stain and culture and sensitivity. When no fluid is obtained, sterile saline may be flushed into the suspected area and withdrawn for culture and gram stain.

Nuclear Medicine Studies

Noninvasively, two nuclear medicine studies appear to demonstrate promise in the localization of soft tissue infection. Gal-

lium-67 citrate is a radiopharmaceutical which localizes in areas of soft tissue infection. The exact mechanism of gallium localization in a foci of infection remains speculative, although it appears that the gallium adheres to the surface of some bacteria and some leukocytes in the presence of infection. Indium-111-labeled leukocytes, on injection, have been shown to migrate to the area of soft tissue abscess, although the utilization of this test remains unproven in the evaluation of foot pathology. Gallium-67 citrate accumulation appears to be a reliable means of detecting radiographically occult infectious disease, although false positive studies may occur in the presence of inflammatory soft tissue disease and some soft tissue neoplasms. False negative studies may also occur.

The bone and joint changes of diabetes mellitus require attention to detail for proper diagnosis. The detection of significant osseous and articular disease is important in the prevention of surgical complications. Delayed healing of osteotomies may result from the consequences of diabetic osteopoenia. Undiagnosed osteolysis may result in post-operative soft tissue and bone changes which mimic osteomyelitis. Neurotrophic joint disease is associated with a higher failure of successful arthrodesis than in the general population. Metatarsal osteotomy performed in the presence of undetected bone infection may result in disastrous consequences.

Osteolysis

Diabetic osteolysis is characterized by the resorption of the distal metatarsals and proximal phalanges. Juxta-articular erosive changes as well as osteolytic disease beyond the confines of the joint typify this entity, which may be mistaken for osteomyelitis or inflammatory joint disease. Chemically, diabetic osteolysis is frequently associated with inflammatory soft tissue pathology. When spotty juxta-articular osteopoenia and inflammatory soft tissues changes are noted in the area of known ulceration, an inferred diagnosis of bone infection is often made. This is especially true when gram stains or cultures demonstrate the presence of bacterial colonization.

Osteolysis may present as a self-limiting disorder, although multiple joint involvement is the general finding. The initial area of bone destruction eventually expands with lysis and fragmentation of the metaphyseal and epiphyseal regions extending through subcortical bone, and eventually destroying the entire bone end, but sparing the central portion of the diaphysis. The end of the remaining metatarsal shaft appears at first ragged and eventually becomes tapered and osteosclerotic, resulting in a "pencil" or "candlestick" deformity. Gouging and broadening of the proximal phalangeal base is also likely to result, with the radiographic presentation of a "pencil in cup" appearance. In the usual case, the joint space is preserved until late in the process.

Table 13.4.
Radiographic and Nuclear Medicine Studies in the Evaluation of Soft Tissue Pathology in the Diabetic Foot

Study	Benefit
Standard radiographs AP, lateral, oblique	Detection of soft tissue defects, air density, vascular calcification, foreign bodies
Air or contrast sinograms	Definition of the limits of sinus tracts, abscess, fascial plane dissection
Diagnostic ultrasound	Anatomical localization of abscess
Tomography; computerized axial tomography	Anatomical localization of abscess and definition of soft tissue destruction in deep tissues
Xeroradiography	Accentuation of soft tissue defects
Gallium-67 citrate scan; indium III-labeled leukocytes	Localization at sites of probable infectious disease
Thallium-201 scan	Predict healing potential of ulcerations
Xenon-133 scan Epicutaneous Intramuscular	

Osteomyelitis

Osteomyelitis is a frequent sequella of the diabetic state, complicating ulcers. As in the nondiabetic, osteomyelitis is dreaded as a complication of foot surgery. Early detection is essential in the post-operative patient, as is differentiation of osteomyelitis from other types of resorptive bone pathology (Table 13.4).

Characteristically, the bone changes of osteomyelitis occur by the introduction of bacteria from the surrounding environment through a wound, or continuity of a soft tissue infection to the contiguous osseous structures. The most common sites for pedal osteomyelitis are the phalanges, metatarsals, and calcaneus, where neurotropic ulceration is very commonly encountered.

Radiographically, the earliest signs of osteomyelitis are presented by increased soft tissue density secondary to the edema produced by the infectious process. Often, a soft tissue defect overlying the ulceration may be seen. Radiographic bone changes associated with osteomyelitis are not present early in the course of the disease, and a minimum of 7–14 days is usually required for detectable characteristic bone changes to appear. The earliest osseous change is that of cortical erosion with surrounding osteoporosis secondary to the intense hyperemia of the inflammatory response. As the infectious process continues, the erosive process enlarges to include greater areas of adjacent cortical bone and cartilage. This progression frequently produces an intense periosteal reaction resulting in new bone formation as an attempt to wall off the infectious process. Roentgenographically, this will appear as a radiodense linear deposition usually parallel to the cortical shaft. Sequestra, which appear as dense, sclerotic fragments separated from the main portion of the bone, represent areas of dead cortical bone, and are seen late in the infectious process. When bacteria reach the medullary bone, progression occurs along the path of least resistance, that being the cortical and haversian canals. The result is that of an osteoporotic shell with a sclerotic periphery representing devascularized bone. With continued progression, an entire osseous structure such as a phalanx may be destroyed, or become radiographically absent.

Radionuclide Evaluation

The differentiation of osteomyelitis from diabetic osteolysis is of major therapeutic consequence. When the radiographic and clinical differentiation of these two clinical entities is equivocal, differential scintography may be of value (Fig. 13.9). A four-phase bone scan is utilized, with technetium-99 methylene disphosphonate, and gallium-67 citrate. As a general rule, the failure of intense focal uptake of gallium corresponding to an area of intense focal technetium accumulation is evidence of noninfective bone disease. Bone scans of patients with diabetic osteolysis will demonstrate diffuse and focal uptake with tech-

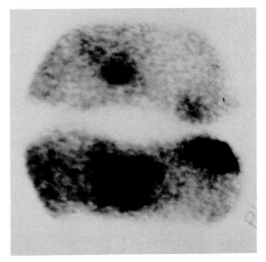

Figure 13.9. Scintigraphy. Osteomyelitis is present involving the entire distal phalanx with some increased uptake in the proximal phalanx. Radionuclide bone imaging may be utilized to determine the extent of infectious osseous disease and to determine the distal "safe" margin for amputation.

netium-99 methylene diphosphonate, but only slightly increased uptake of gallium-67 citrate. In the case of osteomyelitis, both the technetium and gallium scans will typically demonstrate strong diffuse and focal uptake.

Radionuclide imaging is not a substitute for other diagnostic modalities. The value of a scan is dependent on the clinical context in which it is placed. Bone biopsy and culture are far more definitive than scintigraphy for the evaluation of potential osteomyelitis, but are also more invasive.

The triphasic technetium-99 methylene diphosphonate bone scan begins with an intravenous injection of the radiopharmaceutical into the left antecubital fossa. Immediately following injection, a scan that reveals the presence of hyperemia confirms the presence of inflammatory disease. At 5–10 minutes following injection, a second scan is obtained. Because this radiopharmaceutical has an affinity for osseous rather than soft tissue, the delayed post-injection film typically demonstrates some diffuse increased uptake when deep inflam-

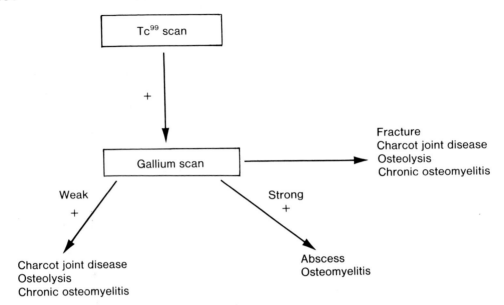

matory disease is present. Two hours following injection, focal uptake of the radiopharmaceutical is consistent with osseous hyperemia and increased bone metabolic activity. On completion of the three-phase scan, the patient is injected with gallium-67 citrate, and scintograms obtained 24 and 48 hours later. At this time, the technetium methylene disphosphonate has been cleared by the body, and any remaining uptake is then attributed to gallium citrate accumulation. While technetium methylene disphosphonate accumulation is nonspecific in terms of etiology, it does localize to the area of bone activity. Gallium citrate is more specific for infectious disease, and will accumulate in both bone and soft tissue. A comparison of the two scans reveals the probability of bone and/or soft tissue infection (108–112).

Osteopoenia

Defective or delayed bone healing may occur in diabetes mellitus as the result of diminished bone matrix. Juvenile diabetes mellitus may be characterized by decreased body stature and associated defective bone formation. Significant loss of bone mineral is frequently associated with the onset of diabetes mellitus, and appears greater in the noninsulin-dependent diabetic patient.

It appears that collagen synthesis and amino acid uptake by bone is increased by the action of insulin.

Spontaneous Dislocation

Spontaneous dislocation involving the foot of a diabetic patient is an entity that is rarely observed. In a foot with normal sensation, dislocations about the tarsus occur only after major trauma, and even then are quite infrequent. It has been stated that the earliest changes in the neuropathic joint involve the soft tissues. Neuropathic changes in the ligamentous structures are such that gross dislocations occur without detectable bone changes. These patients are unaware that they sustain such a form of injury.

Patients who develop spontaneous dislocations follow a certain characteristic pattern concerning their duration and control of diabetes. First, they are known to have had diabetes for only a short time and, secondly, they do not need insulin for control. This is in contrast to most diabetic patients who develop the more common Charcot joint changes of the tarsus where they have diabetes for years and have been on long-term insulin control.

Newman proposed a theory that the ligamentous lesion producing hyperlaxity represented the most early form of neuropathic joint disease which allowed spontaneous dislocation to occur. If allowed to go unrecognized, progressive destructive changes will occur, leading to fracture and eventually reactive new bone formation typical to Charcot joint disease.

Spontaneous dislocations in the diabetic foot most commonly involve the following in descending order: 1) talonavicular joint, 2) Lisfranc tarsometatarsal joints, and 3) ankle joint. The talonavicular dislocations can be either partial or complete. Lisfranc dislocations are common and involve chiefly the homolateral and divergent types. Talocrural dislocations often result in severe deformity and disability and are chiefly posterior in direction (113, 114).

Spontaneous Neuropathic Fractures

Spontaneous fractures complicated by diminished pain sensation and proprioception occurring in the early stages prior to the development of neuroarthropathy have been largely neglected. Charcot, in 1868, noted frequent spontaneous fractures which he attributed to weakened bone. Lippmann et al. (115) pointed out that the first manifestation of diabetic osteopathy was fracture or fragmentation. Also, these fractures are unusual in that they differ from true traumatic fractures in both location and appearance. Common sites of pedal involvement include avulsion fractures of the posterior tubercle of the calcaneus, base of the first and fifth metatarsals, near tendinous insertions of the Achilles tendon, peroneus longus, and brevis muscles, respectively. Metatarsal fractures are a common entity. Other fractures involve compression of the talar dome and body of the calcaneus, often involving the subtalar joint. Though a common belief, there is yet no definite evidence to support the concept of intrinsic bone weakness. The interval between fracture and disorganization of the affected joint can range from 1–13 months before proceeding to frank neuroarthropathy. It is believed that the absence of pain sensation and proprioception leaves the legs without protection from repeated microtrauma in the face of continued activity. Recognition and treatment are paramount as these fractures represent the earliest sign of impending joint derangement and Charcot joint changes (114–118).

Neurotrophic Joint Disease

The incidence of Charcot bone and joint changes has been estimated to be 0.22% at King's College Hospital, 2.5% in a study at another institution of 500 diabetics, and 0.16% at Deaconess Hospital (119–121).

Foster and Bassett (122) were among the first to mention autonomic nervous system lesions having a role in the etiology of diabetic Charcot's joint disease. Diabetic osteopathy, diabetic neuro-osteoarthropathy, and diabetic neuroarthropathy are all terms utilized to describe the joint and bone changes in diabetes in the absence of a primary infective process.

In most studies of Charcot changes observed in diabetic patients, authors have noted varying degrees of impaired sensory, motor, proprioceptive, and reflexive function. Martin (119) discounted the role of autonomic dysfunction because in his study of diabetic arthropathy most patients had some degree of autonomic abnormality. Most authors do not refer to the presence of any vasomotor and/or sudomotor dysfunction. Therefore, it is difficult to assess the contribution of autonomic disturbance directly to the destructive Charcot changes observed in many diabetic patients.

The usual presentation of Charcot disease is found in patients with an average of 12 positive years of diabetic history. Control of hyperglycemia did not seem to correlate with the presence of Charcot changes. The foot and ankle are most commonly involved in the lower extremity in Charcot changes secondary to diabetes mellitus. In some published studies, the metatarsals and/or interphalangeal joints comprise 97% of the bones affected in the diabetic, and up to 50% of the Charcot problems were unilateral.

Periarticular fractures and joint subluxations or dislocations may be noted on clinical and radiographic examination. On radiographic examination, evidence of both destructive and reparative changes may be noted, depending on the stage of the Charcot process. It has been shown in experimental fashion that a pure sensory defect in the posterior column will not create a Charcot joint. A defect in the articulating bones appears to be necessary for the precipitation of events leading to frank Charcot joint changes.

The lower extremity deformities can be divided into several major categories, including ankle, tarsus and/or forefoot disease. Finby (125) describes a Charcot joint type of destructive process affecting the ankle and tarsal bones in which there was fracture, subluxation, and total joint disorganization, often seen in various stages of repair. In the forefoot, the bone absorption processes or mutilating type of Charcot joint disease is often found with osteolysis of the metatarsals and phalanges. This deformity has been described in various terms, including "pencil-cup" or "mortar-pestle" type of deformity.

Sella (123) suggests that the complex of somatic and autonomic nerves that run together in the lower extremity are jointly involved in diabetic disease. This would account for the often observed unilateral intermittent and variable somatic and autonomic lower extremity findings. This motor neuropathy multiplex is thought to be caused by ischemic changes in the vasa nervorum.

The increased bone resorption observed radiographically is facilitated by an auto-sympathectomy, which causes vasodilation and hyperemia to the affected area. Technetium radionuclide imaging will show increased uptake in Charcot joints due to the hyperemia in the initial states. In a small series, technetium scans have been shown as hot areas in diabetics before evidence on conventional radiographs of frank Charcot changes. Utilizing the consideration of hyperemia preceding the Charcot radiographic changes, thermography was found to be useful in the early detection of im-

pending gross Charcot changes in joints. The exact involvement of the autonomic nerve disease in Charcot processes remains unclear and is still one of speculation. The management of Charcot's joints is one of prophylaxis and supportive therapy. Surgical intervention has been advocated by some authors (119, 120, 122–128).

BONE HEALING IN DIABETES MELLITUS

Among the complications which could be reasonably expected in the diabetic population would be an increased rate of delayed union of osteotomies, non-union of osteotomies, or excessively high failure rates for arthrodesing procedures. The etiological considerations for such problems might include reduced osseous, vascular flow secondary to microvascular or macrovascular disease, vasomotor instability associated with previously discussed autonomic neuropathy, or deleterious effects from the multitude of metabolic abnormalities associated with diabetes mellitus.

No specific reviews of the complications of pedal osteotomy or arthrodesing procedures are available for review. The majority of literature presently available, concerning the effects of diabetes mellitus on skeletal healing, concern themselves with fracture healing. Defective fracture healing has been described in diabetic patients by Cozen (129). Levin et al. (130), utilizing photon absorption to measure bone density, was able to demonstrate a significant loss of bone mass in both juvenile and adult onset diabetes, as compared to controls matched for age and sex. Bone loss in the Levin study did not correlate with the duration of diabetes, and was found to be present in patients with diabetes of less than 5 years' duration. The loss of bone substance noted was not related to the severity of diabetes, with insulin-dependent diabetics demonstrating less loss of bone mineral than patients controlled by either diet or oral hypoglycemic agents. McNair and his co-workers (131), also utilizing photon absorption, studied 215 insulin-treated diabetics and concluded that residual insulin secretion and the quality of metabolic control were major factors in determining bone mineral content in insulin-treated diabetic patients. They reported a 20.7% bone loss in patients, demonstrating the poorest metabolic control of their disease. Weiss et al. (132) reported on their findings of abnormal proteoglycan synthesis in the cartilage and bones of streptozotocin-treated rats. These authors found that experimental diabetes is associated with decreased synthesis of proteoglycans, poor and diminished proteoglycan aggregate formation, and decreased molecular weight. Because proteoglycans represent a major constituent for the structural integrity of bone and cartilage, biochemical alterations of this macromolecular structure may be of significant clinical importance. Cerawi (133), Berenson (134), Schneir (135), Golub (136), and Weiss (132), in separate reports, demonstrated a variety of collagen and connective tissue defects associated with glycosylated proteins in experimental diabetes mellitus. The lowered organ tension to an osteotomy or fusion site, which would be expected in the presence of macrovascular or microvascular disease, would certainly be detrimental to bone healing.

The significance of osseous changes from diabetes mellitus, and their potential clinical significance in post-operative healing, remain obscure, particularly with reference to foot surgery. Menezel et al. (137) reported on incidence of proximal hip fractures as 22% in osteopeonic diabetic patients. A number of authors have described an unusually high incidence of spontaneous fracture in diabetics, including Berney (138), Kuhlencordt (139), Forgacs (140), and Neuman (141). Hypercalciuria in diabetic patients has been described by Rifkin and Zeiter (15), and its presence in diabetic subjects confirmed by Heath et al. (142), who were unable to identify diabetes mellitus as a risk factor in skeletal fractures. With the possible exception of medial malleolar fractures, Heath and his co-workers concluded that bone mass reductions in diabetes mellitus were of no practical importance.

Metatarsal osteotomies are a commonly performed surgical procedure for the correction of excessive weightbearing contributing to plantar calluses and neurotrophic ulcers in the diabetic patient. No data is presently available to suggest that this procedure is attended by an unusually high complication rate. Delayed healing of fractures in diabetic patients may be related to a variety of factors, of which peripheral vascular perfusion would appear to be the most important. In a well-controlled diabetic patient, with normal hemoglobin A_{1C} levels, adequate vascular status, and no evidence of marked autonomic neuropathy, it does not appear that metatarsal osteotomy presents an unusual risk. Osteopoenia observed on standard radiographs represents a loss of greater than 30% of bone mineral, as compared to the 20% loss of bone mineral noted in poorly controlled diabetics. When marked osteopeonia is noted on standard radiographs, a search for an etiology other than diabetes should be made.

With regard to arthrodesing procedures, fusion rates are lower in neurotrophic joint disease. This is particulary true in atrophic type neurotrophic joints, in which vasomotor instability produces a paradoxical hyperemia, osteoclast stimulation, and bone resorption.

OSTEOMYELITIS AND DEEP SPACE INFECTION

Osteomyelitis is regarded as a not uncommon complication of ulcerative lesions in the diabetic foot, and usually represents a direct extension of the infectious process from contiguous soft tissue rather than hematogenous in origin. Recent articles have suggested that the evidence of hematogenous osteomyelitis in elderly patients may be greater than previously thought. Osteomyelitis, as any infection, will result in delayed wound healing, and may occur as a complication of surgery.

Early recognition of osteomyelitis is essential for treatment. The role of the four-phase radionuclide imaging in the elucidation of radiographically occult disease has been discussed earlier in this chapter.

Park and his co-workers (143) have demonstrated a sensitivity of 83% and a specificity of 75% of technetium-99 methylene disphosphonate scans for diabetic osteomyelitis, as compared to standard radiographs, which were less sensitive (62%) and less specific (69%). They concluded that the predictive value of technetium scans were 80% as compared to radiographs (47%) for osteomyelitis. Scoles et al. (144) have presented a review of radionuclide patterns in patients with acute osteomyelitis. The early recognition of osteomyelitis in the diabetic patient, whether associated with a post-operative wound or as a complication of ulceration or bacteremia, requires not only a high index of suspicion for osseous disease, but requires differentiation from osteolysis, Charcot joint disease, and other musculoskeletal problems. Although radiographs and gallium-67 citrate scans are useful in this regard, the diagnosis of osteomyelitis is presumptive without bone culture or biopsy, as shown separately by Classen (145) and his co-workers, as well as Eymontt et al. (146). The differentiation of osteomyelitis from degenerative joint disease has been discussed by Park et al. (143).

The medical management of osteomyelitis is difficult under ordinary circumstances, a problem which is aggravated in the patient with poor vascular flow and impaired cellular and humoral response secondary to diabetes mellitus. The problem of treatment is further complicated by the poor penetration of certain antibiotics in bone, and the presence of necrotic tissue deep within the foot.

When osteomyelitis is suspected or presumed to be present, soft tissue cultures and blood cultures are usually obtained. Definitive isolation of the bone pathogen requires a culture from bone, which may be obtained through an open wound such as an ulcer or surgical dehiscence. Morrey (147) and Peterson, Dich et al. (148), and Nade (149) have shown that blood cultures are positive in 50% of the cases of hematogenous osteomyelitis, and when positive appear to obviate the need for bone culture

and biopsy. Bone culture may be obtained by sterile saline flush with a syringe, the flushed material being withdrawn for culture. Following sterile preparation, "flush cultures" may be performed at bedside or under fluoroscopy guidance. The technique of bone aspiration for culture has been described by Mollan and Piggot.

If osteomyelitis is associated with an open wound or draining sinus tract, Mackowiak et al. (150) have shown that gram stains and cultures obtained from the soft tissue wound have very little relationship to organisms isolated at the time of surgery from bone.

Complete discussion regarding the bacteriology of osteomyelitis in the diabetic patient can be found elsewhere, and is beyond the scope of this chapter. Although *Staphylococcus aureus* is a common pathogen, the diminished vascular flow to many diabetic feet results in an unusually high incidence of gram-negative and mixed gram-positive/gram-negative infections. Traumatic puncture wounds of the foot are frequently associated with *Pseudomonas aeruginosa* (151). When post-operative osteomyelitis is suspected, Waldvogel and Vasey (152) recommend confirmatory invasive procedures. Problems such as nonunion of osteotomies addressed at a later time when the infectious process has resolved. Immobilization during treatment may interdict delayed union or non-union in some cases.

Because of diminished blood supply and inadequate response to infection, osteomyelitis in the diabetic must be treated aggressively. Kahn and Pritzner (153) have demonstrated that the presence of necrotic bone represents the major therapeutic problem in osteomyelitis, since it is in the necrotic, devascularized bone that pathogens reside. When the infectious process is acute, and extensive osseous disease is not evident, antibiotic therapy may be sufficient to resolve the problem. Bone vascular flow, as well as osseous penetration of antibiotics and the achievement of therapeutic levels in bone, remain problematic in the diabetic.

With regard to antibiotic therapy, therapeutic blood levels of antibiotics in bone cannot be evaluated in a clinically practical manner. Norden (154) has demonstrated an 80% cure rate of experimental osteomyelitis with 4–6 weeks of appropriate parenteral therapy. Although a variety of antibiotics, including cephalosporins, lincomycin, clindamycin, aminoglycosides, rifampin, penicillin G, and semisynthetic penicillin have been recovered from bone (152), therapeutic levels cannot be assured despite monitoring of serum levels. Studies of oral antibiotic therapy for osteomyelitis, such as that of Cunda (155), have usually been restricted to acute hematogenous osteomyelitis, and do not appear to be applicable to the diabetic patient. Four to six weeks of parenteral antibiotic therapy appear appropriate for most cases, with proper monitoring of serum therapeutic levels, radiographs, and clinical signs and symptoms. A positive technetium-99 methylene diphosphonate scan, and negative gallium-67 citrate scan, or decreasing intensity of technetium scintigraphy, are consistent with resolving acute infection. Quantitative bacteriology may be used to demonstrate resolving infection. Serial cultures and sensitivities should be obtained to monitor the patient for changing bacterial flora, as well as changing antibiotic sensitivity. Patients must be monitored for adverse antibiotic reactions, and evaluated for the potentially hazardous sequellae of many antibiotics, such as nephrotoxicity, a granulocytosis, or pseudomembranous colitis.

Chronic osteomyelitis is characterized by slowly progressive radiographic changes, intermittent wound breakdown, drainage, and sequestration. Deysine (156) has shown that a positive technetium scan and negative gallium scan is consistent with chronic osteomyelitis. With appropriate local wound care, Bell (157) has demonstrated good results with oral antibiotic therapy in chronic osteomyelitis. Becher and Spadaro (158) have demonstrated the use of electrically generated silver ions in the treatment of chronic osteomyelitis.

Necrotic bone supporting bacterial infection in the diabetic patient must be removed. When cellulitis accompanies osteomyelitis, an attempt should be made at parenteral resolution of the soft tissue infection prior to bone resection, since soft tissue infection remains a major cause of wound breakdown. Amputations of severely infected toes or rays may be performed, and left open for drainage. Because patients in bed are supine, efforts to extend incisions dorsally to allow gravity drainage are useful. The wound should be flushed with an appropriate antibiotic or iodophor following deep gram stain, culture and sensitivity, or bone biopsy.

When osteomyelitic bone is resected, a decision must be made whether to pack the wound open, or to close the wound primarily. If the surrounding soft tissues appear healthy, and intra-operative gram stains are negative, the wound may be closed over continuous closed suction irrigation. Again, because the patient will be supine, the ingress tubes should be placed distally while the egress tubes are placed proximally, consistent with the effects of gravity. The major problems encountered with the closed suction irrigation include blockage of the egress tubes and wound maceration. Maceration may be avoided by utilizing the ingress flush on an intermittent, rather than continuous basis. Newer closed suction irrigation systems employ two, rather than one, egress tubes. These must be carefully monitored, and require the cooperation of a concerned and competent nursing and house staff. The tubes should be placed into the wound through separate puncture incisions made with the stylus attached to the tubing. When large stab wounds are made, an airtight system does not develop, and leakage of fluid occurs. Active suction with a Gomco® or wall suction unit are preferred to the usually inefficient power of plastic or vacutainer-type apparatus.

When osteomyelitis is associated with deep abscess, or when drainage and debridement are performed for abscess alone, or when significant soft tissue infection or necrosis is present, the wound should not be closed primarily. Stainless steel sutures may be placed for later closure if a margin of safety exists between infected or necrotic and healthy tissue. Necrotic tissue is debrided and the wound packed with plain gauze. In addition to debridement, iodophor flushing, and repacking should be performed together with appropriate monitoring of bacterial flora and antibiotic levels. With the exception of β-hemolytic streptococci, wounds may be closed when there are 10^5 bacteria per gram of tissue or less.

Deep space infections, or any abscess, must be drained on an emergency basis. Pain, throbbing, or tenderness are signs of abscess. In the case of medial, central, or lateral plantar space abscess, swelling of the arch, dorsal edema, arch tenderness, or swelling and tenderness at the ankle or lower leg may be noted. Aspiration with a large gauge needle may confirm the presence of pus or exudate. Sharp dissection with wide exposure is mandatory. A leukocytosis with a shift to the left, elevated erythrocyte sedimentation rate or C reaction protein, elevated oral temperature, and an elevated serum glucose level may be noted. Because deep infectious processes follow the flexor tendons, extension of dissection along the medial arch, ankle, or lower leg may be necessary. Minimal trauma is desirable, but adequate drainage must be established. Blood cultures should be obtained initially, and at times of febrile episodes, or when evidence of septicemia or bacteremia is present. Resolving local signs and symptoms, decreasing insulin requirements, and decreased serologic and hematologic markers of infection are useful methods of monitoring progress. When evidence of recurrence or non-response to the original procedure is evident, the patient should be reevaluated.

The presence of gas on a radiograph is an ominous sign, particularly when an open lesion through which soft tissue emphysema can occur is not present (Fig. 13.10). When crepitant cellulitis or unexplained gas density on x-ray is present, immediate incision, drainage, and debridement should be performed. Diabetic patients are partic-

ularly prone to infection by facultatively anaerobic bacteria, and obligate spore-forming and non-spore-forming bacteria. MacLennan (159) has defined gas gangrene as an invasive, anaerobic infection of muscle, characterized by extensive local edema, massive tissue necrosis, variable degrees of gas production, and, eventually, toxemia. Acute clostridial myonecrosis has been described by Miskew et al. (160). Altmeir and Culbertson (161) and Drago (162) have described acute nonclostridial crepitant cellulitis. Fisher and McKusick (163) have described gas gangrene associated with *Bacteroides*, while DeHaven and Evarts (164) have described nonclostridial crepitant cellulitis with streptococci.

In most cases, in addition to emergency incision, drainage, and debridement, large

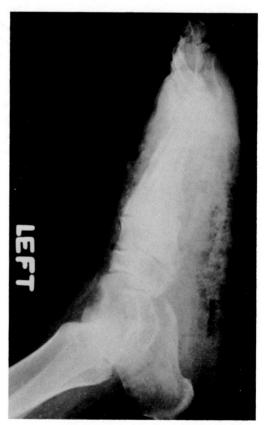

Figure 13.10. Gas density on x-ray. The presence of gas on x-ray, especially when associated with crepitation, and findings of septicemia, fever, local edema, erythema, and pain, is a medical and surgical emergency.

doses of antibiotics are required. The usefulness of hyperbaric oxygen remains controversial (165).

AMPUTATION OF THE DIABETIC FOOT

Local radical amputation of the foot in the diabetic patient is usually performed for osteomyelitis, gangrene, localized ulceration with infection, and less commonly for ischemic rest pain. Root (166) and later McKitterick (167) described successful transmetatarsal amputations in diabetic patients, and asked surgeons to consider more distal amputations in selected diabetic patients. At the time of their original papers, the prevailing philosophy was that the first amputation should be the last, and that an above the knee or below the knee amputation represented definitive treatment for dysvascular foot problems. Twenty-three years later, Sizer and Wheelock (168) reported their 95% success rate in limb salvage of diabetics with digital amputations. Following their report, which was presented to the Twenty-sixth Annual Meeting of the Society for Vascular Surgery, Dr. Jack Cannon stated, in a discussion of their findings (148):

> It is a privilege to discuss this paper. This series reports a success rate in the 90 to 95 percent area. It concerns vascular disease and yet vein grafts, direct arterial surgery, and lumbar sympathectomy have not been involved. Presented, however, are some basic principles the elucidation of which have been a long time in coming. Many of these I first learned of more than 25 years ago. At the same time, I would have a strong feeling that if we sampled around the country for knowledge of these principles, we would not find them applied very frequently or very effectively, and often unheard of, especially amongst our orthopedic colleagues.

In spite of the major advances which have been made in our understanding of peripheral vascular flow and diabetes mellitus, it would appear that Dr. Cannon's observation continues to be correct even today. More than 62,000 amputations are performed every year for arteriosclerotic peripheral vascular disease. A recent review by Kacy et al. (169) of 249 extremity amputations performed between January, 1976 and December, 1980 revealed 23% above knee amputations; 48% below the knee, 22% digital amputations; 6% transmetatarsal amputations, and 1% Syme amputations.

Types of Amputations

Amputations refer to the removal of a portion of an extremity through bone, while disarticulation refers to removal of a portion through a joint. In the case of diabetic patients, amputations are preferred to disarticulations because the relatively avascular cartilage is more susceptible to infection, and contributes very little to stump healing (170).

Four general types of amputations can be performed. In the standard or simple amputation, all tissues down to bone are transected at the same level. Deeper tissues tend to retract proximal to the level of skin incision. Tendons and nerves are appropriately resected, and the bone resected proximal to the level of the skin incision. The wound is closed primarily. Standard or simple amputations have the highest success rate for healing in diabetes mellitus.

The osteomyoplastic and osteomyodesing type of amputation represent two other kinds. In the osteomyoplastic type, antagonistic muscles are sutured to each other in an effort to maintain function and prevent deformity. Osteomyodesing type amputations are characterized by the attachment of tendons directly to bone, again in an effort to maintain function and to prevent deformity. In certain types of amputations, such as the Chopart or Lisfranc type, the typical equinus or equinovarus deformities encountered could be prevented. The osteomyoplastic and osteomyodesing amputations should not be utilized in the average diabetic since they require extra surgical trauma and the potential for healing is less.

The final type of amputation is the open or provisional amputation. Open amputations are typically performed to remove grossly infected or gangrenous tissue, and allow drainage of deep infection. Amputation wounds may be left partially open, or totally open, usually with some form of packing. At times, open amputations may be required as an emergency procedure. Following resolution of the infectious process, with daily local care and appropriate antibiotic therapy, open amputation is followed by secondary closure, reamputation, revision, or plastic repair. When possible, long skin flaps are prepared at the time of the original open amputation, since significant skin retraction and loss of skin mobility from edema or fibrosis may be problematic (169, 171, 172). Open amputations may also be performed without the creation of skin flaps at the time of the original surgery (guillotine amputation). Such "circular" open amputations heal very slowly and require traction on the skin to obtain stump coverage. Undesirable scarring is often the result. When a margin of safety allows, sutures may be placed in skin and into the wound. Stainless steel sutures are preferred. The sutures are not tied, but may be twisted to slightly close the wound over packing or to allow appropriate traction on the soft tissues. Bedside debridement and closure of the wound can then be performed at an appropriate time. Open amputations of the foot have the highest failure rate in the diabetic, requiring a greater blood supply to heal than do closed amputations (170).

Vascular Considerations

The potential for healing of a digital, ray, or transmetatarsal amputation can be difficult to evaluate. Wheelock (173), Goodman (172), and Sizer (168) have shown that pedal pulses do not have to be present for the healing of pedal amputations. Sizer and Wheelock (168), in a review of 692 digital amputations for gangrene, ulceration, or infection in diabetic patients, had a 2.2% failure rate in patients with palpable pedal pulses, and an 11% failure rate with absent pedal pulses. These authors stated that, for

successful digital amputation, "circulation must be adequate but palpable pedal pulses are not a necessity." The 11% failure rate in patients without palpable foot pulses was attributed by the author, in part, to a large number of open amputations within that subgroup. The criteria used for the vascular evaluation of patients for digital and transmetatarsal amputations by Wheelock were the absence of pain except localized to the area of infection or ulceration, minimal or absent rubor of the toes, and a venous filling time of 20 seconds or less (173).

The evaluation of patients without palpable pedal pulses for amputations is difficult. Verta et al. (174) studied forefoot perfusion pressures in minor amputations for gangrene, and concluded that when infection is not present, forefoot perfusion pressure was the most important factor in determining the prognosis for healing. In seven patients, Verta showed healing of digital amputations with ankle pressures of 30 mm Hg or greater, while at ankle pressures of less than 30 mm Hg, all foot amputations failed. Wagner has stated that an ischemic index of 0.45 or greater should be present for healing to be expected from ablative or other surgical procedures in the dysvascular foot. The recommendations of both Verta and Wagner differ from those of Wheelock, who emphasizes the role of the microcirculation in the success of healing. Radionuclide studies and pulse volume recordings offer a more accurate assessment of small vessel flow than do ankle pressures, which are a reflection of medium-size pulsatile arterial flow. A recent study has suggested that isolated patency of the perforating peroneal artery may be sufficient to support pedal wound healing.

Anatomical Considerations

The incision for amputation should never be made through an area of infection, dependent rubor, or gangrene. Digital amputation for gangrene, ulceration, or infectious disease should be distal to the proximal interphalangeal joint. Transmetatarsal amputations should not be performed in the face of gangrene or infection proximal to the web spaces, spreading cellulitis, or when gangrene in ischemic ulcerations is proximal to the proposed incision line (32, 168, 169, 173).

Other Pre-operative Considerations

Infected lymphatics, unrecognized osteomyelitis, and unrecognized or clinically occult deep space infection may result in the failure of digital or transmetatarsal amputations to heal. Appropriate antibiotic therapy and local care often allow for a resolution of cellulitis or infection to a more distal level. Several weeks of intravenous antibiotics, debridement, and appropriate goal-oriented physical therapy may be required prior to amputation. When necessary, incision and drainage or open amputation may be necessary to allow appropriate drainage of abscesses prior to definitive digital, ray, or transmetatarsal amputation.

When the level of amputation remains in question due to equivocal radiographs for osteomyelitis, technetium and gallium scintigraphy may prove of value. Because the radiographically discernable changes of osteomyelitis trail the actual infectious process in bone by 10–21 days, bone scanning is of value in defining the areas of questionable infection.

A large number of variables may play a role in the healing of digital and metatarsal amputations in the diabetic patient. Serum glucose and hemoglobin A_{1C} levels should be within acceptable ranges when time allows. As has been noted earlier, hemoglobin levels of 12 gm/dl or less appear to be associated with an increased healing rate of digital amputations (46). For this reason, normovolemic hemodilution has been suggested in diabetic patients undergoing digital amputation. The seemingly paradoxical effects of hemodilution with regard to wound healing probably represent a compensation for such factors as increased rouleaux formation, decreased erythrocyte deformability, and increased platelet adhesiveness and aggregation which occur in poorly controlled diabetes mellitus. Blood flow through vessels may be expressed in Poiseville's formula;

Blood flow

$$= \frac{\text{Blood pressure} \times \text{vessel radius}^4}{\text{Length of vessel} \times \text{whole blood viscosity}}$$

It can be seen by this formula that hemodilution will result in a decreased whole blood viscosity and, therefore, increased total blood flow. Similarly, the effects of a stenotic lesion (vessel radius^4) in reducing total blood flow are apparent. Normovolemic hemodilution in selected patients has been shown by Yates and co-workers to increase calf perfusion and decrease intermittent claudication. Decreased blood viscosity through hemodilution has been experimentally confirmed by Messner et al. (175). Dormandy (176) was able to demonstrate improvement of claudication symptoms by reducing blood viscosity with a plasma fibrinogen-reducing agent.

A multitude of other factors have been suggested in consideration of wound healing in the diabetic patient, including zinc deficiency (177) and hypomagnesemia (178).

Complications

Because hematoma can delay wound healing and serve as a medium for the growth of pathogens, the use of drains and suction irrigation apparatus has been suggested by some authors. Others have reported increased complications and wound breakdowns from the use of drains. Appropriate hemostasis at the time of surgery will prevent hematoma in the usual case and, with appropriate compression bandaging, obviate the need for such drainage apparatus. Wounds should be inspected in the immediate post-operative period, and any hematoma or seroma promptly and gently aspirated under sterile conditions.

Simple wound dehiscence may be seen in the diabetic patient. Necrosis of the skin edges may occur when excessive tension has been placed on the wound margins. The temptation to early ambulation must be resisted. Similarly, sutures may be left in place for 2–6 weeks in the diabetic with foot amputations. Wheelock, for example, recommended placing transmetatarsal amputees in a light cast for 2–3 weeks, with weightbearing resumed in 4–6 weeks. Small areas of necrosis at the level of stump incision are common, especially at the sites of suture placement. These areas represent positions of increased wound tension. Such areas should be gently and conservatively debrided, and with control of vasospasm, serum glucose, rest, and removal of necrotic tissue, will generally heal uneventfully.

With regard to wound breakdown, the tendency to rush in and cover the dehisced area should be resisted. Although well meaning, impatience on the part of the surgeon is mentioned by both Wheelock (173) and Brown (179), who note that the sight of exposed bone "seems to trigger a compulsion in some surgeons; they believe that the bone must be covered at all costs. Frequently, the cost is great."

In simple dehiscence, time and appropriate goal-oriented therapy remains the key to management. Gram stains and cultures may reveal the presence of bacterial contamination; and may be confused with infection. Most open wounds are colonized or contaminated by bacteria. In the absence of clinical or radiographic signs and symptoms of infection, cultured bacteria should not be regarded as definite evidence of infection. When a serious question arises as to the appropriate course of therapy, a small piece of subcutaneous tissue may be submitted for quantitative bacteriology. If 10^5 bacteria/gm of tissue or more are present, the bacteria may be regarded as contaminants. The exception to this rule include β-hemolytic streptococci and anaerobic cultures growing clostridia species.

When evidence of an abscess appears, it must be drained immediately, with all necrotic tissue removed. Continuous closed suction irrigation is not recommended because of its tendency to cause wound breakdown with maceration in distally performed amputations in which the skin incision encompasses three of the four pedal surfaces.

Infected amputation stumps are debrided and packed open. Gram stains at surgery will give a major indication as to the appropriate initial antibiotic therapy. Aerobic and anaerobic cultures and sensitivities will reveal the definitive choice of antibiotic.

Following transmetatarsal amputations, the foot should be splinted or cast at a right angle to the leg or in very mild plantarflexion, and should not be placed in either varus or valgus. Exercises to strengthen the muscles of the foot, or the use of a muscle stimulator, should be initiated. In the case of a Chopart or Lisfranc type of amputation, poor positioning of the foot may be corrected by appropriate splinting, stretching, or by atraumatic subcutaneous tenotomy of the appropriate deforming muscle tendon unit, as described by Burgess (180) or Zaricznyj (181).

The neurologic complications of amputations include amputation or stump neuroma and phantom limb pain. At the time of surgery, peripheral nerves, like tendon, should be gently pulled distally and cleanly severed and allowed to retract deep into the wound. When the resected end of a nerve becomes entrapped in scar tissue, severe pain may result, often accentuated by attempts to move the foot or bear weight. Weight redistribution, ultrasound, and appropriate shoe modifications may fail to relieve symptoms, in which case neurectomy and neurolysis must be performed. Silastic nerve cuffs have been suggested by some as reducing the incidence of stump neuroma.

Amputation Techniques

Resection of a digit or a portion of a digit may be performed through the distal phalanx (terminal or distal Syme), the distal or proximal interphalangeal joint, the proximal metaphysis of the proximal phalanx, at the metatarsal-phalangeal joint, or with the head of the adjacent metatarsal and appropriate portion of the metatarsal shaft (Fig. 13.11). The exact level of amputation is dependent upon the clinical scenario, with the extent of gangrene or infection,

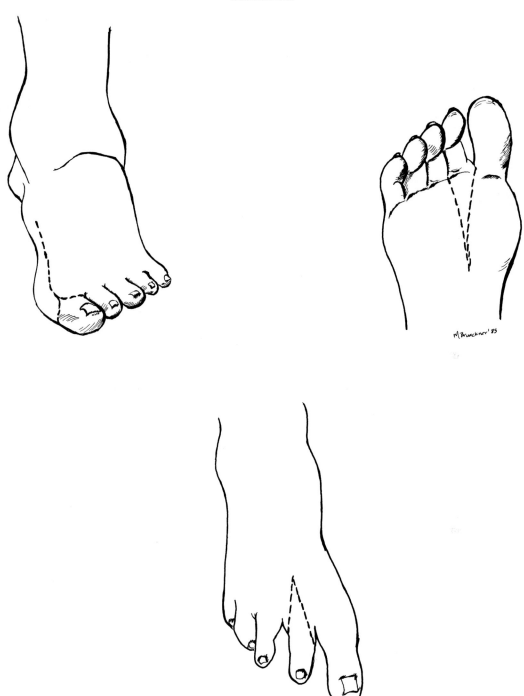

Figure 13.11. Amputation techniques.

and the vascular status of the patient the major determining factors, as was discussed earlier.

A towel clamp or surgical glove is placed so as to limit contact of the surgeon's glove with contaminated and infected tissue. In the usual case, resection through the proximal phalanx is preferred, leaving only the

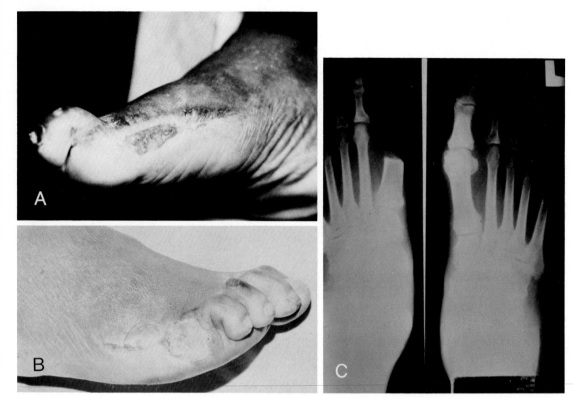

Figure 13.12. Slowly healing first ray amputation (right foot, *A*) and fifth ray amputation (left foot, *B*) are shown. Wound necrosis, dehiscence, and delayed healing may occur even in properly selected patients. Goal-oriented local wound care, together with appropriate control or diabetes, frequently result in a successful but delayed result. In such cases, the surgeon must resist the tendency toward impatience and "rushing in to do something." *C*, radiograph of above.

base of this bone (Fig. 13.12). A variety of skin incisions are suitable, although Wheelock recommends side-to-side flap creation. The flaps should be handled gently, with minimally traumatic soft tissue dissection and sharp instrumentation. Minimal periosteal stripping should be performed, and bone quickly and cleanly resected without leaving spicules. Any irregular bone edges or spicules are remodeled with a rongeur. Tendons and nerves are pulled into the wound, resected cleanly, and allowed to retract.

When clearly avascular, devitalized, or infected tissues are encountered, several options are available. The wound may be debrided and left open to be closed at a later date, or the amputation may be extended to a more proximal level. When hemostasis has been achieved, the skin is closed with simple interrupted sutures of a nonabsorbable suture. Some studies have suggested that surgical stainless steel is the preferred sutures for amputation closure. Extension of the incisions onto the dorsum of the foot is preferable for relaxing the skin flaps, and in allowing surgical drainage when necessary. Sutures are allowed to remain in place for as long as necessary. Excessive manipulation of the skin with forceps is to be avoided.

When digital amputation is combined with resection of a portion of the corresponding metatarsal, two racquet-shaped incisions are combined with a long dorsal incision. For central ray resection, long elliptical incisions are made along both the dorsal and plantar surfaces, and joined in the web spaces. If the amputation is performed for osteomyelitis with soft tissue infection, the wound is either packed open or, if the previously described conditions are present, closed over continuous closed suction irrigation (Fig. 13.13).

Transmetatarsal amputation is performed through an initial transverse dorsal incision (Figs. 13.14 and 13.15). The medial and lateral incisions are extended distally and plantarly. A plantar transverse incision then completes the incision. Sharp dissection is carried to bone, which is resected level or slightly proximal to the dorsal incision. A generous plantar flap should be created initially to alleviate any wound tension. As with other amputations, hemostasis and appropriate resection of tendon and nerves are essential. Simple sutures of a nonabsorbable material are preferred, together with minimal soft tissue handling. The medial flap should be longer (more distal) than the lateral flap to accommodate the thickness of the first metatarsal.

A variety of less commonly performed amputations have been described, including the Lisfranc, Hey, Chaport, Boyd, Piragoff, and proximal Syme. The reader is referred to appropriate references for detailed information of these amputation techniques and the complications attendent to them.

DIABETIC EMERGENCIES
Hypoglycemia

Maintaining plasma glucose levels within relatively narrow boundaries is essential for

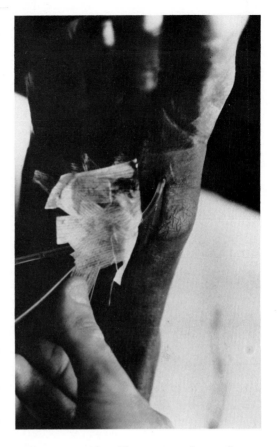

Figure 13.13. Placement of continuous closed suction irrigation apparatus. Two egress tubes are placed through separate wounds proximally, in the dependent portion of the foot. The ingress tube is placed distally.

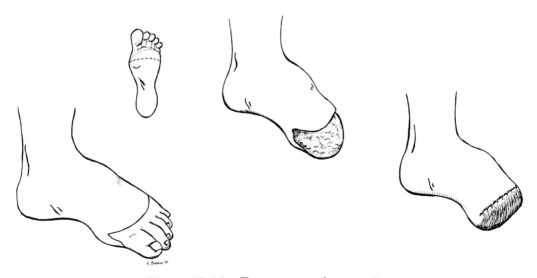

Figure 13.14. Transmetatarsal amputation.

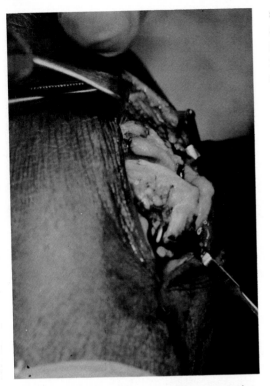

Figure 13.15. Transmetarsal amputation. Wound margins should be carefully closed with a minimum of handling. Stainless steel is preferred. Tendon and nerve should be distracted and the wound cleanly resected and allowed to retract.

proper metabolic function. Hypoglycemia represents a high-risk metabolic abnormality since glucose is the main energy substrate for the brain and nervous system. Its absence may result in loss of tissue function and death if the deficit is prolonged. Accurate diagnosis and prompt treatment are essential. Almost all patients with serious hypoglycemia are diabetics taking insulin or oral hypoglycemics. Common factors which may precipitate hypoglycemia are: decreased or delayed food intake, increased ethanol without increased carbohydrate intake, medication error, excessive insulin, sulfonylurea, or medications which may potentiate effects of sulfonylureas, such as decreasing steroid dosage or the simultaneous administration of salicylates.

The clinical presentation falls into two categories: those symptoms which are as-

sociated with the secretion of epinephrine and those due to dysfunction of the central nervous system. With the release of epinephrine, the patient may experience sweating, tremor, tachycardia, anxiety, and hunger. Central nervous system symptoms include dizziness, headache, clouding of vision, blunted mental acuity, confusion, abnormal behavior, convulsions, and loss of consciousness. Treatment is directed to return serum glucose values to within a normal range. A blood sample is drawn for glucose determination prior to therapy. If the patient is unconscious, 25 gm of glucose (50 ml of dextrose 50 in water IV push) is necessary. If the patient is conscious, oral administration of a rapid-acting carbohydrate will be adequate (orange juice with sugar). Hypoglycemia may require repeated intravenous boluses of glucose, continuous infusion, or repeated oral doses.

Diabetic Ketoacidosis

This condition is a form of metabolic acidosis resulting from insulin deficiency with an increase in ketone bodies and free fatty acids, hyperglycemia, and volume depletion. Ingested glucose is the primary stimulant of insulin release from β cells of the pancreas. Insulin will act on the liver to facilitate the uptake of glucose and the conversion of glucose to glycogen. It inhibits glycogen breakdown (glycogenolysis) by inactivation of the enzyme required for release of glucose from glycogen; and it suppresses gluconeogenesis. The net effect is to store glucose as glycogen. Insulin's action on lipid metabolism is to increase lipogenesis within the liver and the adipose cell and decrease lipolysis. The overall result of insulin's action on lipid metabolism is to convert glucose to a storage form of energy as triglycerides, and increase total fat deposits. The effect of insulin on protein metabolism is to stimulate uptake of amino acids into muscle cells and to mediate incorporation of amino acids into muscle protein. It inhibits the release of amino acids from muscle protein and from hepatic protein sources.

Insufficient insulin results in glycogenolysis. Ketonemia during diabetic ketoacidosis results from increased lipolysis and ketogenesis. Insulin deficiency permits increased breakdown of triglycerides to free fatty acids and glycerol. The fatty acids are assimilated by the liver and are converted to acetyl CoA. Normally, acetyl CoA is converted to oxaloacetate, then to glycogen or citrate for fatty acid synthesis. Both of these steps are inhibited during insulin deficiency. The resultant ketone bodies, β-hydroxybutyrate and acetoacetate, are produced in excessive amounts.

Patients present with evidence of volume depletion, i.e., postural blood pressure changes, tachycardia, and hypotension. Respiration is continuous and deep (Kussmaul) and ketone breath may be detected with pH <7.2. Neurologically, varying degrees of mental status changes may be seen from mild confusion to profound coma. Other signs and symptoms include: polyuria, thirst, dizziness, malaise, anorexia, nausea, vomiting, and abdominal pain. Laboratory analysis yields an increased hematocrit, indicating plasma volume depletion. Electrolytes reflect an increase in sodium due to free water deficit. Serum potassium may be normal, abnormal, or increased; most patients will have a total body potassium deficit, however, Serum glucose is elevated, as are serum ketone levels. Arterial pH and blood gases usually reflect metabolic acidosis with some respiratory compensation.

Therapy is determined by the degree of ketoacidosis. Initially, correction of volume depletion and hyperosmolarity, hyperglycemia, acidosis, and potassium depletion is implemented.

Hyperglycemia Nonketotic Coma

This clinical entity is usually associated with maturity onset noninsulin-dependent diabetics. It is a syndrome of severe dehydration resulting from sustained hyperglycemic diuresis occurring under circumstances where the patient is unable to drink sufficient water to keep up with urinary losses. The patient is usually middle-aged or elderly with no history of diabetes or mild diabetes controlled by diet and/or oral agents. Some factors which may cause or aggravate hyperglycemia are: acute stress, infection, the use of glucocorticoids, thiazide diuretics, or phenytoin sodium. Preexisting renal disease is common.

Clinically, the patient presents with severe hyperglycemia, usually greater than 600 mg/dl, hyperosmolarity, and volume depletion, coupled with central nervous system signs ranging from confusion to coma. Polyuria, polydypsia, malaise, and light headedness are seen. The patient may be tachycardic, with decreased tissue turgor. Seizures of the Jacksonian type are not uncommon. A transient hemiplegia may also be seen. Laboratory analysis reveals an increased hematocrit and sodium value indicative of volume depletion. Serum potassium depletion is invariably present. The BUN and osmolarity are elevated. The serum ketones are usually negative, although sympathetic nervous stimulation of adipose tissue and fatty acid mobilization may result in mild ketonemia. A high index of suspicion for infection should be maintained, and routine blood and spinal fluid cultures are indicated. Therapy is directed to correcting volume depletion, hyperglycemia, potassium depletion and the precipitating disorder.

Septic Shock

Many diabetic infections are caused by organisms which are gram-negative. In an overwhelming infection, bacteremia may result in inadequate tissue perfusion. This results in shock due to septicemia. Although septic shock may be associated with gram-positive infections, namely *Pneumococcus* and *Streptococcus*, it is more common following bacteremia with gram-negative bacilli: *E. coli*, *Klebsiella*, *Enterobacter*, *Pseudomonas*, and *Proteus* being the most common. The shock syndrome is not due to the bloodstream invasion of bacteria per se, but is related to the release of endotoxin, the lipopolysaccharide moiety of the organisms' cell walls into the circulation. Predisposing factors include: diabetes mellitus, granulocytopenia, congestive heart failure, renal insufficiency, leukemia, lymphoma, and antecedent urinary tract or gastrointestinal, as well as wound infection. The endotoxin exerts its major effect on small blood vessels with sympathetic innervation. The intense arterial and venospasm which occurs leads to immobilization of blood in the pulmonary, splanchnic, and renal capillaries, and to hypoxia in these tissues. The activation of Factor VII (Hageman factor) and the release of bradykinin causes peripheral pooling of blood and increased capillary permeability, allowing plasma protein to leak into the interstitium. This effectively lowers circulating blood volume. The ensuing decreases in cardiac output and systemic arterial hypotension stimulate further sympathetic activity, leading to vasoconstriction and selective reduction of blood flow to visceral organs and skin. The kidney and lung are particularly susceptible to the endotoxin. The patient presents clinically with phototension, fever, chills, nausea, vomiting, tachycardia and altered mental status, metabolic acidosis, jaundice, and disseminated intravascular coagulation; renal or pulmonary failure may also complicate the clinical picture. Hypovolemia may be profound due to "third space" losses. The restoration of intravascular volume is essential to maintain adequate tissue perfusion.

Gas Gangrene

Gas gangrene or clostridal organisms including: C. perfringens, C. welchii, C. novyi, and C. histolyticum. These organisms grow on anoxic tissue and produce at least 12 exotoxins. α-Toxin, a lecithinase, is clearly the most important and causes tissue destruction and hemolysis. C. perfringens also produces collagenase, hemolytic theca toxin, hyaluronidase, leukocidin, deoxyinbonuclease and fibrinolysin.

Organisms which must be included in the differential diagnosis due to their ability to produce gas are other anaerobes such as;

Peptostreptococcus and Bacteroides fragilis. Other organisms include E. coli, Klebsiella, β-hemolytic Streptococcus, Streptococcus pyogenes, and Staphylococcus aureus.

The clinical presentation of gas gangrene includes a sudden onset with rapidly increasing wound pain. The incubation period is usually 1–4 days, but may vary from 3 hours to 6 weeks. There is a fall in blood pressure with resultant tachycardia. The patient may be febrile but not proportionate to the severity of the inflammation. The wound becomes edematous, and the surrounding skin is pale as a result of fluid accumulation beneath it. Vesicles or hemorrhagic bullae may appear. The wound drainage is brown to brown-tinged, serous, and foul-smelling. As the process continues, the surrounding tissues change from pale to dusk and deeply discolored. Gas may be palpable in the tissues in advanced cases, but can easily be seen on x-ray or auscultated. Systemic manifestations may also include: anorexia, vomiting, profuse watery or bloody diarrhea, and, eventually, circulatory collapse.

Treatment involving administration of high doses of penicillin (20 million units per day IV) following aerobic and anaerobic cultures, gram staining, and the usual laboratory analyses. Multiple hyperbaric oxygen treatments may reduce the amount of surgical debridement, which will be necessary. A tetanus toxoid booster should also be given.

References

1. Rice, J. Diabetic infection, ulceration, and gangrene. JAPA 64:74, 1974.
2. Barrer, J., and Mooney, V. Neuropathy and diabetic pressure lesions. Orthop. Clin. North Am. 4:45, 1973.
3. Martin, W., Weil, L., and Smith, S. Surgical management of neurotrophic ulcers in the diabetic foot. JAPA 65:365, 1975.
4. Louie, T. J., et al.: Aerobic and anaerobic bacteria in diabetic foot ulcers. Ann. Intern. Med. 85:461–463, 1976.
5. Bailey, C. C., and Root, H. F. Neuropathic foot lesions in diabetes mellitus. N. Engl. J. Med. 236:397, 1947.
6. Rubiow, A., Spark, E. C., and Canoso, J. J. Septic arthritis in a Charcot joint. Clin. Orthop. Relat. Res. 147:203, 1980.
7. Whitehouse, W. M., and Smith, W. S. Osteo-

myelitis of the feet. Semin. Roentgenol. 5:367, 1970.

8. Levin, M., and O'Neal, L. W. *The Diabetic Foot.* C. V. Mosby, St. Louis, 1973.

9. Ellenberg, M. Diabetic foot, N. Y. State. J. Med. 73:2778, 1973.

10. Godinsky, M. A study of the fascial spaces of the foot and their bearing on infections. Surg. Gynecol. Obstet. 39:437, 1929.

11. Coldwell, A. R. Vascular disease in diabetes. Diabetes 14:110, 1965.

12. Dible, J. H. Some pathological adaptions in the peripheral circulation. Lancet 1:1031, 1958.

13. Bloodworthy, J. M. B., Jr. Diabetic microangiopathy. Diabetes 12:9919, 1963.

14. Marble, A. Relation of control of diabetes to vascular sequellae. Med. Clin. North Am. 49:1137, 1965.

15. Rifkin, H., and Leiter, L. *Diabetic Microangiopathy in Clinical Diabetes Mellitus* edited by M. Ellenberg and H. Rifken. McGraw-Hill, New York, 1962.

16. Locke, S. Diabetes and the nervous system. Med. Clin. North Am. 49:1081, 1965.

17. Ellenberg, M. Long-term problems, in *Diabetic Neuropathy in Diabetes Mellitus: Diagnosis and Treatment*, edited by Danowski, T. S. American Diabetes Association, New York, 1964.

18. Spritz, N. Nerve disease in diabetes mellitus. Med. Clin. North Am. 62:787, 1978.

19. Pirart, J. Diabetic neuropathy: A metabolic or vascular disease? Diabetes 14:1, 1965.

20. Dolman, C. L. The morbid anatomy of diabetic neuropathy. Neurology 15:2, 1963.

21. Lippmann, H. I., Perotto, A., and Farrar, R. The neuropathic foot of the diabetic. Bull., N. Y. Acad. Med. 52:1159, 1976.

22. Gray, R. G., and Gottlieb, N. L. Rheumatic disorders associated with diabetes mellitus (literature review). Semin. Arthritis Rheum. 6:19, 1976.

23. Forgacs, S. Stages and roentgenological picture of diabetic osteoarthropathy. Fortschr. Geb. Roentgenstr. Nuklearmed. 126:36, 1977.

24. Sheppe, W. Neuropathic (Charcot) joints occurring in diabetes mellitus. Ann. Intern. Med. 39:625, 1953.

25. Byyny, R. L. Management of diabetics during surgery. Postgrad. Med. 68:191–202, 1980.

26. Levin, C. N., and Deally, F. N. The surgical diabetic: A five-year survey. Ann. Surg. 102:1029–1039, 1935.

27. Galloway, J. A., and Shuman, C. R. Diabetes and surgery: A study of 667 cases. Am. J. Med. 34:177, 1963.

28. Galloway, J. A. *Surgery in Diabetic Patients in Diabetes Mellitus*, 8th ed. Lilly Research Laboratories, Indianapolis, 1980.

29. Meade, J. W., and Mueller, C. B. Major infections of the foot. Med. Times 96:154, 1968.

30. Wagner, F. W., Jr. Amputations of the foot and ankle: Current status. Clin. Orthop. 122:62, 1977.

31. Wagner, F. W., Jr. A classification and treatment program for diabetic, neuropathic, and dysvascular foot problems. Part II: Management of the diabetic, neurotrophic foot. American Academy Orthopedic Surgeons, Instructional Course Lectures. Mosby, St. Louis, 1979, pp. 143–165.

32. Wagner, F. W. The dysvascular foot: A system for diagnosis and treatment. Foot Ankle 2:64–121, 1981.

33. Condon, R. E., and Nyhus, L. M. *Manual of Surgical Therapeutics*, 5th ed. Little, Brown & Co., Boston, 1982, p. 232.

34. Moore, F. D. *The Metabolic Care of the Surgical Patient*, W. B. Saunders, Philadelphia, 1959.

35. Fletcher, J., Langman, M. J. S., and Kellock, T. D. Effect of surgery on blood-sugar levels in diabetes mellitus. Lancet 2:52, 1965.

36. Jones, R. L., and Peterson, C. M. Hematologic alterations in diabetes mellitus. Am. J. Med. 70:339–349, 1981.

37. Alberti, K. G. M. M., Emerson, P. M., Darley, J. H., et al.: Red cell 2,3-diphosphoglycerate and tissue oxygenation in uncontrolled diabetes mellitus. Lancet 2:391, 1972.

38. McMillan, D. E., et al.: Reduced erythrocyte deformability in diabetes. Diabetes 27:895, 1978

Vascular Disease

39. Colwell, J. A., et al.: Vascular disease in diabetes: Pathophysiological mechanisms and therapy. Arch. Intern. Med. 139:139, 1979.

40. Gancia, O. W. Pathogenesis of macrovascular disease in the human diabetic. Diabetes 29:931–939, 1980.

41. Wagner, F. W., Jr. Transcutaneous Doppler ultrasound in the prediction of healing and the selection of surgical level for dysvascular lesions of the toes and forefoot. Clin. Orthop. Relat. Res. 142:110–114, 1979.

42. Pascarelli, E. F., and Bethrand, C. A. Comparison of blood pressures in the arms and legs. N. Engl. J. Med. 270:693, 1964.

43. Verta, M. J., et al.: Forefoot perfusion pressure and minor amputation for gangrene. Surgery 80:729–734, 1976.

44. Raines, J. R., et al.: Vascular laboratory criteria for the management of peripheral vascular disease of the lower extremities. Surgery 79:21–29, 1976.

45. Strandness, D. E., Jr., et al.: Application of a transcutaneous Doppler flowmeter in evaluation of occlusive arterial disease. Surg. Gynecol. Obstet. 122:1039–1045, 1966.

46. Bailey, M. J., et al.: Preoperative hemoglobin as predictor of outcome of diabetic amputations. Lancet 2:168–170, 1979.

47. Kacy, S. S., et al.: Factors affecting the results of below knee amputation in patients with and without diabetes. Surg. Gynecol. Obstet. 144:513–518, 1977.

48. Lassen, N. A., and Holstein, P. Use of radioisotopes in assessment of distal blood flow and distal blood pressure in arterial insufficiency. Surg. Clin. North Am. 54:39–55, 1974.

49. Kostuik, J. P., et al.: The measurement of skin blood flow in peripheral vascular disease by epicutaneous application of Xenon 133. J. Bone Jt. Surg. Am. Vol. 58A:833–837, 1976.

50. Seder, J. J., et al.: Detecting and localizing peripheral arterial disease: Assessment of 201 TI scintigraphy. Am. J. Radiol. 137:373–380, 1981.

51. Siegel, M. E., and Siemsen, J. K. A new non-

invasive approach to peripheral disease: TI 201 leg scans. Am. J. Radiol. 131:827–830, 1978.

52. Sejrsen, P. E. R. Atraumatic local labeling of skin by Xenon 133 for blood flow measurement: Use of Xenon 133 clearance methods in burns. Scand. J. Plastic. Reconstr. Surg. 2:39–43, 1968.

53. Moore, W. S. Amputation level determination by skin blood flow measurement using Xenon 133. Presented at the Twenty-First Scientific Meeting of the International Cardiovascular Society, Toronto, Ontario, Canada, June, 1973.

54. Mayne, E. C., et al.: Platelet adhesiveness, platelet fibrinogen and factor VIII levels in diabetes mellitus. Diabetologia 6:436–440, 1970.

55. Odegard, A. E., et al.: Increased activity of "anti-Willebrand factor" in diabetic plasma. Thromb. Diath. Haemorrh. 11:27–37, 1964.

56. Breddin, K. Experimental and clinical investigations on the adhesion and aggregation of human platelets. Exp. Biol. Med. 3:14–23, 1968.

57. Bagdade, J. D., et al.: Diabetic lipemia: A form of acquired fat-induced lipemia. N. Engl. J. Med. 276:427, 1967.

58. McMillan, D. E. Deterioration of the microcirculation in diabetes. Diabetes 24:944–957, 1975.

59. Siperstein, M. D., et al.: Studies of muscle capillary basement membrane in normal subjects, diabetics, and pre-diabetic patients. J. Clin. Invest. 47:1973–1999, 1968.

60. Kilo, C., et al.: Muscle capillary basement membrane changes related to aging and to diabetes mellitus. Diabetes 21:881–898, 1972.

61. Colwell, J. A. Effect of diabetic control on vascular disease in clinical recognition and treatment of diabetic vascular disease. Charles C. Thomas, Springfield, 1975, pp. 38–48.

62. Spiro, R. G. Investigation into the biochemical basis of diabetic basement membrane alterations. Diabetes 25:909–913, 1976.

63. Dowd, P. M., et al.: Treatment of Raynaud's phenomenon by intravenous infusion of prostacyclin (PGI$_2$). Br. J. Dermatol. 106:81–89, 1982.

64. Willerson, J. T., et al.: Reserpine in Raynaud's disease and phenomenon: Short-term response to intra-arterial injection. Ann. Intern. Med. 72:17–27, 1970.

65. Charles, C. R., and Carmick, S. Skin temperature changes in Raynaud's disease after griseofulvin. Arch. Dermatol. 101:331–336, 1970.

66. Varaai, D. P., and Laurence, A. W. Suppression of Raynaud's phenomenon by methyldopa. Arch. Intern. Med. 124:13–18, 1969.

67. Kety, S. S. Measurement of regional circulation by the local clearance of radioactive sodium. Am. Heart J. 38:321–328, 1949.

68. Thulesius, O. Beurteilung des Schweregrades Arterieller Durchblutungs-storungen mit dem Doppler-Ultraschall Monografie, Gesellschaft fur Angiogie, Schweitz Huberverlag, 1971.

69. Kappert, A. Contribution to the discussion at the Symposium on Peripheral Blood Flow, Blood Pressure, and Metabolism in Control of Surgical and Medical Therapy, Copenhagen, 1972. Scand. J. Clin. Lab. Invest. 31:128, 1973.

70. Ogbuawa, O., et al.: Diabetic gangrene in black patients. South. Med. J. 75:285–288, 1982.

71. Catteral, R. F. C. The surgeon's viewpoint. Postgrad. Med. 44:969–973, 1968.

72. Cameron, H. C., et al.: Amputations in the diabetic outcome and survival. Lancet 2:605–607, 1964.

73. Retief, D. H., and Dreyer, C. J. Effects of neurodamage on the repair of bony defects in the rat. Arch. Biol. 12:1035–1039, 1967.

74. Eloesser, L. On the nature of neuropathic affections of the joints. Ann. Surg. 66:207–207, 1971.

75. Bower, A. C., et al.: Pathogenesis of the neurotrophic joint: Neurotraumatic versus Neurovascular. Radiology 139:349–354, 1981.

76. Schuster, S., and Jacobs, A. Diabetic autonomic neuropathy in the surgical management of the diabetic foot. J. Foot Surg. 21:16–22, 1982.

77. Timperly, W. R., et al.: Clinical and histologic studies in diabetic neuropathy. Diabetilogica 12:237, 1936.

78. Olsson, Y., and Sourander, P. Changes in the sympathetic nervous system in diabetes mellitus. J. Neurovasc. Rel. 31:86, 1968.

79. Asbury, A. R., and Johnson, P. C. Pathology of peripheral nerves, in *Major Problems in Pathology*. W. B. Saunders, Philadelphia, 1978, vol. 9, pp. 96–109.

80. Anderson, J. W. Metabolic abnormalities contributing to diabetic complications. Am. J. Clin. Nutr. 29:402, 1976.

81. Clements, R. S. Diabetic neuropathy. Diabetes 28:604, 1979.

82. Clarke, B. F., et al.: Clinical features of diabetic autonomic neuropathy. Horm. Metab. Res. 9:50, 1980.

83. Goodman, J. I. Diabetic anhidrosis. Am. J. Med. 41:831, 1966.

84. Martin, M. M. Involvement of automatic nerve fibers in diabetic neuropathy. Lancet 1:560, 1953.

85. Barany, F. R., and Cooper, E. H. Pilomotor and sudomotor innervation in diabetes. Clin. Sci. (Lond.) 15:533, 1956.

86. Rundle, R. W. Diabetic neuropathy. Medicine 24:111, 1945.

87. Bruckner, F. E., and Howell, A. Neuropathic joints. Semin. Arthritis Rheum. 2:47–69, 1972.

88. Deanfield, J. E., et al.: The role of autonomic neuropathy in diabetic foot ulceration. J. Neurol. Sci. 47:203–210, 1980.

89. Feldman, F. Neuropathic osteoarthropathy. In *Diagnostic Radiology*. UCSF Press, 1977, pp. 397–418.

90. Norman, A., et al.: The acute neuropathic arthropathy: A rapid, severely disorganizing form of arthritis. Radiology 90:1159–1164, 1968.

91. Shim, S. S. Physiology of blood circulation of bone. J. Bone Jt. Surg. 50A:812, 1968.

92. Faerman, I., et al.: Autonomic nervous system and diabetes. Diabetes 22:225, 1973.

93. Page, M., et al.: Prevention of postural hypotension by insulin in diabetic autonomic neuropathy. Diabetes 25:90, 1976.

94. Bradley, R. F., and Schonfeld, A. Diminished pain in diabetic patients with acute myocardial infarction. Geriatrics 17:322, 1962.

95. Kassander, P. Asymptomatic gastric retention in diabetes. Am. Intern. Med. 48:797, 1958.

96. Campbell, I. W., et al.: Diabetic autonomic neuropathy. Br. J. Clin. Pract. 30:153, 1976.

97. Stewart, I. M., et al.: Esophageal motor changes in diabetes mellitus. Thorax 31:278, 1976.

98. Zimmerman, M. A. The neuropathies of diabetes: Part I. The symmetric polyneuropathy. Minn. Med. 63:119–124, 1980.

99. Lam, S. J. S. A tarsal tunnel syndrome. Lancet 2:1354–1355, 1962.

100. Keck, C. The tarsal tunnel syndrome. J. Bone Jt. Surg. 44A:180–182, 1962.

101. Oloff, L., Jacobs, A. M., and Jaffe, S. Tarsal tunnel syndrome in systemic disease. J. Foot Surg., accepted for publication.

102. Roux, as cited by Lam, S. J. S. Tarsal tunnel syndrome. J. Bone Jt. Surg. 49B:87–92, 1967.

103. Behse, F., Buchtal, F., and Carlseu, F. Nerve biopsy and conduction studies in diabetic neuropathy. J. Neurol. Neurosurg. Psychiat. 40:1072–1082, 1977.

104. Behse, F., Buchtal, F., and Rosenfalck, A. *Sensory Conduction and Quantitation of Biopsy Findings in Studies in Neuromuscular Diseases,* edited by Kunze, K., and Desmedt, J. E. Karger, Basal, 1975, pp. 229–231.

105. LeMont, H., et al.: Sensory conduction studies of the branches of the superficial peroneal nerve. Arch. Physical Med. Rehab. 62:24–27, 1981.

Radiographic and Nuclear Medicine Considerations

106. Gangrene Localized to Lower Extremities in Diabetics-Lithner F., et al, Acta. Med. Scand., 1980, 208 (4):315–320.

107. Infection and Diabetes Mellitus, Wheat, L. J., Diabetes Care, 1980, Jan.-Feb., 3 (1):187–97, (139 ref.).

108. Park, H., et al.: Three phase bone scan in diabetic foot. J. Nuc. Med. 20:602–603, 1979.

109. Park, H. M., et al. Scintigraphic evaluation of diabetic osteomyelitis: Concise communication. J. Nucl. Med. 23:569–573, 1982.

110. Hoffer, P. Gallium and infection. J. Nucl. Med. 21:484, 1980.

111. Raptopoulos, V. et al. Acute osteomyelitis: Advantage of white cell scans in early detection. AJR 139, 1078–1082, Dec., 1982.

112. Lisbona, R., and Rosenthal, L. Observation on the sequential use of 99mTC—phosphate complex and 67GA imaging in osteomyelitis, cellulitis, and septic arthritis. Radiology 123:123–129, April, 1977.

113. Giesecke, S. B. et al. Lisfranc's fracture dislocation: A manifestation of peripheral neuropathy. Am. J. Roentgenol. 131:139, 1976.

114. Newman, J. H. Spontaneous dislocation in diabetic neuropathy. J. Bone Jt. Surg. 61B:484, 1979.

115. Lippman, E. M., et al. Neurogenic arthropathy associated with diabetes mellitus. J. Bone Jt. Surg. 37A:971, 1955.

116. Johnson, J. T. H. Neuropathic fractures and joint injuries. J. Bone Jt. Surg. 49A:1, 1967.

117. Coventry, M. B. et al. Bilateral calcaneal fracture in a diabetic patient. J. Bone Jt. Surg. 61A:462, 1979.

118. El-Khoury, G. Y., and Kathol, M. H. Neuropathic fractures in patients with diabetes mellitus. Radiation 134:313, 1980.

119. Martin, M. M. Neuropathic lesions of the feet in diabetes mellitus. Proc. R. Soc. Med. 47:139, 1954.

120. Lippmann, H. I., et al. The neuropathic foot of the diabetic. Bull. N. Y. Acad. Med. 52:1159, 1976.

121. Bailey, C. C., and Root, H. F. Neuropathic foot lesions in diabetes mellitus. N. E. J. Med. 236:397, 1947.

122. Foster, D. B., and Bassett, R. C. Neurogenic arthropathy associated with diabetic neuropathy. Arch. Neurol. Physiol. 57:173, 1947.

123. Sella, E. J. Diabetic neurosteoarthropathy of the tarsus. Conn. Med. 43:70, 1979.

124. Boehm, H. J. Diabetic Charcot joint. N. Engl. J. Med. 267:185, 1962.

125. Finby, N. et al. Diabetic osteopathy of the foot and ankle. Am. Family Phys. 14:90, 1976.

126. Kraft, E., et al. Neurogenic disorders of the foot in diabetes mellitus. Am. J. Roentgenol. 124:17, 1975.

127. Friedman, S. A., and Rakow, R. B. Osseous lesions in the foot in diabetic neuropathy. Diabetes 20:302, 1971.

128. Wolf, D. S., et al. Charcot's joint in a juvenile onset diabetic. JAPA 67:201, 1977.

129. Cozen, L. Does diabetes delay fracture healing? Clin. Orthop. 82:134–140, 1972.

130. Levin, M. E. et al. Effects of diabetes mellitus on bone mass in juvenile and adult onset diabetes. N. Engl. J. Med. 294:241–244, 1976.

131. McNair, P. et al. Bone loss in diabetes: Effects of metabolic state. Diabetologia 17:283–286, 1979.

132. Weiss, R. E. et al. Abnormalities in the biosynthesis of cartilage and bone proteoglycans in experimental diabetes. Diabetes 30:670–677, 1981.

133. Cerawi, A., et al. Role of nonenzymatic glycosylation in the development of the sequelae of diabetes mellitus. Metabolism 28:431–437, 1979.

134. Berenson, A. S., et al. Acid mucopolysaccharide changes in diabetic kidneys. Diabetes 19:161–170, 1970.

135. Schneir, M., et al. Response of rat connective tissues to streptozotocin diabetes: Tissue-specific effects on collagen metabolism. Biochem. Biophys. Acta 583:95–102, 1979.

136. Golub, L. M. et al. Inflammatory changes in gingival collagen in the allozan-diabetic rat. J. Periodontal Res. 12:402–418, 1977.

137. Menezel, J., et al. Prevalence of diabetes mellitus in Jerusalem: Its association with presenile osteoporosis. Isr. J. Med. Sci. 8:918–919, 1972.

138. Berney, P. W. Osteoporosis and diabetes mellitus. J. Iowa Med. Soc. 42:10–12, 1952.

139. Kuhlencordt, H., et al. Dtsch. Med. Wochenschr. 91:1913–1917, 1966.

140. Forgacs, S., et al. Bone changes in diabetes mellitus. Isr. J. Med. Sci. 8:782–783, 1972.

141. Neuman, H. W., et al. Occurrence of diabetes mellitus in 201 patients with femoral neck fractures and spinal compression. Zentralbl. Chir. 97:831–836, 1972.

142. Heath, H., et al. Diabetes mellitus and the risk of skeletal fracture. N. Engl. J. Med. 303:567–570, 1900.

143. Park, H. M., et al. Scintigraphic evaluation of diabetic osteomyelitis: Concise communication. J. Nucl. Med. 23:569–573, 1982.

144. Scoles, P. V., et al. Bone scan patterns in acute

osteomyelitis. Clin. Orthop. Relat. Res. 153: 210–217, 1980.

145. Classen, J. N., Rolley, R. T., Carneiro R., et al. Management of foot conditions of the diabetic patient. Ann. Surg. 42:81–88, 1976.

146. Eymontt, M. J., Alavia Dalinka, M. K., et al. Bone scintography in diabetic osteoarthropathy. Radiology 140:475–477, 1981.

147. Morrey, B. F., and Peterson, H. A. Hematogenous pyogenic osteomyelitis in children. Orthop. Clin. North Am. 6:935–951, 1975.

148. Dich, V. Q., et al. Osteomyelitis in infants and children: A review of 163 cases. Am. J. Dis. Child. 129:1273–1278, 1975.

149. Nade, S. Choice of antibiotics in management of acute osteomyelitis and acute septic arthritis in children. Arch. Dis. Child. 52:679–682, 1977.

150. Mackowiak, P. A. et al. Diagnostic value of sinus tract cultures in chronic osteomyelitis. JAMA 239:2772–2775, 1978.

151. Johnson, P. H. Pseudomonas infections of the foot following puncture wounds. JAMA 204:262, 1968.

152. Waldvogel, F. A., and Vasey, H. Osteomyelitis: The past decade. N. Engl. J. Med. 303:360–368, 1980.

153. Kahn, D. S., and Pritzner, K. D. H. The pathophysiology of bone infection. Clin. Orthop. 96:12–19, 1973.

154. Norden, C. W. Experimental osteomyelitis: I. A. description of the model. J. Infect. Dis. 122:410–418, 1970.

155. Cunda, B. A., et al. The penetration characteristics of cefazolin, cephalothin, and cephradine into bone in patients undergoing total hip replacement. J. Bone Jt. Surg. 59:856–859, 1977.

156. Deysine, M., et al. Acute hematogenous osteomyelitis: An experimental model. Surgery 79:97–99, 1976.

157. Bell, S. M. Further observations on the value of oral penicillins in chronic staphlococcal osteomyelitis. Med. J. Aust. 2:591–593, 1976.

158. Becher, R. B., and Spadaro, J. A. Treatment of orthopaedic infections with electrically generated silver ions. J. Bone Jt. Surg. 60A:871–880, 1978.

159. MaClennan, J. D. The histotoxic clostridial infections of man. Bacteriol. Rev. 26:177, 1962.

160. Miskew, D. B. et al. Clostridial myonecrosis is in a patient undergoing oxacillin therapy for exacerbation of chronic foot ulcers and osteomyelitis. Clin. Orthop. Relat. Res. 138, 1979.

161. Altmeir, W. A., and Culbertson, W. R. Acute non-clostridial crepitant cellulitis. Surg. Gynecol. Obstet. 87:206, 1948.

162. Drago, J. J. Emphysematous cellulitis in diabetes. JAPA 72:201–203, 1982.

163. Fisher, A. M., and McKusick, V. A. Bacteroides infections: Clinical, bacteriological, and therapeutic features of fourteen cases. Am. J. Med. Sci. 225:253, 1953.

164. DeHaven, K. E., and Evarts, C. M. The continuing problems of gas gangrene: A review and report of illustrative cases. J. Trauma 11:12, 1971.

165. Fischer, B. H. Treatment of ulcers on the legs with hyperbaric oxygen. J. Dermatol. Surg. 55–58, 1978.

166. Root, H. F. Factors favoring successful transmetatarsal amputation in diabetics. (1948), N. Engl. J. Med. 239:453, 1948.

167. McKitterick, L. S., and Drisley, T. S. Ann. Transmetatarsal amputation for infections and gangrene for patients with diabetes mellitus. Ann. Surg. 130:826–842, 1949.

168. Sizer, J. S., and Wheelock, F. C., Jr. Digital amputations in diabetic patients. Surgery 72:980–989, 1972.

169. Kacy, S. S., et al. Factors affecting the results of below knee amputation in patients with and without diabetes. Surg. Gynecol. Obstet. 155:513–518, 1982.

170. Pertracelli, R. C. Amputations of the lower extremity. Orthop. Rev. 10:113–114, 1981.

171. Baddeley, R. W., and Fulford, J. L. A trial of conservative amputations for lesions of the feet in diabetes mellitus. Br. J. Surg. 52:000, 1965.

172. Goodman, J., et al. Risk factors in local surgical procedures for diabetic gangrene. Surg. Gynecol. Obstet. 143:587–591, 1976.

173. Wheelock, F. L., Jr. Transmetatarsal amputations and arterial surgery in diabetic patients. N. Engl. J. Med. 264:316–320, 1976.

174. Verta, M. J., Jr., et al. Forefoot perfusion pressure and minor amputation for gangrene. Surgery 30:729–734, 1900.

175. Messner, K., et al. Acute normovolemic hemodilution. Eur. Surg. Res. 4:55–70, 1972.

176. Dormandy, J. A., et al. Treatment of severe intermittent claudication by controlled defibrination. Lancet 1:625–626, 1977.

177. Tucker, B., et al. Zinc deficiency (remarks). JAMA 235:2399, 1976.

178. Mather, M., et al. Hypomagnesaemia in diabetes. Clin. Chim. Acta 95:235–242, 1979.

179. Brown, P. The fate of exposed bone, presented at the fifty-ninth annual meeting of the New England Surgical Society, 1978.

180. Burgess, E. Wound healing amputation. Effects of controlled environment: A preliminary study. J. Bone Jt. Surg. 60A:245–246, 1978.

181. Zaricznyj, J. B. Correction of equinus deformity following midtarsal amputation by tibiotalar arthrodesis. Clin. Orthop. Relat. Res. 160:222–227, 1981.

Suggested Readings

Vascular Complication (WHO Multinational Study of Vascular Disease in Diabetics)

Arenson, D. J., et al. Neuropathy, angiopathy and sepsis in the diabetic foot. II. Angiopathy. JAPA 71:661–665, 1981.

Jarrett, R. J. et al. General description. Diabetes Care 2:175–186, 1979.

Jarrett, R. J., et al. Microvascular disease. Diabetes Care 2:196–201, 1979.

Keen, H., et al. Macrovascular disease prevelance. Diabetes Care 2:187–195, 1979.

Infection

Arenson, D. J., et al. Neuropathy, angiopathy, and sepsis in the diabetic foot: III. Sepsis. JAPA 72:35–40, 1982.

Frankle, D. R., et al. Gangrene in the diabetic foot: Its implications and consequences. J. Foot Surg. 17:112–117, 1978.

Murphy, D. P., et al. Infectious complications in diabetic patients. Primary Care 8:695–714, 1981.

Rayfield, E. J., et al. Infection and diabetes: The case for glucose control. Am. J. Med. 72:439–450, 1982.

West, K. M. Infection and diabetes mellitus. J. Med. 130:515–521, 1979.

Wheat, L. J. Infection and diabetes mellitus. Diabetes Care 3:187–197, 1980.

Radiology

Geoffrey, J., et al. The feet in diabetes: Roentgenologic observation in 1501 cases. Diagn. Imaging 48:286–293, 1979.

Glynn, T. P., Jr. Marked gallium accumulation in neurogenic arthropathy. J. Nucl. Med. 22:1016–1017, 1981.

Reinhardt, K. The radiological residua of healed diabetic arthropathies. Skel. Rad. 7:167–172, 1981.

Resnick, D. R. *Niwayama diagnosis of bone and joint DK orders.* W. B. Saunders, Philadelphia, 1981, chapt. 60, pp. 2042–2129.

Hyperglycemic Nonketotic Coma

McCurdy, D. K. Hyperosmolar hyperglycemic nonketotic diabetic coma. Med. Clin. North Am. 54:683–699, 1970.

Podolsky, S. Hyperosmolar nonketotic coma in the elderly diabetic. Med. Clin. North Am. 62:815–828, 1978.

Author. *Manual of Surgical Therapeutics.* Little, Brown, & Co. Boston, 1981, pp. 231–234.

Gas Gangrene

Bessman, A. N., and Wagner, W. Nonclostridial gas gangrene. JAMA 233:958, 1975.

Darke, S. G., et al. Gas gangrene and related infection. Port. J. Surg. 64:104, 1977.

Drago, J. J., et al. Emphysematous cellutis in diabetes. JAPA 72:210, 1982.

Weinstein, L., and Barza, M. A. Gas gangrene. N. Engl. J. Med. 289:1129, 1973.

Amputation

Petrucelli, R. C. Amputations of the lower extremity. Resident Rev. #27, Orthop. Rev. Vol. X, No. 6, June, 1981.

Sizer, J. S., and Wheelock, F. C. Digital amputations in diabetic patients. Surgery 72:980–989, 1972.

Wheelock, F. C. Transmetatarsal amputation and arterial surgery in diabetic patients. N. Engl. J. Med. 264:316–320, 1964.

Robson, M. C., Edstrom, L. E. The diabetic foot: An alternative approach to major amputation. Surg. Clin. North Am. 57, 1977.

Gram-negative Sepsis

Anderson, E. P., et al. Antimicrobial synergism in the therapy of gram-negative rod bacterium. Chemotherapy 24:45–54, 1978.

Kreger, B., et al. Gram-negative bacteremia: III. reassessment of etiology, epidemiology and ecology in 612 patients. Am. J. Med. 68:332–343, 1980.

Kreger, B., et al. Gram-negative bacteremia: IV. Reevaluation of clinical features and treatment in 612 patients. Am. J. Med. 68:344–355, 1980.

Schumer, W. Steroids in the treatment of clinical septic shock. Ann. Surg. 184:333–334, 1976.

Young, L. S., et al. Gram-negative rod bacteremia: Microbiology, immunologic and therapeutic considerations. Ann. Intern. Med. 86:456–471, 1977.

Osteomyelitis

Waldvogel, F. A., and Vasey, H. Osteomyelitis: The past decade. N. Engl. J. Med. 303:360–369, 1980.

Scoles, D. V., et al. Bond scan patterns in acute osteomyelitis. Clin. Orthop. Relat. Res. 153:210–217, 1980.

Park, H.-M., et al. Scintographic evaluation of diabetic osteomyelitis: Concise communication. J. Nucl. Med. 23:569–573, 1982.

Diabetic Ketoacidosis

Harrison, T. R. *Principles of Internal Medicine*, 1900, pp. 1746–1749.

Eisenberg, M., and Copass, M. *Emergency Medical Therapy*, 2nd ed. 1900, pp. 49–53.

Alberti, O., and Kamm Nattrass, M. Severe diabetic ketoacidosis. Med. Clin. North Am. 62:799–814, 1978.

Surgical Anatomy of the Diabetic Foot

Kamel, R., and Sakla, F. B. Anatomical compartments of the sole of the human foot. Anat. Rec. 140:57, 1961.

Feingold, M. L., Resnick, D., Niwayama, G., and Garetto, L. The plantar compartments of the foot, a roentgen approach: I. Experimental observations. Invest. Radiol. 12:281, 1977.

Rao, V. R., and Kini, M. G. Infections of the foot, an anatomical and experimental study of the fascial spaces and tendon sheaths with clinical correlations of certain types of infections of the foot. Indian Med. Res. Memoirs 37:1, 1957.

Diabetic Emergencies

Alberta, K. G. M. M., and Hockaday, T. D. R. Diabetic coma: A reappraisal after five years. J. Clin. Endocrinol. Metab. 6:421–455, 1977.

Alberta, K. G. M. M., and Nattrass, M. Severe diabetic ketoacidosis. Med. Clin. North. Am. 62:799–814, 1978.

Arieff, A. L., and Kleeman, C. R. Studies on mechanisms of cerebral edema in diabetic comas. J. Clin. Invest. 52:571–583, 1973.

Beigelman, P. M. Potassium in severe diabetic ketoacidosis. Am. J. Med. 54:419–420, 1973.

Beigelman, P. M. Severe diabetic ketoacidosis (diabetic "comma"). Diabetes 20:490–500, 1971.

Felig, P. Diabetic ketoacidosis. N. Engl. J. Med. 290:1360–1363, 1974.

Felig, P. Pathophysiology of diabetes mellitus. Med. Clin. North Am. 55:821–834, 1971.

Felts, P. W. *Coma in the Diabetic.* Upjohn, Kalamazoo, 1974.

Gerich, J. E., Lorenzi, M., Bier, D. M. et al. Prevention of human diabetic ketoacidosis by somatostatin; Evidence for an essential role of glucogon. N. Engl. J. Med. 292:985–989, 1975.

McGarry, J. D., and Foster, D. W. Ketogenesis and its regulation. Am. J. Med. 61:9–13, 1976.

Newman, J. H., Neff, T. A., and Ziporin, P. Acute respiratory failure associated with hypophosphatemia. N. Engl. J. Med. 296:1101–1103, 1977.

Posner, J. B., and Plum, F. Spinal fluid pH and neurologic symptoms in systemic acidosis. N. Engl. J. Med. 277:606–613, 1967.

Rosenfeld, M. G. ed. *Manual of Medical Therapeutics*, 20th ed. Little, Brown and Co., Boston, 1971, p. 376.

Skillman, T. G. Diabetic ketoacidosis. Heart Lung 7:594–602, 1978.

Soler, N. G., Bennett, M. A., Fitzgerald, M. G., et al. Intensive care in the management of diabetic ketoacidosis. Lancet 1:951–954, 1900.

Unger, R. H. The essential role of gluagon in the pathogenesis of diabetes mellitus. Lancet 1:14–16, 1975.

Neuropathy

Clements, R. S., Jr., et al. Diabetic neuropathy: Peripheral and autonomic syndrome. Postgrad. Med. 71:50–52, 55–57, 60–67, 1982.

Deanfield, J. E., et al. The role of autonomic neuropathy in diabetic foot ulceration. J. Neurol. Sci. 47:203–210, 1980.

Jacobs, R. L., et al. Office care of the insensitive foot. Foot Ankle 2:230–237, 1982.

Julsrud, M. E., Diabetic neuropathy. JAPA 71:318–322, 1981.

Kaplan, W. E., et al. Diabetic peripheral neuropathies affecting the lower extremity. JAPA 71:356–362, 1981.

Porte, D., Jr., et al. Diabetic neuropathy and plasma glucose control. Am. J. Med. 70:195–200, 1981.

Charcot Joints (Neurogenic Arthropathy)

Frykberg, R. G., et al. Neuropathic arthropathy in the diabetic foot. Am. Family Phys. 17:105–113, 1978.

Kristiansen, B. Ankle and foot fractures in diabetics provoking neuropathic joint changes. Acta. Orthop. Scand. 51:975, 1980.

Weissman, S. D., et al. Diabetic neurotrophic osteoarthropathy (Charcot joint): A case report. JAPA 70:196–200, 1980.

Zaafan, A., et al. Neuro-arthropathy (Charcot joints) occuring in diabetes mellitus. J. Egypt. Med. Assoc. 60:437, 1977.

Hypoglycemia

Eisenberg, M., and Copass, M. *Emergency Medical Therapy*, pp. 55–57.

Fajans, S. S., and Floyd, J. C. Jr. Fasting hypoglycemia in adults. N. Engl. J. Med. 294, 1975.

Krupp, M., et al. Current Med. Diagnosis and Treatment, pp. 749–771, 1980.

Medical Management

Berstein, R. E. Glycosylated hemoglobin and monitoring of diabetic control (letter). Ann. Intern. Med. 93:380, 1980.

Brownlee, M. Insulin treatment of diabetes. Hosp. Pract. 14:95–94, 1979.

Byyny, R. L. Management of diabetics during surgery. Postgrad. Med. 68:191, 198, 200, 1980.

Jones, R. L., et al. Hematologic alterations in diabetes mellitus. Am. J. Med. 70:325, 1981.

Walts, L. F., et al. Perioperative management of diabetes mellitus. Anesthesiology 55:104, 1981.

Surgical Management

Bryant, R. L. Forefoot amputation (letter). Arch. Surg. 115:889, 1980.

Gibbons, G. W., et al. Predicting success of forefoot amputations in diabetics by non-invasive testing. Arch. Surg. 114:1034, 1979.

Goodson, W. H., et al. Wound healing and the diabetic patient. Surg. Gynecol. Obstet. 149:600, 1979.

Newman, J. H. Management of the diabetic foot (letter). Ann. R. Coll. Surg. Engl. 61:485, 1979.

Whitehouse, F. W. Saving a foot and salvaging a limb. Diabetes Care 2:453, 1979.

Dermatology

Gouterman, I. H., et al. Cutaneous manifestations of diabetes. Outis 25:45–84, 1980.

Huntley, A. The cutaneous manifestations of diabetes mellitus. J. Am. Acad. Dermatol. 7:427, 1982.

CHAPTER 14

Current Concepts in the Management of Ankle Repair

CHARLES J. GUDAS, D.P.M.

Ankle fractures are among the most common orthopedic injuries. Emmett and Breck (28), who studied 10,768 fresh bone fractures over a 19-year period, found that fractures of the ankle occurred most often with a relative frequency of 8% (827/10,768). Nilsson (70) reported that the annual incidence of ankle fractures was 10–15/10,000 in a rigidly defined population. Garraway et al. (31, 32) studied the incidence of limb fractures in a demarcated population and found that, among 2,519 limb fractures which occurred during a 3-year period, ankle fractures occurred at a rate of 60.5/100,000 in males and at a rate of 41.8/100,000 in females. If these figures were extrapolated to the population of the United States in 1980, the overall number of ankle fractures would approach 158,000–200,000 per year. It is apparent from these statistics that adequate treatment of such a common traumatic injury is of vital importance.

Treatment methods for the reduction of ankle fractures vary widely and are often related to the type of injury. Malka and Tillard (59) found that open reduction gave anatomically correct results in 80–85% of fractures, and that closed reduction gave good or excellent results in 56% of the cases studied. They stated that open reduction and internal fixation of ankle fractures produced a higher number of anatomic reductions than did a technique of closed reduction with plaster. They considered it impossible to maintain good reductions with casting techniques. They also pointed out that the type of fracture is of paramount importance for the result. They found that fractures due to pronation with external rotation gave particularly bad results, regardless of the treatment utilized. Cedell (16, 17) studied the results of operative treatment for 100 supination-external rotation injuries and obtained good results in 88% of the cases. For patients with the most severe injuries (stage IV), he obtained good results in 83.6% of the cases.

Bistrom (4) used closed reduction in the treatment of 183 ankle fractures, with good results in 60% of the cases. Klossner (44) followed 167 patients who had been treated with closed reduction and found that 65% had good results. In 70 patients with closed reduction, Kristensen (45, 46) reported 64% good results. By using open reduction in the treatment of severe fracture dislocations, Voronfsov (44) obtained 77% good results, and Cretskaja (44) achieved good results in 60% of cases by using open reduction for 88 ankle fractures with displacement of the talus. Brown (44) followed 34 patients who had severe fracture-dislocations of the ankle treated with closed reduction and observed good results in 53%, whereas Willenegger (101–103) using rigid fixation techniques, obtained 81% good results in the treatment of bi- and trimalleolar fractures. It is apparent from a review of the literature that the success rate for severe bi- and trimalleolar fractures is greatest when open reduction with internal fixation is utilized.

HISTORICAL SURVEY

Active investigation into the causative force and classification of ankle fractures began in the modern era with a description by Percival Pott in 1769 (78). Pott recognized that the fibula provides an important support for the ankle joint. He stated that fracture of the fibula may result in loss of support of the ankle, and thus in abnormal foot movements. He portrayed a primary, nearly transverse fracture of the fibula with a "partial dislocation" of the ankle joint internally, and he pictured the fibula as breaking in the "weak" portion 2–3 inches above its lower extremity. The fractured end of the fibula was described as falling inward, with a rupture of the ligaments below the internal malleolus and with a partial dislocation of the tibia inward. Pott ascribed the causative force to "leaping or jumping," which disrupted the perpendicular bearing of the tibia upon the astralagus and its firm connection with the fibula. In 1922, Ashurst (1) claimed that such a fracture did not exist. It must also be noted that Pott denied the existence of a medial malleolar fracture in his description.

Dupuytren (26), in 1839, combined the teachings of early pioneers such as Pott (78), Bazille (6), Bromfield (9), and Pouteau (79). He was one of the first to distinguish ankle fractures from lesions which had previously been thought of as dislocations. In 1819, Dupuytren (26) published an essay, "The Fracture of the Lower End of the Fibula," in which he proposed theories on the mechanism of injury and on fracture types, based on clinical observation. He was the first to state that the mechanism of injury as described by the patient was unreliable, and that the actual type of fracture would give a clue as to the cause. Dupuytren concurred with Pott in describing lower fibular fractures (1), although his description of the actual site of the fracture and of the cause was unclear. He stated that the lesion was a "fracture of

the fibula, rupture of the tibiofibular ligaments, and an upward displacement of the astralagus along the fibular side of the tibia."

Cooper (21), in 1822, became the first surgeon to classify and describe the major type of ankle fractures. He outlined three major groups of lesions:

1. "Simple Dislocation of the Tibia Inward"—In this case there is a fracture of the fibula, two inches above its tip, carrying with it an attached fragment of the tibia; the lower end of the upper fragment of the fibula rests on top of the astralagus and the tibia with the internal malleolus intact descends on the medial surface of the astralagus." This fracture seems to correspond to that currently classified as the supination-external rotation type of fracture."

2. "Simple Dislocation of the Tibia Forward"—In this case there is a fracture of the fibula three inches above its tip; the internal lateral ligament is partly lacerated. The tibia and upper fragment of the fibula advance forward and the tibia rests on the upper surface of the scaphoid and internal cuneiform. In partial dislocation of the tibia forward, the articular surface of the tibia is divided in two; the anterior part rests on the scaphoid and the posterior on the astralagus." In Cooper's drawing, the fibular fracture runs obliquely upward from anterior to posterior and is at the level of or slightly above the syndesmosis. Cooper was also the first to describe a posterior fracture of the tibia in association with the other disorders.

3. "Simple Dislocation of the Tibia Outward"—The internal malleolus is obliquely fractured and separated from the shaft of the bone; the fractured portion sometimes consists only of the malleolus; at other times, the fracture passes obliquely through the articular surface of the tibia, which is thrown forward and outward on the astralagus before the external malleolus. The astralagus is sometimes fractured, and the lower extremity of the fibula is broken into sev-

eral splinters. The external and internal lateral ligaments are usually intact; but if the fibula is not broken, the external lateral ligaments are ruptured." Here Cooper appears to describe a supination fracture. He was the first to describe a fracture of the medial malleolus in combination with adduction.

Maisonneuve (58) (1840) was one of the first investigators to carry out anatomic experiments on ankle fractures. He accurately described adduction and abduction fractures, and he proposed another mechanism of injury which, he believed, explained the production of the most common type of ankle fracture, namely, outward deviation or external rotation of the foot around a vertical axis. He deduced this injury by observing a necropsy specimen with an oblique fibular fracture which he reproduced by externally rotating the foot. He theorized that this fracture always occurred following external rotation of the foot, and that there was no injury to the ligaments. Maisonneuve believed that continued external rotation would rupture the deltoid ligament, or that a pull-off fracture of the medial malleolus would occur. He stated that a second type of fibular fracture was produced when the anterior tibiofibular ligament was ruptured. This, he postulated, created a diastasis of the inferior tibiofibular joint. If external rotation continued, the fibula was fractured 3–4 inches above the tip of the lateral malleolus. In some instances, a subcapital fracture of the fibular neck was produced, which is commonly known today as a Maisonneuve fracture. Ashurst and Bromer (1) contended that Maisonneuve's chief contribution was his recognition of the oblique fracture of the lower end of the fibula as the initial stage of a fracture that affects the medial malleolus and/or deltoid ligament. Maisonneuve realized in 1840 what has been proved today, that the supination-external rotation fracture is the most common type of ankle fracture seen in general orthopedic practice.

Tillaux (95) performed experiments on cadavers in which he abducted the foot in combination with external rotation. He found that this maneuver produced a rupture of the internal lateral ligament (deltoid) or a tearing off of the internal malleolus. If the force was continued, a fibular fracture occurred 6–7 cm above the tip of the lateral malleolus. Tillaux described a fragment of bone torn from the lateral border of the tibia by the inferior tibiofibular (anterior tibiofibular) ligament. Today, this fracture in pediatric patients is often described as a Tillaux fracture, even though it was described by Cooper (21) 50 years earlier.

Honigschmied (38) studied the mechanism of injury of ankle fractures in 1877 and described the effects of certain foot movements in relation to the fracture produced and to the ligamentous injury. He reproduced dorsiflexion, plantarflexion, supination, pronation, and internal and external rotation of the foot. Honigschmied theorized that the oblique fibular fracture caused by external rotation of the foot was actually a ligamentous pull-off fracture of the "posterior" portion of the anterior tibiofibular ligament, rather than a talar-impact fracture as reported by Maisonneuve.

Destot (24), in 1911, devised a classification system in which ankle mortise and pilon fractures were delineated. He was the first to analyze ankle fractures with the use of roentgenographic interpretation. Quenu (80) disagreed with Destot's classification and put forth his own, in which fractures were grouped as uni- or bimalleolar. Tanton (94) divided fractures of the malleoli into isolated medial or lateral fractures and associated fractures of the malleoli which included low bimalleolar, low Dupuytren's, typical Dupuytren's (Pott's), and Maisonneuve fractures.

Ashurst and Bromer (1) examined 300 ankle fractures and stated that three abnormal movements, i.e., external rotation, abduction, and adduction, were responsible for 95% of fractures about the ankle. They found the following percentages of incidence: external rotation, 61%; abduction, 21%; and adduction, 13%. They further grouped external rotation fractures into first-degree (lower end of the fibula only); second-degree (lower end of the fibula plus rupture of the internal lateral ligament (deltoid), or fracture of the medial malleolus); and third-degree (fracture of the medial malleolus and lower end of the tibia). Complications of fractures caused by external rotation included posterior malleolar fracture and generation of an intermediate fracture fragment.

They divided abduction fractures into first-degree (fracture of the medial malleolus below the tibial plafond without displacement) and second-degree (rupture of the deltoid ligament or fracture of the medial malleolus, followed by a fracture of the fibula either alone or below the inferior tibiofibular joint). The majority of the fibular fractures occurred above the syndesmosis. Finally, adduction fractures were divided into three stages, which include fractures of the medial malleolus below the tibial plafond without displacement) and second first-degree (a transverse fracture of the external malleolus below the tibial plafond), second-degree (fracture of the lateral malleolus plus fracture of the medial malleolus below the tibial plafond, or fracture of the medial surface of the tibia), and third-degree (fracture of the fibula above the syndesmosis plus fracture of the tibia above the ankle joint).

Ashurst and Bromer were the first clinicians to use anatomic, surgical, and radiographic studies in a large series of ankle fractures in order to arrive at a genetic classification.

Lauge Hansen (50, 51) performed a series of experiments on freshly amputated specimens in which he determined the exact mechanism, pathologic anatomy, genetic-roentgenologic diagnosis, and genetic reduction of ankle fractures. He established the following groups of ankle fractures.

Supination-Adduction

Stage I. A pull-off transverse fracture of the distal fibula below the syndesmosis.

Stage II. A fracture of the medial malleolus, or rupture of the deltoid ligament.

Supination-Eversion (External Rotation)

Stage I. The anterior tibiofibular ligament is detached from the anterior tubercle of the tibia (Chaput (18)) with a small sheet of bone.

Stage II. If continued force is exerted, a fracture of the distal fibula occurs which runs from anterior-inferior to posterior-superior at the level of the syndesmosis.

Stage III. If eversion is continued after a distal fibular spiral fracture, avulsion of a triangular fragment from the posterio-lateral surface of the tibia occurs.

Stage IV. Rupture of the deltoid or fracture of the medial malleolus takes place.

Pronation-Abduction

Stage I. When the foot is maximally pronated, a disruptive moment of force causes a horizontal pull-off fracture of the medial malleolus.

Stage II. Continued pressure causes a rupture with a flake of bone of the anterior and posterior tibiofibular ligaments.

Stage III. Continued pronation-abduction of the foot causes an oblique fracture of the fibula, localized slightly above the articular surface of the tibia at the level of the syndesmosis. The fracture runs from medial-inferior to lateral-superior.

Pronation-Eversion (External Rotation)

Stage I. This fracture is the same as a pronation-abduction fracture; that is, a pull-off transverse fracture of the medial malleolus.

Stage II. After fracture of the medial malleolus, stress is placed on the anterior tibiofibular ligament, which ruptures. This is followed by a disruption of the interosseous membrane 6–7 cm above the syndesmosis.

Stage III. Continued eversion (external rotation) causes the talus to impact on and twist the fibula. The syndesmosis and interosseous membrane will rupture. The "torsional tension" of the fibula is exceeded, and an oblique fracture of the fibula occurs 8–9 cm above the tip of the lateral malleolus.

Stage IV. Continuation of this force causes pressure from the talus against the posterior lateral corner and the posterior lip of the tibia, which causes a fracture of this segment. This fracture is a combination of an impaction fracture and a ligamentous (posterior tibiofibular ligament) pull-off lesion of the tibia.

An exact reproduction of ankle fractures allowed Lauge Hansen to understand the mechanism of injury. By using this knowledge, he was able to reverse the injurious force and achieve a non-operative reduction in 95% of all ankle fractures.

Hendelburg (36) and Magnusson (56) disagreed with Lauge Hansen's staging of supination-eversion fractures. These authors thought that a medial malleolar fracture was produced before a posterior tibial fracture (stage III). Magnusson also believed that poorly healed anterior tibiofibular ligaments increased the occurrence of arthrosis deformans of the ankle joint (56, 57). Subsequently, Danis (23) divided ankle fractures into four groups, depending on the position of the fibular fracture in relation to the syndesmotic ligaments. Using another approach, Bonnin (7) classified "outward rotation" injuries according to three degrees of severity in relation to the site of the fibular fracture and the rupture of the syndesmosis, causing "diastasis." Cedell (17), who studied the long-term effects of supination-outward rotation injuries and the formation of osteoarthrosis of the ankle joint, concurred with Magnusson concerning poor healing of stage I injuries with later onset of arthrosis deformans. He advocated open reduction and internal fixation of the posterior malleolar fragment if it exceeded one-fourth of the articular surface.

Danis' classification was expanded by Weber (99, 103) who categorized the fracture types according to the level of the

disruption, i.e., above or below the syndesmosis. Burwell and Charnley (13) advocated the use of the Lauge Hansen genetic classification and the use of rigid internal fixation for successful reduction of ankle fractures and for prevention of later complications.

Further contributions were made by Riede (102) who demonstrated that a 2-mm displacement of the lateral malleolus may reduce the articular contact between the talus and tibia by 50%, thus leading to increased arthrosis of the joint. Lambert (47) outlined the weightbearing function of the fibula, and Ramsey and Hamilton (81) studied changes in the tibiotalar area in relation to lateral shift. In 1976, Pankovich (75) classified five stages in the formation of a Maisonneuve fracture, and he found that this fracture occurred at a much higher rate (5%) than previously thought. Pankovich (73, 74) further classified proximal fibular lesions and postulated that there are three mechanisms of injury: supination-external rotation, pronation-abduction, and pronation-external rotation. Yde (107) reaffirmed Lauge Hansen's classification; in a study of 488 ankle fractures, he concluded that 98.8% of these fractures could be classified according to Lauge Hansen's method.

The classifications used today are hybrid forms of the systems devised by Ashurst and Bromer, Lauge Hansen, Danis and Weber. About 98% of all ankle fractures can be classified according to the bony disturbance and the accompanying ligamentous disruption. The classifications of Lauge Hansen and Ashurst and Bromer place heavy emphasis upon the effect of ligamentous disturbance on the formation of the fracture, whereas the Danis-Weber classification is concerned mainly with the level of the fracture, i.e., whether it lies above or below the syndesmosis of the ankle joint.

CLASSIFICATION OF ANKLE FRACTURES
Modified Lauge Hansen System

As mentioned above, Lauge Hansen (51) utilized cadaver, roentgenographic, and surgical studies in order to determine the exact mechanism of foot placement and rotation in the production of ankle fractures. He found that four main mechanisms produce 98% of all ankle fractures: supination, supination-external rotation, pronation-abduction, and pronation-external rotation. (In this modified classification the terms "abduction" and "eversion" have been changed to "external rotation.")

SUPINATION FRACTURES

Supination fractures are divided into two stages. In stage I, if the foot is loaded excessively while in a supinated position, a pull-off ligamentous transverse fracture is produced below the syndesmosis of the ankle joint. If supination is continued, a push-off fracture of the medial malleolus occurs (Fig. 14.1). Some authors consider medial malleolar fractures as stage I and lateral malleolar fractures as stage II (Fig. 14.2). In Yde's study (107), 80.1% of all supination fractures were stage I fractures of the lateral malleolus. Approximately 70% of these were pull-off (transverse) fractures and were located below the syndesmosis (Fig. 14.3).

Of stage I fractures, 26.5% are chip of avulsion fractures at the origin of the calcaneofibular ligament (107). The type of stage II fracture is usually related to the direction of impact of the talus against the

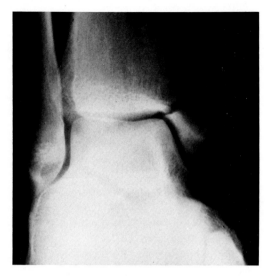

Figure 14.2.   Supination stage II without lateral malleolar fracture.

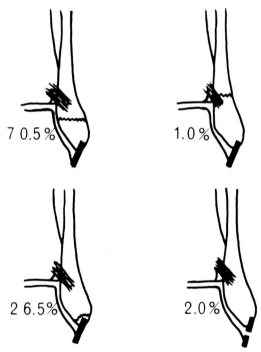

Figure 14.3.   Supination stage I: types and frequency according to Yde.

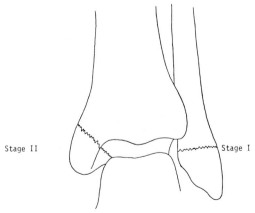

Figure 14.1.   Supination ankle fractures: stages I and I.

medial internal margin of the tibia. The fracture can involve a large portion of the posterior-medial portion of the tibia.

It is often difficult to ascertain the overall percentage of supination ankle fractures because such fractures are commonly combined with all type A lesions in the Danis-Weber classification. Lauge Hansen (50, 51) in his roentgenographic study, found a 36/228 (16%) rate of occurrence of supination fractures, with the two stages occurring with similar frequency. Solonen and Lauttamus (88) reported that 45 of 589 ankle fractures fell into the supination I and II categories with the majority of these fractures in stage II. Malka and Taillard (59), in a follow-up study of 50 ankle fractures, found a 16% incidence of supination injuries, with five of eight fractures in stage I. Yde (107), in his study of 488 ankle fractures over an 8-year period, found that 20.1% were supination fractures, with the majority (80.6%) in stage I. In our survey of ankle fractures in St. Gallen, Switzerland, we found supination stage I fractures in 79 of 803 cases, or approximately 10%. Stage II lesions made up 64% of the supination fracture series.

SUPINATION-EXTERNAL ROTATION (SER) FRACTURES

These are divided into four stages. If the supinated foot is subjected to an external rotational stress, the following sequential disruptions occur (Fig. 14.4).

Stage I

A tear of the anterior tibial tubercle of fibular ligament with or without a flake of bone from the anterior tibial tubercle occurs (18) (Fig. 14.5). According to Weber (99), in one-half of the cases, the anterior tibiofibular ligament is actually ruptured. This injury is rarely isolated and is usually associated with stage II, III, or IV fractures.

Stage II

This occurs with continued supination-external rotation. It is an oblique spiral fracture of the lateral malleolus which runs anterior-inferior to posterior-superior at the level of the syndesmosis (Fig. 14.6). This is the most common form of ankle fracture according to Lauge Hansen (51). Yde (107), Magnusson (56, 57), and Cedell (16, 17). Stage II injuries make up from 50–60% of all SER lesions. Most SER II fractures extend from approximately 1.0 cm below the ankle joint to 1.5 cm above the

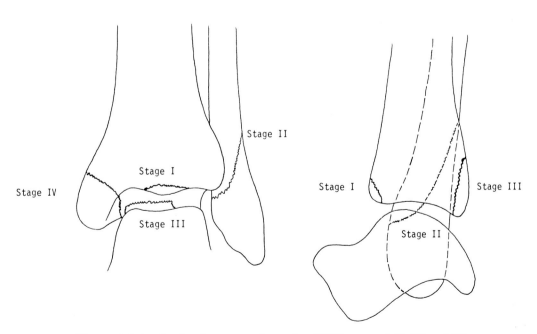

Figure 14.4. Supination external rotation (SER) stages I, II, III, and IV.

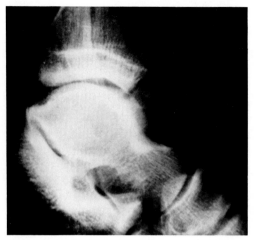

Figure 14.5. Supination external rotation (SER) stage I fracture.

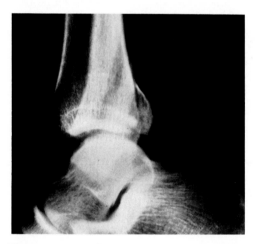

Figure 14.6. Supination external rotation (SER) stage III with characteristic stage II fibular fracture.

articular surface (107) (Fig. 14.7). Because the syndesmosis is kept intact, instability is rarely noted. Lauge Hansen (51) theorized that this fracture occurred in a weak portion on the medial surface of the fibula which has no ligamentous attachments and which is therefore less resistant to torsional forces.

Stage III

This occurs after the stage II disruption, which causes increased outward malleolar rotation. The talus is dislocated laterally;

in this position, only the dorsolateral corner and the dorsal margin of the tibia rest on the talus. This causes a considerable tightening of the posterior tibiofibular ligament. When the stress exceeds the tensile strength of the ligament, bony disruption occurs. Fracture of the posterior malleolus can involve up to one-half of the articular surface of the tibia (Fig. 14.8). In only 14% of Yde's cases (107) did the posterior fragment include more than 25% of the joint surface (Fig. 14.9). The fractures are rarely the end-stage in an SER injury. In the St. Gallen series, it occurred in only 16 of the 803 fractures. In Yde's analysis, the fracture was present as an end-stage SER fracture in 4% of the cases.

Stage IV

Supination-external rotation stage IV injuries are the second most common type of ankle injury, comprising approximately 20–25% of all ankle fractures. It is not necessary for a fracture of the posterior margin to be present before stage IV sets in. Of 193 SER IV fractures studied in St. Gallen, 59 went to stage IV without evidence of bony disruption. Stage IV occurs when outward rotation of the talus around a vertical axis is limited only by the deltoid ligament and the medial malleolus. When the force ex-

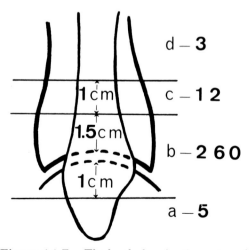

Figure 14.7. The level of supination external rotation (SER) stage II fractures in relation to the syndesmosis according to Yde.

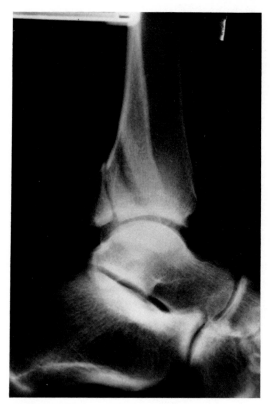

Figure 14.8. Supination external rotation (SER) stage III involving 25% of tibial articular surface.

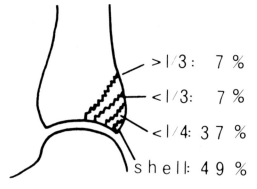

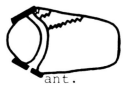

Figure 14.9. Frequency and size of the posterior fragment in supination external rotation (SER) stage III fractures according to Yde.

ceeds the strength of the bone or ligament, the medial malleolus fractures or the deltoid ligament ruptures. In about 50% of the cases, the deltoid ruptures without an obvious medial malleolar fracture (Fig. 14.10). When the medial malleolus fractures, the fracture is usually transverse, which indicates a pull-off deltoid fracture (Fig. 14.11). Between 15 and 20% of medial malleolar fractures are oblique, indicating impact from the talus. Females tend to fracture the medial malleolus approximately twice as often as males.

Overall, SER fractures are the most common ankle fractures in the Lauge Hansen classification; Lauge Hansen (50, 51) found a 71% incidence in his radiographic analysis of 228 cases. Solonen (88) found a 50% incidence in 238 ankle fractures. Yde (107) classified 57.4% of 488 ankle fractures as SER injuries. Analysis of the 803 ankle fractures in St. Gallen, Switzerland, over 8

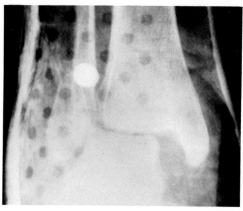

Figure 14.10. Supination external rotation (SER) stage IV with deltoid rupture.

years revealed that 441/803 fractures (54.9%) were SER fractures. Therefore, one can assume that approximately one-half of all ankle fractures are caused by supination-external rotation.

PRONATION DISRUPTIONS

Pronation disruptions are grouped in three stages (Fig. 14.12). The cause is pronation of the foot, which stresses the del-

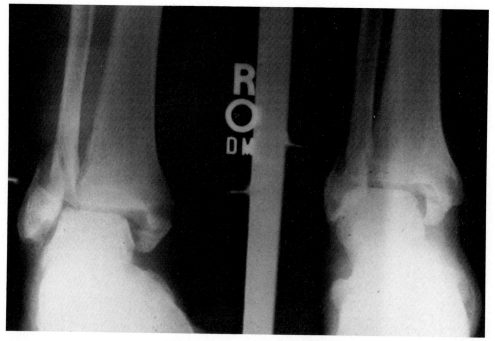

Figure 14.11. Supination external rotation (SER) stage IV with transverse pull-off medial malleolar fracture.

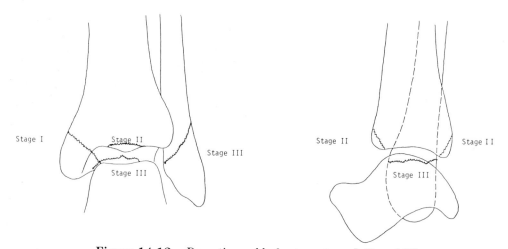

Figure 14.12. Pronation ankle fracture stages I, II, and III.

toid-medial malleolar complex, resulting in either a deltoid rupture or a fracture of the medial malleolus.

Stage I

Approximately 40–50% of stage I pronation injuries are deltoid injuries (Fig. 14.13). Medial malleolar fractures are either avulsion-transverse pull-off, chip, or oblique in nature. The oblique fracture may be caused by wedging of the wider anterior portion of the trochlear surface when the foot is in a pronated position. According to Lauge Hansen, the same mechanism of injury is responsible for pronation and for pronation-external rotation injuries.

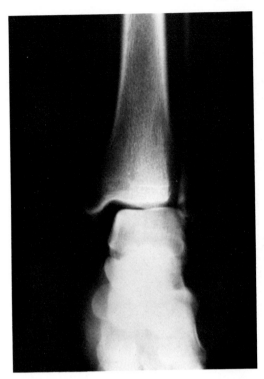

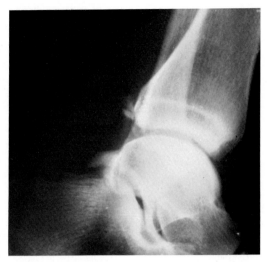

Figure 14.14. Pronation stage II posterior injury.

Figure 14.13. Pronation stage I deltoid injury.

Stage II

After medial release occurs following deltoid rupture or medial malleolar fracture, stress is placed on the anterior and posterior tibiofibular ligaments simultaneously, causing rupture of the ligaments with or without a flake of bone (Fig. 14.14). In some instances, a large posterior malleolar fragment involving more than one-fourth of the articular surface is noted. Stage II accounts for approximately 30–50% of all pronation injuries. With continued pronation, stage III sets in.

Stage III

This is a characteristic fracture of the lateral malleolus from medial to lateral in a superior direction at the level of or slightly superior to the syndesmosis (Fig. 14.15). This is caused by impaction to the lateral superior border of the trochlea of the talus when the wider anterior portion is locked in dorsiflexion and pronation.

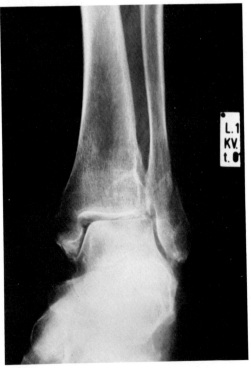

Figure 14.15. Pronation stage III fibular fracture.

Lauge Hansen found only 11 pure pronation fractures among 228 cases (52). Yde (107) reported a 1.96% incidence after combining all pronation I and II fractures with pronation-external rotation stage I and II injuries. Pure pronation fractures are extremely rare fractures, occurring in less than 5% of all ankle fractures.

PRONATION-EXTERNAL ROTATION (PER) FRACTURES

These fractures are classified into four stages (Fig. 14.16).

Stage I

If the foot is pronated and externally rotated, the deltoid malleolar complex undergoes strain until either a deltoid ligament rupture occurs or the medial malleolus is fractured. This injury is similar to a pronation stage I injury and is radiographically indistinguishable from it. The fracture sequence usually does not stop with stage I because of the force involved. In PER injuries, the foot is in maximal ground contact, thus imparting a high transverse-plane torque in a joint designed for sagittal-plane motion (Fig. 14.17).

Stage II

Continued PER causes a rupture of the anterior tibiofibular ligament with or without a shell of bone. This, in turn, initiates a rupture of the interosseous ligament and interosseous membrane to a variable height above the ankle joint (Fig. 14.18).

Stage III

With rupture of the interosseous ligament, a fracture of the fibula occurs approximately 3 inches above the joint (Fig. 14.19). It may be a short simple transverse, long or short spiral oblique, or comminuted fracture with one or more butterfly fragments (Fig. 14.20). The fracture of the fibula is found in the border region between the surgical neck and the shaft of the fibula.

Yde (107), in his analysis of 30 stage III fractures, found that no fracture occurred less than 2.5 cm above the tibiotalar joint; about 75% were located 1–3 inches above the ankle joint, with a fracture line running from the anterior fibular margin in a dorsodistal direction (Fig. 14.21). According to Lauge Hansen (51, 52) the fracture occurs at the level of the interosseous ligament and is accompanied by a membrane rupture.

Pankovich (74) who studied 36 cases of fibular fractures proximal to the syndesmosis, concluded that high fibular fractures can have three mechanisms of injury: 1) supination-external rotation, which creates a spiral oblique fibular fracture extending

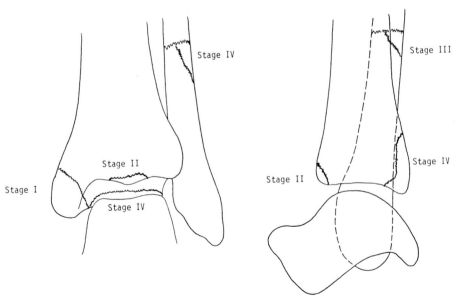

Figure 14.16.   Pronation external rotation (PER) ankle fractures stages I, II, III, and IV.

rupture of the anterior tibiofibular ligament and disruption of the interosseous ligament and membrane. The Maisonneuve fracture is frequently overlooked because of the proximal fibular fracture (Fig. 14.22). Pankovich (74) reported that this fracture comprised about 5% of all ankle fractures seen in the Cook County Hospital emergency room. In the St. Gallen study, Maisonneuve fractures occurred in 4.73% of the 803 ankle fractures studied over an 8-year period.

Stage IV

After the stage III fibular fracture, the posterolateral corner and posterior surface of the talus will impact on the tibia, causing a rupture of the posterior tibiofibular ligament or a fracture of the posterior malleolus. If the posterior malleolus is driven off with great force, a fracture involving up to one-half of the articular surface of the tibia may occur.

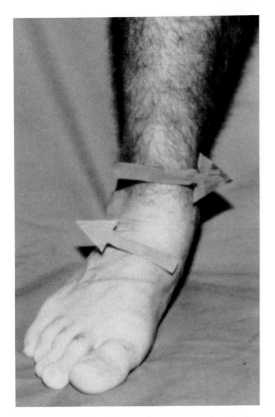

Figure 14.17. Pronation external rotation impact force.

from the anterior edge in a posterior superior direction. The fracture is usually located 4 cm or more proximal to the distal tip of the fibula; 2) pronation-external rotation, which causes a characteristic short, oblique fibular fracture extending from the anterior edge in a posterior-inferior direction; or 3) pronation-abduction, causing an oblique fracture of the fibula which extends from the lateral surface in a inferomedial direction. It is usually located 6 cm from the tip of the lateral malleolus. Rupture of the syndesmosis combined with a fibular fracture may cause diastasis and a severely unstable ankle joint.

Maisonneuve Fracture

Maisonneuve (58), in 1840, described a set of experiments in which he determined that an external rotational force produces a high proximal fibular fracture if there is

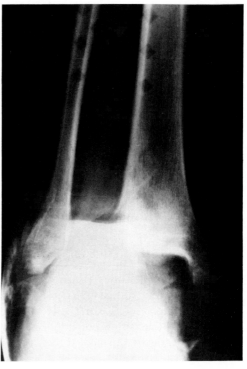

Figure 14.18. Pronation external rotation (PER) stage II with interosseous membrane rupture.

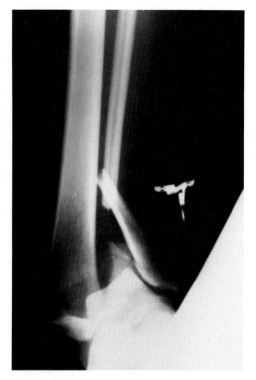

Figure 14.19. Pronation external rotation (PER) stage III.

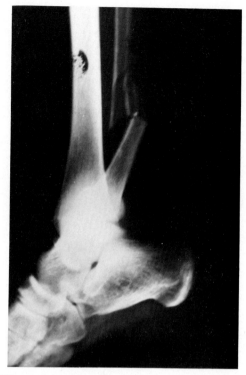

Figure 14.20. Pronation external rotation (PER) stage III fibular fracture with a butterfly fragment.

Danis-Weber Classification

This classification is based on the location of the fibular fracture and its relation to the syndesmosis. According to this system, there are three main types of fractures: A, B, and C, and one subtype, C_2 (99, 103, 68, 35) (Fig. 14.23).

Type A is a fracture of the fibula either at the level of or distal to the talotibial articulation. The syndesmosis of the ankle is intact. Anatomically, the tibiofibular syndesmosis is a form of articulation in which closely opposed bony surfaces are bound together by an interosseous ligament, affording a small degree of movement between adjoining bones (in man, the inferior tibiofibular joint). This joint is between the rough convex surface on the medial side of the lower end of the fibula and the rough concave surface of the fibular notch below the tibia. Below, these surfaces are separated over a distance of about 4 mm by an upward prolongation of the synovial membrane of the talocrural joint. The

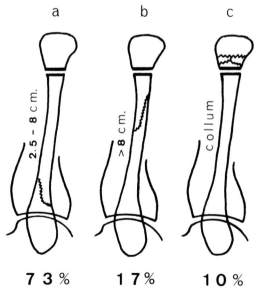

Figure 14.21. Location and frequency of the stage III pronation external rotation (PER) fibular fracture according to Yde.

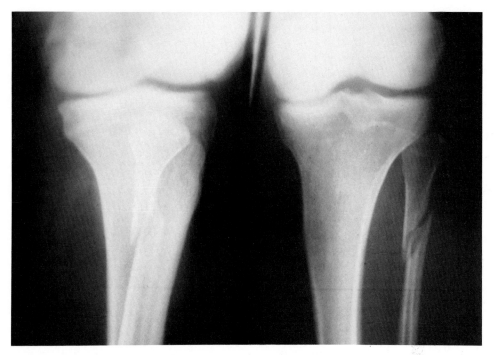

Figure 14.22. Maisonneuve fracture.

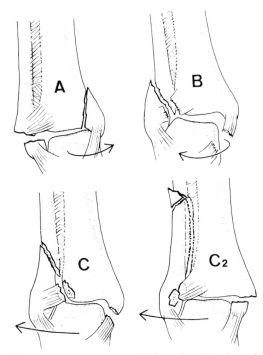

Figure 14.23. Danis-Weber classification of ankle fractures.

main ligaments involved in the syndesmosis are the anterior tibiofibular, posterior talofibular, inferior transverse, and interosseous ligaments. The type A fracture corresponds to supination stages I and II in the Lauge Hansen classification (61).

In Type B lesions, the fracture of the fibula is at the level of the syndesmosis, which is sometimes ruptured. Type B fractures correspond to supination-external rotation fractures, stages I–IV, and to pronation fractures, stages I–III, in the Lauge Hansen classification (61).

Type C fractures usually are located 1–3 inches above the syndesmosis, but may occur in the upper third of the fibular shaft (Maisonneuve) and are then referred to as type C_2. In most instances, the syndesmosis has ruptured, causing marked instability in the ankle joint. Type C and C_2 fractures correspond to pronation-external rotation lesions in the Lauge Hansen system (61) (Fig. 14.24).

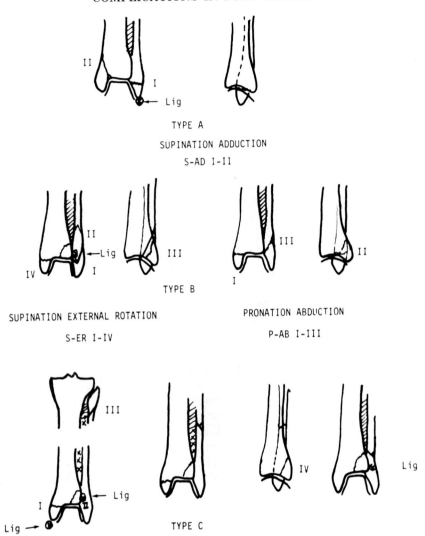

Figure 14.24. Combined Lange-Hansen Danis-Weber classification according to Mast and Teipner (61).

GENERALIZED AND LOCAL ASSESSMENT OF ANKLE FRACTURES

Radiographic Analysis

Standard radiographs should be taken which include AP, lateral, and 15° internal rotational views. If a high fibular fracture is suspected, radiographs of the entire tibia and fibula should be obtained. In severe bi- and trimalleolar fractures, radiographic analysis of the opposite side will provide an excellent frame of reference for anatomic reduction. Stress views of the medial malleolus are sometimes indicated so that a grade II or III disruption of the deltoid complex can be ruled out. These views are best obtained while the injury forcing the external rotation of the foot is being recreated. The stress view is considered positive if a medial clear space of 3–5 mm between the talus and medial malleolus is noted.

Some authors state that the indication for a stress view is rare because the current trend is toward non-operative treatment of the deltoid complex (35, 39). Arthrography as advocated by Cooperman (22) may be helpful in ruling out complex or difficult to classify ankle fractures. It is important to try to obtain standard radiographic views on a reproducible basis. This may be done by fabrication of a jib or alignment device which holds the foot and ankle in the desired position. Such reproducibility is especially helpful in the evaluation of the maintenance of operative and non-operative reduction.

Certain radiographic criteria should be used when the physician evaluates whether open or closed reduction should be utilized (44). 1) The medial clear space should be less than 2 mm wider than the space between the tibial plafond and the talus. 2) There should be less than a 2-mm displacement of the medial malleolus in any direction. 3) There should be less than 2 mm of lateral distal fibular displacement at the fracture. 4) Posterior displacement of the fibula should be less than 3 mm. 5) Less than one-fourth of the tibial articular surface as seen on the lateral view is disrupted. 6) There should be no malposition of the talus. These six criteria can be utilized before reduction, after reduction, or during follow-up, and for evaluation of the success of open reduction with internal fixation.

General and Local Assessment of Ankle Fractures

Ankle fractures often occur in combination with other serious injuries that may need attention before repair or manipulation of the ankle lesion can begin. These include; abdominal injuries, internal hemorrhage, traumatic chest injuries, and head injuries, all of which must be stabilized before attempts at reduction can begin. First, the neurovascular status of the dorsalis pedis and posterior tibial complex should be assessed. The pulses may be palpated or, if gross edema is present, it may be necessary to perform a doppler ultrasound study. If the circulatory status is in doubt, immediate manipulation becomes necessary. The foot must be pulled distally and rotated internally for reestablishment of the neurovascular status. The area of injury must be palpated for evaluation of the type and extent of the disruption. The entire shaft of the fibula should be palpated so that a Maisonneuve high fibular fracture can be ruled out.

NON-OPERATIVE TREATMENT OF ANKLE FRACTURES

The criteria for non-operative treatment of malleolar fractures depend on the type of fracture and on the radiographic interpretation. Lauge Hansen designed the genetic classification system (50–52) in order to be able to reverse the mechanism of injury and produce improved closed treatment results. From his observations, it becomes apparent that fractures localized to one malleolus with an intact or minimally disturbed syndesmosis are best treated non-operatively. Such fractures include most SI, SII (Danis-Weber type A), PI, II, PER I, II, and SER I, II (Danis-Weber type B) lesions. A comparison of operative and nonoperative results for type A fractures by the AO group shows a rating of good to very good for 74% of nonoperatively treated type A fractures. With operative treatment, this rating increased to 80.5%. They concluded that a type A unimalleolar fracture could be treated adequately with closed reduction and immobilization (61).

Bi- and trimalleolar fractures caused by external rotation gave mixed results with non-operative treatment. Hughes (39) found that non-operative treatment of type B fractures yielded a 38% good to very good success rate, whereas operative treatment gave good to very good results in 77% of the cases. Among type C (Lange Hansen PER II–IV) injuries, in only 29% were the results rated as good to very good with closed reduction and immobilization. With AO operative treatment, 74% good to very good results were obtained (Fig. 14.25).

Malka and Taillard (59) found that open reduction and internal fixation of SER and

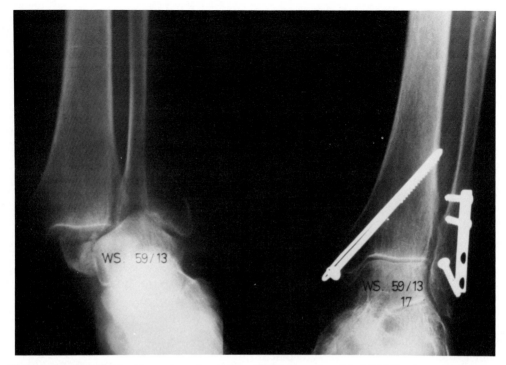

Figure 14.25. Supination external rotation (SER) fracture with ASIF fixation techniques.

PER fractures gave better results than did closed reduction. Wilson and Skilbred (104) compared displaced bimalleolar fractures receiving open and closed treatment. They concluded that most of the excellent results were obtained by open treatment; but when they compared excellent and good results, the results following closed reduction were slightly better. Solonen and Lauttamus (88) felt that SER stages II–IV and PER stages II–IV were best treated operatively. When Magnusson (56) examined post-reduction results for 211 external-rotation fractures with 118 unimalleolar fractures, he found radiographic evidence of arthritis deformans in 29% of the unimalleolar fractures, compared to 82% in bi- and trimalleolar external-rotation injuries. He also found that unimalleolar SER II (type B) fractures had a significantly higher incidence of arthritis deformans when there was an injury to the anterior tubercle (Chaput) and to the accompanying anterior tibiofibular ligament. He found that rupture of the ligament resulted in a partial widening of the inferior tibiofibular joint, causing later complications. Cedell (16, 17) advocated operation for all supination-external rotation injuries, with particular attention focused on repair of the anterior tibiofibular ligament. Klossner (44) compared operative and non-operative treatment and found a 60% success rate with closed reduction. However, when he used operative methods he fixed only the medial malleolus.

Technique of Closed Reduction

Routine radiographs are taken which show the type and extent of the injury. Before radiography, the patient's neurovascular status should be checked and if there is no contraindication, the patient is given systemic medications (IV Valium®, Demerol®, Nubain®) prior to reduction. Next, an intraarticular injection of 1–2% lidocaine mixed with bupivicaine is given.

The aim of closed reduction in bi- and trimalleolar fractures is to replace the talus in an anatomic position in the ankle mortise. This is best achieved by reversal of the mechanism of injury to "unlock" the fragments. The mechanism of injury is reversed in three steps: 1) distal traction (Fig. 14.26), 2) internal rotation and supination of the rearfoot (Fig. 14.27), and 3) pronation and dorsiflexion of the forefoot so that the midtarsal joint is locked (Fig. 14.28). A below the knee (BK) cast is then applied. While the plaster is solidifying, lateral stress should be applied just above the medial malleolus, combined with inversion stress on the talus and calcaneus just below the lateral malleolus. This helps maintain the rearfoot in the proper amount of internal rotation and supination. The foot is held in a dorsiflexed and pronated position by the assistant or by hooking of tube gauze through the third and fourth toes and having the patient pronate the foot (Fig. 14.29). If a large posterior malleolar fragment is present, it may be necessary to plantarflex the foot; dorsiflexion may cause this fragment to dislocate.

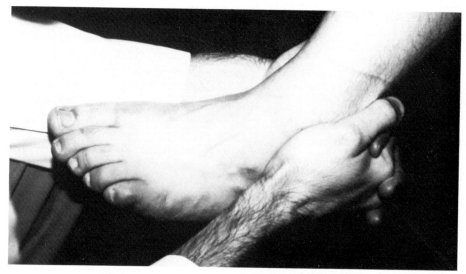

Figure 14.26. Closed reduction: distal traction.

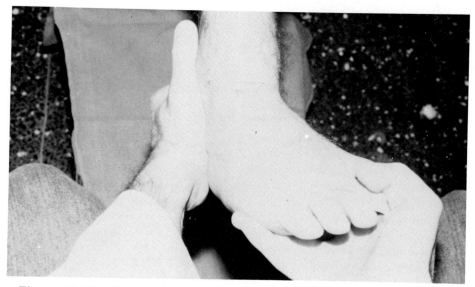

Figure 14.27. Closed reduction: supination and internal rotation of the rearfoot.

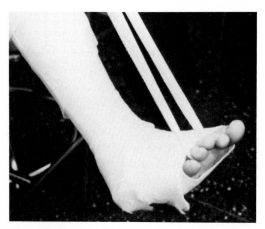

Figure 14.28. Closed reduction: pronation and dorsiflexion of the forefoot.

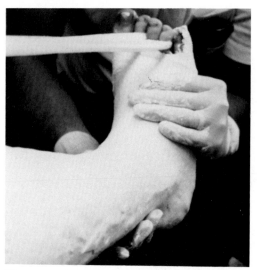

Figure 14.29. Closed reduction: BK cast application.

Care should be taken to obtain the best possible reduction of the lateral malleolus and to restore it to its original length if at all possible. The casting should be completed with application of an above the knee (AK) cast with the knee in 30° of flexion (Fig. 14.30). The superior portion of the cast should be applied to the gluteal fold. Application of the AK segment negates the force of the gastrocnemius complex and eliminates the possibility of displacement of the reduced malleolar fragments.

For nondisplaced type A (SI, II, SER II) fractures, a BK cast may be used for 4–6 weeks, with minimal manipulation. For this type of fracture, the patient does not need to be hospitalized. For SER III, IV and PER III, IV lesions, however, the patient should be hospitalized after closed reduction has been performed. Admission orders should include elevation in a splint or hanging traction; AP, lateral, and 15° internal rotation radiographs of both the injured and uninjured sides for comparison; and administration of diuretics (Diuril®, 500 mg b.i.d.) and ASA (10 gr. b.i.d.). The postreduction radiographs should be judged according to the criteria outlined above. If the reduction is adequate, the patient will be allowed to ambulate with a walker or crutches after the edema subsides. No weightbearing should be permitted on the affected side.

Radiographs should be repeated after the initial cast change and up to 6 weeks to show whether any reduction has been lost. Any loss in alignment may be an indication for remanipulation or for open reduction with internal fixation (Fig. 14.31). An AK cast is then used for an additional 6 weeks. If the reduction has been maintained, however, a BK cast is applied. The patient is kept non-weightbearing for 2 weeks, followed by gradual weightbearing for an additional 2 weeks. The cast is usually discarded after 10 weeks. The patient is taught

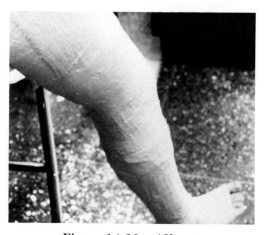

Figure 14.30. AK cast.

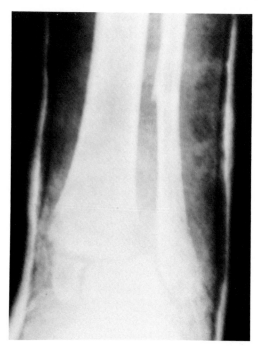

Figure 14.31. Residual malalignment after closed reduction.

active and passive ankle exercises. Physical therapy is beneficial during the first month after cast removal.

Complications of Non-operative Treatment

Bi- and trimalleolar ankle fractures usually cause considerable ligamentous damage, as well as bony disruption subcutaneously. This may lead to two main complications—interruption of the neurovascular status and formation of fracture blisters (epidermal fluid-filled spaces) with massive edema. Marked displacement of malleolar fragments or talar malposition may cause the fragments to impinge on the posterior tibial or anterior tibial arteries. Tissue anoxia occurs after 2 hours; therefore, it is mandatory that the circulatory status be checked as soon as the patient is examined. Failure to do so may result in amputation of the leg. Severe infection can occur after the formation of fracture blisters (Fig. 14.32). The treatment centers around elevation of the extremity to decrease the edema and the application of a long-leg cast to immobilize the fracture and protect the skin from further damage.

Another common complication of non-operative therapy is a position change of the fragments after cast changes (56). If severe edema is present initially, a large, soft compressive AK cast should be applied. After the edema subsides, the position of the fragments often changes, necessitating re-reduction or open reduction with internal fixation. In bi- and trimalleolar fractures, anatomic reduction is difficult to achieve, as outlined by Magnusson (56), Solonen (88), and others. This may be due to ligamentous damage, soft-tissue interposition (posterior tibial tendon), or the position of the fragments. Poor anatomic reduction has been found to cause increased joint arthrosis, but it is difficult to correlate clinical and roentgenographic studies. Attempts to correct malunion are almost impossible with closed reduction, perhaps because of the shape and complex configuration of the ankle joint and the tendency for the fibula to shorten after injury. Repair of

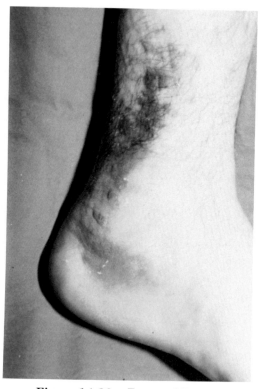

Figure 14.32. Fracture blisters.

ligament injury is impossible with closed reduction. Lauge Hansen (51, 52), Cedell (16, 17), and Willenegger (101–103) have stressed the importance of syndesmotic repair to maintain the integrity and alignment of the ankle joint.

A major complication of non-operative treatment is prolonged immobilization (10 weeks), which results in arthrosis and increased joint stiffness. Salter and others (85) have proved that prolonged immobilization causes rapid degeneration of articular cartilage. Other complications include non-union, especially of the medial malleolus, dislocation and subluxation of the posterior malleolar fragment, and widening of the ankle mortise (Fig. 14.33).

Generally, closed reduction should be utilized for 1) SER I and II fractures with less than 2 mm of lateral clear space present, 2) P-PER I and II fractures with minimal or less than 2-mm displacement, and 3) S I or II unimalleolar fractures with less than 2-mm displacement. These injuries can be treated with little or no manipulation, and with application of a BK walking cast for 4–8 weeks. These patients need not be hospitalized. Non-operative therapy is also reserved for debilitated patients who are unable, for medical reasons or because of trauma, to undergo any type of surgical procedure.

OPERATIVE TREATMENT OF ANKLE FRACTURES

There has been much controversy concerning open versus closed treatment of ankle fractures. In the 1940s, authors such as Magnusson (56), Lauge Hansen (50, 51), Palmer (72), and Danis (23) argued the advantages and disadvantages of each technique. In the 1950s, Vasli (97) published the first detailed comparison of open reduction and internal fixation with the closed genetic methods of Lauge Hansen. He noted that improvement was seen in postoperative radiographic studies with open reduction and internal fixation of severely displaced malleolar fractures. In the 1960s, detailed studies of the operative treatment of ankle fractures were performed by Klossner (44), Burwell and Charnley (13), So-

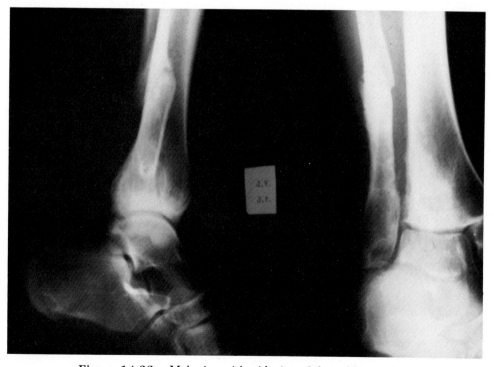

Figure 14.33.   Malunion with widening of the ankle mortise.

lonen and Lauttamus (88), Cedell (16), and Malka and Taillard (59).

Open reduction with internal fixation was common in the mid-1960s in the European centers, where the results were greatly improved over those with closed techniques (23, 99, 101–103). This method was first introduced in the United States in the early to mid-1970s, based on the principles of the AO technique as described by a group of 15 Swiss general and orthopedic surgeons (68). In 1958, these Swiss surgeons met to discuss the poor results obtained with both operative and non-operative treatment of fractures in Switzerland. Dr. Maurice Muller proposed the meeting after studying with Danis, for he was impressed by Danis' concept of rigid internal fixation followed by early pain-free motion. He was intrigued by Danis' principle of primary bone healing in which little or no external callus was formed following rigid fixation of fractures (23). In this meeting, the founders of the AO (Arbeitsgemeinschaft für Osteosynthesefragen) and ASIF (Association for the Study of Internal Fixation) study groups formulated four basic principles that were accepted as working hypotheses: 1) anatomic reduction, 2) rigid internal fixation, 3) a traumatic technique on soft tissue as well as bone, and 4) early pain-free mobilization during the first 10 post-operative days (68). Through 1979, more than 50,000 cases of internal fixation had been analyzed at the documentation center in Berne, Switzerland. The AO group enlisted the aid of metallurgists, engineers, and manufacturers and devised more than 1400 devices for use in the surgery of fractures (68).

Willenegger (101–103) and Weber (99) have extensively studied the effect of rigid internal fixation in the treatment of malleolar fractures and are able to achieve 80% good to excellent results, based on clinical and radiographic data, with this technique in bi- and trimalleolar fractures. This technique has been used at the University of Chicago since 1974, with excellent results. Thus, the results achieved by surgeons skilled in this technique make the AO-ASIF method the treatment of choice for operative reduction of bi- and trimalleolar fractures in the 1980s (Fig. 14.34).

The operative treatment, aftercare, and complications will be outlined for each fracture type according to Lauge Hansen's classification. This system is utilized because of the important role of ligamentous repair in the overall treatment. The Lauge Hansen classification will be correlated with the Danis-Weber system, which specifies the area of the fibular fracture in relation to the syndesmosis.

Timing of the Operation and Metal Removal

The AO group suggests that the optimum time for operative reduction of an ankle fracture is within the first 6–8 hours after surgery if the formation of fracture blisters is to be avoided (68). If blisters occur, the surgery must be postponed by 4–6 days. When a fracture occurs, the skin must be protected with elevation and a cast.

When small lag screws are utilized, their removal may not be necessary. Plates and tension-banding implants must be removed (35, 68). This constitutes a potential complication because anesthesia and a second operative procedure are necessary. In all cases, the metal should be left in place for at least 6 months. Removal of cancellous screws becomes extremely difficult after 6 months, because of bony ingrowth around the wide screw threads. The limb should be protected from extreme activity for 6 weeks, after which normal ambulation can be tolerated.

Incisions

Double incisions are usually indicated for the repair of bi- or trimalleolar fractures. The incision for the lateral malleolus and fibula should be centered over the midportion and gently curved anteriorly or posteriorly, lying sufficiently distal so that the surgeon can inspect the lateral collateral ligaments and the syndesmosis. Care should be taken to avoid damage to the intermediate dorsal cutaneous branch of

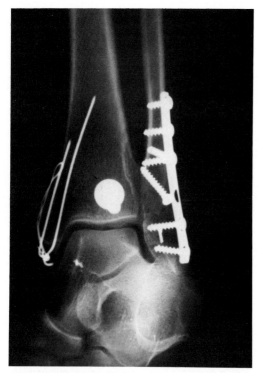

Figure 14.34. ASIF fixation techniques in a supination external rotation (SER) stage IV injury.

the superficial peroneal nerve and the sural nerve.

There are two basic types of medial malleolar incisions. If there is no posterior fracture, the incision commences at the anteromedial distal aspect of the tibia, inferior to the malleolus, and ends at the posterior talocalcaneal joint. If a posterior fragment is present and needs reduction, a curved incision is made on the posteromedial border of the lower distal tibia, ending slightly proximal to the talonavicular joint. If a difficult posterior malleolar fracture is to be reduced, a curved posterolateral incision may be made between the tibia and fibula.

General AO Fixation Techniques

A number of basic principles of ankle fracture fixation as advocated by the AO group must be outlined for a full understanding of the method and sequence of fixation (68, 69).

Reconstruction of the fibula and its connection to the tibia has the highest priority in the successful reduction of a displaced malleolar fracture. Reports by Lambert (47), Yablon (106), and Ramsey (81) outlined the importance of the lateral malleolus in the reconstruction of a displaced ankle lesion. A lateral fibular shift of 1–2 mm can cause loss of contact in up to 50% of the talotibial articulation (81). If untreated, this may result in a high incidence of post-traumatic arthrosis (Figs. 14.35 and 14.36). The exact length of the fibula must be reproduced, and the bone must be repositioned into the fibular notch of the tibia. In addition, the integrity of the tibiofibular ligaments must be maintained. This is achieved by exact repair of the anterior syndesmotic (tibiofibular) ligament, the posterior syndesmotic (tibiofibular) ligament, and the interosseous ligament and membrane. In general, fractures which disrupt the syndesmoses (PER fractures) are prone to cause complications if exact ana-

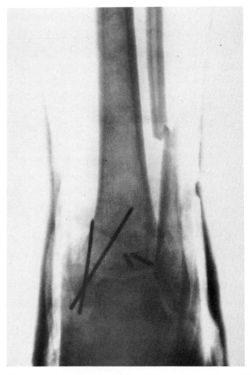

Figure 14.35. ORIF with malposition 24 hours after surgery.

tomic and ligamentous repair is not produced (71, 101–103).

According to Heim and Pfeiffer (35), the shape and structure of the lower fibula must be considered when different types of AO fixation are used. The outer portion of the lower fibula is suitable for a small plate, as there are no muscular insertions. At the level of the articular surface, the fibula widens considerably and has a double bend which requires special attention (35). Small plates must be bent into this "S" shape. At 2–3 cm above the ankle joint, the fibula has a lateral prominence which widens proximally; this causes a posterior rotation. Care must be taken to reproduce the exact rotation in the plate so that a rotational deformity is avoided. Torsional, long oblique fractures of at least twice the width of the bone are stabilized with interfragmentary screws by means of the lag technique. The fracture zone is then protected by a neutralization plate which protects the screw fixation by conducting forces around the fracture site (Fig. 14.37).

According to Mast and Teipner (61), fractures of the fibula caused by bending moments are usually comminuted on the compression side of the lesion. In these cases, a neutralization plate serves to buttress and maintain length in the fibular fracture. Interfragmentary compression may be utilized to hold the comminuted fragments through the plate or at a right angle to the comminuted segments. Chip and distal avulsion fractures of the distal tibia and fibula are best treated with the use of a tension band system or with one or two 3.5-mm cortical screws, 4.0-mm cancellous screws, or a single malleolar screw (Fig. 14.38).

Rupture of the anterior syndesmosis requires exact reduction; otherwise, the integrity of the ankle joint will be lost. Usually, the ends of the ligaments can be sutured with 00 Dexon or vicryl sutures. In some instances, the ligament may be severely shredded, and it must be protected by a transosseous suture which is anchored on the tibia through two small connecting holes drilled at a 45° angle to each other. The suture should be attached to the fibula by being anchored to the screw, plate, or tension band used in the reduction of the fibular fracture. Avulsion fractures of the anterior tibial tubercle (Chaput) can usually be fixed to the tibia with a small cancellous 4.0-mm screw or 3.5-mm cortical screw, or with one or two K-wires that have been bent back upon themselves and driven into the tibia (35, 68). (Fig. 14.39).

In PER fractures, rupture of the interosseous membrane may cause gross instability of the ankle joint to occur. The interosseous membrane usually ruptures from the tibial surface. One syndesmotic protection screw can usually be inserted 2–3 inches above the ankle joint. This should be a 3.5- or 4.5-mm cortical screw which is inserted through both fibular cortices and through the lateral cortex of the tibia. Care should be taken to avoid compressing the tibia and fibula together in a lag screw effect since this may tighten the articulation and result in severe joint deformity (Fig. 14.40).

An alternate method of fixation is Willenegger's technique (101–103). Two oblique 30–45° K-wires are driven through the fibula into the tibia 2–3 inches above

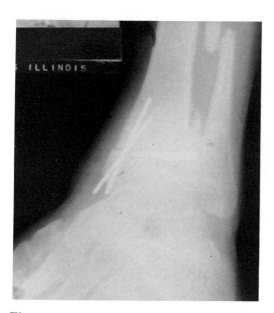

Figure 14.36. Same patient one year later with severe degeneration of ankle joint.

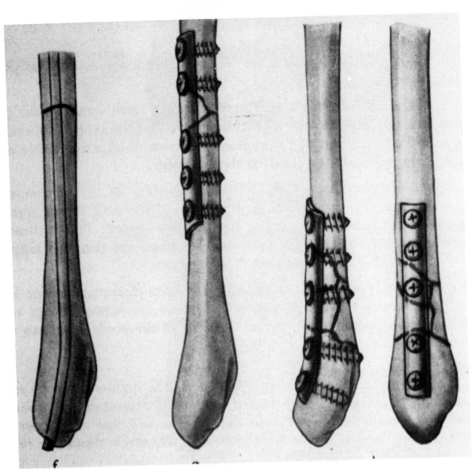

Figure 14.37. ASIF fixation of the fibular with lag screws and neutralization plates.

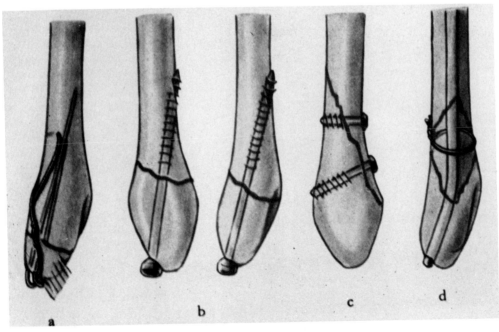

Figure 14.38. Various ASIF fixation techniques for distal fibular fractures.

the ankle joint. Either K-wires or a screw may be inserted through a neutralization plate. Maisonneuve fractures require the insertion of two parallel 4.5-mm cortical screws 2–3 inches above the ankle joint through four cortices, without the lag effect. This is accomplished by tapping of all four cortices. All transfixation screws should be removed after 6–8 weeks, before active weightbearing begins.

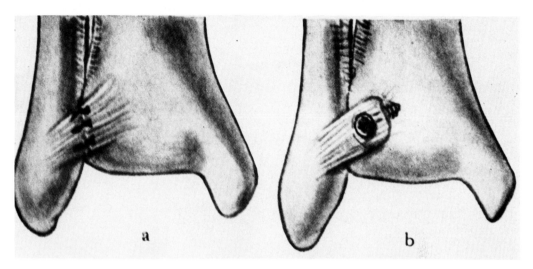

Figure 14.39. ASIF fixation of the anterior tibial tubercle (Chaput).

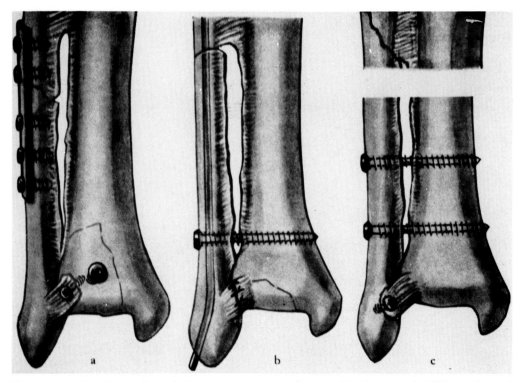

Figure 14.40. Protection of the interosseous membrane with the use of ASIF syndesmotic protection screw(s).

Posterior malleolar fractures are usually not stabilized unless the lateral width exceeds one-fourth of the weightbearing articular surface. In most cases, stable fixation of the fibular fracture reduces the posterior lateral fragment. If the fragments are large, a medial approach is utilized and the fracture is fixed according to Weber's (99) technique. Forceps or K-wires hold the fracture in position; this is followed by anterior-to-posterior fixation of the fragment with two 4.0-mm cancellous screws (Fig. 14.41). A posterior lateral approach may also be used for more accurate reduction of the fragment.

The medial malleolus is usually fixed after the lateral malleolus, although it may first be checked for any soft tissue interposition. In osteoporotic bone or with small fractures, the tension band technique is the procedure of choice. With larger medial malleolar fragments, two 4.0-mm cancellous or 3.5 cortical screws may be utilized for fixation of the fracture. The use of a single screw should be avoided because it allows rotation to take place (Fig. 14.42).

According to Hughes (40), there are four lesions of the medial malleolus that require open reduction and internal fixation. These are: 1) dislocation of the medial malleolus beneath the skin, which compromises the very fragile blood supply to the skin of this area; 2) a displacement of the medial mal-

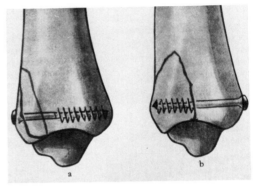

Figure 14.41. Weber fixation of the posterior malleolar fragment.

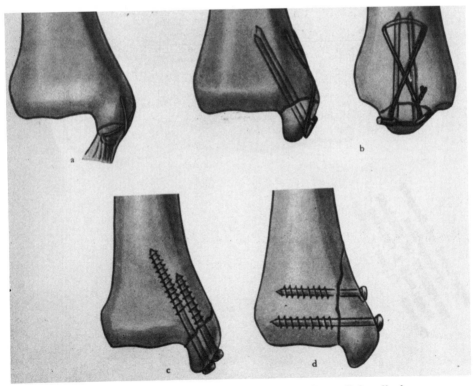

Figure 14.42. ASIF fixation techniques for the medial malleolus.

leolus, either anteriorly or laterally, that cannot be reduced by closed methods; 3) a painful pseudoarthrosis of the medial malleolus; 4) a fracture of the medial malleolus that is associated with small bone fragments within the joint. Ruptures of the deltoid ligament may or may not be sutured, depending upon the stability of the joint after the lateral malleolus is stabilized. Small chip fragments or fragments of the joint surface should be removed so that future disability and pain caused by loose bodies in the joint can be prevented.

Specific Fixation Techniques According to the Lauge Hansen Classification

SUPINATION FRACTURES

Supination stage I and II injuries (type A) most often are unimalleolar, but occasionally may involve both malleoli. The fracture does not disrupt the syndesmotic ligaments. In rare instances, a posteromedial tibial fracture occurs. In the St. Gallen series, there were 79 S I and II fractures. In our opinion, if such a fracture is unimalleolar and nondisplaced, it rarely needs internal fixation. Bimalleolar fractures, however, may need open reduction with internal fixation.

Fixation of the lateral malleolus depends on the fracture type. The most common type of fibular fracture is a transverse pull-off. The fixation in this fracture type is usually accomplished with a 4.5-mm malleolar screw, inserted from the distal tip of the lateral malleolus across the fracture, with the tip of the screw just piercing the medial cortex of the fibula 1–2 inches above the fracture site (68). If the fragment is small, tension banding may be utilized. In approximately 25% of the fractures, a distal fibular avulsion may occur (107). This may be treated with tension band fixation or with four Kirschner wires driven obliquely from the distal to the proximal side. A medial malleolar fracture is usually oblique because of the impact of the talus. This

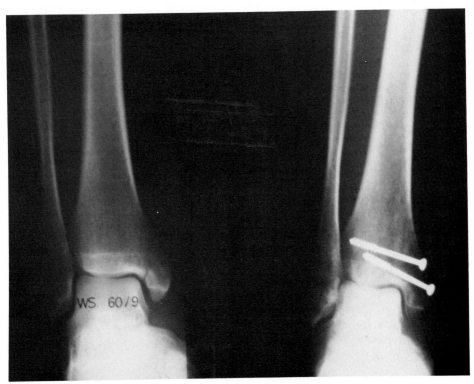

Figure 14.43.   Type A fracture fixed with 4.0-mm cancellous screws.

injury can be fixed with two 4.0-mm parallel cancellous screws passing from medial to lateral, parallel to the articular surface (Fig. 14.43). Alternatively, if the fragments are small, a 4.0-mm cancellous screw and a Kirschner wire are inserted obliquely and parallel to each other, with the Kirschner wire bent on itself and driven into the bone (Fig. 14.44).

Complications include infection, non-union of the smaller medial malleolar fragments, and malunion of the fracture surfaces secondary to small or large cancellous defects caused by impaction and resulting in joint incongruity.

As mentioned before, in most type A fractures excellent results are achieved with non-operative treatment.

SER FRACTURES

Supination external rotation stage I (type B) fractures may be uni-, bi-, or tri-malleolar. A stage I SER fracture is usually seen only with involvement of a higher stage, although external-rotation stress views may show a widening and incongruity

of the distal fibular talar joint. These injuries, if suspected, can be treated adequately with a low-leg walking cast applied for 4–6 weeks. Rarely, if ever, is open reduction with internal fixation indicated.

The most common type of ankle fracture is the SER II fracture. There is considerable controversy concerning treatment of this fracture in two areas. The first is rupture of the anterior tibiofibular ligament. The second area of contention is whether open reduction with internal fixation is indicated for this type of unimalleolar fracture. European surgeons, including Willenegger (101–103), Weber (99), and Mueller (68, 69), feel that a 1-mm lateral-posterior displacement of the distal fibula may result in instability. In Europe, therefore, most SER II fractures are treated with open reduction and internal fixation, with success rates approaching 90% (68). (Fig. 14.45). Surgeons in the United States are more reluctant to reduce SER II unimalleolar fractures operatively, especially if the anterior syndesmosis is not ruptured. In our institution, all SER II fractures are treated with a BK walking cast for 4–6 weeks. Our

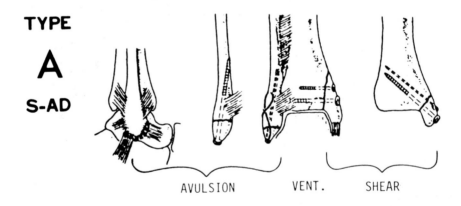

TYPE

A

S-AD

AVULSION   VENT.   SHEAR

FIBULA FRACTURE
BELOW SYNDESMOSIS

- FIBULA
  Lag Screw
  Tension Band Wiring
- Medial Malleolus
  Lag Screws

DORS.
POSTEROMEDIAL FRAGMENT

Figure 14.44. ASIF fixation techniques for type A fractures according to Mast and Teipner (61).

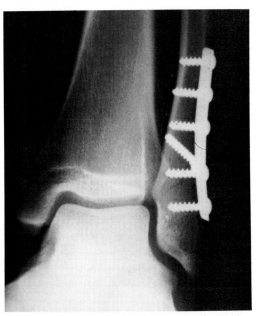

Figure 14.45. Supination external rotation (SER) stage II with ASIF fixation.

success rate approaches 95%. Little or no manipulation is necessary.

Operative reduction with internal fixation of the SER II fracture can be achieved in a variety of ways. The fracture runs from anterior-inferior to posterior-superior on the fibula, with an average length of about 2.5 cm (107). This is a long, oblique fracture having approximately 2–2.5 times the width of the bone, and thus it provides an excellent indication for two 3.5-mm cortical screws in cortical bone and 4.0-mm cancellous screws in the distal fibular cancellous bone. The Swiss presently use 3.5-mm cortical screws in cancellous bone because they consider the design of the 3.5-mm cortical screw to be much more suitable than the 4.0-mm cancellous screw for cancellous-bone fixation. A complication in their method is protrusion of the screw(s) into the lateral talofibular articulation. Weber

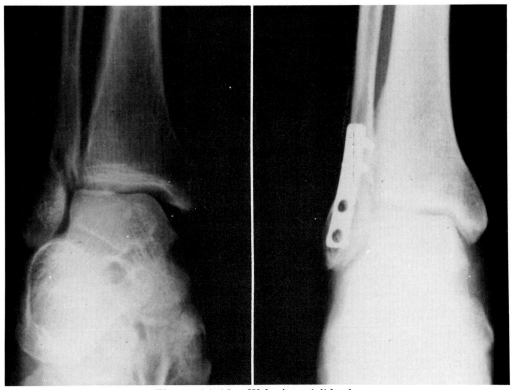

Figure 14.46. Weber's antiglide plate.

has devised a unique method of dealing with this complication. He applies a 3- or 4-hole one-third tubular plate to the posterolateral side of the fibula, with two or three holes superior and one or two holes inferior to the lesion. The superior portion of the plate is fixed with 3.5-mm cortical screws. With this maneuver, the tip of the distal fragment is pressed securely against the proximal fragment. Weber refers to this as an anti-glide plate (Fig. 14.46). A separate lag screw may be utilized which provides interfragmental compression.

Alternative methods of stabilizing SER II fractures include the use of a single malleolar screw driven from the distal tip of the lateral malleolus through the medial cortex of the lower third of the fibular shaft. If the anterior tibiofibular ligament has been ruptured, it must be repaired. This can be achieved by a Dexon® suture anchored in the tibia, and by fixation implants which stabilize the fibula (35, 68). Chaput fractures or small anterolateral tibial or anteromedial fibular avulsion frac-

tures may be fixated with a small cancellous or 3.5-mm cortical lag screw. An alternative technique employs a Kirschner wire which is bent upon itself and driven into the bone.

The third stage of an SER fracture is a rupture of the posterior tibiofibular ligament or a fracture of the posterior aspect of the tibia. This is referred to as a Volkmann fracture in most publications, although von Volkmann (98) described an anterior tibial fracture. It is usually an intermediate stage of an SER fracture, with only 4–6% seen in the isolated stage. The decision concerning fixation is usually based on the amount of tibial articular disruption as visualized on a lateral radiograph. If the fracture exceeds one-fourth the posterior tibial articular surface, open reduction with internal fixation is indicated. Approximately 14–20% of all SER fractures exceed one-fourth the posterior tibial articular surface (16, 44, 51, 52, 107).

Fixation of the so-called von Volkmann fracture is usually achieved by a long, curved medial incision. Reduction forceps

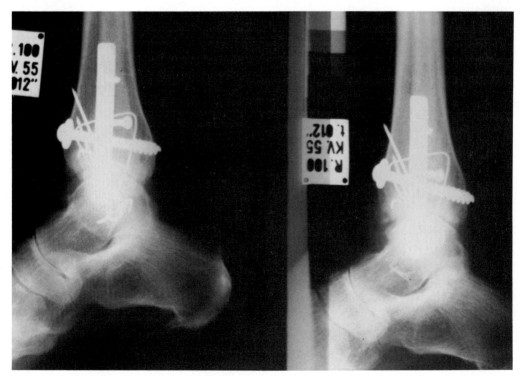

Figure 14.47.   ASIF fixation of the posterior malleolar fracture.

are applied to hold the fracture after fixation of the lateral malleolus. Either two 4.0-mm cancellous screws or a mixture of 4.0- and 6.5-mm cancellous screws are inserted from anterior to posterior to secure the fragment (Fig. 14.47). The fragment should first be stabilized with K-wire, and intraoperative radiographs should be taken as a check of the reduction. Occasionally, a posterolateral incision may be used for the same purpose. Fragments that include less than one-fourth the articular tibial surface are usually reduced after rigid fixation of the lateral malleolus.

The fourth stage is the end-stage of the SER fracture. In 50% of the cases, this stage is a rupture of the deltoid ligament, an avulsion fracture, or a transverse pull-off or oblique impact fracture of the medial malleolus (107). According to Heim and Pfeiffer (35), these types of medial malleolar fractures are seen in a small avulsion

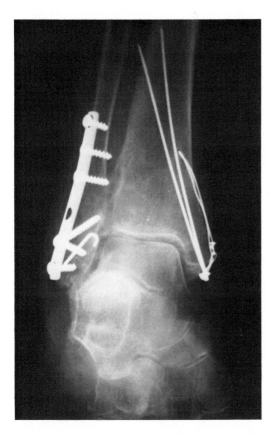

Figure 14.48. Tension band fixation of the medial malleolus.

fracture, a large anterior fracture, or a posterior semicircular fracture. Deltoid ruptures need not be explored and sutured unless there is a large posterior fracture and medial exposure is necessary, or unless a suspected interposition of soft tissue interferes with adequate reduction. According to the AO group (35, 68), most medial malleolar fractures should be fixed. If the fragment is small or the bone is osteoporotic, tension band fixation is the procedure of choice (Fig. 14.48). Larger fragments may be fixed with two parallel 4.0-mm cancellous screws, or with a single malleolar screw and Kirschner wire, which may be bent into the cruciate head of the screw. These screws should not be countersunk because the bone is soft and because manual tension is usually enough to bury the screw head in the bone so that its impingement on subcutaneous tissue is avoided.

Wound closure should include the use of a small Hemovac® drain on both the medial and lateral sides, exiting posteriorly so that gravity helps drainage. The drain can be removed after 24–48 hours. An anterior or posterior splint is applied to facilitate dressing changes and passive range-of-motion exercises. For SER II fractures, a BK walking cast is applied immediately and is left in place for 6 weeks. Patients with SER III and IV fractures remain non-weight-bearing for 10–14 days, during which passive range-of-motion exercises are performed. A BK walking cast is applied for an additional 4–6 weeks. If the bone is osteoporotic, or if the stability of a fracture is questionable, a BK non-weightbearing cast should be utilized for 6 weeks, followed by 4 weeks with a BK walking cast. For reduction of pain and edema, physical therapy and elastic support are utilized for 1 month after cast removal.

Complications of this procedure include unstable fixation because of early weight-bearing. This may result in disintegration of the fixation, with a resultant nonstable talotibial joint. Infection rates following ankle fractures are currently less than 1% when nontraumatic techniques and prophylactic IV antibiotics are used. A deep infection leading to osteomyelitis can be disastrous and may lead to multiple surgeries, including the possibility of an eventual below the knee amputation. In a study performed by the author of 15 complications of ankle fracture fixation, one necessitated a below the knee amputation secondary to a severe infective process.

The most common complication is the formation of a post-traumatic arthrosis, which leads to pain and instability of the ankle joint. This complication is thought to be caused by non-anatomic fixation of the fibular fracture. Klossner (44) found evidence of arthrosis after open reduction with internal fixation in 13% of men and 27% of women with ankle fractures after an average follow-up period of 4 years. Severe post-operative edema may be present after open reduction with internal fixation and may affect 30% of the patient population, depending upon the patient's age and vascular status. Marked limitation of the ankle may be present in approximately 25% of the patients (16, 17, 41, 44–46, 61).

Malposition of the ankle, with a varus or valgus attitude, may be present after surgery and lead to increased pain and disability. Antalgic gait is another potential complication, occurring in up to 5% of openly reduced ankle fractures. Post-operative flattening of the arch may occur in 5–10% of the patients. According to Cedell (16, 17), displacement of the posterior tibial fragment accounts for a high incidence of arthritis deformans following open reduction and internal fixation of SER fractures. Post-operative atrophy of the calf may occur in up to 25% of the cases (16). Pseudo-arthrosis of the medial malleolus is rare because of the rigid AO fixation of the fibula and medial malleolus.

PRONATION FRACTURES

The first stage of a pronation (type B) fracture is a unimalleolar pull-off fracture of the medial malleolus or a rupture of the deltoid ligament. The medial malleolar fracture, which may be transverse or oblique, constitutes approximately 40% of all ankle fractures. As stated before, the treatment of choice for a non-displaced unimalleolar fracture is the application of a BK cast for 4–6 weeks. Ruptures of the deltoid can also be treated in this manner. When the medial malleolar fracture is displaced, open reduction with internal fixation may be considered. Small fragments can be fixed best with tension banding. Larger fragments can be stabilized with two 4.0-mm cancellous screws or with a malleolar screw and Kirschner wire. The end of the Kirschner wire is bent upon itself and inserted into the cruciate head of the screw or driven into the bone.

In stage II pronation fractures, both the anterior and posterior talofibular ligaments rupture. If the posterior fracture exceeds one-fourth the lateral distal tibial surface, anterior-to-posterior fixation as described by Weber (99) is necessary.

Post-operative care of this fracture depends on the stage of the fracture. Nondisplaced unimalleolar fractures are treated with a BK walking cast for 6 weeks. Bimalleolar P II and P III fractures are protected against weightbearing for 10–14 days, followed by application of a BK walking cast for an additional 4–6 weeks. If the fixation is questionable, a BK non-weight-bearing cast should be applied for 6 weeks, followed by a BK walking cast for 4 weeks. As in all ankle fractures, physical therapy and edema control are of prime importance during the first month after cast removal.

Complications of this fracture type are similar to the complications outlined for SER fractures.

PRONATION-EXTERNAL ROTATION FRACTURES

Pronation-external rotation fractures (type C) account for approximately 20% of all ankle disturbances. The prognosis is worse for this type of ankle fracture because there is partial or complete disruption of the syndesmosis and interosseous membrane. Open reduction of this fracture requires great skill if the surgeon is to avoid the many complications associated with malunion or non-union. According to Malka et al. (59), the prognosis for PER fractures is unfavorable regardless of whether open or closed reduction is utilized. They found that, despite a high rate of anatomic reductions (80%), excellent objective results were achieved in only 54% of the cases. They postulated that this might be due to the extensive ligamentous damage that accompanies the fractures. Mast and Teipner (61) had poor results in 12.5% of PER fractures after open reduction with internal fixation. The same procedure when used for SER fractures yielded only a 4% complication rate.

In our study of ankle fusion techniques, we found that, in six of eight cases, ankle fusions were necessary when poor results were obtained with ORIF of PER III and IV fractures.

It must be emphasized that, although the repair is described in the sequence in which the fracture occurs, reduction and fixation of the fibula always take precedence in the fixation sequence. Fixation techniques for stage I medial malleolar fractures are similar to the methods utilized for PER I lesions. The medial malleolus may be fixed with tension banding, two 4.0-mm cancellous screws, or a malleolar-screw and K-wire combination.

The stage II fracture involves rupture of the anterior syndesmosis and interosseous membrane, which usually precedes stage III. This is a rare injury which is repaired with sutures, stainless steel wire, and small cancellous or 3.5-mm cortical screws. Repair of the stage III portion of the fracture presents many difficulties. Complete repair demands exact and perfect anatomical reduction of the anterior syndesmosis, sometimes combined with protection and repair of the interosseous membrane. When stages III and IV occur, exact anatomic restoration of the fibula is mandatory and should be performed first so that congruity of the ankle joint is reestablished. According to Yde (107), 73% of PER stage III fractures occurred from 2.5–8 cm above the ankle joint. If the fracture is transverse, a

mini-DC plate or ⅓ tubular five- to six-hole plate should be utilized with 3.5-mm cortical lag screw fixation (Fig. 14.49). Care must be taken when the DC plate is applied. Excessive compression can cause shortening or angulation of the distal fibula and thus result in incongruity. This plate is thicker than the normal ⅓ tubular plate. It should be placed in an area where sufficient soft-tissue coverage is available.

Oblique fractures with or without a butterfly fragment are stabilized with a five- to eight-hole ⅓ tubular plate that is contoured to the shape of the fibula (Fig 14.50). Lag screw fixation can be applied either through the plate or independent of the implant. The anterior syndesmosis should be repaired with meticulous care in an attempt to stabilize the bony fixation. The repair can be achieved with sutures of figure eight stainless steel wire (35). A transsyndesmotic screw should be utilized only in rare instances for protection of the

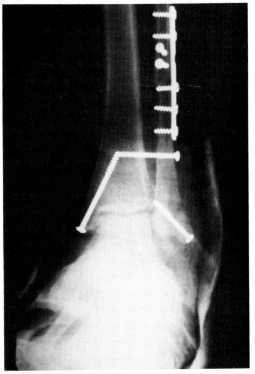

Figure 14.49. ASIF repair of a stage III pronation external rotation (PER) fracture.

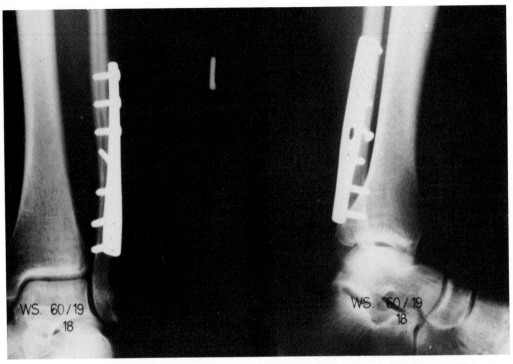

Figure 14.50.   Tubular plate fixation of a pronation external rotation (PER) stage III fracture.

interosseous membrane (35, 68). Usually, stable fixation of the anterior syndesmosis will provide enough rigidity to allow the interosseous membrane to heal.

In the opinion of Heim (35) and Willenegger (101–103) transsyndesmotic screw fixation is used too often for reduction of PER III and IV fractures. If repair of the anterior syndesmosis is incomplete and stabilization is not assured, the use of a transsyndesmotic stabilization screw may be indicated. The screw is usually inserted 3–5 cm above the ankle joint through three cortices—two fibular and one tibial—without compression. A gliding hole should not be made through the fibula; otherwise, a lag effect will occur which causes compression of the malleolar fork of the ankle joint. The screw can be applied either through the plate or inferior to the semitubular implant (Fig. 14.51). Before transfixation of the tibia and fibula, and after syndesmotic repair, the fibula should be pulled distally and rotated internally and fixed with a K-wire. Intra-operative radiographs should be taken at all angles and compared

to those of the unaffected ankle so that one can determine whether an anatomic reduction has been achieved. If the length of the fibula is correct and the joint is congruous, transfixation is achieved with a 3.5- or 4.5-mm cortical screw. Temporary fixation should be carried out with the ankle in full dorsiflexion so that the 2.2-mm increase in the width of the anterior trochlear surface of the talus can be accommodated. If this precaution is not taken, dorsiflexion may be severely limited.

Stage IV consists of a disruption of the posterior syndesmosis or a fracture of the posterolateral surface of the tibia. If the posterior malleolar fragment exceeds one-fourth the lateral width of the joint, anterior-to-posterior or posterior-to-anterior fixation may be necessary (Fig. 14.52). This is achieved according to Weber's technique (99), with the cancellous screws directed from anterior to posterior. A medial and lateral suction drain should be inserted and removed after 1–2 days. An anterior cross splint or a posterior V splint is applied immediately after surgery and kept in place

To check the alignment, one may use temporary K-wire fixation and control radiographs.

If the joint is congruous and the fibular length is normal, transfixation can be carried out in the following manner. Two 4.5-cm cortical screws are inserted parallel to the ankle joint, 3–5 cm above the articular surface (Fig. 14.53). All four cortices of the tibia and fibula are tapped; this avoids compression by the lag effect. These screws are used as stabilizing screws rather than compression screws. This type of fixation also prevents proximal displacement of the lower fibula. The fixation should be performed with the foot in maximal dorsiflexion. Meticulous repair of the anterior syndesmosis is necessary because it helps to stabilize the ruptured interosseous ligaments. If a posterior malleolar fracture occurs that involves more than one-fourth the articular surface, it should be repaired at

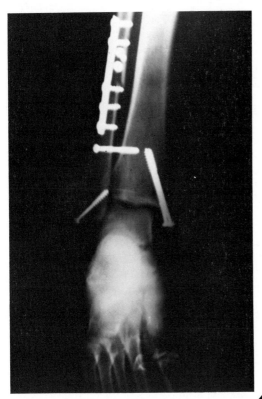

Figure 14.51. Transfixation ASIF (non-gliding) screw applied below the plate.

for 7–10 days. The splint can easily be removed for drain removal and passive range-of-motion exercises. A BK non-weightbearing cast is applied for 4–6 weeks after splint removal. The dorsal surface of the cast on the foot and ankle can be removed for passive range-of-motion exercises. If a transsyndesmotic screw has been inserted, it should be removed after 8 weeks before active weightbearing is allowed. A walking cast is applied for an additional 3–4 weeks. Active physical therapy and control of edema are of prime importance in the post-operative regimen.

According to Pankovich (75), Maisonneuve fractures account for up to 5% of the total ankle fracture rate. Because this is a high fibular fracture, it is often misdiagnosed. Fixation must be specific, otherwise, severe dislocation of the ankle joint will occur. The fibula should be pulled down and rotated internally into the fibular notch with a medium or large bone hook.

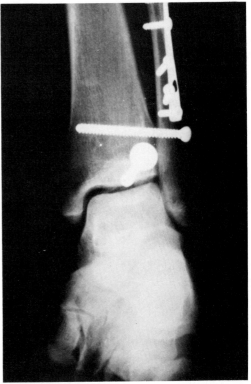

Figure 14.52. Fixation of the posterior malleolar fracture in a pronation external rotation (PER) fracture.

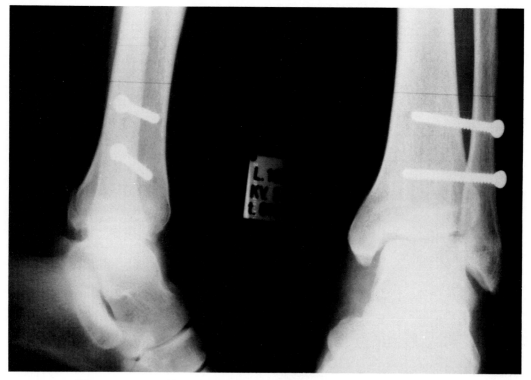

Figure 14.53. Two 4.5-mm screw fixation of a Maisonneuve fracture.

this time. According to the techniques previously mentioned, repair of the deltoid or medial malleolus is indicated. One or more Hemovac® drains are inserted and are removed 2 days post-operatively. The extremity is protected from weightbearing for 8 weeks or until the transfixation screws are removed. Walking in a BK cast is permitted for another 4 weeks. Vigorous physical therapy, consisting especially of dorsiflexion exercises, is encouraged so that the patient can regain maximal use of the joint. Edema control with the use of compression dressings and diuretic agents is indicated.

Because of the wide disruption of the ligaments of the syndesmosis, the post-trauma arthrosis rate is higher in this type of fracture. The arthrosis may occur for the following reasons: 1) mechanical injury to the joint cartilage, 2) a nutritional disturbance of the cartilage, 3) a trauma-induced incongruity resulting in step formation in the articular surface of the tibia, and 4) faulty weightbearing. If the fibula is not reduced exactly in the fibular notch,

shortening and backward displacement of the distal fibula occur, creating a loss of talotibial contact with eventual formation of a post-traumatic arthrosis. Compression of the malleolar fork leads to lack of dorsiflexion, with the production of an antalgic equinus gait. External rotation and valgus positions of the foot are seen with less-than-adequate reduction of the fracture.

OPEN FRACTURES OF THE ANKLE JOINT

In the study of 803 ankle fractures over a 7-year period at the Kantonsspital in St. Gallen, it was found that there were 25 open fractures, an incidence of 3.11%. The Mayo Clinic (31, 32) reported similar findings (4%).

The AO group classified open fractures according to three degrees (68). In first degree fractures, the skin is pierced from within by sharp fragments, with a skin opening of less than 1 cm. In second degree fractures, the skin is disrupted and crushed from without, with extensive soft-tissue damage. The rupture exceeds 1 cm in length. In third degree fractures, the injury is severe, with extensive skin, subcutaneous, and muscle necrosis. Third-degree fractures are often associated with injury to vessels and nerves and with damage to soft tissue. According to Anderson (108), 81% of 520 open fractures analyzed at Hennepen County Medical Center were grade I and II, whereas 19% were grade III.

The treatment of open ankle fractures is centered around the avoidance of infection. Chapman (110) states that grade I malleolar fractures can be fixed with no greater risk than incurred in closed fractures. Grade II and III injuries require great skill if further wound contamination, infection, and osteomyelitis are to be avoided. According to the AO group (68), only one-third of open fractures are contaminated with pathogenic material at the time of hospital admission. Contrasting statistics were reported at the Hennepen County Medical Center, where bacteriologic studies revealed 70.3% contamination at the time of admission or at wound closure (108). The AO group states that antibiotics are of little use in open fractures, whereas American surgeons utilize bacteriocidal broad spectrum antibiotics given intravenously. Cephalosporins and aminoglycosides are the antibiotics of choice for open wound contamination. The duration of antibiotic therapy usually is related to the type of wound closure. When the wound is closed primarily, the antibiotics are given for 3 days. When secondary closure of the wound is used, antibiotics are continued for at least 6 days or until the threat of infection has been averted.

Wound contamination can be tested by a variety of means; however, the most sensitive test is one in which a portion or portions of the deep wound are analyzed bacteriologically according to the method of Robson et al. (113, 114). Wound contamination is considered present if the bacteria count exceeds 10^5. Slides can be prepared for culture immediately, which is of great advantage for the treatment of an open wound.

Debridement of grade II and III injuries is extremely important. Extensive removal of foreign material and of necrotic soft tissue (ligaments, muscle, etc.) must be carried out. Skin debridement should be held to a minimum, with extensive incisions utilized instead of skin removal. Non-viable flaps should be removed. One can test the viability of a flap by utilizing intravenous fluorescein and a Wood's lamp. Contaminated tissue and deep fascia have a poor blood supply and must be debrided radically. The viability of muscle should be tested by pinching with forceps or by electrical stimulation, rather than on the basis of bleeding and color. Debridement of bone, like that of skin, should be conservative. Soft tissue attachments to bone should be preserved if at all possible.

It must be emphasized that copious irrigation of the wound with lactated Ringer's solution is indicated. Studies have shown that doubling the quantity of the irrigating solution may be a factor in decreasing wound contamination. At least 8 liters of solution should be utilized. It is advisable to employ a Water Pic® or Surgilav® to achieve maximum penetration into the wound.

The type of internal fixation utilized depends upon the nature of the wound. Generally, the normal type of internal fixation can be utilized for grade I open ankle fractures. For grade II and III fractures, minimal internal fixation protected by external fixation is the procedure of choice, followed by open packing of the wound. More rigid fixation can be applied after delayed primary closure has been completed. Soft-tissue healing usually is adequate after 3 months (110). In some severe grade II or III ankle injuries, ankle fusion after primary closure is the procedure of choice. Autogenous cancellous bone grafting should be performed after 3–6 months if active callus formation is absent.

ANKLE FUSION

If primary open or closed reduction fails, the ankle joint may become so painful or deformed that a secondary procedure is necessary. The two options available today are ankle fusion and implantation of a total-joint prosthesis. To date, the long-term results of total ankle replacement have been disappointing. The procedure of choice is fusion of the ankle. Six ankle fusions were performed at our institution because of failure of ankle fracture reductions; four of these failures occurred after PER fractures (Fig. 14.54).

More than 40 different fusion procedures for the ankle joint are available. A survey of published data indicates that, regardless of the procedure used, the average healing time for an ankle fusion is 5.2 months. The most common type of fusion performed at our institution over the last 5 years was external fixation with a 2 or 3-pin compression system. In 16 attempts, only four fusions proceeded without complications. Problems encountered were non-union (32%) (Fig. 14.55), infection leading to os-

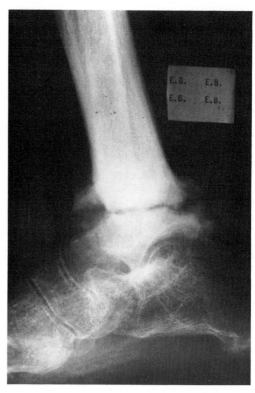

Figure 14.55. Hypertrophic non-union secondary to external fixation or lack of external fixation.

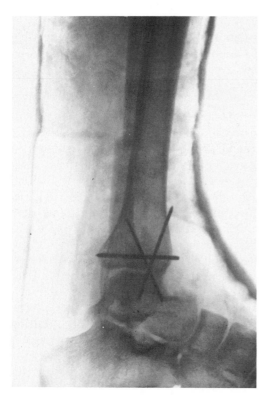

Figure 14.54. Inadequate fixation technique in a pronation external rotation (PER) fracture leading to later post-traumatic arthritis.

teomyelitis (26%), malposition, and the need for amputation.

Because of these complications, a procedure was tested which utilizes internal instead of external fixation. Over the last 2 years, all fractures have been stabilized internally with two or three 6.5-mm cancellous screws (Fig. 14.56). We believe that internal fixation offers distinct advantages over external fixation in that it avoids pin tract infections which can lead to chronic bone infection. The results of this type of fusion have been encouraging, especially when this technique has been used secondarily for cases in which ankle fusions failed with external fixation. To date, five of six fusions have occurred with this procedure in an average of 18 weeks, as confirmed by radiography. If the fusion of the joint fails, a below-knee amputation must be considered.

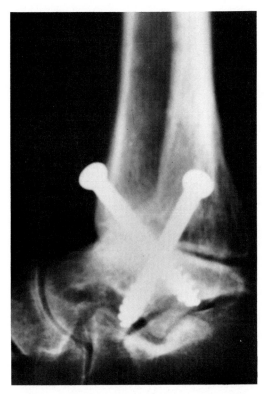

Figure 14.56. Ankle fusion with 6.5-mm cancellous screw fixation 6 months post-operatively.

CHILDREN'S ANKLE FRACTURES

Ankle fractures in children can be classified according to either radiographic interpretation or causative force.

Radiographic Interpretation

In this method, injuries are grouped according to the radiographic disturbance of the epiphyseal plate and its surrounding structures. The epiphyseal plate is a cartilagenous segment interposed between the epiphysis and the metaphysis of a long bone, i.e., the distal ends of the tibia and fibula (3). The epiphyseal plate is divided grossly into two zones. One of these is the cartilage production zone, which causes growth of the long bone. This region lies closest to the epiphysis and can be further subdivided into the zone of small cartilage cells and the zone of cell columns. The zone of small cells is thought to produce matrix for the germinal cells located in the zone of cell columns, which cause longitudinal growth (Fig. 14.57).

Many factors affect the growth rate of long bones, including the blood supply, as well as the effects of estrogen, testosterone, and growth hormone, and any disease or trauma which influences growth patterns. Degeneration and calcification occur in the zone of transformation which lies close to the metaphysis (the zone of hypertrophic cell formation). Vascular infiltration, osteogenesis, and remodeling occur in the metaphysis of a growing long bone.

Epiphyseal plate separation usually occurs in the zone of hypertrophic cell formation (111, 112) between the calcified and uncalcified layers. Separation of the epiphyseal plate is also termed epiphysiolysis, whereas separation or disruption of the plate and metaphysis can be called a fracture of the adjoining metaphysis or epiphysis.

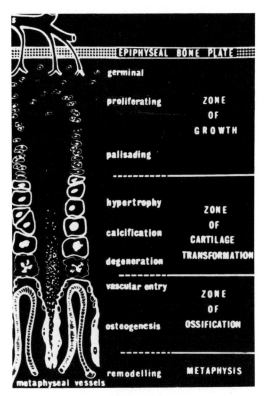

Figure 14.57. Epiphyseal plate zones according to Rang (112).

Two main classifications are in use today. Poland's (111) classification differentiates between partial and complete plate separation, combined with fractures of the epiphysis or of the metaphyseal-diaphyseal area. The most common classification of epiphyseal plate injury is the grouping according to Salter and Harris (86), who placed epiphyseal plate injuries in five categories. In type I injuries, the plate separates without fracture of either the metaphysis or the epiphysis (Fig. 14.58). In type II injuries, there is a partial separation of the epiphyseal plate, combined with a fracture of the metaphysis (Fig. 14.59). In type III injuries, there is a separation and vertical fracture of the epiphysis (Fig. 14.60). In type IV injuries, there is a vertical fracture through the epiphysis, epiphyseal plate, and metaphysis (Fig. 14.61). In type V injuries, the epiphyseal plate may be compressed or crushed; this may result in permanent, partial, or total arrest of growth (Fig. 14.62).

In general, type I epiphyseal injuries to the ankle joint can be treated non-operatively, i.e., by casting for 3–6 weeks (111). The prognosis for type II, III, IV, and V fractures depends on the anatomic regions, as will be seen when each specific fracture is examined.

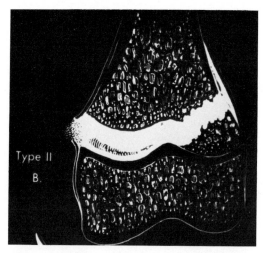

Figure 14.59. Salter II epiphyseal plate injury.

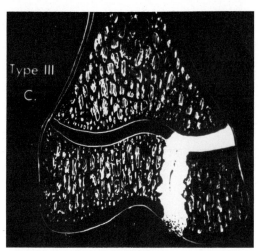

Figure 14.60. Salter III epiphyseal plate injury.

Causative Force

In the second method, the force causing a specific disturbance is analyzed. The ankle is, for the most part, a hinge joint whose motion is primarily in the sagittal plane, with very little transverse movement. The ankle joint is supported by ligamentous structures on its anterior, posterior, medial, and lateral margins. In addition, the joint is highly congruous with constantly changing contact points throughout the gait cycle. Any violent force which causes abnormal transverse-plane motion of the ankle

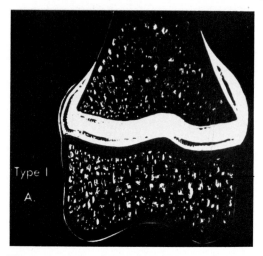

Figure 14.58. Salter I epiphyseal plate injury.

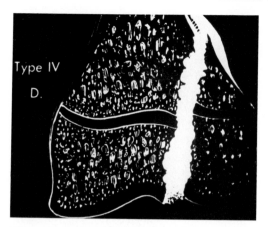

Figure 14.61. Salter IV epiphyseal plate injury.

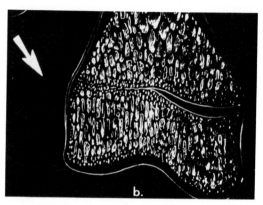

Figure 14.62. Salter V epiphyseal plate injury.

or in combination with a medial corner (Salter III) disturbance of the ankle joint (Fig. 14.65). In a study by Spiegel et al. (90), this injury compromised 7.6% of the

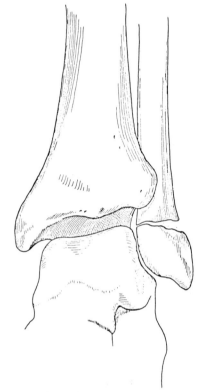

Figure 14.63. Salter I fibular fracture diagram.

joint may result in a fracture. Most ankle injuries occur when the foot is forced into extreme pronation or supination, with or without external rotation of the foot. In children, dorsiflexion or plantarflexion may accentuate the injury.

Classification and Treatment

The presence of the epiphyseal plate permits grouping of juvenile ankle fractures into specific types according to the cause of the injury.

SALTER TYPE I FIBULAR
FRACTURES (Figs. 14.63 and 14.64)

The cause of this type of fracture is supination. It can occur as an isolated injury

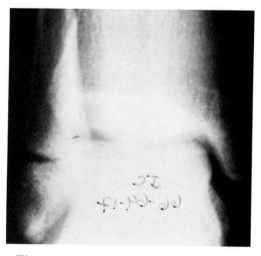

Figure 14.64. Salter I fibular fracture.

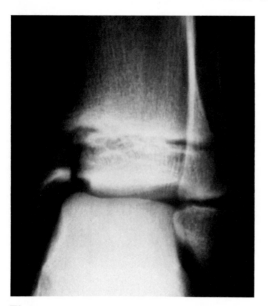

Figure 14.65. Salter I fibular injury with a Salter III medial corner tibial injury.

cases. It may be difficult to diagnose without comparative radiographic views of the unaffected ankle, an estimate of the amount of soft-tissue edema lateral to the epiphyseal plate as seen radiographically, and an associated clinical finding of pain. Generally, when the diameter of the ankle with soft-tissue edema exceeds that on the unaffected side by 5 mm or more, a Salter I fibular fracture can be suspected. Complications of this type of fracture are rare. Malposition, asymmetry, and shortening (90) are among the post-fracture disturbances that can occur. The treatment of choice is a BK walking cast for 3 weeks. Open reduction with internal fixation is rarely indicated. Care should be taken to rule out a medial corner (Salter III or IV) tibial injury.

SALTER II FIBULAR FRACTURE
(Fig. 14.66)

The mechanism of injury in this fibular fracture is pronation with external rotation of the foot. This is a rare injury, making up only 3–5% of all pediatric ankle fractures. Complications are infrequent. Treatment of this injury consists of a BK cast for 4 weeks.

SALTER TYPE I TIBIAL FRACTURE
(Figs. 14.67 and 14.68)

The mechanism of this injury also is pronation with external rotation of the foot. This type of disorder places the fibula under high torque, and in 25% of the cases (90) a spiral or transverse fracture of the fibular shaft occurs (Fig. 14.69). The fracture is located 2–3 inches above the syndesmosis. Fractures of the fibula above the syndesmosis constitute about 15% of all childrens' ankle fractures (111). These fractures can be displaced or non-displaced and are diagnosed on the basis of edema, pain, and tenderness along the tibial epiphyseal plate line. Edema may be minimal; therefore, comparison radiographs are important for evaluation of the extent of the injury. Complications are infrequent; they include overgrowth or growth stimulation on the affected side, premature closure of the dis-

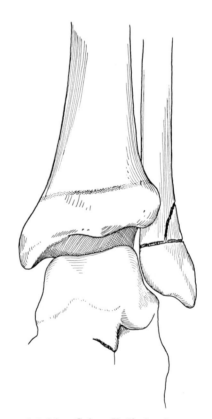

Figure 14.66. Salter II fibular fracture diagram.

tal epiphyseal plate, and, in rare instances, a residual angular deformity. Treatment consists of closed reduction, if needed, followed by immobilization in a non-weight-bearing long-leg cast for 3 weeks, and then 3 weeks in a BK walking cast.

SALTER II TIBIAL FRACTURE (Figs. 14.70 and 14.71)

This is the most common distal-epiphyseal-plate injury encountered in children (90, 111, 112). These fractures are caused by three main mechanisms, namely, pronation, external rotation, and plantarflexion. Because of the high shear torque associated with this injury, a high fibular fracture occurs in approximately 25% of the cases (Fig. 14.72). This fracture can be spiral, transverse, or greenstick in nature. Complications include premature closure of either the medial or the lateral portion of the plate, causing an angular deformity. Spiegel (90) stated that any non-reduced angular deformity may eventually lead to a

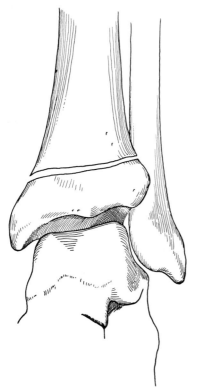

Figure 14.67. Salter I tibial injury diagram.

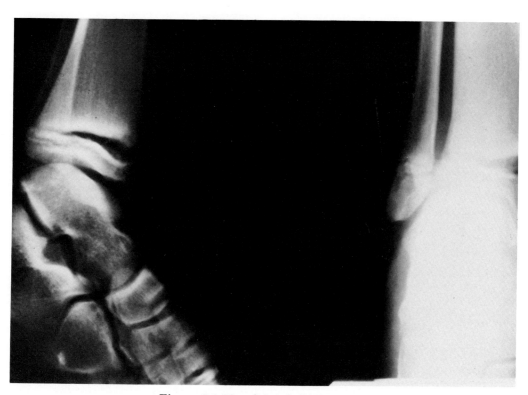

Figure 14.68. Salter I tibial fracture.

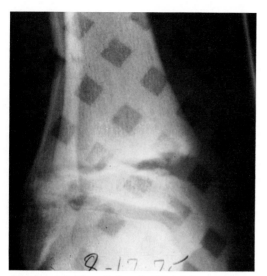

Figure 14.69. Salter I tibial injury with an associated fibular fracture.

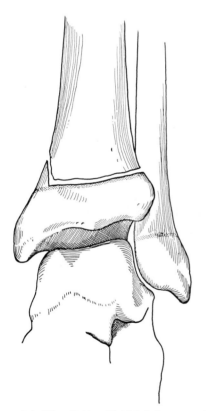

Figure 14.70. Salter II tibial fracture diagram.

residual deformity. He found that the Salter II tibial injury had a 16.7% complication rate. The treatment consists of reversing the mechanism of injury by providing ade-

quate immobilization. Excessive manipulation should be avoided so that the germinal cells are protected from further damage. After adequate reduction, these fractures should be held in a long-leg nonweightbearing cast for 3 weeks, followed by a walking cast for an additional 3 weeks.

SALTER III TIBIAL FRACTURES

There are three types of Salter III tibial injuries: a medial corner injury, a vertical fracture, and a vertical-lateral (Tillaux) fracture. Each fracture has a different etiology and requires a different treatment regimen; they will be discussed separately.

The medial corner Salter III injury (Fig. 14.73) is caused by supination, which may create a pull-off fracture of the distal fibular epiphyseal plate (Fig. 14.74) in about 25% of the cases. The medial corner of the talus impacts against the inner corner of the medial malleolus. The displacement of the medial malleolus is proportional to the

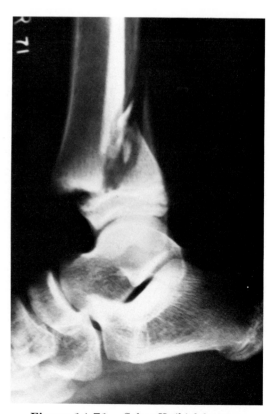

Figure 14.71. Salter II tibial fracture.

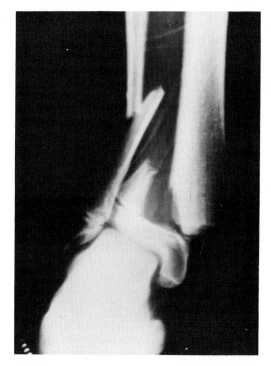

Figure 14.72. Salter II tibial fracture with associated fibular fracture.

force involved and, if excessive, may cause displacement of the fragment (Figs. 14.75 and 14.76) or produce a Salter IV medial corner injury. Complications of this type of fracture occur when displacement is excessive (more than 2 mm). If this fracture heals in malposition, angular deformities may result. Premature plate closure with widening and asymmetry of the ankle joint may also occur.

Treatment of this fracture depends upon the amount of displacement. If displacement is less than 2 mm, the patient must be immobilized by a long-leg non-weight-bearing cast for 3 weeks, followed by a BK walking cast for an additional 3 weeks. If the displacement exceeds 2 mm, an open reduction with internal fixation should be performed. It is important to take an internal oblique radiograph of the ankle for clear visualization of the inner medial surface of the tibia, so that the amount of displacement can be judged accurately. Approximately 20% of all Salter III medial corner injuries require open reduction and internal fixation (90). Open reduction is best achieved by two parallel K-wires or two parallel 3.5-mm cortical or 4.0-mm cancellous screws (Fig. 14.77). Care must be taken

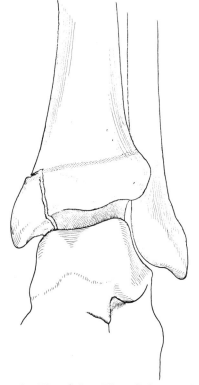

Figure 14.73. Salter III medial corner injury diagram.

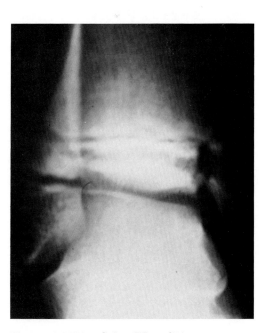

Figure 14.74. Salter III medial corner injury combined with a Salter I fibular fracture.

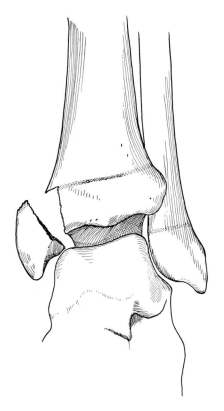

Figure 14.75. Displaced Salter III medial injury diagram.

not to enter the epiphyseal plate region with the screws, for this may cause premature plate closure and poor results.

Another type of Salter III injury is an intra-articular vertical fracture through the epiphysis and plate (Figs. 14.78 and 14.79). The mechanism of injury is impaction with dorsiflexion or plantarflexion. These fractures occur in the central portion of the epiphyseal plate just prior to plate closure. They occur at about the same age as a Tillaux (lateral Salter III) fracture (see below), at 13 years, and are caused by direct impact rather than by a shearing or rotary force. A good internal oblique radiograph is necessary for the diagnosis; it may be helpful to use tomograms for confirmation (22). These are rare fractures, occurring in less than 2% of the cases of ankle fractures. Complications are unusual but may include premature closure of the distal tibial epiphyseal plate (90). Treatment of a central

Salter III fracture consists of 3 weeks in an AK non-weightbearing cast, followed by 3 weeks in a BK walking cast.

The third type of Salter III distal tibial fracture encountered is the Tillaux fracture (95), a vertical fracture localized in the anterolateral corner of the distal tibial epiphysis and plate (Fig. 14.80 and 14.81). This is the last portion of the distal tibial epiphyseal plate to close. Final closure occurs first in the central portion, then in the medial portion, and then laterally (111). The ligamentous attachments of the anterior tibiofibular ligament are localized in the anterior-lateral portion of the epiphysis and plate. The causative force is plantarflexion with external rotation, which allows the talus to impact on the lateral side of the tibia. It has also been theorized that this injury may involve a pull-off fragment of the anterior tibiofibular ligament. This fracture constitutes approximately 10% (14) of all Salter III fractures (90). It may be displaced if the anterior tibiofibular attachment is not ruptured. Any displacement of more than 2 mm requires open reduction and internal fixation with small screws or K-wires for reattachment of the anterior portion of the lateral ankle syndesmosis (Fig. 14.82).

Complications include residual rotatory instability and articular incongruity. Nonoperative treatment is designed to negate future rotatory instability by reversing the mechanism of injury. This is achieved by internal rotation of the foot and by a long-leg non-weightbearing cast for 6 weeks. If the fragment is displaced by more than 2 mm, open reduction with internal fixation must be initiated, followed by 6 weeks of an AK non-weightbearing cast in internal rotation.

SALTER IV TIBIAL FRACTURE (Figs. 14.83 and 14.84)

The mechanism of injury for this fracture is supination, which causes the trochlear surface of the talus to impact on the medial anterior corner of the distal tibia, thus initiating a disruption of the medial malleolus

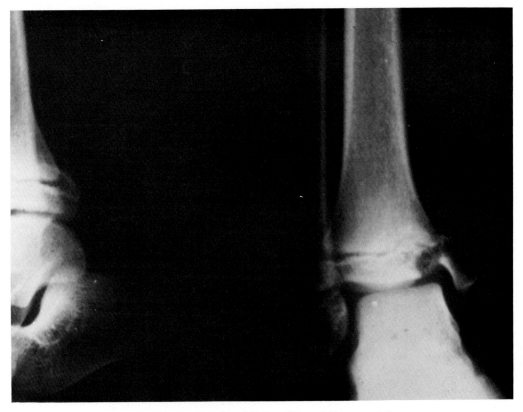

Figure 14.76. Displaced Salter III medial corner injury.

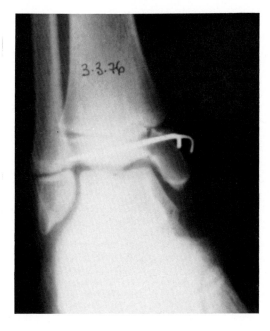

Figure 14.77. Displaced Salter III medial corner injury with internal fixation.

which extends through the epiphyseal plate into the metaphysis. If sufficient force is generated, the fracture may be displaced by more than 2 mm. Such a displacement may result in a loss of congruity to the ankle joint, leading to a higher incidence of osteoarthritis and thus to disability in later life. Potential complications of malunion in this type of fracture include growth arrest of the plate, which causes a discrepancy in limb length; varus angulation; and incongruity of the ankle joint. Non-operative treatment of the disruption necessitates the use of an AK non-weightbearing cast for 3 weeks, followed by a BK walking cast for 3 weeks. If the medial corner is disrupted by more than 2 mm, open reduction with internal fixation is necessary so that the normal congruity of the ankle joint can be maintained. This is best achieved by the use of two small K-wires or one or two 4.0-mm cancellous or 3.5-mm cortical screws

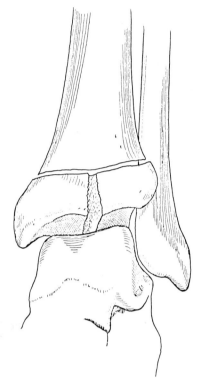

Figure 14.78. Central Salter III vertical tibial fracture diagram.

placed parallel to the epiphyseal plate. Care must be taken to avoid crossing the plate with the screws. The trauma caused during surgery must be minimized so that premature closure of the epiphysis does not occur.

TRIPLANE FRACTURE (Salter I–IV)
(Figs. 14.85 and 14.86)

This fracture occurs across all three body planes: frontal, transverse, and sagittal. Radiographically, such a fracture is seen on the AP view as a central Salter III and on the lateral view a Salter II type with an attached portion of the metaphysis. There has been some conjecture as to the actual configuration of the fracture. Marmor (60) performed an open reduction of an apparently nonreducible type II fracture and observed a distal tibial fracture in three parts: the tibial shaft, an anterolateral epiphyseal fragment, and a combination of the remainder of the epiphysis and an attached posterior metaphyseal fragment. Cooperman (22) used tomograms to determine the three-dimensional configuration and found

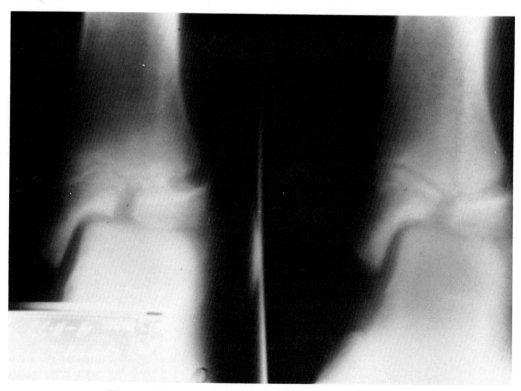

Figure 14.79. Central Salter III vertical tibial fracture.

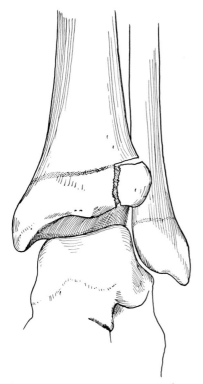

Figure 14.80. Tillaux fracture diagram.

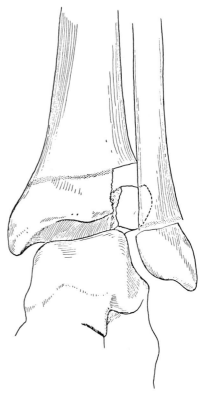

Figure 14.82. Displaced Tillaux fracture diagram.

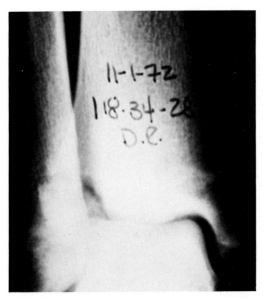

Figure 14.81. Tillaux fracture (non-displaced).

a two-part fracture which consisted of a medial fragment that included the tibial shaft, the medial malleolus, and the anteromedial part of the epiphysis. The lateral fragment included the remainder of the epiphysis, together with a piece of the posterior metaphysis and the attached fibula.

The mechanism of injury can only be postulated; it may consist of loading of the foot in plantarflexion, combined with an external rotation force. Proper radiographic evaluation, including tomograms, is necessary if this injury is suspected. These fractures are often missed on routine radiographs. Complications of this injury include joint incongruity and premature closure of the epiphyseal plate. Cooperman et al. (22) performed a CT scan on a triplane fracture and found that the bone was minimally displaced medially, with a large displacement laterally. In their opinion, a poor reduction could lead to joint incongruity or to potential complications in later life. Premature closure of the plate is a less serious problem because most of the fractures occur in children who are near skeletal maturity, at about 13½ years, and because they leave little residual deformity.

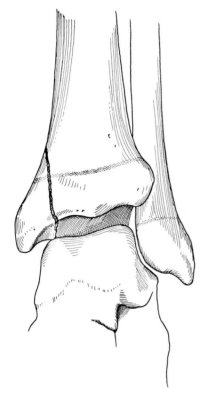

Figure 14.83. Salter IV tibial fracture diagram.

thought to be a major cause of this disturbance. Therefore, it is necessary to rotate the foot internally so that the lateral gap is closed properly and the fragments are realigned. Non-operative treatment is generally successful if there is a gap of less than 2 mm between the anterior and posterior fragments. The internal position of the talus and foot should be held in a nonweightbearing AK cast for at least 6 weeks. If the gap exceeds 2 mm, open reduction with internal fixation is indicated. This is best achieved by the use of small 3.5-mm cortical or 4.0-mm cancellous screws or interfragmentary K-wires.

SALTER V FRACTURES

These fractures are caused by severe axial loads across the epiphyseal plate (Fig. 14.87). This type of force is generated from falls which cause supination-external rotation injuries to the ankle joint. Often both the tibia and fibula are comminuted (Fig. 14.88). This is a rare injury, seen in less than 1% of cases. The major complication

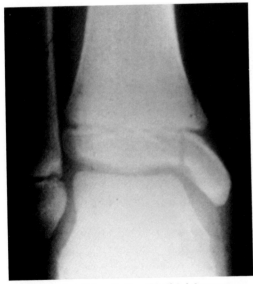

Figure 14.84. Salter IV tibial fracture.

Non-operative treatment is aimed at reversing the causative force. CT scans and laminograms show a wider lateral than medial displacement. External rotation is

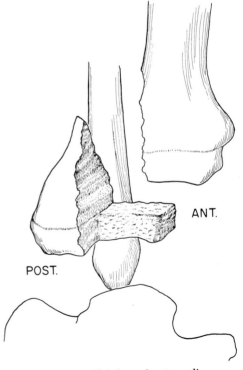

Figure 14.85. Triplane fracture diagram as outlined by Cooperman et al. (22).

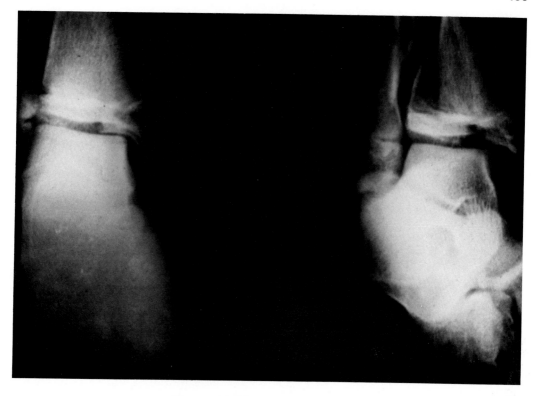

Figure 14.86. Triplane fracture.

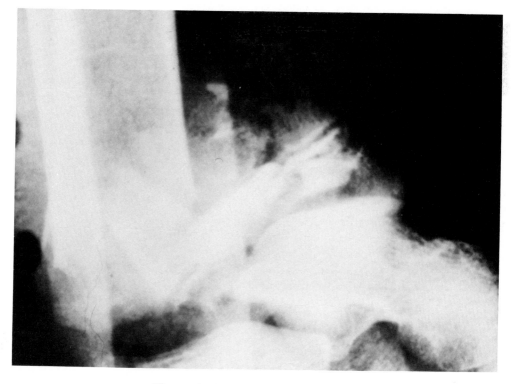

Figure 14.87. Salter V crush injury.

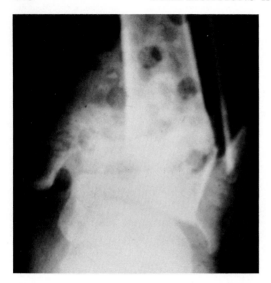

Figure 14.88. Comminuted Salter V distal tibial injury.

is partial or complete premature closure of the physis. Premature arrest of longitudinal growth may result from destruction of the germinal cells of the physis, or the formation of a bony bridge between the metaphysis and epiphysis. An osseous bridge may occur throughout the entire epiphyseal plate, the central portion, or any section of the peripheral portion (111). Complete premature plate closure leads to an age-dependent limb length discrepancy (Fig. 14.89). Partial early closure causes asymmetry and angulation of the distal tibia or fibula, and thus future disability (85, 86). Treatment of this severe injury depends upon the degree of associated soft-tissue trauma and the amount of plate damage and comminution. If soft-tissue injuries are severe, external fixation or traction may be the treatment of choice. If soft-tissue injuries are minimal, open reduction with internal fixation may be indicated. In some instances, it may be judicious to apply gentle manipulation with cast immobilization. The goal of all forms of treatment is to minimize the effect of premature closure of the distal tibia and fibula.

Miscellaneous Epiphyseal and Periepiphyseal Ankle Injuries

From 4–8% of all ankle injuries in juve-

nile patients consist of fractures involving the peripheral region of the growth plate (89, 90) pull-off or separation fractures of the epiphysis or metaphysis, and isolated posterior malleolar fractures. The causes are varied and can include direct impact, twisting forces, angulated impact, as well as plantarflexion and dorsiflexion injuries. Potential complications are the formation of osteochondral fractures, osteocartilagenous exostosis formation, perimeter osseous bridging, and incongruity of the joint. Treatment of these injuries should be individualized and should be directed toward the prevention of any permanent disability.

Fractures of the distal tibia and of fibular growth centers are among the most frequent injuries in children. Spiegel et al. followed 184 patients with such fractures for 28 months after injury (90). They defined a group of complications, including shortening of the leg, angular deformity of bone, or incongruity of the joint, which have the potential of leading to future dis-

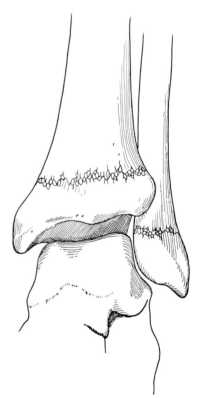

Figure 14.89. Salter V tibial injury with resultant limb length discrepancy.

ability. They then analyzed Salter I–V fractures of the ankle in order to pinpoint high-risk types of fractures which may result in specific complications. These studies indicate that the incidence of complications was lowest in type I fibular fractures, type I tibial fractures, type III or IV nondisplaced tibial fractures, and epiphyseal avulsion injuries. For patients having Salter II tibial fractures, the outcome was unpredictable. A high-risk group of patients was identified, which included patients with displaced Salter III and IV tibial fracture, displaced Tillaux fracture, triplane fractures, and Salter V crushing injuries. Oh et al. (71) studied 162 epiphyseal injuries and concluded that in Salter II injuries, a significant discrepancy and distortion of bone growth had occurred.

In general, Salter I and II tibial and fibular fractures should be reduced to within 10% of anatomic reduction. Salter III and IV injuries should be reduced to anatomic status; this will limit the potential complications of malunion leading to joint incongruity or premature growth plate closure, which causes asymmetry and limb length discrepancy.

The treatment of ankle fractures is a complex and fascinating art. The introduction of the AO technique has greatly changed the outcome for bi- and trimalleolar fractures. Following studies in the future should provide information on the long-term success rate of these procedures.

References

1. Ashurst, A. P. C., and Bromer, R. S. Classification and mechanism of fractures of the leg bones involving the ankle. AMA Arch. Surg. 4:51, 1922.
2. Berridge, F. R., and Bonnin, J. G. The radiographic examination of the ankle including arthrography. Surg. Gynecol. Obstet. 79:383, 1944.
3. Bishop, P. A. Fractures and epiphyseal separation fractures of the ankle. Am. J. Roentgenol. 28:49, 1932.
4. Bistrom, O. Conservative treatment of severe ankle fractures. A clinical and follow-up study. Acta Chir. Scand. Suppl. 168:4–36, 1952.
5. Bolin, H. The fibula and its relationship to the tibia and talus in injuries of the ankle due to forced external rotation. Acta Radiol. 56:439, 1961.
6. Bazille: Mem, sur les sujets proposes pour le prix de l'Acad. Roy. de Chir. Paris 4:563, 1778.
7. Bonnin, J. G. Injuries to the Ankle. William Heinemann, London, 1950.
8. Bonnin, J. G. Injury to the ligaments of the ankle. J. Bone Jt. Surg. 47B:609, 1965.
9. Bromfield, W. Chirurgical Observations and Cases. T. Cadell, London, 1773.
10. Brostrom, L. Sprained Ankles. Diss., Stockholm, 1966.
11. Brostrom, L., Liljedahl, S.-O., and Lindvall, N. Isolated fracture of the posterior tibial tubercle. Aetiologic and clinical features. Acta Chir. Scand. 128:51, 1964.
12. Brostrom, L., Liljedahl, S.-O., and Lindvall, N. Sprained ankles. II. Arthrographic diagnosis of recent ligament ruptures. Acta Chir. Scand. 129:485, 1965.
13. Burwell, N. H., and Charnley, A. D. The treatment of displaced fractures at the ankle by rigid internal fixation and early joint movement. J. Bone Jt. Surg. 47B:634, 1965.
14. Edmonson, A. S., and Crenshaw, A. H., eds. Campbell's Operative Orthopaedics, 6th ed. C. V. Mosby, 1980, pp. 552–565.
15. Cave, E. F. Complications of the operative treatment of fractures of the ankle. Clin. Orthop. 42:13, 1965.
16. Cedell, C. A. Outward rotation-supination injuries of the ankle. Clin. Orthop. 42:97, 1967.
17. Cedell, C.-A., and Wilberg, G. Treatment of eversion-supination fracture of the ankle (2nd degree). Acta Chir. Scand. 124:41, 1962.
18. Chaput, V. Les Fractures Malleolaires du Cu-depieds et Les Accidents du Travail. Masson and Cre, Paris, 1907.
19. Charnley, J. Closed Treatment of Common Fractures. Livingston, Edinburgh, 1957.
20. Close, R. J. Some applications of the functional anatomy of the ankle joint. J. Bone Jt. Surg. 38A:761, 1956.
21. Cooper, A. P. A Treatise on Dislocations and on Fractures of the Joints. 353–375, London, 1822.
22. Cooperman, D. R., Spiegel, P. G., and Laros, G. S. Tibial fractures involving the ankle in children. The so-called triplane epiphyseal fracture. J. Bone Jt. Surg. 60:1040–1046, 1978.
23. Danis, R. Les fractures malleolaires, in Theorie et Pratique de L'osteosynthese. Masson, Paris, 1949.
24. Destot, E.: Diastasis et fracture des malleoles. Rev. Chir. Paris 27:279, 1907.
25. Dias, L. S., and Tachdjian, M. O. Physeal injuries of the ankle in children: classification. Clin. Orthop. 136:230–233, 1978.
26. Dupuytren: Ann. Mid-chir. Hop. Hosp. Civ. Paris, 1819.
27. El Banna, S., DeLauwer, M., and Raynal, L. Fracture of the ankle (review of 136 cases). Acta Orthop. Belg. 44:402–415, 1978.
28. Emmett, J. E., and Breck, L. W. A review and analysis of 11,000 fractures seen in a private practice of orthopedic surgery, 1937–1956. J. Bone Jt. Surg. 40A(#5): October, 1958.
29. Fahey, J. J., Schlenker, L. T., and Stauffer, R. C. Fracture dislocation of ankle with fixed displacement of fibula behind tibia. Am. J. Roentgenol. 76:1102, 1956.
30. leFort, L. Note sur une variete indecrite de la fracture verticale de la malleole externe par ar-

rachement (quoted by Lauge Hansen). Bull. Gen. Therap. Med. Chir. 110:193, 1886.

31. Garraway, W., Stauffer, R., Kurland, L., et al. Limb fractures in a defined population. I. Frequency and distribution. Mayo Clin. Proc. 54:701–707, 1979.

32. Garraway, W., Stauffer, R., Kurland, L., et al. Limb fractures in a defined population. II. Orthopedic treatment and utilization of health care. Mayo Clin. Proc. 54:708–713, 1979.

33. Warwick, R., and Williams, P., eds. *Gray's Anatomy*, 35th British Edition. W. B. Saunders, Philadelphia, 1973, p. 460.

34. Harris, E. J. Epiphyseal plate injuries in pediatric ankle traumatology. J. Foot Surg. Fall 20:145–147, 1981.

35. Heim, V., and Pfeiffer, K. M. *Small Fragment Set Manual.* Springer Verlag, Heidelberg, 1974.

36. Hendelberg, T. The roentgenographic examination of the ankle joint in malleolar fractures. Acta Radiol. 11:411–444, 1946.

37. Hirsch, C., and Lewis, J. Experimental ankle joint fractures. Acta Orthop. Scand. 36:408, 1965.

38. Honigschmeid, J. Leichenexperimente uber die Zerreissungen der Bander im Sprunggelenk mit Rucksicht auf die Enstehung der indirecten Knochelfracturen. Dtsch. Z. Chir. 8:239, 1877.

39. Hughes, J. The medial malleolus in ankle fractures. Orthop. Clin. North Am. 11:649–660, 1980.

40. Hughes, J. L., Weber, H., Willenegger, H., and Kuner, E. H. Evaluation of ankle fractures: Nonoperative and operative treatment. Clin. Orthop. 138:111–119, 1979.

41. Jergesen, F. Open reduction of fractures and dislocations of the ankle. Am. J. Surg. 98:136, 1957.

42. Kleiger, B. The mechanism of ankle injuries. J. Bone Jt. Surg. 38A:59, 1956.

43. Kleiger, B. The treatment of oblique fractures of the fibula. J. Bone Jt. Surg. 43A:969, 1961.

44. Klossner, O. Late results of operative and nonoperative treatment of severe ankle fractures. Acta Chir. Scand. Suppl. 293:123–131, 1962.

45. Kristensen, T. B. Treatment of malleolar fractures according to Lauge Hansen's method. Preliminary results. Acta Chir. Scand. 97:362, 1949.

46. Kristensen, T. B. Fractures of the ankle. VI. Follow-up studies. AMA Arch. Surg. 73:112, 1956.

47. Lambert, K. L. The weightbearing function of the fibula. J. Bone Jt. Surg. 58A:3, 1976.

48. Lambotte, A. The operative treatment of fractures. Br. Med. J. 4:1530, 1912.

49. Lane, W. A. Method of procedure in operations on simple fractures. Br. Med. J. 4:1532, 1912.

50. Lauge Hansen, N. Ankelbrud. I. Genetisk diagnose og reposition. Diss. Munksgaard, Kobenhavn, 1942.

51. Lauge Hansen, N. "Ligamentous" ankle fractures. Acta Chir. Scand. 97:544, 1949.

52. Lauge Hansen, N. Fractures of the ankle. III. Genetic roentgenologic diagnosis of fractures of the ankle. Am. J. Roentgenol. 71:456, 1954.

53. Lauttamus, L., and Solonen, K. A. Treatment of malleolar fractures. Acta Orthop. Scand. 36:321, 1965.

54. LeRoy, L. *De la Fracture Marginale Anterieure de la Malleole Externe.* Paris, 1887.

55. Lindblom, K. Arthrography. J. Fac. Radiol. Lond. 3:151, 1952.

56. Magnusson, R. On the late results in non-operated cases of malleolar fractures. I. Fractures by external rotation. Acta Chir. Scand. Suppl. 84:98–116, 1944.

57. Magnusson, R. Ligament injuries of the ankle joint. Acta Orthop. Scand. 36:317, 1965.

58. Maisonneuve, J. G. Recherches sur la fracture du perone (quoted by Bonnin). Arch. Gen. Med. 7:165, 1840.

59. Malka, J. S., and Taillard, W. *Clinical Orthopedics.* 1969, pp. 67–159.

60. Marmor, L. An unusual fracture of the tibial epiphysis. Clin. Orthop. 73:132, 1970.

61. Mast, J. W., and Teipner, W. A. A reproducible approach to the internal fixation of adult ankle fractures: Rationale, technique, and early results. Orthop. Clin. North Am. 11:661–679, 1980.

62. Mau, H. Die Osteochondrosis dissecans und frei Korper des Sprunggelenkes. Ztschr. Orthop. 91:582, 1959.

63. Mazur, J. M., Schwartz, E., and Simon, S. R. Ankle arthrodesis. Long-term follow-up with gait analysis. J. Bone Jt. Surg. 61:964–975, 1979.

64. McLaughlin, H. L., and Ryder, C. T. Open reduction and internal fixation for fractures of the tibia and ankle. S. Clin. North. Am. 29:1523, 1949.

65. Meyer, T. L., Jr., and Kumler, K. W. ASIF technique and ankle fractures. Clin. Orthop. 150:211–216, 1980.

66. Mitchell, W. G., Shaftan, G. W., and Sclafani, S. J. Mandatory open reduction. Its role in displaced ankle fractures. J. Trauma 19:602–615, 1979.

67. Mueller, M. E., Allgoewer, M., Schneider, R., and Willenegger, H. *Manual of Internal Fixation*, 2nd ed. Springer-Verlag, Heidelberg, 1979, pp. 282–299.

68. Mueller, M. E., Allgoewer, M., and Willenegger, H. *Technique of Internal Fixation of Fractures.* Springer Verlag, Heidelberg, 1965, pp. 114–145.

69. Muller, G. M. Fractures of the internal malleolus. Br. Med. J. 11:320, 1945.

70. Nilsson, B. E. R. Age and sex incidence of ankle fractures. Acta Orthop. Scand. 40:122–129, 1969.

71. Oh, I., et al. Cerclage of the lateral malleolus in displaced fractures of the ankle. Orthopedics 1:374–379, 1978.

72. Palmer, I. Arthritis deformans, etiologi och behandling. II. Frakturer och arthrosis deformans. Nord. Med. 21:103, 1944.

73. Pankovich, A. M. Adult ankle fractures. J. Cont. Med. Ed. Orthop. 3:17–40, 1979.

74. Pankovich, A. M. Fractures of the fibula proximal to the distal tibio fibular syndesmosis. J. Bone Jt. Surg. 60A:221, 1978.

75. Pankovich, A. M. Maisonneuve fracture of the fibula. J. Bone Jt. Surg. 58A:337–342, 1976.

76. Pennal, G. E. Subluxation of the ankle. Can. Med. J. 49:92, 1943.

77. Phillips, W. A., and Spiegel, P. G. Symposium. Rigid internal fixation of fractures. Evaluation of ankle fractures. Non-operative vs. operative. Clin. Orthop. 138:17–20, 1979.

78. Pott, P., *The Chirugical Works.* Haives, London, 1775.

79. Pouteau, G. *Oeuvres Posthumes.* Paris 1783.

80. Quenu, E. Du diastasis de l'articulation tibio-peroniere inferieure (quoted by Lauge Hansen). Rev. Chir. Paris 1:897 and 36:62, 1907.

81. Ramsey, P. L., and Hamilton, W. Changes in the tibiotalar area of contact caused by lateral shift. J. Bone Jt. Surg. 58A:356, 1976.

82. Reckling, F. W., McNamara, G. R., and DeSmet, A. A. Problems in the diagnosis and treatment of ankle injuries. J. Trauma 21:943–950, 1981.

83. See Ref. 54.

84. Ruth, J. C. The surgical treatment of the fibular collateral ligaments of the ankle. J. Bone Jt. Surg. 43A:229, 1961.

85. Salter, R. B. *Textbook of Disorders and Injuries of the Musculoskeletal System.* Williams & Wilkins, Baltimore, 1970, pp. 417–422.

86. Salter, R. B., and Harris, W. R. Injuries involving the epiphyseal plate. J. Bone Jt. Surg. 45A:587–622, 1963.

87. Ogden, J. A., ed. *Skeletal Injury in the Child.* Lea & Febiger, Philadelphia, 1982, pp. 555–620.

88. Solonen, K., and Lauttamus, L. Acta Orthop. Scand. 39:223–237, 1968.

89. Spiegel, P. G. Distal tibial intra-articular fractures (editorial). Clin. Orthop. 138:17, 1979.

90. Spiegel, P. G., Cooperman, D. R., and Laros, G. S. Epiphyseal fractures of the distal ends of the tibia and fibula. A retrospective study of 237 cases in children. J. Bone Jt. Surg. 60A:1046, 1978.

91. Staples, O. S. Injuries to the medial ligaments of the ankle. J. Bone Jt. Surg 42A:1287, 1960.

92. Stimson, L. A. Pott's fracture at the ankle. N. Y. Med. J. 55:701, 1892.

93. Staples, O. S. Ligamentous injuries of the ankle joint. Clin. Orthop. 42:21, 1965.

94. Tanton, R. *Fractures du Membre Inferieur.* Paris, 1916.

95. Tillaux, P. Recherches cliniques et experimentales sur les fractures malleolaires, rapport par Gosselin. Bull. Acad. Med. (Paris) 21:817, 1872.

96. Vahvanen, V., and Aalto, K. Classification of ankle fractures in children. Arch. Orthop. Trauma Surg. 97:1–5, 1980.

97. Vasli, S. Operative treatment of ankle fractures. Acta Chir. Scand. Suppl. 226, 1957.

98. Von Volkman, R. Beitrage zur Chirurgie, Leipzig, Breitkopf. u. Hortel, 1875, pp. 105.

99. Weber, B. G. Die Verletzungen de oberen Sprunggelenkes, In *Aktuelle Probleme in der Chirurgie, 3.* Verlag, Bern, 1966.

100. Wheelhouse, W. W., and Rosenthal, R. E. Unstable ankle fractures: Comparison of closed versus open treatment. South Med. J. 73:45–50, 1980.

101. Willenegger, H. Fragen der operativen Frakturenbehandlung. Arch. Klin. Chir. 276:173, 1953.

102. Willenegger, H. Di Behandlung der Luxationsfrakturen des oberen Sprunggelenkes nach biomechanischen Gesichtspunkten. Helv. Chir. Acta 28:225, 1961.

103. Willenegger, H., and Weber, B. G. Malleolarfrakturen, in *Technik der operativen Frakturenbehandlung.* Springer-Verlag, Berlin, 1963.

104. Wilson, F., and Skilbred, A. Long-term results in the treatment of displaced bimalleolar fractures. J. Bone Jt. Surg. 48A:1065, 1966.

105. Wolff, A. Artrografi av ankelled. Nord. Med. 8:2449, 1940.

106. Yablon, I. G., Heller, F. G., and Shouse, L. The key role of the lateral malleolus in displaced fractures of the ankle. J. Bone Jt. Surg. 59A:169, 1977.

107. Yde, J. The Lauge Hansen classification of malleolar fractures. Acta Orthop. Scand. 51:181–192, 1980.

Suggested Additional Readings

108. Anderson, J. T., and Gustilo, R. B. Immediate internal fixation in open fractures. Orthop. Clin. North Am. 11:569–577, 1980.

109. Brunner, C. H., and Weber, B. G. *Special Techniques in Internal Fixation.* Springer-Verlag, Berlin, 1982.

110. Chapman, M. W. The use of immediate internal fixation in open fractures. Orthop. Clin. North. Am. 11:579–591, 1980.

111. Ogden, J. A. *Skeletal Injuries in the Child.* Lea and Febiger, Philadelphia, 1982, pp. 555–620.

112. Rang, M. *Children's Fractures.* J. B. Lippencott, 1974, pp. 198–209.

113. Robson, M. C., Duke, W. F., and Krizek, T. J. Rapid bacterial screening in the treatment of civilian wounds. J. Surg. Res. 14:426, 1973.

114. Robson, M. C., Krizek, T. J., and Heggers, J. P. Biology of surgical infection. Curr. Probl. Surg. Chap. 3, 62, 1973.

CHAPTER 15

Sports-related Surgery

STEVEN I. SUBOTNICK, D.P.M., M.S.

A. Soft Tissue

NAILS

Among the most successful procedures in digital nail surgery are those utilizing the method of Suppan (1). When doing a Suppan-type nail procedure, surgical excision of the matrix and removal of all remnants with a rongeur is recommended. There is very little disability and sutures are not necessary.

If a subungual exostosis is symptomatic and associated with nail pathology, it is removed through a dorsal transverse distal incision. Utilizing a rongeur and rasp, the spur is easily excised. One or two sutures are necessary for closure (2).

INTERDIGITAL NEUROMAS

Neuromas may be in any interspace, but are quite rare in the fourth interspace, and are less common in the first interspace. When in the first interspace, they may be associated with a hypertrophic or dystrophic fibular sesamoid. This should be ruled out radiographically and clinically.

Neuromas may respond to injection therapy with combinations of cortisone, local anesthetics, and vitamin B_{12}. Ultrasound and transverse friction, as well as mobilization, is utilized following the injections. Accommodative orthoses are helpful. Success rate may range between 60 and 80% utilizing this method. At times, what may be a neuroma is actually a capsulitis or bursitis or some form of fibrositis (3, 4). This may account for the high success rate. Despite the high success rate, there may be as high as 20–30% recurrence of neuroma symptoms within 1 or 2 years.

Neuromas may occur in more than one interspace at the same time. Symptoms existing in both interspaces may be due to the fact that the neuroma in the third interspace is actually coming from beneath the neck of the third metatarsal (Fig. 15A.1).

Neuromas appear to be as common in the second as in the third interspaces in athletes. This may be due to a long second metatarsal with a hypermobile first ray. Excessive pressure on the second metatarsal, as well as shearing taking place in the interspace, may predispose to neuromas. The third metatarsal usually has a greater sagittal plane range of motion than the second, and this may place more soft tissue and bony pressure upon the nerve, thereby predisposing to traumatic neuroma. There can be little doubt that neuromas are associated with excessive plantar trauma, twisting, and compressive forces of the metatarsals. Thus, excessive motion, poor biomechanics, and compression from footgear all contribute to posttraumatic neuromas (5).

The diagnosis is relatively simple. The nerve can be impinged upon the bone and readily palpated. There is a corresponding painful sensation from the patient as the clicking is felt. (Mulder's sign) (6).

Multiple neuromas are best treated with injection therapy, padding, or accommodative orthoses. If this works, then more permanent orthoses are indicated to help prevent recurrence. At times, multiple neuromas will need excision. A dorsal approach is preferred, although plantar approaches are acceptable. Plantar incisions often-

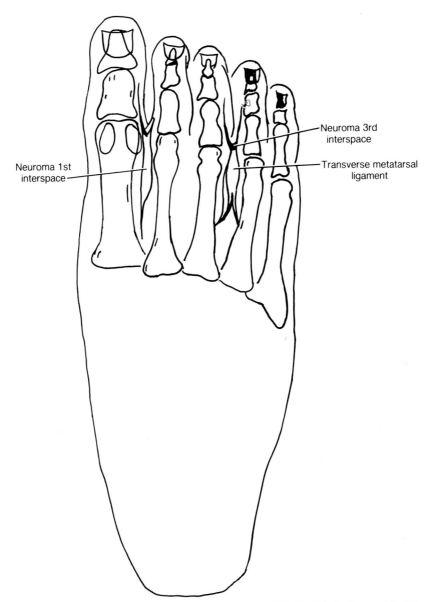

Figure 15A.1. Interdigital neuroma. (From Subotnick, S. I. *Podiatric Sports Medicine*. Futura, Mt. Kisco, NY, 1975, p. 134, with permission.)

times leave a scar if made directly beneath a weightbearing area (Fig. 15A.2).

Whenever forefoot neuropathy is present, one must rule out tarsal tunnel syndrome, generalized neuropathy, bursitis, and other forms of soft tissue trauma. The use of anti-inflammatory medications may therefore be helpful. If there is any joint stiffness, laboratory tests should be utilized to rule out autoimmune disease. Screening

for arthritis and gout should be carried out if there is a high index of suspicion of either disorder. Radiographs should be utilized to rule out bony prominences and/or narrowing of joint spaces.

Recurrent neuromas, despite meticulous surgical technique, are possible. They may be as high as 1–2%. In one series, when the transverse metatarsal ligament was not sectioned, there was a 7% recurrence of neu-

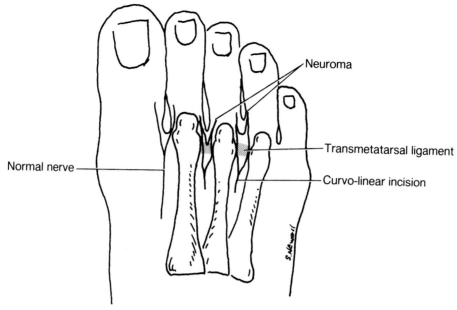

Figure 15A.2. Dorsal incision for adjacent neuromas in interspaces 2 and 3. (From Subotnick, S. I. *Podiatric Sports Medicine.* Futura, Mt. Kisco, NY, 1975, p. 151, with permission.)

romas (7). If the neuroma recurs, it should be treated with injection therapy utilizing slow-acting steroids on the neuroma stump. If entrapment occurs, injection therapy with physical therapy should be utilized. Oral anti-inflammatory medications may be helpful. In the event that re-operation is necessary, the patient should be informed that there is a chance that relief will only be temporary. There is a much higher rate of failure with re-operation on recurrent neuromas than with the primary procedure. At re-operation, a longer incision should be made and the proximal normal nerve should be excised. The nerve should then be removed from the wound from proximal to distal. When possible, a sympathectomy nerve clamp is placed on the normal portion nerve prior to sectioning.

Neuromas may be associated with plantar keratomas and plantar-flexed metatarsals. If a neuroma is present in the second and third interspaces and there is an associated keratoma under the third metatarsal, an osteotomy of the third metatarsal is recommended. The neuromas are not normally excised. By raising up a plantar-flexed metatarsal, the neuroma will be decompressed and vascular compromise of

the toe or excessive numbness following excision of a neuroma may not be necessary.

It is important to note that an osteotomy at the metatarsal neck associated with excision of a neuroma may render the osteotomy site unstable, and a transfer lesion or malrotation of the osteotomy distally may occur. Fixation should be considered in these instances.

TARSAL TUNNEL SYNDROME

The medial tarsal tunnel syndrome may be functional or anatomical. If it is functional in nature, it may be secondary to compression of the tarsal tunnel following prolonged pronation. This condition will usually respond to orthotic control, injection therapy, and physiotherapy. Abnormal electromyographic nerve conduction studies have been reversed simply by utilizing the above procedures. A neurological consultation is usually helpful. One must rule out generalized neuropathy and/or radiculopathy. The association of peripheral neuropathy with endocrine disease may necessitate a medical follow-up (8–10) (Fig. 15A.3).

Posterior tarsal tunnel syndrome is ini-

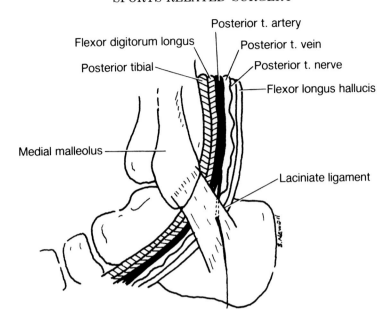

Posterior t. artery

Flexor digitorum longus

Posterior t. vein

Posterior tibial

Posterior t. nerve

Flexor longus hallucis

Medial malleolus

Laciniate ligament

Figure 15A.3. Tarsal tunnel syndrome. (From Subotnick, S. I. *Podiatric Sports Medicine.* Futura, Mt. Kisco, NY, 1975, p. 135, with permission.)

tially treated conservatively. If extreme pain is present and neurologic consultation reveals that there is no serious damage to the nerve, cast immobilization for 3–6 weeks may be helpful. A tarsal tunnel syndrome usually becomes far less symptomatic with neutral foot position cast immobilization. If, however, pain persists, despite the fact that conservative treatment has been carried out, a neuroplasty with decompression is indicated. Clinically, there is a positive Tinel sign. There may or may not be delayed nerve conduction velocity. There will be clinical evidence of a tarsal tunnel with pain directly over the tunnel radiating proximally and distally (Vallieux phenomenon). This pain may worsen with athletic endeavors (11, 12) (Fig. 15A.4).

Complications

Tarsal tunnel surgery is not always successful. It may initially relieve symptoms for (1–2) years, but slight recurrence can occur after this amount of time. Recurrence is as high as 5–10%. Some sources quote a 20% recurrence rate (13). Incomplete release or small incisions may predispose to recurrence. Meticulous dissection and hemostasis, may reduce post-operative fibrosis and recurrence of symptoms. Orthotic foot control for the pronated foot is essential in the total rehabilitative program.

Anterior Tarsal Tunnel Syndrome

An anterior tarsal tunnel syndrome is a compression of the deep peroneal (anterior tibial) nerve. It occurs beneath the extensor retinaculum and may be associated with post-traumatic compression and underlying bone spurs. A positive Tinel sign is usually present. This condition may respond to conservative treatment, especially if there is pronatory dorsal jamming occurring at the tarsal-midtarsal joints. Decompression with resection of underlying spurs is indicated if conservative therapy fails. This procedure usually works quite well and there appears to be less re-occurrence than with the posterior tarsal tunnel syndrome. Adequate bone must be resected with raw bone surfaces being concave. The retinaculum is not sutured (14).

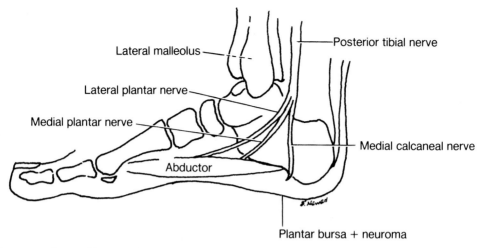

Figure 15A.4. Plantar adventitious bursitis with nerve entrapment. (From Subotnick, S. I. *Podiatric Sports Medicine.* Futura, Mt. Kisco, NY, 1975, p. 133, with permission.)

SUPERFICIAL NERVE COMPRESSION

Superficial nerves, including the sural, saphenous, and superficial peroneal, may need surgical attention (9, 11, 12, 15–18). Oftentimes, a sprained ankle or excessive inversion of the foot will result in a sural nerve traction neuropathy. Excessive pressure on the dorsal aspect of the foot and/or exostoses may result in nerve entrapment. Excessive pressure beneath the medial aspect of the hallux may result in Joplin's compression neuropathy. Neuroplasty may fail in thin individuals and result in entrapment neuropathy which may later necessitate a neurectomy. If the patient has more abundant subcutaneous fat, a neuroplasty or neurolysis is usually successful.

FASCIITIS

Plantar fasciitis is a common problem and usually responds to conservative treatment with orthoses and heel lifts. Oral anti-inflammatory medication and a complete work up for autoimmune diseases should be carried out with resistant cases of plantar fasciitis (19–21) (Figs. 15A.5). In the face of resistant plantar fasciitis, a fascial release may be necessary. The plantar fascia should be released as far proximal from the calcaneal tubercle as possible. In a ca-

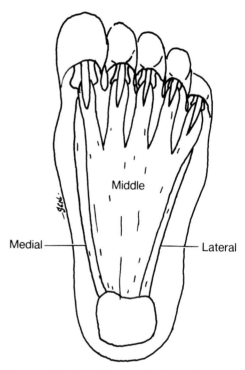

Figure 15A.5. Plantar fasciitis. (From Subotnick, S. I. *Podiatric Sports Medicine.* Futura, Mt. Kisco, NY, 1975, p. 132, with permission.)

vus foot with plantar fasciitis and/or abductor myositis, the first plantar layer of intrinsic foot muscles should be gently stripped from the periosteum and released at the time of surgery. Post-operatively, the foot should be placed in a cast, with the forefoot dorsiflexed on the rearfoot, for a period of at least 3 weeks. This allows for the plantar fascia to heal elongated. Weightbearing should be delayed for 1–3 weeks.

Complications occur when an osteotome is utilized to remove heel spurs associated with plantar faciitis, and a cut is carried into the calcaneus which results in excessive damage to the bone. Release of the plantar fascia, distal rather than proximal, results in bleeding of intrinsic musculature, and the resulting hematoma must be evacuated to allow for normal healing. If a heel spur syndrome is present with the triad of plantar fasciitis, medial calcaneal nerve entrapment, and heel spur, all must be surgically inspected and treated appropriately.

TENDINITIS

Achilles Tendinitis

The Achilles tendon is the most common tendon afflicted in the lower extremity. There appears to be three distinct possibilities when discussing a damaged Achilles tendon. It can be injured secondary to a spontaneous sudden force, or may become chronically injured due to repetitive stress which occurs in an overuse syndrome. Biomechanical malpositioning and abnormality of the lower extremity may predispose various portions of the tendon to more stress than would be present in a normal functioning foot. A pronated foot tends to have more strain on the medial aspect of the Achilles tendon. The lateral aspect of the Achilles may be injured secondary to a sudden inversion sprain or chronic overuse in a cavus-type foot. Degeneration of the tendon itself appears to parallel generalized degeneration of the body itself. Patients with arteriosclerosis or generalized breakdown of connective tissue of the body tend to have a higher incidence of tendon pathology. Classification of Achilles tendinitis is as follows: 1) peritendinitis; 2) tendonosis; and 3) a combination of peritendinitis and tendonosis.

Peritendinitis is an inflammation of the paratenon. The normal space between the visceral and parietal portions of the paratenon becomes occluded. Adherence between the paratenon and the tendon results. This is the common presenting complaint with overuse injury of the Achilles tendon (22–24).

Tendonosis presents when there is degeneration of the tendon itself. This may occur secondary to overuse and/or partial rupture. As degeneration of the tendon occurs, metaplasia may take place with the end result being intra-tendinous calcification. Tendonosis by itself may be asymptomatic (25), but when combined with peritendinitis, symptoms are evident.

CLINICAL FINDINGS

When there is a great deal of soft tissue edema, it is usually a result of a swollen paratenon. Thus, peritendinous swelling is associated with tendinitis, but not necessarily tendonosis. When there is a thickening of the tendon itself without associated swelling of the surrounding paratenon, one may assume damage to the tendon. If both situations exist, there is usually peritendinitis, as well as tendonosis.

Achilles problems should be treated as conservatively as possible, yet aggressively. Anti-inflammatory measures should be carried out, as well as stretching over ice. Ultrasound, with fluorinated steroid creams through the process of phonophoresis does have an effect upon the inflamed peritendinous structures. Utilization of phonphoresis versus injection therapy appears to be much safer. Injections are to be discouraged in as much as they cause central necrosis of the tendon itself and may predispose to rupture. Oral anti-inflammatory medication may be utilized along with the ultrasound and ice massage. Antagonistic muscles should be strengthened and stretched.

BIOMECHANICAL CONSIDERATIONS

The anterior equinus foot with a dropped forefoot responds to an orthoses with a heel lift. This allows for contact on the ball of the foot without excessive overload of the Achilles tendon. A cavus foot with lateral instability may need a heel lift, as well as a lateral flare or a perpendicular rearfoot post to prevent excessive inversion of the heel. When forefoot valgus is present, a lateral forefoot post is helpful to prevent supinatory compensation.

A pronated foot responds to an orthotic to prevent abnormal pronation which places additional strain on the medial posterior fibers of the tendo Achilles. A heel lift is also helpful to relieve abnormal pressure on the tendon. Heel lifts must be used bilaterally to prevent iatrogenic limb length discrepancy. When Achilles pathology is present, as with all overuse injuries, limb length discrepancy should be ruled out.

If crepitation is present, the Achilles tendon should be immobilized by placement in a posterior splint or unna boot for 2–3 weeks, depending upon the severity of the crepitation. Systemic anti-inflammatory medication may be necessary. Most forms of acute Achilles tenosynovitis respond well to physiotherapy when followed with appropriate biomechanical treatment. When tendonosis or chronic Achilles tenosynovitis is present, the prognosis is not as encouraging.

Chronic Achilles Tenosynovitis

Achilles tenosynovitis unresponsive to therapy for 6–12 months requires surgical intervention. Conservative treatment should consist of periods of rest, physiotherapy, ice massage, stretching and strengthening exercises, and a biomechanical approach if applicable. When conservative therapy fails, the athlete will go from an asymptomatic situation, following rest, to recurrence of symptoms as athletic activity resumes. Prior to surgery, explain to the athlete that there can be peritendinitis, tendonosis, or a combination of both. The athlete should be informed that if tendonosis is present, the prognosis is less favorable. The surgery should be performed to allow for excision of abnormal tissue and migration into the tendon of healthy fibroblasts from the surrounding fat so that metaplasia and healing can take place.

Nonsurgical Approach to Achilles Peritendinitis, Tendonosis, or Peritendinitis with Tendonosis

The nonsurgical approach consists of instructing the athlete to rest until all symptoms have disappeared, and then having him return to a graduated program of walking and, finally, running. Conservative measures to decrease inflammation, including oral anti-inflammatory drugs, ultrasound, ice massage, and gentle stretching exercises, should be utilized. Stretching over ice, especially with resistance, is helpful. If crepitation is present, a cast can be utilized for 1–3 weeks. If a partial rupture is suspected, cast immobilization for 4 weeks, followed by physiotherapy is the treatment of choice. In the event that conservative treatment has been exhausted and the patient has rested for prolonged periods of time only to find that the pain returns when activity is resumed, surgery is the treatment of choice. There are some who feel that when tendonosis is present, surgery should be carried out to allow for surgical healing of the tendon which otherwise may not properly heal.

SURGERY

The success is dependent upon findings at the time of surgery and the actual amount of damage to the tendon. If the tendon is normal and the sheath itself is damaged, prognosis is quite good. If there is central necrosis and degeneration of the tendon itself, the prognosis is less favorable, although better than if surgical intervention was not undertaken. Athletes should be informed that depending upon their age and activity, it may take from 2 months to 1 year to fully recuperate from the surgery and regain the pre-injury athletic level of activity.

SURGICAL CONSIDERATIONS

Longitudinal tendon incisions are not closed so that it will be possible for the fibroblasts from surrounding fat to migrate into the tendon to allow for proper healing. If there is bony metaplasia of the tendon at the attachment to the calcaneus, then a midline incision through the tendon is made and abnormal bone is removed. This defect may be sutured; and the tendon may need to be attached more securely to the tendo Achilles through drill holes with nonabsorbable suture. A Jones compressive cast dressing is applied and left intact for 7–10 days. Following this, the cast is removed and the patient is started on gentle active and passive range of motion exercises. These are gradually increased so that at the end of the 3 weeks, the patient is walking comfortably and is able to stand on his toes. A walking-jogging program is started at the 4th post-operative week. Physical therapy is instituted until there is no evidence of inflammation or tenderness about the Achilles tendon.

If there is considerable degeneration of the tendon, a below-knee walking cast with the foot held in moderate gravity equinus position is utilized for 4 weeks. In the event that a partial rupture is found, then the cast is utilized for 6 weeks. When the patient is taken out of this cast, a ¼-inch felt heel lift is utilized for an additional month. This heel lift is gradually reduced as the tendon lengthens.

Retrocalcaneal Exostosis with Intratendinous Calcification

If there is intratendinous calcification at the insertion of the Achilles tendon, then a greater extent of surgery is required. The tendon should be incised longitudinally at its central portion and the calcification removed. A retrocalcaneal exostosis or hyperostosis is removed by releasing the Achilles tendon medially and laterally and then resecting the bone. If the Achilles tendon is damaged or a bony procedure is performed, the foot should be placed in gentle gravity

equinus for 4–6 weeks. Non-weightbearing for the first 2 weeks is recommended. Following cast removal, appropriate physiotherapy for muscle strengthening is utilized.

POST-OPERATIVE FAILURE

Post-operative failure occurs from incomplete tenolysis or incomplete excision of abnormal tendon sheath. Failure to utilize post-operative physiotherapy from the 7th to 10th days may decrease the optimal results. Ultrasound and gentle stretching over ice is recommended. If adhesions are present or excessive inflammation is present, dynawave and whirlpool may be helpful. If the tendon is damaged, failure may result simply from the amount of damage present. Surgical error can result in trading one scar for another, and the adhesions that result may reduce the optimal results of surgery. Even in the best hands, complications or recurrence develop due to autoimmune diseases such as rheumatoid arthritis or gout.

Chronic periostitis may occur secondary to the repetitive stresses of sports. It appears as though certain sports activities predispose to spur formation and/or periostitis.

Peroneal Tendinitis

Peroneal tendinitis may be secondary to sprained ankles, ski injuries, or forceful dorsiflexion of the foot upon the ankle during a forward fall. The peroneal tendons may dislocate over the fibular malleolus. Chronic peroneal tendinitis and dislocations usually respond to conservative treatment, but surgery may be necessary to reform the retinaculum (26–28). It is unnecessary to do bony procedures for corrections of this problem. Chronic peroneal tendinitis responds to a tenolysis. At times, there may be a chronic peroneal cuboid syndrome (pain plantar to the cuboid) secondary to peroneus longus tendonopathy and/or bony abnormalities. A tenolysis with a regrooving of the peroneal groove may be performed. Unstable plantar-flexed cuboids may respond to a cuboid ostectomy (29).

Posterior Tibial Tendinitis

Posterior tibial tendinitis may be chronic and secondary to tenosynovitis and/or tendonopathy. There may be granulomatous changes within the posterior tibial sheath which requires surgical attention. If sclerosing tendonopathy is present, a surgical emergency exists and immediate decompression should be implemented. As in all cases of soft tissue problems in the lower extremity, physiotherapy and biomechanial control should be attempted prior to surgery.

Partial or complete ruptures of the tendons of the lower extremity may exist and may require cast immobilization and/or surgical repair, depending upon the severity and the circumstances.

Extensor tendinitis usually responds to conservative treatment. Tenolysis is rarely required. Usually, tendonopathy is secondary to underlying spurs which need surgical attention if there is a failure of conservative treatment (30).

References

1. Suppan, R. J., and Ritchlin, J. D. A non-debilitating surgical procedure for "ingrown toenail." JAPA 52:900–902, 1962.
2. Sandel, R. K. Subungual exostosis: A simplified surgical procedure. JAPA 48:57–58, 1958.
3. Bossley, C. J., and Cairney, P. C. The intermetatarsophalangeal bursa—its significance in Morton's metatarsalgia. J. Bone Jt. Surg. 62b:184, 1980.
4. Reed, R. J., and Bliss, B. O. Morton's neuroma: Regressive and productive intermetatarsal elastofibrositis. Arch. Pathol. 95:125, 1973.
5. Morton, T. G. A peculiar and painful affection of the fourth metatarsophalangeal articulation. Am. J. Med. Sci. 71:37, 1976.
6. Subotnick, S. I. Podiatric Sports Medicine. Futura, Mt. Kisco, NY, 1975, p. 134.
7. Sokoloff, T. Recurrent Neuromas: Levine residency class. Personal communication, 1979.
8. Subotnick, S. I. Podiatric Sports Medicine. Futura, Mt. Kisco, NY, 1975, p. 135.
9. Carrel, J., and Davidson, D. Nerve compression syndromes of the foot and ankle. JAPA 65:332, 1975.
10. Edvards, W. G., Lincoln, C. R., Bassett, F. H., III, and Goldner, J. L. The tarsal tunnel syndrome. JAMA 207:716, 1969.
11. Rask, M. Medial plantar neuropraxia (Jogger's foot). Clin. Orthop. Relat. Res. 134:193, 1978.
12. Sidney, J. D. Weak ankles: A study of common peroneal entrapment neuropathy. Br. Med. J. 3:623, 1969.
13. Scurran, B. Recurrent tarsal tunnel. Personal communication, 1982.
14. Subotnick, S. I. Anterior impingement exostosis of the ankle. JAPA 66:958–963, 1976.
15. Lemont, H. The branches of the superficial peroneal nerve and their clinical significance. JAPA 65:310, 1975.
16. Haimovici, H. Peroneal sensory neuropathy entrapment syndrome. Arch. Surg. 105:586, 1972.
17. Copell, H. P., and Thompson, W. A. L. Peripheral entrapment neuropathies of the lower extremity. N. Engl. J. Med. 56:262, 1960.
18. Subotnick, S. I. Podiatric Sports Medicine. Futura, Mt. Kisco, NY, 1975, pp. 134–137.
19. Weller, R. O., Bruckner, F. E., and Chamberlain, M. A. Rheumatoid neuropathy: A histological and electrophysical study. J. Neurol. Neurosurg. Psychiatry 33:592, 1970.
20. Furey, J. G. Plantar fascitis. The painful heel syndrome. J. Bone Jt. Surg. 57a:672, 1975.
21. Subotnick, S. I. Podiatric Sports Medicine. Futura, Mt. Kisco, NY, 1975, p. 132.
22. Subotnick, S. I. Achilles tendon injury in sports: A comprehensive approach. Sports Med. Part II:47–53, 1980.
23. Snook, O. A. Achilles tendon tenosynovitis in long distance runners. Med. Sci. Sports Exerc. 4:155, 1972.
24. Clancy, W. G., Neithart, D., and Brand, R. L. Achilles tendinitis in runners: A report of five cases. Am. J. Sports Med. 4:46, 1976.
25. Burry, H. C., and Pool, C. J. Central degeneration of the Achilles tendon. Rheumatol. Rehabil. 12:177–181, 1973.
26. Earle, A. A., Mortiz, J. E., and Tapper, E. H. Dislocation of the peroneal tendons at the ankle: an analysis of twenty-five ski injuries. N. W. Med. 71:180, 1972.
27. Kelly, R. E. An operation for chronic dislocation of peroneal tendons. Br. J. Surg. 7:502, 1920.
28. Savastino, A. A. The treatment of recurrent dislocations of the common peroneal tendons. Presented at the Eighth Annual Meeting of the American Orthopedic Foot Society, Dallas, 1978.
29. Grumbine, N. Personal communication, 1982.
30. Subotnick, S. I. Podiatric Sports Medicine. Futura, Mt. Kisco, 1975, pp. 28–131.

B. Surgical Considerations and Complications of Bony Procedures of the Lower Extremity in the Athlete

As with the soft tissue problems of the lower extremity, bony problems require an analysis of etiological factors. The specific sport, the biodynamics of injury, and rehabilitation are of paramount importance. The general rule for bony procedures is to provide stability. Thus, when a bunion procedure is performed on an athlete, osteotomies are oftentimes utilized to assure congruent joints. Rigid internal fixation is preferred. Early range of motion exercises are necessary to prevent contracture of joint structures.

FOREFOOT PROCEDURES

Subungual Exostoses

Subungual exostoses are problematic in athletes. They may be caused by excessive pressure secondary to tight footgear or from running downhill. Likewise, direct trauma, which may occur in football or soccer, can cause subungual exostoses and/or hematomas. When they are symptomatic, they should be surgically removed, preferably a dorsal distal transverse skin incision (Fig. 15B.1).

Failures occur when less than meticulous surgery is carried out and damage is done to the nail bed. There have been failures with closed surgical techniques whereby a power drill cuts through the exostosis but the exostosis itself is not removed. Closed surgical techniques for subungual exostosis, as in almost all instances, should be avoided in the athlete since direct visualization of pathology and careful disection is mandatory for best results.

Subhallux Sesamoids

Subhallux sesamoids are present with hyperextension of the hallux and there may be burning pain and callus associated with this sesamoid. These problems may respond to orthotics which decrease the amount of hallux limitus present and decrease the hyperextension of the interphalangeal joint. If orthotics are unsuccessful, surgical excision can be performed quite simply from a medial plantar approach. Failure or complication results when damage is done to the long flexor tendon. Inasmuch as this is an intra-capsular procedure, damage can be done to the joint with less than meticulous dissection (Fig. 15B.2).

Exostoses and Osteochondromas

These bony prominences on toes can be removed surgically if symptomatic.

Hammertoes

Hammertoes in athletes can be bothersome. Conservative treatment consists of utilizing crest pads. Flexible hammertoes may respond to a biomechanical balancing of the foot. When surgery is necessary, an arthroplastic procedure is usually recommended. If interphalangeal contracture is present, Kirshner wire fixation may be necessary. When the second toe is unstable and there is an associated hallux valgus, an arthrodesis of the toe should be considered.

If contracture is present at the metatarsophalangeal joint as well as in the toes, a complete dorsal release of the metatarsophalangeal joint is recommended. Releases of the long flexor tendon through the incision utilized for the arthroplasty may be helpful if excessive contracture is present. A flexor set procedure at the distal interphalangeal joint may be necessary in conjunction with an arthroplasty at the proximal interphalangeal joint, to completely reduce a claw toe deformity. If the joint is arthritic, an arthrodesis may be carried out. If flexion is necessary, then a digital implant may be utilized (Fig. 15B.3 and 15B.4).

Failures occur when there is inadequate fixation of arthrodesed toes. Inadequate release of metatarsophalangeal joints may

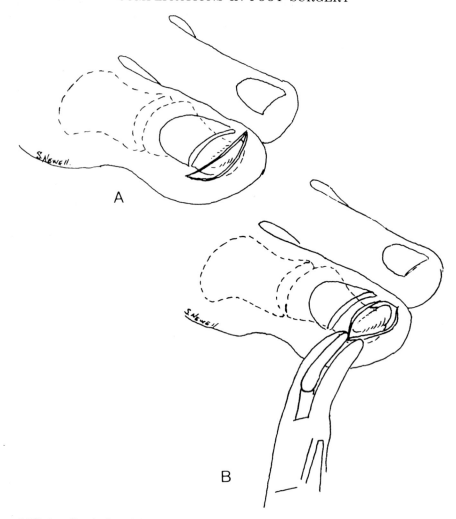

Figure 15B.1.   Surgical excision—exostectomy. Surgical excision, subungual exostectomy without nail procedure. *A,* nail plate is cut back carefully to allow a transverse dorsal wedge resection of skin to be taken, exposing the subungual exostosis and distal tuft of the hallux. *B,* distal tuft of the hallux and subungual exostosis is resected with a rongeur, smoothed with a rasp, and then the wound is flushed with normal saline and closed with simple interrupted 5-O Dexon.

result in failure to completely resolve a contracted toe. If too little bone is resected, then arthritis and/or abnormal ankylosis may be the end result. Failure to reattach the extensor apparatus may result in a floppy or plantar-flexed toe. It is essential to stabilize the toes for a period of 6–8 weeks to allow for proper healing in an anatomical position. It is always best to stabilize an unstable toe following an arthrodesis or arthroplasty with the Kirschner wire when in doubt (Case 1).

CASE 1 (Fig. 15B.5)

C.L. is a 16-year-old high school woman basketball star. Chief complaint is that of clawing of the toes and tailor's bunions.

Hallux Valgus with Bunion Deformity

Hallux valgus and bunion deformity in the athlete may be a cause of disability and pain. Careful planning before carrying out surgical procedures is necessary. It is important to evaluate the foot type, the amount of metatarsus adductus, the amount of metatarsus primus adductus, positioning of the sesamoid, the proximal and distal facet angles, and the needs of the athlete, as well as the stresses going through the first metatarsophalangeal joint. The presence or absence of arthritis, either systemic or post-traumatic, and the mobility of the first ray, are important considerations (Case 2). Whether or not the

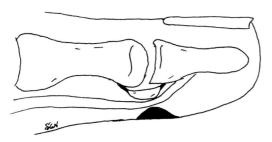

Figure 15B.2. Subhallux sesamoid—interphalangeal joint hallux. The plantar subhallux sesamoid is intracapsular. Care must be taken to retract the long flexor tendon from the capsular structures when dissecting this sesamoid. The sesamoid is usually associated with hyperextension of the interphalangeal joint and a plantar callus underlying the bony prominence.

foot can be controlled post-operatively with an orthoses must be taken into account. The relative length of the first metatarsal in relationship to the adjacent second metatarsal is also an important factor. The type of capsule and soft tissue procedures, likewise, should be considered inasmuch as hypermobile feet have a tendency to do poorly with soft tissue procedures (2–17).

McBride Procedure

McBride procedure or modification of the McBride procedure is carried out for positional deformity. Careful attention should be paid to the criteria before performing this procedure or any other hallux valgus correction (2, 4, 7, 14).

CASE 2 (Fig. 15B.6)

This is a hallux limitus in a 37-year-old long distance runner. Patient had pain with dorsiflexion.

If the extensor brevis tendon is a deforming factor, it should be sectioned. If additional medial stability is necessary, or metatarsus primus adductus is present, and

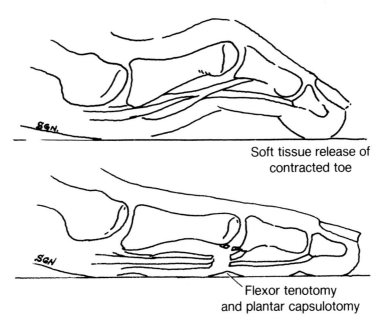

Soft tissue release of
contracted toe

Flexor tenotomy
and plantar capsulotomy

Figure 15B.3. Digital deformities. (From Subotnick, S. I. *Podiatric Sports Medicine.* Futura, Mt. Kisco, New York, 1975, p. 158, with permission.)

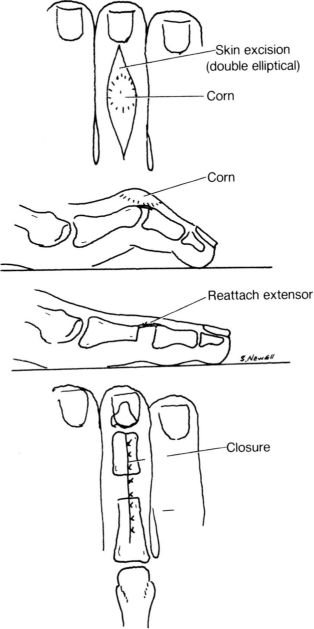

Figure 15B.4. Arthroplasty for digital deformities. (From Subotnick, S. I. *Podiatric Sports Medicine*. Futura, Mt. Kisco, New York, 1975, p. 159, with permission.)

it is elected not to do an osteotomy of the first metatarsal, the extensor brevis may be transpositioned underneath the extensor longus. This helps decrease the intermetatarsal space and, adds to the stability of the medial capsulorrhaphy by utilizing an overlay tendon graft.

In the athlete, it must be remembered that the full dorsal surface of the first metatarsal head is utilized during the push-off phase of running and this portion should not be disturbed surgically. In the event that there is excessive dorsal bone, or metatarsus primus elevatus is present with some degree of hallux limitus, some form of osteotomy plantar-flexing the first meta-

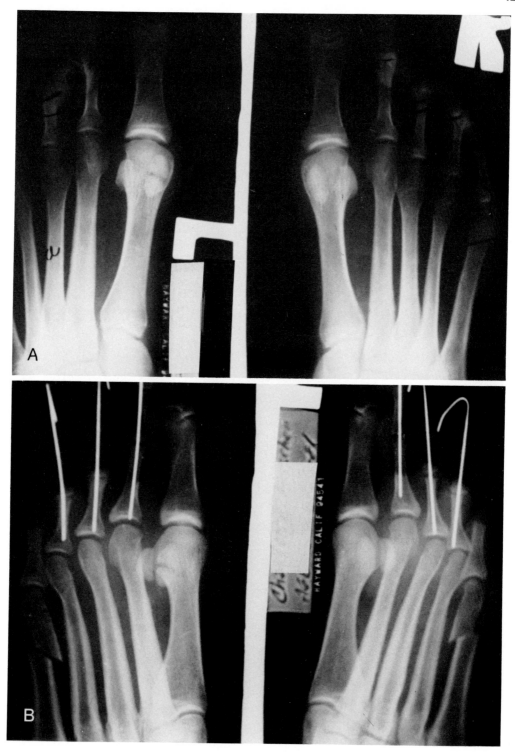

Figure 15B.5. *A*, AP view of the feet showing contracture of the proximal interphalangeal joints on toes two through five and a splaying of the fifth metatarsal head and neck. *B*, post-op arthroplasty with DIP and MPJ release, with K-wire. Osteotomies on fifths were too proximal yet healed uneventfully.

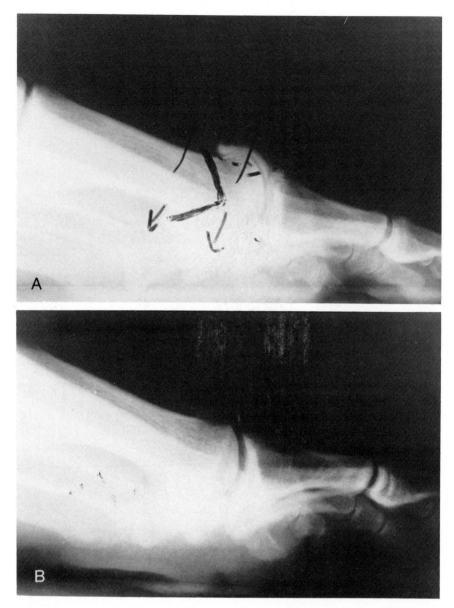

Figure 15B.6. *A,* pre-op arthrogram. Note fracture dorsal base proximal phalanx outlined by dye. Joint space appears normal. *B,* post-op excision and debridement of joint. Implant was unnecessary as predicted by arthrogram.

tarsal is indicated. A McBride procedure in itself will ultimately result in failure.

POST-OPERATIVE CARE FOR MCBRIDE PROCEDURE

Following the removal of the foot cast, the patient is started on active and passive range of motion of the first metatarsophalangeal joint. Dynawave and whirlpool, three times a week, are utilized for the first 2 weeks. Following this, ultrasound is utilized if there is any capsular inflammation or stiffness. Active and passive range of motion exercises are continued. The patient, at 3 weeks post-op, starts a walking program and then advances to a walking-jogging program. Strengthening exercises of the flexors and extensors about the great toe are initiated at the 3rd post-operative week. This is enhanced by utilizing elastic tubing to offer resistance to the flexors and extensors when exercises are performed.

FAILURES WITH MCBRIDE PROCEDURE

Failures occur when pronatory forces cannot be dealt with post-operatively. This is especially true when the soft tissue lacks sufficient strength to maintain correction. When this exists, osteotomies are preferred. It is essential to position the first metatarsal back over the sesamoids (Case 3). Interphalangeal valgus cannot be corrected with a modified McBride procedure (Case 4).

CASE 3 (Fig. 15B.7)

This is a case of a middle-aged woman who complained of painful bunion with overlapping second toe. She had pain consistent with neuromas of second and third interspaces.

CASE 4 (Fig. 15B.8)

A 38 year old active woman with complaints of bilateral hallux valgus and keratomas under second metatarsal heads. Correction obtained with an Akin osteotomy, proximal phalanx of the right great toe, and an Austin osteotomy of the neck of the first metatarsal.

CASE 5 (Fig. 15B.9)

Case 5 is a 16-year-old who had juvenile hallux valgus, corrected by a modified McBride procedure initially, and then a second operation consisting of a modified Mitchell was caried out, with iatrogenic hallux varus being the end result. The patient now has almost no function of the right first metatarsophalangeal joint and constant pain. She has recurrent hallux valgus on the left foot, follow-

ing the McBride procedure. (COMMENT: Juvenile hallux valgus oftentimes responds best to appropriately planned osteotomies.)

Complications such as hallux hammertoe or hallux varus will result if an osteotomy is performed and a negative intermetatarsal angle results. The same may result due to excessive resection of the medial plantar plateau of the first metatarsal head, (Case 5). Dorsal adhesions and a limited range of motion may be the end result of excessive resection of bone dorsally. Dorsal bunions reveal hypermobility or dorsiflexion of the first ray. A plantar flexory osteotomy would be preferred to correct the biomechanical etiology of the problem (Case 6).

CASE 6 (Fig. 15B.10)

Case 6 is in a 37-year-old marathon runner complaining of persistent pain of the first metatarsophalangeal joint. Evaluation showed limited range of motion of the first metarsophalangeal joint, as well as metatarsus primus elevatus with a hypermobile first ray (3, 5, 9).

Hallux hammertoe is a complication that will resut when both of the short flexor tendons are transected. This would occur if both sesamoids were removed at the same time or if the short flexor tendons are inadvertently transected at the time of surgery. Hallux varus may also result from excessive medial capsulorrhaphy.

Narrowing of the first metatarsal phalangeal joint is also a contraindication in a soft tissue bunion correction. An osteotomy to decompress the joint is preferred. In an athlete, the osteotomy is preferred over an implant unless the joint is involved in such advanced arthritis that no form of shortening and remodeling will render the joint asymptomatic (3, 5, 8, 9, 11, 12) (Case 6).

A modified Austin-Reverdin procedure can be utilized to achieve a congruous joint. It appears as though this procedure may

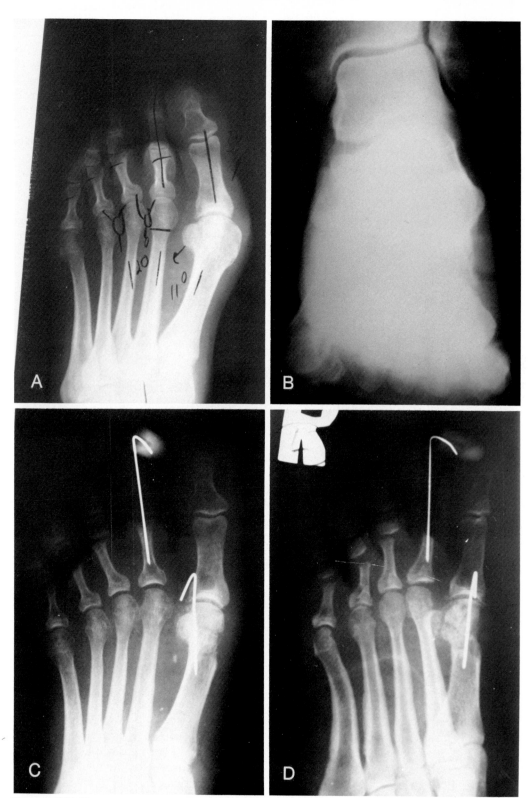

Figure 15B.7. *A,* pre-op. Note mild narrowing of joint. *B,* axial view showing sesamoid rotation and subluxation. *C,* modified Austin. Note relocation of sesamoids with opening at joint space. *D,* oblique view shows plantar-flexion of first metatarsal head held with K-wire fixation; second toe arthrodesed.

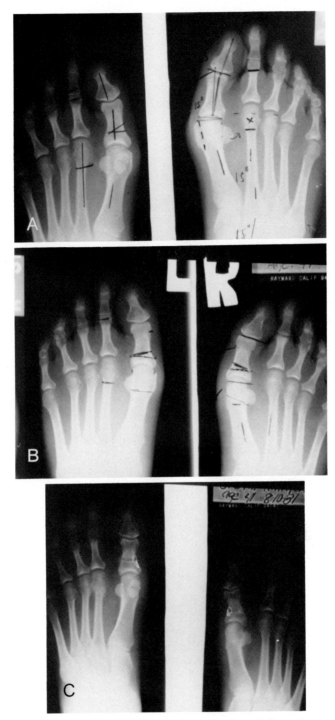

Figure 15B.8. *A,* pre-op. *B,* McBride procedure, right foot: failure due to persistent valgus deviation. *C,* Austin-Reverdin and Akin, right foot. Akin, left foot: V-osteotomy, for second metatarsal.

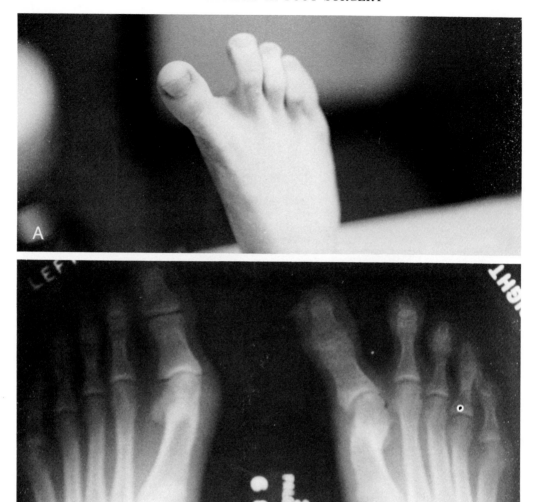

Figure 15B.9. *A*, hallux varus of the right foot with spasm of the abductor hallucis. *B*, x-ray of the right foot with osteotomy at the first metatarsal neck being evident. There has been a negative intermetatarsal angle created by the angulation of the osteotomy with secondary subluxation of the great toe in the direction of varus. The exessive negative intermetatarsal angle resulted in the eventual dislocation of the tibial sesamoid and hallux varus deformity. The left foot shows a deviated proximal facet angle but persistent hallux valgus following a McBride procedure.

prevent advanced arthritis and the need for an implant in the future with athletes (Fig. 15B.11).

A McBride procedure has a particularly high failure rate when performed on a female athlete who also wears dress footwear. The deforming forces of fashionable shoes are difficult to be tolerated by soft tissue procedures. Bony procedures with exact realignment of the proximal and distal facets as well as the sesamoids are preferred (2, 4, 7, 14).

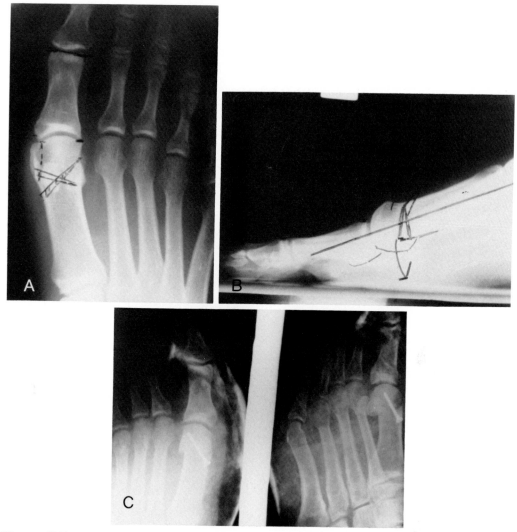

Figure 15B.10. *A,* narrowing of the first metatarsal phalangeal joint, yet no obvious arthritis. The angle of the osteotomy cut is outlined as is the placement hole for the bone screw. *B,* metatarsus primus elevatus with a dropped hallux in relation to the first metatarsal head. The osteotomy is outlined at the first metatarsal neck. A wedge will be taken which will plantar-flex the first metatarsal head and relocate the first metatarsophalangeal joint. *C,* Austin-Reverdin osteotomy at opening of first MPJ and A-O screw fixation.

MCBRIDE PROCEDURE WITH OSTEOTOMY OF THE FIRST METATARSAL BASE

When metatarsus primus adductus is present and there is a soft tissue deformity of the first metatarsophalangeal joint, accommodation of a closing wedge osteotomy of the first metatarsal and a McBride procedure may be carried out successfully (2, 7, 10, 13, 17). It is important to make sure

that when performing this type of procedure, the proximal facet is not deviated to such an extent that the McBride procedure cannot be performed (2). If this is the case, a double osteotomy would be necessary (13). This is accomplished utilizing a closing wedge osteotomy of the first metatarsal with an Aiken osteotomy of the proximal phalanx of the great toe (Fig. 15B.12).

Failures with osteotomies result when there is less than perfect fixation of the

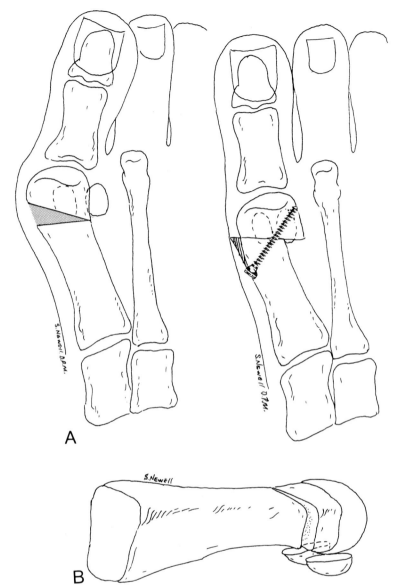

Figure 15B.11. Subotnick modification of Austin-Reverdin procedure with AO fixation. *A,* anterior-posterior view of foot showing oblique wedge resection and transpositioning and fixation with AO cortical screw. Note realignment of normal proximal facet angle. Re-establishment of normal sesamoid pattern and mild shortening of first metatarsal to decompress joint. *B,* lateral view of same foot showing plantar flexory wedge resection. First metatarsal head is transpositioned laterally and plantar-flexed to allow for first metatarsal weightbearing pattern and stability of joint.

osteotomy site. Osteotomies angled from dorsal to plantar usually compress dorsally and allow for the occurrence of metatarsus primus elevatus. This is especially true after abductory osteotomies of the first metatarsal. A plantar approach for the osteotomy of the first metatarsal base may eliminate this post-operative complication. Internal fixation with bone screws help maintain osseous alignment. A negative intermetatarsal angle following an osteotomy oftentimes leads to hallux varus or hallux hammertoe (Case 5).

When metatarsus adductus is present

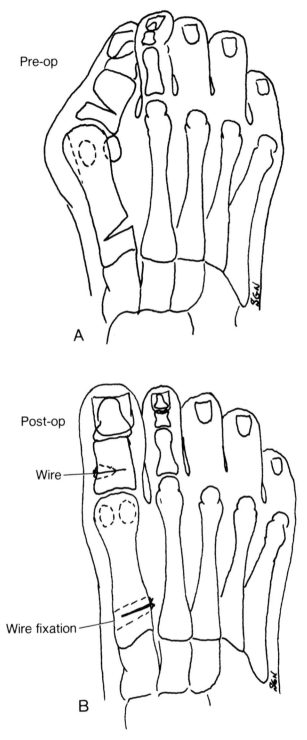

Pre-op

A

Post-op

Wire

Wire fixation

B

Figure 15B.12. *A,* osteotomies to correct metatarus primus adductus with hallux valgus. *B,* closing wedge: Akin-McBride procedure. (From Subotnick, S. I. *Podiatric Sports Medicine.* Futura, Mt. Kisco, New York, 1975, p. 175, with permission.)

and a closing wedge osteotomy of the first metatarsal base is performed, a negative intermetatarsal angle may be the end result. A distal osteotomy is preferred in these instances (Case 7).

CASE 7 (Fig. 15B.13)

Case 7 is a 32-year-old laborer who enjoys jogging. Chief complaint of bilateral hallux valgus and limitus.

Excessive dorsiflexion of first metatarsal osteotomies may be prevented by having the patient non-weightbearing in a cast for three to four weeks. First metatarsal base osteotomies may result in shortening and relative dorsiflexion of the first metatarsal. This may eventually lead to hallux limitus or dorsal bunions. It is important to have the plantar aspect of these sesamoids on the same relative level as the second metatarsal for appropriate stability. When the first metatarsal is considerably shorter than the second metatarsal, additional plantar flexion may be necessary. Excessive plantar flexion may lead to chronic sesamoiditis or a keratoma beneath the first

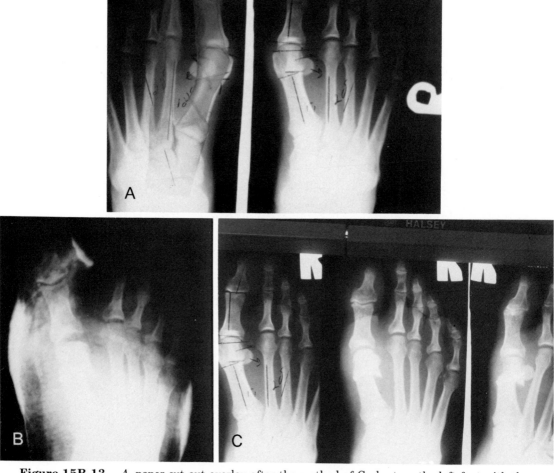

Figure 15B.13. *A,* paper cut-out overlay after the method of Gerbert on the left foot with the right foot demonstrating metatarsus adductus, metatarsus primus adductus, and hallux valgus. *B,* post-op with case immobilization showing an osteotomy of the metatarsal neck, oblique in nature, with three-plane correction. The first metatarsophalangeal joint has been opened by the shortening of the first metatarsal. *C,* post-op x-ray shows the angulation of the osteotomy with the A-O screw fixation. The relative plantar flexion of the first metatarsal head is noted on the oblique view.

metatarsal head. Rigid internal fixation with the first metatarsal in anatomical realignment may prevent these complications (Case 8).

CASE 8 (Fig. 15B.14)

Case 8 is a 36-year woman who had an intractable keratoma under the fourth metatarsal. A dorsal wedge osteotomy at mid-metatarsal with internal wire fixation was carried out with resolution of the lesion. Three years later, the patient developed a painful callus under the fifth metatarsal head and, had persistent pain under

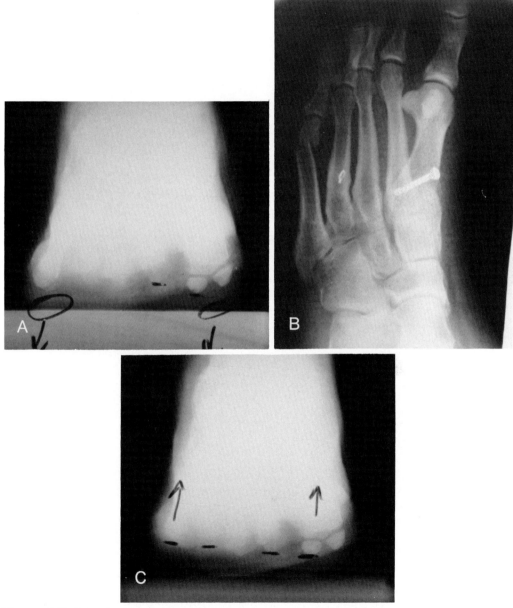

Figure 15B.14. *A,* pre-op plantar-flexed first and fifth metatarsals. *B,* post-op dorsal wedge osteotomy of the first metatarsal with A-O screw fixation. and angular osteotomy of the fifth metatarsal neck. The wire fixation for the previous osteotomy of the fourth metatarsal is seen. *C,* post-op axial view.

both sesamoids associated with a
large keratoma secondary to a
plantar-flexed first metatarsal.
This had been treated previously
with an accommodative orthosis.

Distal Osteotomies, First Metatarsal

Osteotomies of the first metatarsal neck
are utilized to correct a deviated proximal
facet angle. Among the most common pro-

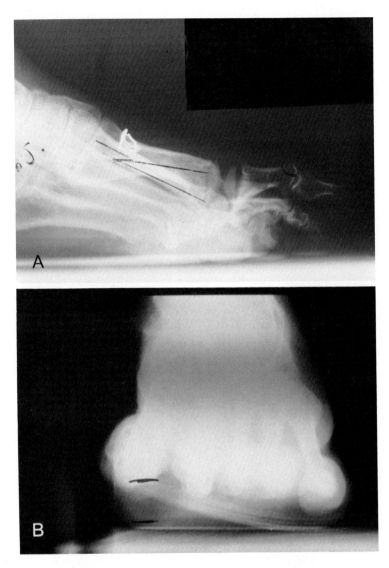

Figure 15B.15.   *A,* lateral view of the foot with excessive dorsiflexion of the first metatarsal, as
well as a total joint replacement in place. *B,* excessive dorsiflexion of the first metatarsal on axial
view. *C,* AP and oblique views of the foot demonstrates mild hallux hammertoe as well as hallux
valgus. The patient has some hypertrophic changes taking place around the Dacron mesh total
joint replacement. *D,* post-op lateral of the foot showing a plantar flexory osteotomy of the first
metatarsal base with K-wire fixation and a replacement of the total joint prosthesis with a Dow-
Corning double-stemmed hinged great toe prosthesis. *E,* post-op oblique and AP view with Dow-
Corning double-stemmed prosthesis in place and fixation of the osteotomy, first metatarsal base.
An osteotomy of the second metatarsal neck was necessary, as well as an arthroplasty of the
proximal interphalangeal joint of the second toe.

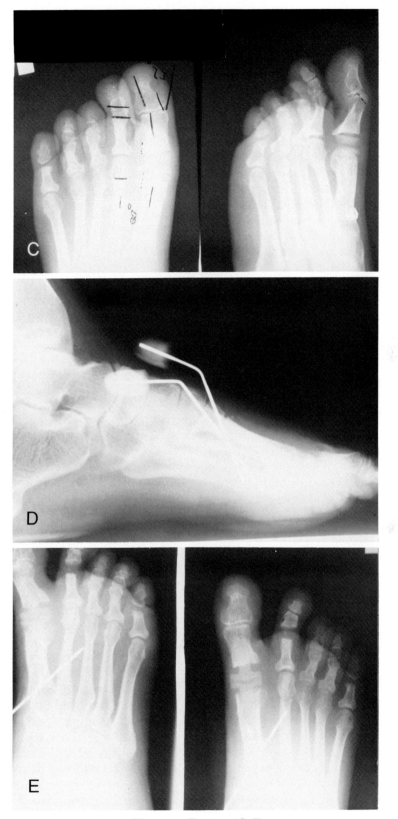

Figure 15B.15. (*C–E*)

cedures are the Austin and/or Reverdin osteotomies. This provides for a stable first metatarsophalangeal joint and repositions the first metatarsal head over the sesamoids, thus providing for dynamic stability of the joint. Internal screw fixation or Kirschner wire fixation is usually indicated (Cases 3, 6, and 7). Following cast removal, physical therapy is initiated. Dynawave, along with whirlpool and active and passive range of motion at the joint, is initiated as soon as possible. Osteotomies require at least 6 weeks for healing and athletic activity is initiated between the 6th and 7th post-operative week with a walking program which is gradually increased to a walking-jogging program. A minimum of 3 months before returning to minimal athletic activity is required. Full activity may not be reached for 4–5 months.

Failure with distal osteotomies may result from inadequate fixation as well as inadequate osteotomy cuts, and failure to adequately realign the joint.

SESAMOIDITIS

A problem utilizing the Reverdin osteotomy alone is that of sesamoiditis. This can be remedied by the Green modification of the Reverdin or by utilization of the Austin-Reverdin procedure. In this way, a plantar shelf is left above the sesamoids to avoid injury (Case 6 and 7).

MALUNION

A potential problem with many osteotomies is that of malunion. It may occur secondary to inadequate fixation or interposition of soft tissue. Metabolic problems may also predispose to this complication.

Double Osteotomy, First Metatarsal

A double osteotomy in the first metatarsal (base plus head or neck) may be necessary when there is excessive metatarsus primus adductus, as well as a deviated proximal facet angle (2, 13). The surgeon must guard against excessive shortening of the first metatarsal. At times, an opening wedge osteotomy of the first metatarsal base combined with a closing wedge osteotomy of the first metatarsal neck will solve this problem. There may be a higher incidence of malunion when two osteotomies on the same bone are performed which can be remedied with rigid internal fixation or adequate placement of cross K-wires and nonweightbearing for 6 weeks.

Deviated Distal Facet Angle (Interphalangeal Abductus)

When the distal facet angle exceeds 11–15°, a closing wedge adductory osteotomy of the proximal phalanx is indicated (Akin) (6). Complications occur if the osteotomy is too close to either the proximal or distal joint with fracture occurring through the joint. Hallux varus may result if overcorrection results. If internal wire fixation is utilized, a circlage technique is preferred over the common practice of utilizing wire through two dorsal holes on adjacent sides of the osteotomy.

CASE 9 (Fig. 15B.15)

Case 9 demonstrates dorsal displacement of a dorsal wedge osteotomy, of the first metatarsal, with failure of mesh total joint replacement. This is a 33-year-old young woman who is active jogging and walking. She presented with a plantar-flexed first metatarsal and an associated hallux limitus. She had a dorsal wedge osteotomy of the first metatarsal with fixation from the dorsum which led to eventual excessive dorsiflexion of the first metatarsal. The dacron mesh failed, and the patient had to have a revision. She now has a functional foot and is able to partake in jogging and walking. (COMMENT: This case demonstrates the need for Kirschner wire or screw fixation of dorsal wedge osteotomies of the first metatarsal. Non-weightbearing for 3–6 weeks

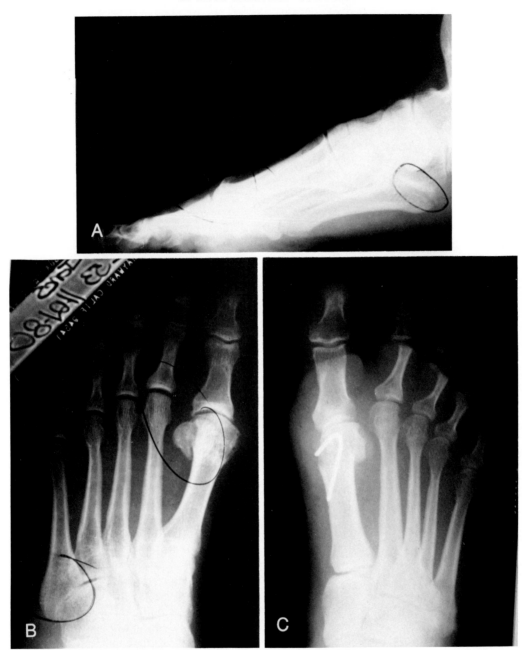

Figure 15B.16. *A,* lateral view of the foot with dorsal bunion and spur formation evident. The patient also has recently sustained a fracture of the base of the fifth metatarsal while playing tennis. *B,* dysplastic fibular sesamoid with a proximal spur. The first metatarsal head protrudes dorsally and medially. The joint space is somewhat narrow. *C,* Austin bunion procedure with K-wire fixation. The deviated proximal facet angle has been corrected, the first metatarsal shortened slightly to decompress the joint, and the hallux itself straightened to relatively lengthen the first ray. The fibular sesamoid has been excised. Arthroplasties of lesser toes have been carried out.

is suggested. Fixation with wire at the dorsal aspect of the dorsal wedge osteotomy may lead to excessive dorsiflexion. If compression is necessary, then closed K-wires should be utilized first to maintain the relative level of elevation, and then compressive wires may be utilized to allow for primary bone healing. A-O fixation is an alternative method.)

Hallux Limitus and Hallux Rigidus

Hallux limitus and hallux rigidus most often occur when there is a Jack syndrome. This is described as a hypermobility or dorsiflexion of the first ray (Case 6). In these instances, the first metatarsal head is elevated above the level of the proximal phalangeal base. When dorsiflexion occurs, jamming results at the dorsal aspect of the first metatarsal head, which results eventually in hallux limitus and finally hallux rigidus. Excessive pronation may cause a functional hallux limitus.

FIRST M-P SPURS

Hallux limitus or hallux rigidus oftentimes shows a dorsal spur which is similar ion appareance to a heel spur (Case 10). This spur may be due to traction. Traction is secondary to the dorsiflexion of the first metatarsal and relative plantar flexion of the hallux causing tension on the dorsal capsular tissue with the spur being the end result.

CASE 10 (Fig. 15B.16)

Case 10 is a 53-year-old woman who enjoys jogging, golf, and tennis. She complained of hallux limitus and bunion deformity, as well as pain beneath the fibular sesamoid.

Osseous spurs occur secondary to traction or compression. Spurs as a result of compression are formed when there is excessive jamming in the joints and appear to be the body's attempt to limit motion. Spurs resulting from traction occur secondary to soft tissue pulling on bone with subsequent subperiosteal bleeding and new bone formation. It may be reasonable to assume that one must correct surgically, or biomechanically, these abnormal forces in order to have long-term results when correcting hallux limitus or hallux rigidus. Hallux limitus normally indicates a dorsal spur and some limited range of motion in dorsiflexion at the first metatarsophalangeal joint. Hallux rigidus indicates extreme limits of motion at the first metatarsophalangeal joint and the utilization of implants is often necessary (15–17).

With mild hallux limitus a biplane Reverdin procedure to plantar-flex the first metatarsal and decompress (open) the joint is preferred (Case 6). When arthritis is present, an implant is necessary. A double-hinged implant for hallux limitus or hallux rigidus is preferred over a hemi-implant (Cases 11 and 12). When implants are utilized in athletes, it is recommended not to remove any of the first metatarsal head (15). This has the advantage of minimal shortening of the first metatarsal, and sesamoid function may be preserved. If the implant is rejected for any reason, one is left with a Keller procedure. This procedure, therefore, has the advantages of the hemi-implant arthroplasty and the added advantage of less chance for wearing out of the hemi-implant and/ or abnormal rotational deformities which occur when utilizing a hemi-implant (Case 13).

In the event that a hemi-implant is utilized, it is essential to have adequate correction of the deviated proximal facet angles. In the event that a total joint replacement is utilized, it is important to reduce the cartilage on the first metatarsal head. This reduces the possibility of hypertrophic osteoarthritic changes (Case 11).

CASE 11 (Fig. 15B.17)

Case 11 is an arthritic forefoot in a 42-year-old active individual who enjoys golfing and gentle jogging.

CASE 12 (Fig. 15B.18)

This is a 46-year-old marathon runner who, despite deformity of first metatarsal phalangeal joints, was able to run three marathons. The pain in the feet was severe, causing compensatory gait changes at the knees and hips with overuse injury. The patient had bilateral total joint replacement, first metatarsophalangeal joints, with excision of both sesamoids on one foot. He recovered uneventfully and 4 weeks following surgery was jogging three miles a day. Six weeks following surgery, he was jogging 7–8 miles per day.

CASE 13 (Fig. 15B.19)

Case 13 is G.R., a middle-aged golfer with post-traumatic arthritis, first and second metatarsophalangeal joints. Patient had implant arthroplasty, first and second metatarsophalangeal joints, with eventual failure of the implant in the first metatarsophalangeal joint. The implant was removed and the patient continued to function well following what was, in effect, a Keller procedure. Total joint replacement for the second MPJ was successful.

CASE 14 (Fig. 15B.20)

Case 14 is a 38-year-old marathon runner who had had a modified Silver procedure for hallux limitus which failed. He then had

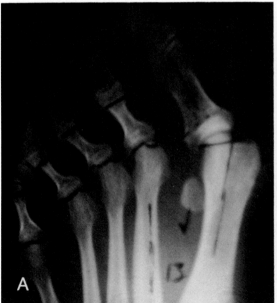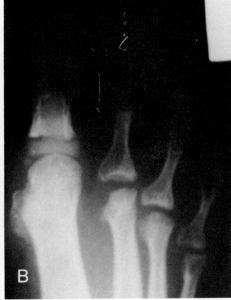

Figure 15B.17. *A*, AP view of the foot showing subluxation of metatarsophalangeal joints and a high degree of hallux valgus. *B*, post-op hemi-implant arthroplasty with panmetatarsal partial head resection. There has been gentle remodeling of the first metatarsal head carried out to afford a congruous joint. Patient returned to full activity and sports.

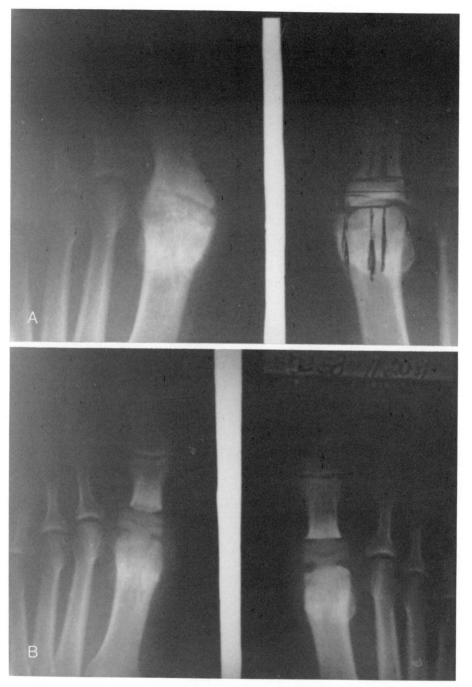

Figure 15B.18. *A*, pre-op views of left and right foot, patient A.C. Marked hallux rigidus with arthritis first metatarsophalangeal joint left and narrowing of joint with arthritis, first metatarsophalangeal joint right. *B*, post-op AP view showing total hinged Swanson first metatarsophalangeal joint replacement arthroplasties. Note that sesamoids on left foot had been removed due to arthritis and effusion. This was necessary to allow normal range of motion of first MPJ. Note that the first metatarsal head length has been maintained with resection of bone being obtained from base of proximal phalanx. Right foot shows normal first metatarsal head with a total joint replacement in place, sesamoids in normal position.

a hemi-implant which, likewise, failed due to impingement of the implant upon the bone. Following the implant arthroplasty, the joint was too tight with eventual failure. The patient then had a total joint replacement and was able to again run at the marathon level.

COMPLICATIONS

When complications with implant arthroplasty of the first metatarsophalangeal joint occur, the implants can be replaced or removed. Hemi-implants should be utilized only when there is a congruous joint. When total joint replacement is utilized, it is preferable to resect as little of the first metatarsal headas possible. Resecting the frontal plane of the first metatarsal head may result in the implant compressing into the capsulous bone and/or medullary canal of the first metatarsal. If this does occur, the failed implant can be removed and the first metatarsal head repaired with bone cement, following which a new total implant may be inserted. An articulating total joint replacement and bone cement may work in the nonathlete, but this type of implant may fail in the athlete due to the excessive torque taking place in various sports (Case 15).

CASE 15 (Fig. 15B.21)

Case 15 is an 18-year-old woman who enjoys jogging and running. She has Charcot neuropathy, right first metatarsophalangeal joint, with absent vibratory sensation. A Keller procedure was carried out inasmuch as it was felt that the patient lacked proper proprioceptive protective responses to protect an implant arthroplasty. The Keller worked quite well and the patient was able to participate unimpeded in all sports activities (18).

If both sesamoids are arthritic and need to be removed, a total joint replacement is indicated (Case 12). Failure to utilize a total joint replacement when both sesamoids are removed will result in a hallux hammertoe. When excessive metatarsus primus adductus is present, a closing wedge osteotomy is necessary prior to utilizing a hemi- or total implant.

Utilization of the double-stemmed flexible type with Dow-Corning HP material appears to be well suited for the athlete inasmuch as it provides for stability and does not rely upon a perfect articulation between the implant concavity and the first metatarsal head convexity. Thus, excessive shearing or wearing out of the implant during the various motions taking place at the first metatarsophalangeal joint during sports is avoided.

Arthritic Hallux Interphalangeal Joint

The arthritic interphalangeal joint in an athlete may either be fused or treated with a flexible total joint replacement. If fusion is preferred, screw fixation is best. If the athlete requires a flexible interphalangeal joint for sports, then total joint replacement with a silastic HP implant may be utilized (Case 16).

CASE 16 (Fig. 15B.22)

Case 16 is a young woman with a post-surgical arthritis of the interphalangeal joint of the great toe. Patient had prior surgery for a painful pinched callus under the plantar medial aspect of the interphalangeal joint. This resulted in eventual arthritis of the joint due to overzealous resection of bone. The patient desired a flexible great toe and, therefore, a total joint replacement was carried out. The patient now has considerable improvement in flexibility and is able to participate in sports without pain.

Lesser Metatarsophalangeal Joints

Metatarsophalangeal joints may be contracted and in need of soft tissue release.

The joints may be arthritic and in need of debridement and/or implant arthroplasty. At times, when plantar, painful keratotic lesions are present, a decision must be made as to a release of the contracted metatarsophalangeal joint and/or osteotomy of the metatarsal neck or base. Oftentimes, when there is a contracted toe with dorsal con-

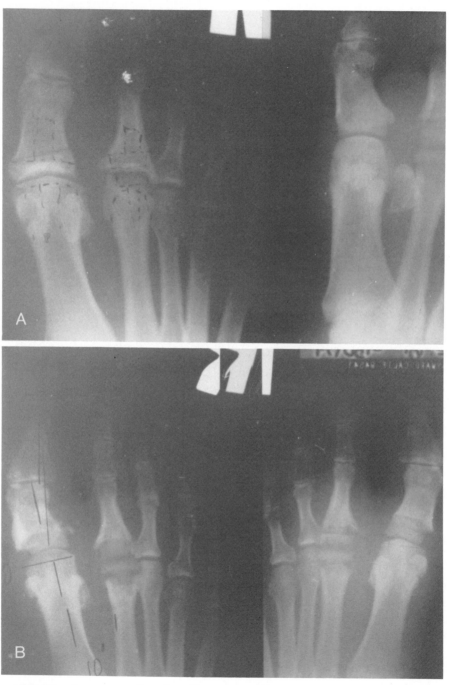

Figure 15B.19. *A*, pre-operative view. *B*, post-operative view. *C*, post-operative failed hemi-implant. *D*, implant failed.

tracture of the metatarsophalangeal joint, soft tissue release of the metatarsophalangeal joint with arthrodesis or arthroplasty of the toe will allow sufficient relaxation of the retrograde force in the metatarsal head to effectively reduce the pressure on the keratotic lesion.

Soft Tissue Release, Metatarsophalangeal Joints

When a metatarsophalangeal joint is in need of release, it is best to do a longitudinal incision over the joint and completely section the long and short extensor tendon apparatus. A transverse capsulotomy allows for the dorsally displaced proximal phalanx of the toe to be released and returned to a more anatomical position.

Metatarsal Head Resection

At times, there may be an excessively long metatarsal with a painful arthritic metatarsophalangeal joint and a plantar lesion. A resection of the metatarsal head may result in a normal parabola and resolution of the lesion, as well as the arthritic joint. If the metatarsophalangeal joint is arthritic yet the metatarsal itself is not long, then a total implant arthroplasty would be preferred. If the metatarsal head resection has been performed and there is regrowth of the head or recurrence of ar-

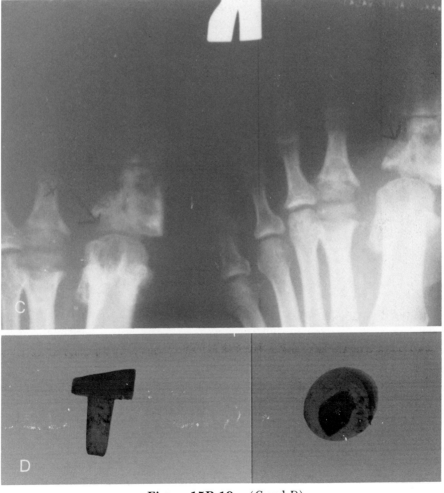

Figure 15B.19. (*C* and *D*)

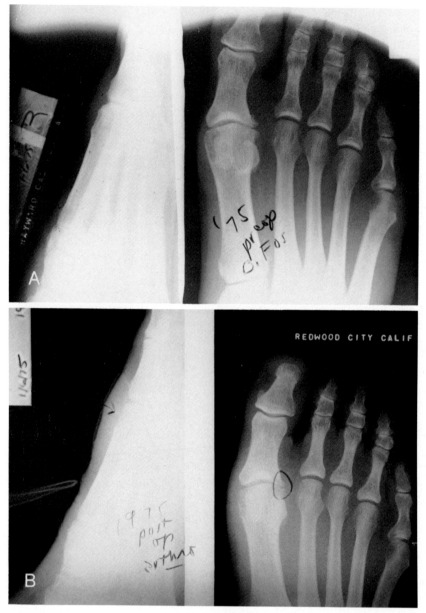

Figure 15B.20. *A*, AP and lateral view, 1975. Lateral view of narrowing of the joint. AP view of bone spur, lateral aspect, base of proximal phalanx and adjacent surface, head of first metatarsal. *B*, immediate post-op x-ray following modified Silver procedure with removal of dorsal aspect, head of first metatarsal, and attempts at repositioning hallux. Note that the hypertrophic bone at the lateral aspect of first metatarsophalangeal joint has not been resected. Narrowing of joint persists. *C*, failure of hemi-implant for correction of persistent hallux limitus. Note sinking of hemi-implant into proximal phalanx medullary canal with hypertrophic changes medially. Note mild osteone-crosis, head of first metatarsal, secondary to abnormal pressure. *D*, 1 year post-op, total joint replacement for failed hemi-implant. Note that total joint replacement is allowing relatively normal length of great toe and anatomical alignment. Patient has pain-free range of motion and is able to run marathons with total joint replacement.

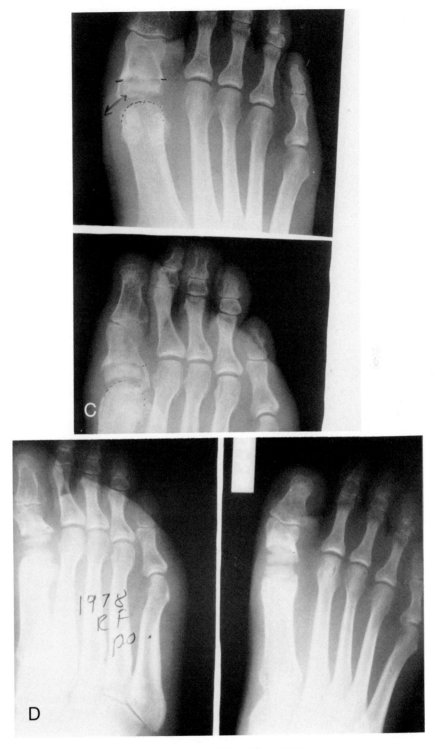

Figure 15B.20. (*C* and *D*)

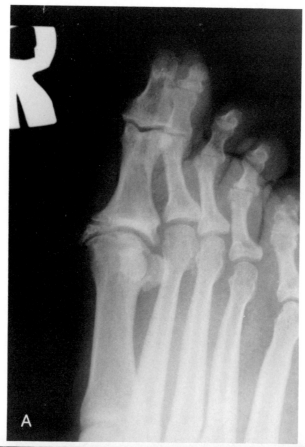

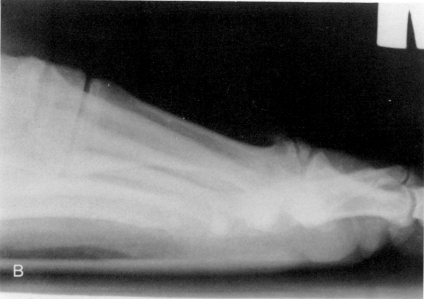

Figure 15B.21. *A* and *B*, pre-op hallux limitus with Charcot neuropathy and fracture. *C* and *D*, post-op Keller with remodeling head.

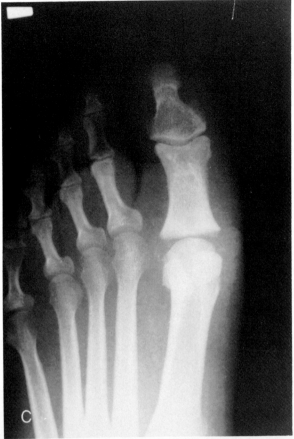

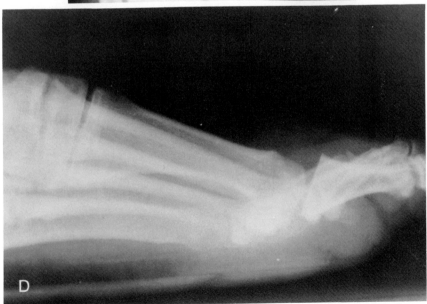

Figure 15B.21. (*C* and *D*)

thritis, an implant arthroplasty is preferable (Case 17).

CASE 17 (Fig. 15B.23)

Case 17 is a 44-year-old jogger, hiker, and hunter with complaints of a painful second metatarsophalangeal joint, left foot.

Sesamoids

Sesamoid dysplasia and/or fractures about the first metatarsophalangeal joint

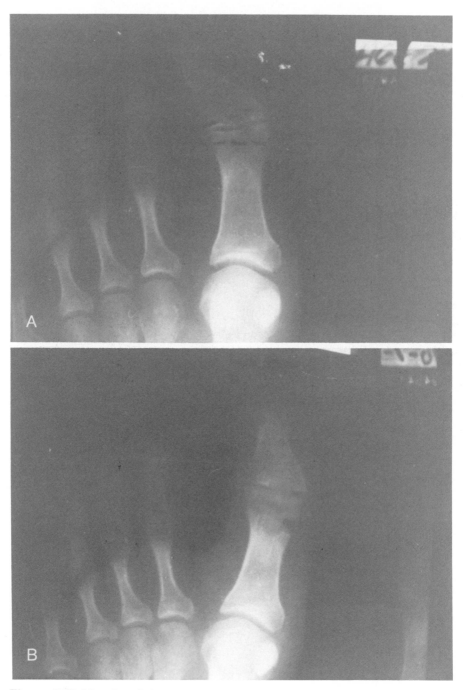

Figure 15B.22. *A*, arthritis of the interphalangeal joint. *B*, total joint replacement.

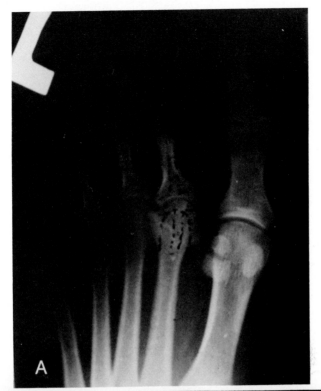

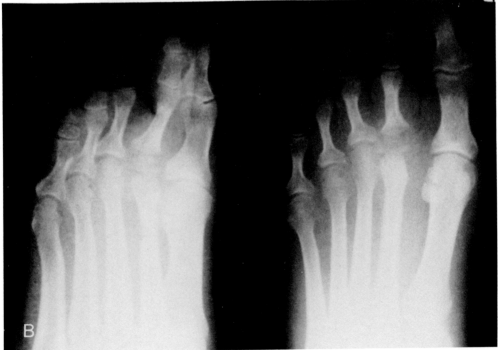

Figure 15B.23. *A*, narrow arthritic second metatarsophalangeal joint. *B*, post-op total Swanson-hinged joint replacement.

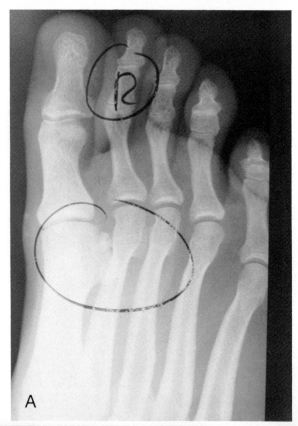

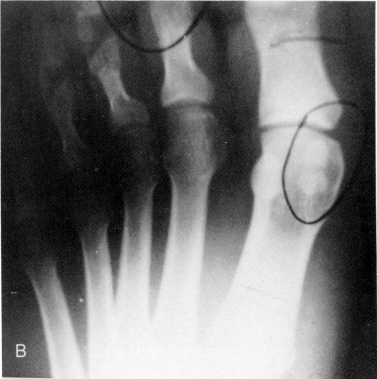

Figure 15B.24. *A*, fractured tibial sesamoid with dysplasia of the fibular sesamoid. *B*, AP view of fractured tibial sesamoid. *C*, axial view showing mild relative plantar-flexion of the first metatarsal. *D*, post-operative views showing the osteotomy of the first metatarsal base with fixation.

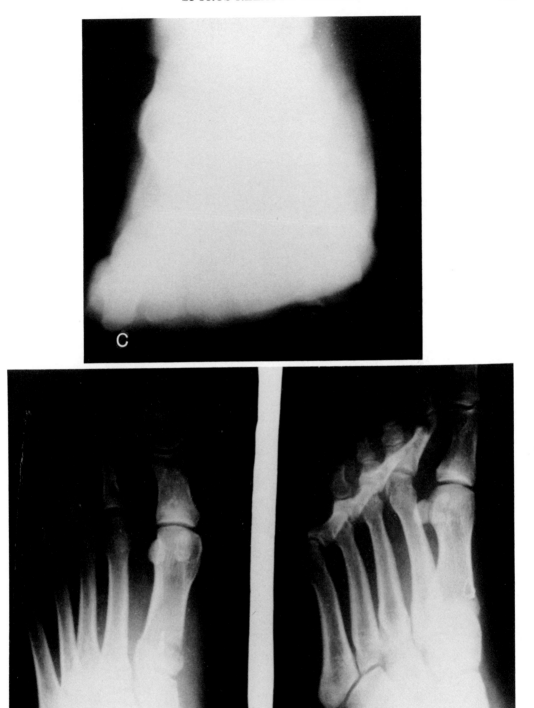

Figure 15B.24.   (*C* and *D*)

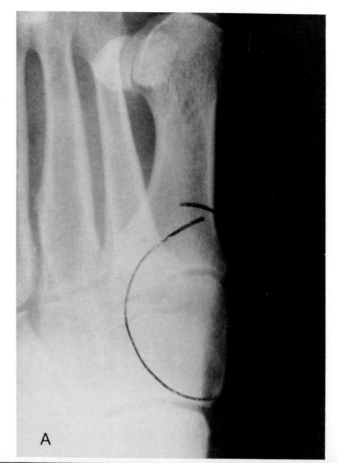

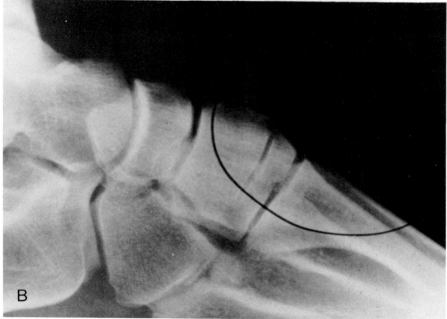

Figure 15B.25.   *A*, pre-op. *B*, post-op excision of exostosis.

are problematic to both the athlete and the treating physician. Dystrophic sesamoids may be difficult to differentiate from stress fracture. When fracture is suspected, cast immobilization for 3–4 weeks may result in complete union without the sequella of malunion and the need for eventual surgical excision. If sesamoid dysplasia is present and there has been failure to respond to conservative treatment, surgical excision may be necessary.

The sesamoids plantar to the first metatarsophalangeal joint have the same range of pathological conditions as the patella. There can be chondromalacia as well as medial or lateral subluxation. When the first metatarsal goes into adductus, the sesamoids are relatively laterally subluxed. In addition, the sesamoids may be involved with medial subluxation, and a hallux varus or hallux hammertoe may be the end result. Maltracking of the sesamoid with eventual chondromalacia may occur. A plantar-flexed metatarsal results in chondralgia sesamoid secondary to abnormal forces. A fracture may result. A hypermobile first ray may result in maltracking of the sesamoids with dystrophic changes and/or chondromalacia.

When chondralgia of the sesamoids of the first metatarsophalangeal joint are present, simple biomechanical realignment of the first metatarsophalangeal joint may suffice in lessening the symptoms and reversing an eventual progressive deformity (Case 18).

CASE 18 (Fig. 15B.24)

Case 18 shows a fractured tibial sesamoid with chronic fibular sesamoiditis in an 18-year-old young woman active in sports. Biomechanical exam revealed a mild relatively plantar-flexed first metatarsal. Patient had a tendency toward hallux valgus. Procedure of choice was a dorsiflexory wedge osteotomy of the first metatarsal base with cast immobilization for 6 weeks. This allowed the sesa-

moids to heal uneventfully and the patient resumed participation in sports pain-free. (COMMENT: When the first metatarsal is plantar-flexed and there are dystrophic or fractured sesamoids, a dorsal wedge osteotomy may be the treatment of choice without excision of the sesamoids. Non-weightbearing for 6 weeks following this procedure may allow for healing of the sesamoids.)

The loss of the medial dynamic stabilizer, which occurs after excision of a dystrophic tibial sesamoid, often results in hallux val-

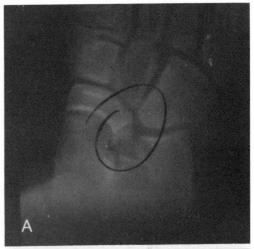

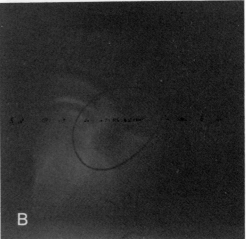

Figure 15B.26. *A*, oblique view with coalition. *B*, post-op excision of coalition.

gus; bony stability and a congruent joint are essential for athletic performance. If there are dystrophic changes under both sesamoids and a long and/or plantar-flexed first metatarsal is present, you may have success utilizing a dorsal wedge osteotomy of the first metatarsal base. A-O fixation assures saggital plane stability without concurrent excessive dorsiflexion of the first metatarsal (Cases 7, 8, and 17).

Tailor Bunion

Hyperostosis of the fifth metatarsal, or tailor bunion, is usually corrected by a sliding osteotomy of the fifth metatarsal neck. This osteotomy should be carried out as far distal as possible as it will allow for primary bone healing (Case 1). A more proximal osteotomy may result in malunion. Theosteotomy should be angled from lateral distal to proximal medial and from dorsal distal to proximal plantar. In this way, the metatarsal head is transpositioned medially and somewhat dorsally (Case 8).

Plantar Keratomas

Plantar keratomas under metatarsal heads usually respond to conservative treatment utilizing orthoses. In the event that orthoses are not completely successful, a "V" or transverse osteotomy of a depressed metatarsal may be carried out. Complications with osteotomies are that of malunion, pseudo-arthrosis, or transfer le-

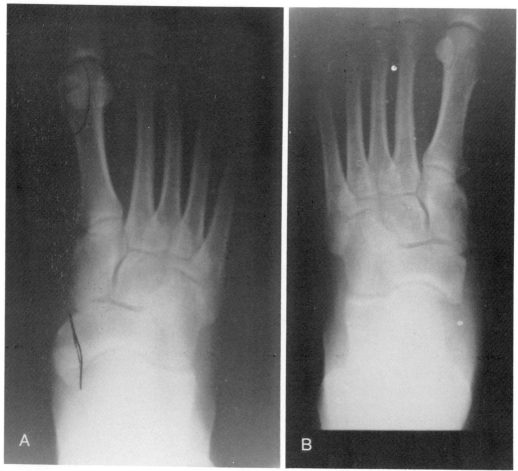

Figure 15B.27. *A*, pre-op view with the os navicularis and fractured tibial sesamoid. *B*, post-op excision of the os navicularis and the medial tubercle of the navicular. Tibial sesamoid has been resected and medial capsulorrhaphy performed.

sions. Lack of proper bone healing can be minimized by utilizing a proper osteotomy site and post-op stabilization for 3–4 weeks. When performing distal metatarsal osteotomies, it is important to leave the collateral ligaments intact so that malrotation of the distal aspect does not occur.

Midtarsal Joint Exostoses

An exostoses at the dorsal aspect of the first metatarso-cuneiform joint may be problematic in an athlete. This can occur secondary to excessive hypermobility of the first ray which causes a jamming of the first metatarso-cuneiform joint with a reactive hyperostosis being the end result. When the hyperostosis is resected a dell should be left. Failure to do so may result in recurrent hyperostosis (Case 19).

CASE 19 (Fig. 15B.25)

J.J., a middle-aged gentleman who hikes and jogs, with dorsal exostosis, first metatarsocuneiform joint.

Midtarsal Coalitions

Coalitions of the midtarsal joint will produce symptoms in the athlete. This may have occurred with a twisting motion and a synostosis may have been fractured. Most often, a coalition is found between the navicular and the calcaneus. There can, however, be coalitions in other portions of the midtarsal joint. If radiographs are negative, tomograms may be necessary to delineate the bony bridge. Conservative treatment with injection therapy and mobilization, as well as orthoses, should be utilized before surgery is considered.

The surgical approach for midtarsal joint coalitions involves a dorsolateral incision where the extensor brevis tendon is detached to expose the midtarsal joint (19). Failure results due to incomplete excision of the coalition or when an extensor brevis arthroplasty is not utilized. In the event that there is long-standing calcaneal valgus associated with the midtarsal joint coali-

tion, a calcaneal osteotomy may be necessary (20). If peroneal tightness or spasm is present with the deformity, excessive postoperative physical therapy will be necessary. Orthoses may be indicated as well (Case 19).

Fifth Metatarsal Base Problems

The fifth metatarsal base may be involved with a nonunion fracture. If this is the case, bone grafts may be necessary with fixation. Hyperostotic fifth metatarsal bases may need surgical resection.

Os Navicularis

Os navicularis or a hypertrophic navicular tubercle may be symptomatic. There may be chronic recurrent posterior tibial tendinitis associated with this problem. Pain over the bony protuberance occurs most commonly in skiing and ice-skating. Sprinters have been known to avulse the os navicularis from its fibrous attachment to the main body of the navicular. When this occurs, surgery is indicated. The hypertrophic medial tubercle should be excised flush with the medial cuneiform (Case 20). The Kidner procedure should be avoided in the athlete to avoid post-operative tendinitis (21). When chronic posterior tibial tendinitis is present, a tenolysis is recommended. The tendon sheaths should then be very loosely sutured to prevent the possibility of tenosynovitis.

CASE 20 (Fig. 15B.26)

Case 20 is a teenager with pain at the midtarsal joint, secondary to midtarsal coalition.

Dorsal Navicular Pathology

Dorsally, the navicular may be involved with a fracture secondary to jumping or excessive running forces. Traumatic arthritis of the navicular cuneiform and talar navicular articulations are common. When arthralgia is present with dorsal spurring, arthroplasties with debridement are recommended. If there has been a true fracture, the free-floating body must be excised (Case 21).

CASE 21 (Figs. 15B.27 and 15B.28)

Case 21 is a young woman with complaints of pain over the os navicularis. The tibial sesamoid has been fractured and is also symptomatic.

Peroneal Cuboid Syndrome

Peroneal cuboid syndrome presents with pain where the peroneus longus passes beneath the cuboid in the peroneal groove. Cuboid subluxation may be present. Failure of conservative treatment may necessitate surgical intervention. Successful surgery requires decompression of the peroneus longus tendon and the formation of a new groove to be fashioned in the cuboid (Case 22).

CASE 22 (Fig. 15B.29)

Case 22 shows a post-traumatic fracture of the proximal dorsal aspect of the navicular in a teenager who ran track. She had persistent pain at the dorsal aspect of the joint, especially when on the ball of her foot. (COMMENT: The patient returned within 4 weeks to pain-free athletic endeavors.)

REARFOOT PROCEDURES
Calcaneal Spurs

Plantar calcaneal spurs usually respond to conservative treatment, consisting of injection therapy, physiotherapy, taping, rest, and orthoses. At times, cast immobilization is utilized. Bone scans may be necessary to rule out bone lesions and/or stress fractures. Systemic diseases should be ruled out with appropriate lab tests. In the event that all conservative treatment fails, and pain is still present, surgery is indicated.

In addition to bone resection, the plantar fascia should be released as far proximal as possible. There is usually a triad of symp-

toms, including medial calcaneal neuritis, plantar fasciitis, and heel spur syndrome with or without adventitious bursitis. All of these anatomical relationships should be explored at the time of surgery (Figs. 15B.30–15B.32) (Case 23).

TECHNIQUE

Complications occur with entrapment of the medial calcaneal nerve, incomplete release of the plantar fascia, or inadequate resection of the hyperostosis of the calcaneus.

Retrocalcaneal Exostosis and Posterior Calcaneal Pathology

Retrocalcaneal exostoses, as well as posterior calcaneal hyperostosis, may be bothersome (Fig. 15B.31). There may be intratendinous calcification of the Achilles. If

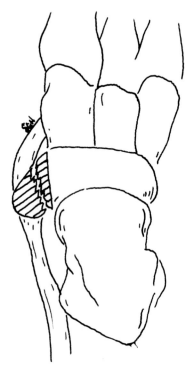

Figure 15B.28. Os navicularis. (From Subotnick, S. I. *Podiatric Sports Medicine.* Futura, Mt. Kisco, New York, 1975, p. 175, with permission.)

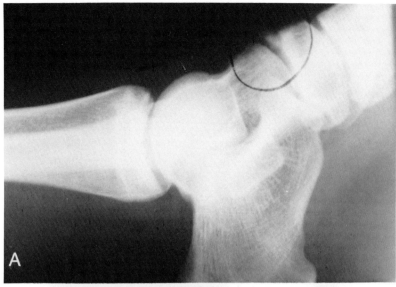

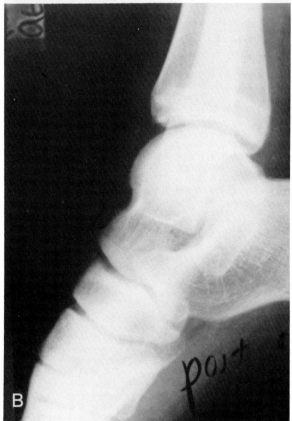

Figure 15B.29. *A*, pre-op: note fractured fragment. *B*, post-op.

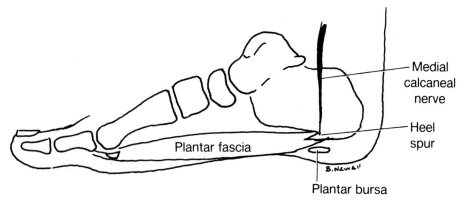

Figure 15B.30. Heel spur. (From Subotnick, S. I. *Podiatric Sports Medicine.* Futura, Mt. Kisco, New York, 1975, p. 145, with permission.)

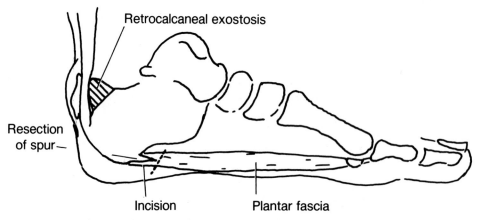

Figure 15B.31. Calcaneal spurs and retrocalcaneal exostosis. (From Subotnick, S. I. *Podiatric Sports Medicine.* Futura, Mt. Kisco, New York, 1975, p. 170, with permission.)

conservative treatment is unsuccessful, surgery may be indicated (Case 23).

CASE 23 (Fig. 15B.32)

Case 23 is that of a heel spur.

Physical therapy is essential during the post-operative course. Ultrasound, dyna-wave, and passive-resistive exercises, followed by active-resistive exercises allow for proper flexibility and strength of the posterior musculature.

Failures are associated with chronic periostitis, bone regrowth, or repetitive chronic stress resulting in a recurrence of posterior calcaneal pathology. Autoim-

mune diseases may be present which predispose to posterior calcaneal or plantar calcaneal pain, even after surgical procedures have been performed. In these instances, reoperation may be required.

Os Trigonum and Posterior Talar Shelf Pathology

An os trigonum may be fractured with a sudden plantar flexory force to the foot and ankle. The posterior shelf of the talus may become arthritic by chronic repetitive excessive plantar flexion or by a single traumatic incident. If this is the case, cast immobilization may be indicated, followed by

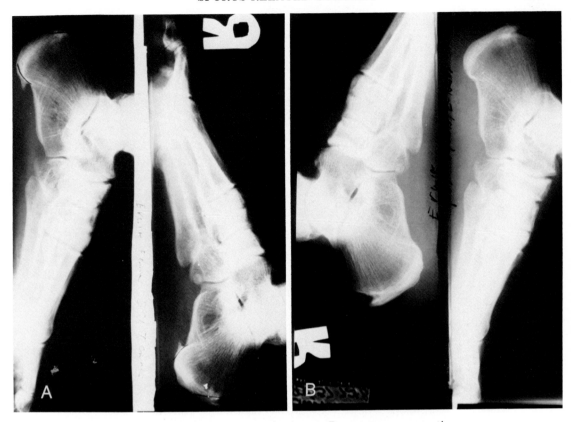

Figure 15B.32. *A*, pre-op heel spur. *B*, post-op spur resection.

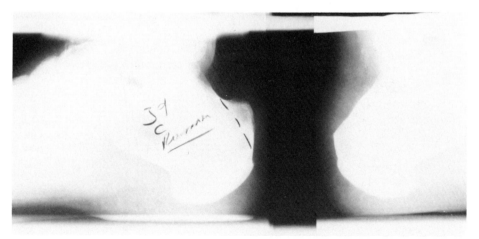

Figure 15B.33. Retrocalcaneal exostosis: *left*, pre-op; *right*, post-op bone resection.

physiotherapy and injection therapy. If symptoms persist, surgery is indicated. Care should be taken not to injure the medial flexor tendon group (Fig. 15B.34).

CASE 24 (Fig. 15B.33)

Pre-op and post-op x-rays of a 39-year-old caucasian runner who had symptomatic retrocalcaneal exostosis, refractory to conservative treatment. Pre-op x-ray is on the left. Post-operative radiograph (*right*) shows post-resection retrocalcaneal hyperostosis and exosto-

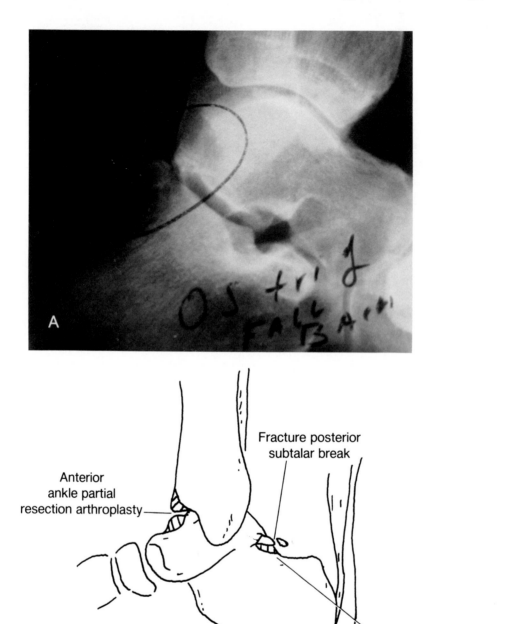

Figure 15B.34. *A*, removal of os trigonum. *B*, extension of talar posterior process beyond subtalar joint. Pre-operative os trigonum and impingement exostosis-anterior ankle with post-fracture arthritic posterior STJ shelf. (From Subotnick, S. I. *Podiatric Sports Medicine.* Futura, Mt. Kisco, New York, 1975, pp. 174–175, with permission.)

sis. The patient returned to symp-
tom-free running 6 weeks following
surgery.

CASE 25 (Fig. 15B.35)

Case 25 is a 29-year-old caucasian female who injured the poste-

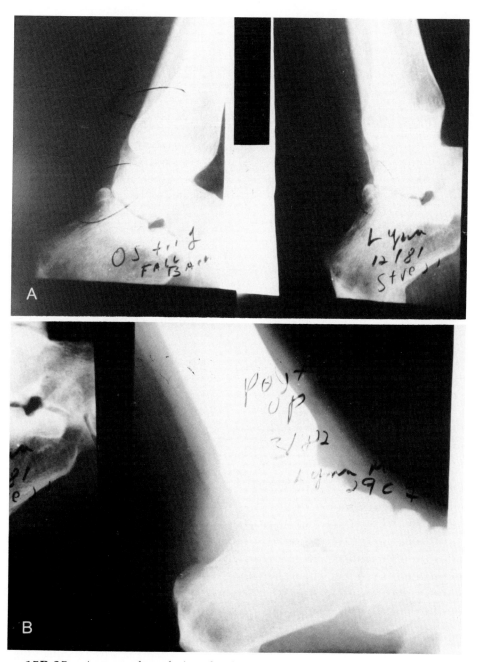

Figure 15B.35. *A*, pre-op lateral view showing the os trigonum. *B*, post-op view of the foot
showing excision of the os trigonum with minimal remodeling, posterior aspect, posterior facet of
the subtalar joint.

rior aspect of her subtalar joint while falling from a ladder, landing on her heels, and then rocking back as she fell on her posterior buttocks. This injury caused acute plantar flexion at the ankle and subtalar joint and the os trigonum abutted against the tibia causing its fracture. The patient developed a chronic pain syndrome and eventually had excision of the os trigonum with full recovery.

CASE 26 (Fig. 15B.36)

M.H., young woman who had subtalar joint arthritis. She eventually had a triple arthrodesis which was carried out with the heel in varus. This caused lateral instability and strain at the ankle joint, with considerable callus formation and pain under the lateral aspect of the heel and fifth ray. This was eventually resolved with a Dwyer osteotomy.

Talar Neck Spurs

Dorsal talar neck impingement exostosis may cause pain about the anterior aspect of the ankle joint. These spurs can be surgically excised. If there is concurrent hyperostosis on the anterior leading edge of the tibia, excision of this spur is recommended.

MAJOR DEFORMITIES OF THE FOOT
Cavus Foot

Cavus foot in the athlete may require surgical intervention. When an anterior cavus deformity is present, an osteotomy of the first metatarsal, together with a plantar fascial release may suffice. In the presence of a posterior cavus deformity, a Dwyer osteotomy may be required (Case 26). When a total cavus deformity is present, a midtarsal joint osteotomy is necessary. Although anterior cavus deformities are relatively easy to correct, total cavus deformities usually result in a foot which is less

than optimal for athletic performance. Posterior cavus deformity does respond well to osteotomy procedures of the calcaneus, and a fairly normal functional foot for athletic endeavors will be the end result.

Flatfoot

Many athletes have various degrees of flatfoot deformity. These usually respond to orthotic foot devices. At times, the flatfoot deformity is so severe that the athlete or would-be athlete cannot participate. Utilization of extra-articular subtalar joint arthroeresis are recommended for the young athlete (Case 27). If there is excessive tightness of the posterior structures, a posterior release or tendo Achilles lengthening may be indicated. When excessive calcaneal valgus is present, a calcaneal osteotomy is indicated (Case 28).

A medial talo-navicular joint desmoplasty may be the procedure of choice if excessive midtarsal joint deformities are associated with the flatfoot (Case 29).

Neuromusculature Problems of the Lower Extremity

There will be times when there are neuromusculature imbalances of the lower extremity in the athlete. Rossi-Levi syndrome, a variant of Charcot-Marie-Tooth disease, peroneal atrophy, and associated cavus foot deformity can successfully be treated with osteotomy of the first metatarsal and plantar fascia release. Jones suspension and Dwyer osteotomy were utilized with some success (Case 30).

CASE 27 (Fig. 15B.37)

Case 27 is a young man in his early thirties with persistent pain secondary to cavus foot deformity. This was eventually treated with a Dwyer osteotomy and a dorsal wedge osteotomy of the first metatarsal with plantar fascial release. The patient tolerated the surgery well and had an excellent functional and cosmetic result. Addi-

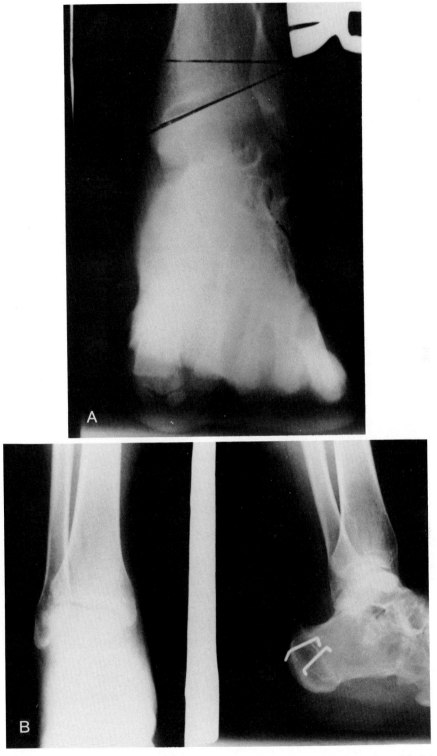

Figure 15B.36. *A*, pre-operative maximum pronation taking place at the right ankle joint with persistent plantar flexion of the lateral column of the foot. *B*, post-operative lateral following Dwyer osteotomy.

tional dorsiflexion was gained by allowing the distal fragment to dorsiflex upon the proximal fragment prior to fixation.

CASE 28 (Fig. 15B.38)

Case 28 is an 11-year-old child with persistent painful calcaneal valgus foot. He responded well to a stay peg extra-articular subtalar joint procedure for calcaneal valgus. The patient was ambulatory one day following the surgery without a cast and was able to return to pain-free sports participation within 3 months.

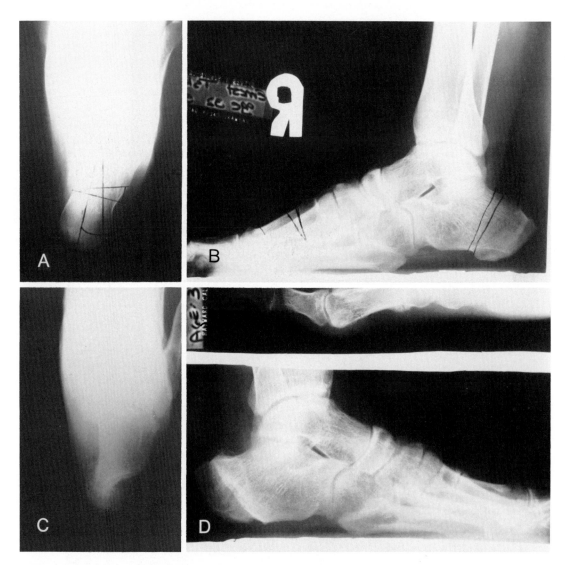

Figure 15B.37. *A*, pre-op calcaneal axial view showing a significant amount of calcaneal varus. *B*, pre-op stress lateral showing dorsiflexion of the plantar-flexed first ray. *C*, post-op calcaneal view showing reduction of calcaneal varus with a Dwyer osteotomy. *D*, post-op lateral view showing Dwyer osteotomy at the calcaneus and dorsal wedge osteotomy, first metatarsal base. Note relative lowering of the longitudinal arch with some dorsal displacement, as desired, of the posterior aspect of the calcaneus.

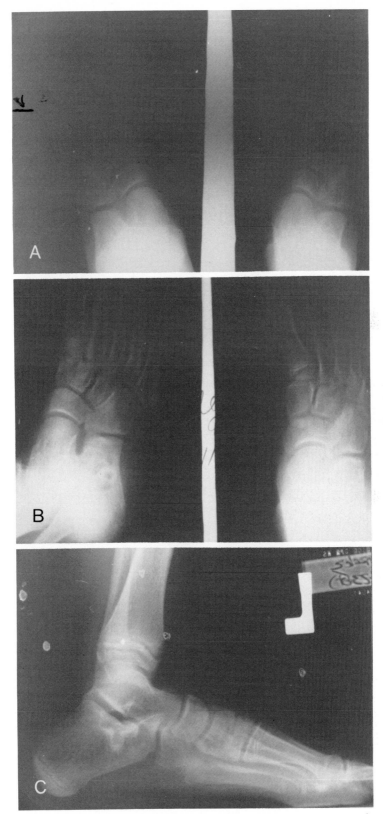

Figure 15B.38. *A*, pre-op anterior posterior view of the feet showing very wide talo-calcaneal angle with anterior medial protrusion of the talar head and neck and lateral subluxation of the forefoot. *B*, post-op AP view showing relocation of talonavicular joint following arthrroresis. *C*, lateral view of patient, 3 years post-op, arthrroresis at the sinus tarsi.

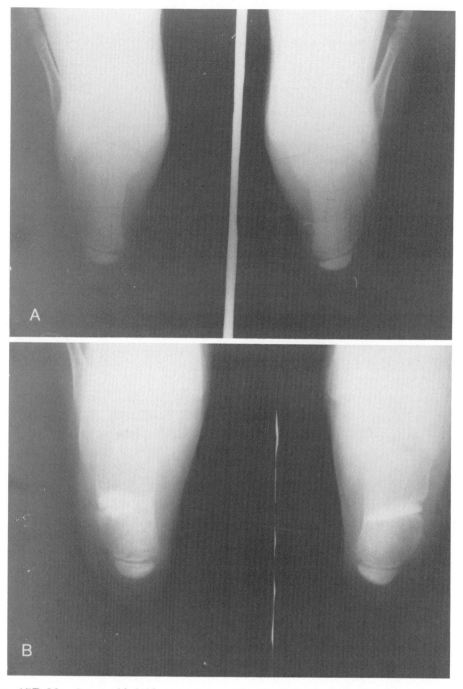

Figure 15B.39.   8-year-old child complaining of hypermobile flat feet with calcaneal valgus and medial declination of subtalar joint. *A*, calcaneal axial views showing medial slant of posterior facet of subtalar joint. *B*, post-op calcaneal opening wedge osteotomy showing realignment of subtalar joint and calcaneus. Patient is currently 4 years post-op and asymptomatic with relatively normal alignment of feet being maintained.

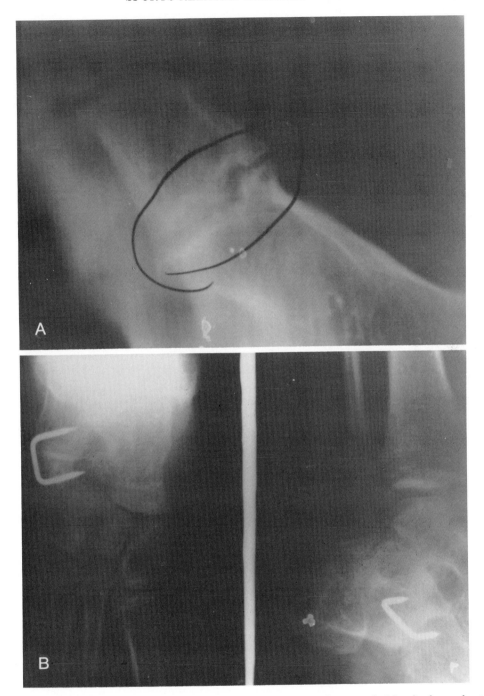

Figure 15B.40. *A,* pre-op tomogram of the foot. Note significant arthritis of calcaneal articulation. *B,* post-op fusion of mid-tarsal joint. Note staple across calcaneal cuboid joint where fusion has taken place.

CASE 29 (Fig. 15B.39)

Eight-year-old child complaining of hypermobile flat feet with calcaneal valgus and medial declination of subtalar joint.

CASE 30 (Fig. 15B.40)

Case 30 is a young man with post-traumatic arthritis of the midtarsal joint, which eventually was resolved with a midtarsal joint fusion. At time of fusion, appropriate wedges were taken to restore a more normal arch in the foot.

References

1. Subotnick, S. I. *Podiatric Sports Medicine.* Futura, Mt. Kisco, NY, 1975, pp. 158–159.
2. Gerbert, J., Mercado, O. A., and Sokoloff, T. H. *The Surgical Treatment of Hallux-Abducto-Valgus and Allied Deformities.* Futura, Mt. Kisco, NY, 1973.
3. Austin, D. W., and Leventen, E. O. A new osteotomy for hallux valgus. Clin. Orthop. Relat. Res. 157:25–30, 1981.
4. Mann, R. A., and Coughlin, N. J. Hallux valgus—Etiology, anatomy, treatment, and surgical considerations. Clin. Orthop. Relat. Res. 157:31–41, 1981.
5. Pelet, D. Osteotomy and fixation for hallux valgus. Clin. Orthop. Relat. Res. 157:42–46, 1981.
6. Aiken, O. F. Treatment of hallux valgus: A new operative procedure and its results. Med. Sentinel 33:678, 1925.
7. Helal, B. Survey for adolescent hallux valgus. Clin. Orthop. Relat. Res. 157:50–62, 1981.
8. Wilson, J. N. Oblique displacement osteotomy for hallux valgus. J. Bone Jt. Surg. 45B:552, 1963.
9. Reverdin, J. Anatomie et operation de l'hallux valgus. Int. Med. Cong. 2:408, 1918.
10. Trethowan, J. Hallux valgus, in Choice, C. C. (ed): *A System of Surgery.* P. B. Ober, New York, 1927, p. 1046.
11. Peabody, C. W. The surgical cure of hallux valgus. J. Bone Jt. Surg. 13:273, 1931.
12. Mitchell, C. L., et al. Osteotomy-bunionectomy for hallux valgus. J. Bone Jt. Surg. 40A:41, 1958.
13. Logroscino, D. Il Trattamento Chirurgico dell'alluce Valgus. Chir. Organi Mov. 32:81, 1948.
14. McBride, E. D. A conservative operation for bunions. J. Bone Jt. Surg. 10:735, 1928.
15. Cracchiolo, A., Swanson, A., and Swanson, G. D. The arthritic great toe metatarsal phalangeal joint: A review of flexible silicone implant arthroplasty from two medical centers. Clin. Orthop. Relat. Res. 157:64–69, 1981.
16. Swanson, A. B., et al: Silicone implant arthroplasty of the great toe. Clin. Orthop. 141:30, 1979.
17. Subotnick, S. I. *Podiatric Sports Medicine.* Futura, Mt. Kisco, NY, 1975, pp. 160–169.
18. Keller, W. L. The surgical treatment of bunions and hallux valgus. N. Engl. J. Med. 80:741–742, 1904.
19. Cowell, H. R. Extensor brevis arthroplasty. J. Bone Jt. Surg. 52A:820, 1970.
20. Koutsogiannis, E. Treatment of mobile flatfoot by displacement of osteotomy of calcaneus. J. Bone Jt. Surg. 53B:96, 1971.
21. Kidner, F. C. The prehallux in relation to flatfoot. JAMA 101:1539, 1933.

C. Ankle Joint Surgery in the Athlete

INTRODUCTION

The most common lower extremity sports injury is an inversion sprain of the ankle. The ankle joint may be involved in a myriad of acute or chronic conditions which reduce the athlete's ability to participate in or enjoy sports. At times, these injuries require surgical intervention. Surgery is considered successful if the athlete has full return to the pre-injury level of athletic involvement.

Complications may result secondary to the surgeon's failure to understand the demands of the specific sport in which the athlete is engaged. Failure to consider appropriate biomechanical pre-operative considerations can lead to less than optimal surgical results. Since all athletic injuries result in loss of mobility, strength, and function, post-operative physical therapy is essential to assure maximum rehabilitation. Failure to appropriately utilize physical therapy modalities, integrated with a well-planned return to full activity, may result in surgical failure. Failures may also be associated with inappropriate procedures, inadequate stabilization or immobilization, or post-operative infections. There will be instances where the damage to the ankle joint is of such severity that it precludes, even with the best surgical techniques, full return to active sports. It is imperative for the athlete to understand the limitations of surgery, as well as the expected results. Acute as well as chronic repetitive stress can eventually compromise the results of any surgical procedure. Thus, the consequences of repeated athletic involvement upon the long-term integrity of the ankle joint are to be understood by the surgeon as well as the athlete.

BIOMECHANICAL CONSIDERATIONS

The ankle joint is a hinge joint which provides motion in the sagittal plane. Dorsi- and plantar-flexion occur along an axis which is slightly curved. There is a small component of inversion associated with these motions. The ankle joint works in harmony with the subtalar joint. The subtalar joint may be considered the inferior ankle joint (1). The primary motion taking place at the ankle joint is, therefore, dorsi- and plantar-flexion with pronation and supination taking place at the subtalar joint. Any condition which decreases the range of motion of the subtalar joint places additional stresses on the ankle joint. It is well known that subtalar joint arthritis or coalition may lead to an unstable ankle joint. This is oftentimes the long-term sequela of triple arthrodesis.

There are biomechanical foot types that influence the function of the ankle joint. The cavus foot with an anterior equinus (dropped forefoot) has a functional limitation of dorsiflexion. The need for additional dorsiflexion in this type of foot may lead to excessive anterior impingement and eventual spur formation.

The anterior equinus foot with a plantar-flexed first metatarsal and forefoot valgus may lead to supinatory compensation and additional lateral stress to the ankle joint. This may eventually cause lateral instability of the ankle joint and may be a factor in recurrent lateral ankle sprains.

The pronated foot is associated with chronic synovitis about the ankle joint in athletes.

Subtalar joint varus or tibia varum may contribute to lateral sprains or instability of the ankle joint. Tibia or rearfoot valgus may contribute to medial strain about the ankle joint.

Excessive external rotation of the foot or leg contributes to lateral instability of the ankle joint. Excessive internal rotation of the leg or foot contributes to medial strain about the ankle joint.

The ankle joint, due to the shape of the trochlear surface of the talus, becomes most unstable in plantar-flexion. There is a higher degree of frontal plane mobility of the ankle joint when the foot is plantar-flexed (2). Conversely, repeated dorsiflexion of the foot upon the ankle joint results in anterior impingement exostosis or anterior synovitis (3). A sudden dorsiflexory eversion strain to the ankle joint may lead to chronic anterior periostitis about the ankle and/or anterior instability to the ankle. Anterior instability of the ankle may also contribute to lateral instability of the ankle.

It becomes readily apparent that an understanding of the biomechanics of the foot and its inter-relationship to the ankle is imperative for proper surgical planning. In addition, the post-operative course may include orthotic foot control to help stabilize the foot and the ankle (4–7).

Anterior Ankle Joint Pathology

The anterior aspect of the ankle joint can be involved in soft tissue inflammatory processes. With the anterior capsule becoming inflamed secondary to underlying exostoses (3), chronic traction on the capsule of the ankle joint may cause capsulitis. The traction itself may cause spurring from the adjacent anterior aspects of the tibia and/or talus. These spurs characteristically follow the lines of the capsular tissue. Spur formation may also result secondary to an acute dorsiflexory injury. Dorsiflexion and eversion usually result in diastasis at the ankle joint with rupture of the inferior anterior tibiofibular ligament. The syndesmosis between the tibia and fibula may become chronically strained with rupture of the inter-osseous ligament, resulting in an anterior periostitis.

Soft tissue injuries about the ankle joint respond to treatment with anti-inflammatory medications and physical therapy. Orthotic foot control, when indicated, should be prescribed. Injection therapy with slow-acting steroids is helpful in protracted cases. When chronic soft tissue pain is secondary to underlying spurs, these spurs should be excised. Most often, the ankle joint itself is not affected with an arthritic process when anterior impingement exostoses is present.

Anterior Impingement Exostosis

Anterior impingement exostosis may be present secondary to traction or compression. Chronic traction occurs in jumping sports and is prevalent in ballet and gymnastics (8). Compression of the talar neck upon the tibia occurs with forceful dorsiflexion and eversion (3). This has been called lineman's or footballer's ankle (9). These spurs become symptomatic and dorsiflexion becomes limited. Surgical excision is usually required. Repeated trauma of the type that originally caused the spurs often cause recurrence of this condition (Cases 1 and 2).

CASE 1 (Fig. 15C.1)

Patient M.W., 34-year-old soccer player, is a post-traumatic anterior ankle exostosis following boot-top lower leg fracture which occurred during skiing (A). He complained of anterior ankle pain during walking and, more severely, during sports. B is a pre-operative lateral of the ankle. The ankle joint is narrow. Anterior hyperostosis of the talus and tibia is evident. The spur is secondary to a combination of traumatic impingement, traction, and prolonged cast immobilization following the fracture. The joint space narrowing is consistent with cast immobilization. C is a 3-month post-operative lateral x-ray of the ankle and foot. Note resection at the anterior ankle.

CASE 2 (Fig. 15C.2)

M.D., 24-year-old male runner and soccer player. Lateral x-ray of the ankle shows anterior traction tendon exostosis, as well as symptomatic os trigonum, both following acute ankle sprains.

Anterior Tarsal Tunnel

Anterior tarsal tunnel results when the neurovascular bundle is compressed be-

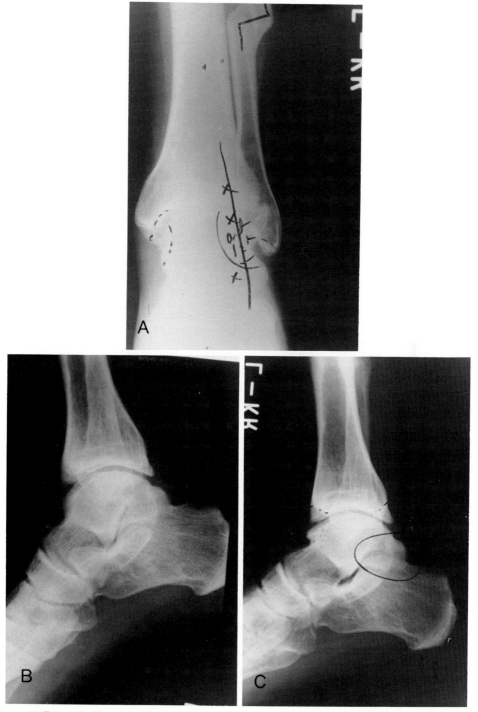

Figure 15C.1. *A*, X-ray ankle A.P. *B*, pre-operative lateral view of ankle. *C*, post-operative 3 months.

tween underlying spurs and inflamed soft tissue. At times, there may be an extensor tendinitis and associated neuropathy of the forefoot secondary to tight shoelaces. This generally resolves rapidly to such simple measures as ice massage and tying the

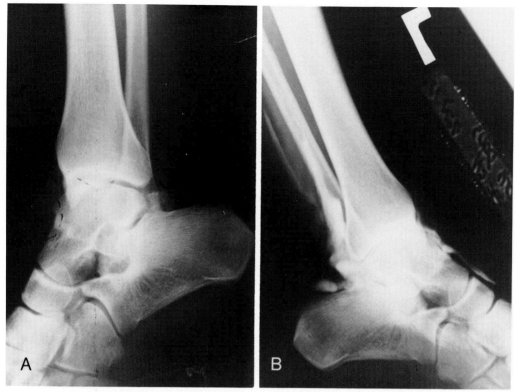

Figure 15C.2. *A*, lateral x-ray of the ankle shows anterior traction tendon exostosis as well as symptomatic os trigonum, both following acute ankle sprains. *B*, lateral x-ray of ankle which shows arthrogram following inversion plantar-flexory sprain. Note dye leakage anterior which is consistent with anterior capsular rupture. Posterior lateral dye leakage is secondary to complete rupture of the fibular talar ligament with capsular tear near the middle fibular-calcaneal ligament. Note dye escaping along the peroneal sheath.

shoes over a piece of felt, or arranging the shoelaces in such a way that they do not cross the inflamed area. At times, steroid injections followed by ultrasound or other forms of physical therapy are necessary.

A true anterior tarsal tunnel syndrome is present when there is a positive Tinel's sign upon palpation of the neurovascular bundle. Resultant numbness occurs on the dorsal aspect of the foot extending to the first interspace. The pain can be diminished markedly with steroid injections. If the condition recurs, x-rays are indicated and almost always show underlying spur formation. They are usually associated with anterior impingement exostoses. When symptoms persist, it is necessary to do an anterior arthroplasty along with excision of the adjacent spurs. The spurs must be excised

in a concave fashion so that when bony defects fill in during healing, new spurs do not form. The anterior tarsal tunnel must be meticulously decompressed.

When a true anterior tarsal tunnel syndrome is present, the extensor retinaculum should not be reapproximated since this may cause neurovascular compression. The same principle is applicable to the posterior tarsal tunnel concerning the lacinate ligament.

When an anterior arthroplasty of the ankle is performed for anterior tarsal tunnel syndrome, an anterior midline incision is preferred. When most of the spur formation is lateral, an anterior lateral incision is indicated. This affords excellent visualization of the ankle joint and avoids the neurovascular bundle. The only major structures to be encountered are the superficial peroneal nerves and the large branch of the lesser saphenous vein which must be ligated. When performing decompression of the neurovascular bundle, the tourniquet should be released prior to closure. This insures proper hemostasis and eliminates the possibility of any bleeding from the neurovascular bundle.

Post-operative care consists of a Jones cast for 10 days. Weightbearing to tolerance is permitted. After cast removal, physical therapy is initiated with passive and, then, passive and active range of motion. Physiotherapy is utilized to reduce post-operative inflammation and increase local profusion. The athlete can begin more strenuous activity 3 weeks following surgery.

Anterior Ankle Arthroplasty

Anterior ankle arthroplasties are differentiated from excision of impingement anterior exostosis of the ankle by the extent of hypertrophic spurring as well as the limitation of motion. In general, an anterior ankle arthroplasty is indicated for a limited range of motion with spurring evident at the anterior, as well as the lateral and/or medial aspect of the ankle joint. The pathology may be secondary to acute trauma or the sequella of accumulated microtrauma. Instability of the ankle joint with repeated sprains may lead to anterior arthritis as well as hypertrophic changes about the talar malleoli interface. Anterior anthroplasty with resection of excessive bone at the anterior medial and/or lateral aspects greatly improves the range of motion while decreasing symptoms. An arthroplasty rather than a fusion may not render the athlete entirely asymptomatic, but will reduce symptoms to allow continuance of athletics. This is not to say that repeated stress on the operated ankle will not lead to the necessity of a repeat anterior arthroplasty in 3–5 years following the initial procedure.

POST-OPERATIVE CARE

When an anterior ankle arthroplasty is performed, post-operative care with a semi-weightbearing cast for 10 days is sufficient. Following cast removal, passive range of motion, along with physiotherapy 2–3 times a week, is initiated. At the 2nd–3rd post-op week, more active range of motion is encouraged. Return to athletic training is usually allowed between the 3rd and 4th post-op week, starting a walking program, and then graduating to a walking-jogging program. Full strength and balance must be achieved before the athlete can return to full athletic participation (Case 3).

CASE 3 (Figs. 15C.3 and 15C.4)

Case 3 involves anterior talar head and neck impingement exostosis following an acute sprain of the ankle and midtarsal joint.

Osteochondritis Dissecans

Osteochondritis dissecans is a result of acute trauma to the talar dome. In most instances, the anterior medial corner of the talus is sheared off from the adjacent surface of the tibia. Occasionally, it may be present at the central or anterior lateral portion of the talus. When ankle joint pain persists following an acute sprain, x-rays should be taken and one should suspect osteochondritis dissecans. At times, tomograms are necessary to detect the lesion. If a lesion is found, it is necessary to do an anterior ankle arthroplastic approach with excision of the loose fragment of bone. Kirschner wires may be buried through the fragment if it appears that the loose body can be salvaged. When excision of the loose body is carried out, it is necessary to place small drill holes in the raw bone bed to allow for fibrocartilage to form.

Attempts have been made to visualize ankle joints with an arthroscope when arthritis or osteochondritis dissecans is suspected. The arthrogram may be helpful in delineating the fragment and noting whether the body is attached or loose.

Medial Instability of the Ankle Joint

Medial instability of the ankle joint occurs secondary to an acute inversion injury.

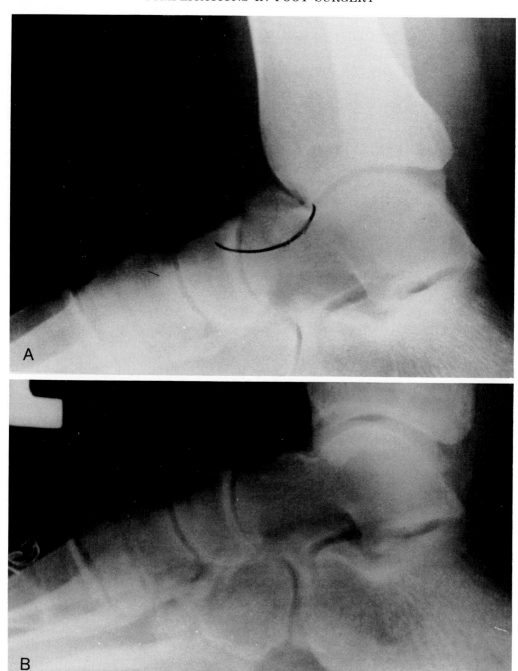

Figure 15C.3. *A*, X-ray shows a stress lateral of the foot and ankle. The talar neck and head exostosis is impinging upon the anterior distal aspect of the tibia, limiting dorsiflexion. There is also exostotic change between the dorsal aspect of the navicular and talus causing bony impingement and pain at this joint. *B*, the stress lateral of the foot and ankle post-operatively. There has been a dorsal wedge osteotomy of the first metatarsal for anterior local cavus foot. There also has been resection of the exostosis of the talar neck and head, as well as an arthroplasty of the talonavicular joint.

Often there is a fracture associated with the rupture of the deltoid ligament. When medial instability is present, surgical repair of the deltoid ligament is indicated. When fractures are present, internal stabilization is required.

In cases of chronic medial instability, it may be necessary to do a surgical repair utilizing a portion of the posterior tibial tendon for stability (13). Non-operative treatment of medial instability may be aided by orthotic foot control.

There have been cases of medial ankle pain associated with subtalar joint arthritis, coalition, or flexor tendinitis beneath the sustentaculum tali. There have also been incidences of medial ankle joint exostoses causing medial ankle pain. These cases have responded relatively well to surgical excision.

Posterior Ankle Joint Pathology

Posterior ankle joint injury may be soft tissue or osseous. Soft tissue problems include Achilles tenosynovitis, retrocalcaneal bursitis, retrocalcaneal exostoses, and flexor or peroneal tendon pathology. The posterior capsule of the ankle joint may become strained during trauma. Generalized synovitis about the ankle joint may be secondary to overuse injury as occurs in jogging. These soft tissue problems generally respond to biomechanical and physical therapy treatment.

Osseous posterior ankle joint problems include an avulsed os trigonum and a hypertrophic or arthritic posterior talar shelf. With these conditions, there will be accentuated pain upon plantar-flexion as the posterior superior surface of the talus abutts the tibia. With plantar-flexion and inversion, the os trigonum will become stressed with the end result acute pain (Case 2).

When an os trigonum is present, pain occurs at the posterior lateral aspect of the heel over the posterior surface of the talus. Pain occurs upon plantar-flexion and inversion. An injection of cortisone and a local anesthetic over the os trigonum usually stops the pain until the effects of the injection wear off. At times, however, steroid injections followed by physical therapy will alleviate the problem. If there is a protruding posterior shelf of the talus interfering with subtalar joint motion, then surgical excision of the offending bone may be necessary. An arthrodesis is almost never indicated when this pathology is present (14).

When an os trigonum is symptomatic, surgical excision is recommended (Fig. 15C.5).

Chronic soft tissue problems such as tendinitis may require decompression. In cases of chronic posterior tibial tendinitis, at the time of tenolysis, inflammatory material has been found within the posterior tibial sheath. Removal of this chronic inflammatory material resolves the problem. Villonodular synovitis about the ankle joint is associated with lateral instability. Cases of ganglionic cysts at the posterior and posterior medial aspect of the ankle joint also respond well to surgical excision.

Subluxing Peroneal Tendons

Peroneal tendons may sublux with a forceful dorsiflexion injury. When this occurs, the peroneals move forward over the fibula and may avulse a portion of bone. The superior peroneal retinaculum is either ruptured or avulsed from the fibula (15). This has been termed the lateral margin avulsion syndrome. Subluxing peroneal tendons are not uncommon in ski injuries where the ski becomes fixated and the skier continues falling downhill with a forceful dorsiflexion injury to the ankle joint. This same mechanism may cause rupture of the tendo Achilles and anterior impaction injury to the ankle joint (16) (Case 4). When rotation takes place, this mechanism will cause fractures.

CASE 4 (Fig. 15C.6)

This is a lateral x-ray of the foot and ankle showing lateral margin avulsion syndrome of the fibula in

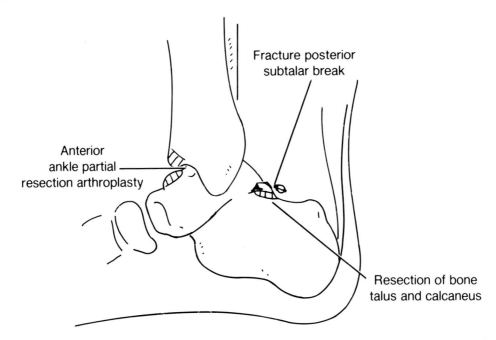

Figure 15C.4. Impingement exostosis: anterior ankle with post-fracture arthritic posterior STJ shelf. (From Subotnick, S. I. *Podiatric Sports Medicine*. Futura, Mt. Kisco, New York, 1975, p. 175, with permission.)

a young cross-country skier with a forceful dorsiflexion injury at the ankle joint causing anterior sub-luxation of the peroneals with sub-sequent avulsion and rupture of the superior peroneal retinaculum.

Subluxing peroneal tendons present with tenderness in the sheath and/or tendon. If subluxation persists and is not controlled by neutral orthotic foot control or an ankle brace, surgery may be required. Surgery involves reapproximating the retinaculum to the fibula through several small drill holes. The new retinaculum may be fash-ioned out of surrounding soft tissue (17, 18). It is usually unnecessary to utilize other bony procedures when repairing the peroneal retinaculum (14). When lateral stabilization procedures are performed, an unstable peroneal tendon superior retinac-ulum may be found. In these instances, a repair is mandatory.

There have been reports of subluxing peroneal tendons secondary to a shallow peroneal groove not associated with acute trauma. This form of pathology seldom re-quires surgery inasmuch as there is only minimal symptomatology. Orthotic foot control to stabilize the heel and keep the peroneal tendons seated behind the fibular malleolus usually suffices. If surgery is in-dicated, utilization of soft tissue procedures usually prove successful. Post-operative care consists of 3 weeks in a below-the-knee walking cast. Following cast removal, physiotherapy is initiated for strength, flexibility, and range of motion. Balancing exercises are indicated since ankle sprains or tendon subluxation about may result in loss of proprioception, and this must be re-established if total rehabilitation and ath-letic involvement are to be appreciated.

Lateral Sprains and Ruptures of the Ankle Joint

The most common athletic injury about the ankle joint is a sprain or rupture of the

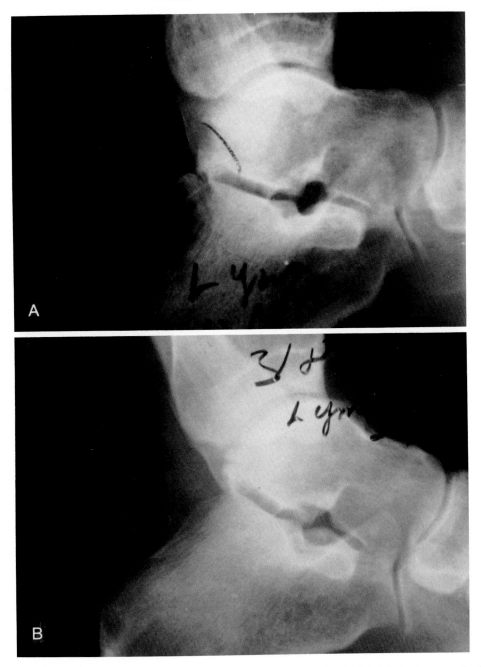

Figure 15C.5. *A,* Extension of talar posterior process beyond subtalar joint. *B,* removal of os trigonum. (From Subotnick, S. I. *Podiatric Sports Medicine.* Futura, Mt. Kisco, New York, 1975, p. 174, with permission.)

anterior talofibular ligament (20). Garrick has pointed out that sprains constitute 85% of the injuries to the ankle and that no fewer than one-sixth of all time-loss injuries in organized sports are ankle sprains.

The typical mechanism of injury is that

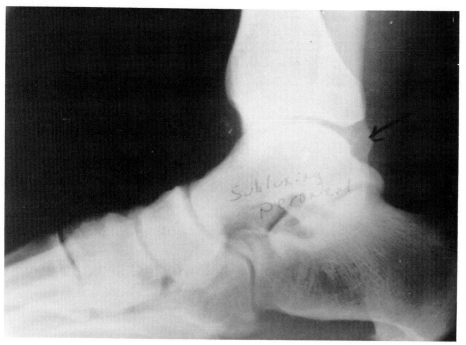

Figure 15C.6.   Lateral margin avulsion syndrome of the fibula, lateral view.

of plantar-flexion of the ankle and inversion of the foot, initiated by the shoe-surface fixation or an angled shoe-surface orientation. Garrick has shown that there are 50% more ankle sprains and knee injuries utilizing the football shoes with 7 cleats versus the football shoes with the shallower wider 14 cleats. A significant mechanism involves the fixation of the toe portion of multi-cleated shoes in artificial turf with the ankle in plantar-flexion. An anteriorly directed force is applied to the posterior aspect of the heel, thereby forcibly inverting the ankle.

The inversion plantar-flexory injury places the majority of strain over the anterior collateral ligament. With inversion stress, and the ankle more neutral, the calcaneal-fibular ligament is strained. With the foot plantar-flexed and inverted, after rupture of the anterior collateral ligament, the middle collateral ligament becomes strained and then ruptured. Following rupture of the anterior collateral ligament, if the unprotected ankle is again involved in

a plantar-flexory inversion injury, the middle as well as posterior lateral collateral ligaments may be ruptured, and a totally unstable ankle may be the end result. Chronic repetitive ankle sprains lead to the long-term sequella of arthritis of the ankle joint. Osteochondritis dissecans may be the sequella of an acute ankle sprain.

When the anterior aspect of the calcaneal fibular ligament is lax or has been ruptured, instability leads to chronic lateral instability of the ankle joint. Bosien reports that one-third of acute ankle injuries treated conservatively will become chronic ankle instability problems (21). Although this is a relatively high percentage, it becomes obvious that ankle sprains must be carefully evaluated and appropriate treatment instituted.

Examination—Acute Ankle Sprain

If an acute ankle injury can be evaluated within the first couple of hours following injury, much can be learned from the physical examination versus examination 1 or 2 days following injury. Immediately, treatment consists of icing the injured area. The rule of RICE (rest, ice, compression, and elevation) is important. Tape should not be removed from the ankle during the first few hours inasmuch as this adds to the compression. Following ice, elevation, and compression for 20 minutes, if difficulty walking persists, appropriate evaluation and treatment is indicated. X-rays may be necessary.

ANTERIOR DRAWER TEST

When the foot is plantar-flexed, the heel is pulled forward as the tibia is pushed backward, and there will be a noticeable slip of the talus forward on the ankle (Fig. 15C.7). This occurs when the anterior calcaneal fibular ligament has been ruptured. This ligament is normally taut when the foot is plantar-flexed and inverted in the uninjured state. An x-ray of the anterior drawer test will show greater than a 3-mm displacement when compared with the opposite normal side. This is indicative of anterior lateral talar instability.

STRESS INVERSION TEST

If there is a great deal of stress inversion on the involved ankle compared to the uninvolved ankle, it must be assumed that an anterior as well as middle collateral ligament rupture has occurred. The stress test is usually greater than 5° on the involved side than the uninvolved side and indicates at least anterior lateral collateral instability. When the test is greater than 15°, it may be assumed that there is also rupture of the middle collateral ligament. There are, however, anatomical variations and the uninvolved side may show increased inversion stress. At times, on inversion stress, a noticeable talar tilt will be absent, yet there is increased stress at the subtalar joint. This is indicative of subtalar joint instability with middle collateral ligament rupture or stretching.

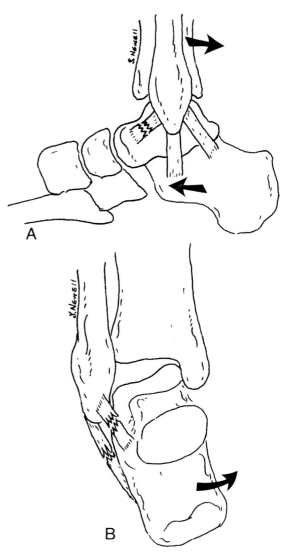

Figure 15C.7. *A*, positive anterior drawer sign. Anterior collateral ligament has been ruptured. This ligament prevents forward slippage of the talus and foot from the ankle mortis. *B*, frontal plane inversion stress view. The anterior and middle collateral ligaments have been ruptured, thus allowing for over 15° of talar tilt.

DIASTASIS TEST

The calcaneus and talus are pushed laterally against the fibula while the leg itself is maintained in a stable position with the palm of the opposite hand. If there is a lateral protuberance of the fibula, diastasis may be present. This is more easily recognized when an arthrogram is performed and there is dye leakage in the interosseous space. When diastasis has occurred, there will be lateral motion of the fibula when the calcaneus is pushed laterally against it. (Fig. 15C.7B)

STRESS X-RAYS

Significant information can be obtained by doing stress views. It is often necessary to do a peroneal nerve block prior to performing the stress test to allow for cessation of pain and elimination of peroneal muscular contraction and guarding. Prior to doing stress views, standard radiographs should be taken to rule out fracture. The inversion stress test will help confirm complete rupture of the anterior collateral ligament. It will also give information as to the status of the middle collateral ligaments.

Watson-Jones has described interpretations of these stress x-rays (22). He suggests that 30% of the adult population has a physiological talar tilt up to 5°. In 20% of the adult population, a variation of talar tilt between individual ankles exists. Watson-Jones felt that an increase of 5–15° of inversion talar tilt over the normal ankle indicates anterior talofibular ligament tear. Talar tilt of 15–30° is indicative of tears of both the anterior talofibular and the calcaneal fibular ligaments. Over 30° of talar tilt indicates a tear of all three ligaments. Anderson and Le Cocq (23) felt that increased talar tilt was due only to rupture of the calcaneal fibular ligament; stress lateral x-ray was need to confirm anterior talofibular ligament tear (Case 5).

CASE 5 (Fig. 15C.8)

Anterior posterior inversion stress test of the ankle on a 26-year-old male; acute inversion plantar-flexory sprain of left ankle. This patient demonstrates a 25° talar tilt. He has obvious disruption of the anterior lateral collateral ligament and middle collateral ligament. The anterior drawer test appears positive. The contrast air dye arthrogram is carried out and dye leakage is present along the lateral aspect of the ankle joint. The dye travels along the course of the peroneal tendons. There is obvious rupture of the capsule and the arthrogram confirms anterior and middle collateral ligament rupture.

Examination of Acute Ankle Sprain in Late Stages

Often, an athlete will visit the doctor several days following a sprain. In this instance, the ankle is edematous, making it difficult for a physical examination. Arthrograms are then excellent for diagnosis. An arthrogram can be carried by utilizing a 10-cc injection of 60% Renographin. This radiopaque dye is utilized with a contrast media injection technique. A mixture of 2 cc Renographin 60%, 2 cc of 2% Xylocaine (plain), 2 cc of 0.5% Marcaine (plain), 0.5 cc of Decadron, and 1.5 cc of air is utilized. This contrast air dye arthrogram is then injected into the anterior capsule of the ankle joint. Following injection, an x-ray is taken (Case 6).

Interpretation of Arthrogram

Lateral leakage of the dye is suggestive of lateral rupture of the ankle joint and ankle joint capsule. When the dye travels along the peroneal tendon, it is suspected that the middle collateral ligament has been ruptured and there has been escape from the capsule to the ligament to the tendon. There may be a false-positive as some individuals will have dye leakage along the peroneal tendons without rupture of the lateral ligaments of the ankle joint. Normally, when a great amount of dye leaks laterally, an ankle joint capsular and ligamentous rupture has occurred. When anterior capsular rupture occurs, there will be

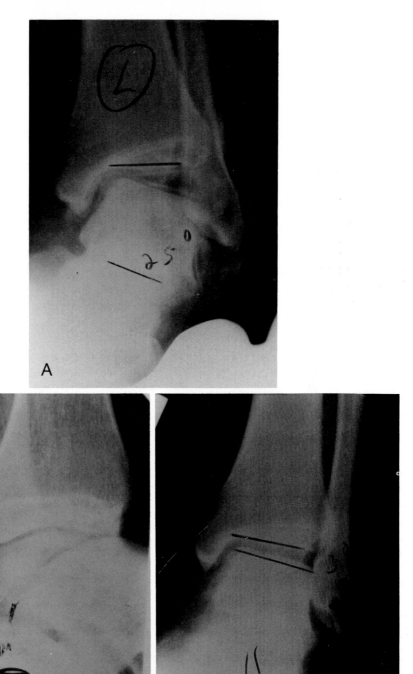

Figure 15C.8. *A,* eversion ankle stress (AP). *B,* anterior drawer test with contrast arthrogram. Dye leakage is seen along peroneal tendons. There is a 10-mm gap as the talus and foot are subluxed anteriorly at the ankle joint from the tibia. This is conclusive evidence of a ruptured middle and anterior collateral ligament. *C,* AP stress view of the ankle 11 weeks following lateral stabilization with a modified Chrisman-Snook technique. There is a 3° talar tilt showing a stable ankle from the previous 25° talar tilt noted pre-operatively.

an anterior dye leakage in a characteristic pattern (Case 6).

CASE 6 (Fig. 15C.9)

AP of ankle joint showing a contrast air-dye arthrogram. Positive arthrogram, inversion sprain.

Treatment of Acute Ankle Sprains

When an acute ligamentous rupture of the ankle joint has occurred and this is the first incident of rupture, decisions as to cast immobilization versus surgical repair of the ligament must be made. For the recreational athlete, cast immobilization followed by a physical therapy program is indicated, while in college or professional athletes, surgery must be given primary consideration.

Surgical Repair—Acute Ankles

Prior to surgery the ankle must be elevated until the edema subsides. The ruptured anterior collateral ligament is reapproximated and, if need be, additional tissue from the bifurcate ligament is utilized to help act as a strut for this ligament. The middle collateral ligament is inspected and repaired surgically. The athlete is maintained in a below-the-knee walking cast for 6 weeks. Following cast removal, physiotherapy is initiated. The athlete is taken through a graduated program of running; first, in a straight line, and then doing figure-eights, going from a large figure-eight to, finally, a very small figure-eight. When adequate strength, flexibility, and agility has been demonstrated, the athlete is able to return to full, unlimited competition.

Chronic Instability of the Ankle Joint

Chronic lateral instability of the ankle joint may be the sequella of repeated sprains. The majority of lateral ankle sprains, when treated with proper initial immobilization, and then a well-planned physical therapy and rehabilitation program, do not end up with lateral instability. Recurrent sprains, however, will cause repeat rupture of partially healed ligaments. The anterior lateral collateral ligament is often lax and, then, the middle collateral ligament ruptures. When this occurs, considerable lateral instability is the end result. The lateral instability may be aggravated by biomechanical deformities such as forefoot valgus or anterior equinus. When this is the case, orthotic foot control, as well as physical therapy, should be utilized. Peroneal strengthening exercises may help. If the peroneals appear to be weak, a neurological examination should be carried out to rule out peroneal weakness secondary to neuromuscular disease. In the event that orthotics taping, lace-up braces, and physical therapy fail to maintain stability, surgical secondary repair is indicated (24).

COMMENTS ON CHRISMAN-SNOOK PROCEDURE

Surgical errors result when the calcaneus is forced into maximum eversion and held there with a lateral stabilization procedure. Some supination is necessary for normal function and taking the heel from maximum eversion back into 4–6° of inversion assures adequate range of motion. Even though it is true that the tenodesis repair may stretch out with time, surgical compli-

---

Figure 15C.9. *A,* positive arthrogram, inversion sprain. There is massive dye leakage from the lateral joint capsule extending along the peroneal tendons. This is indicative of rupture of the lateral collateral ligaments, including the anterior and middle portions. *B,* positive arthrogram, lateral view. Photo shows lateral view of the same ankle with the contrast air dye arthrogram. There is dye leakage at the posterior lateral aspect of the ankle joint. The anterior aspect of the ankle joint appears normal with the dye outlining the anterior ankle joint capsular pouch.

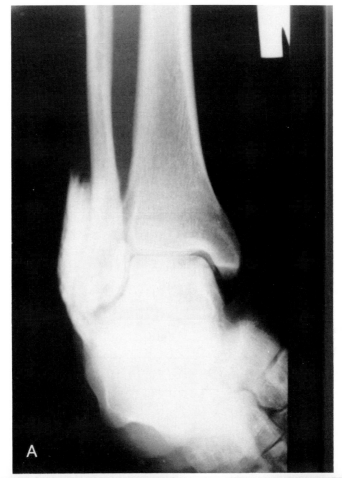

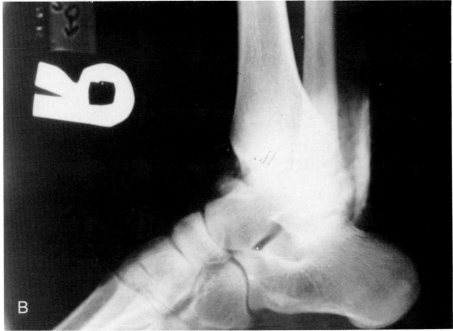

Figure 15C.9. (*A* and *B*)

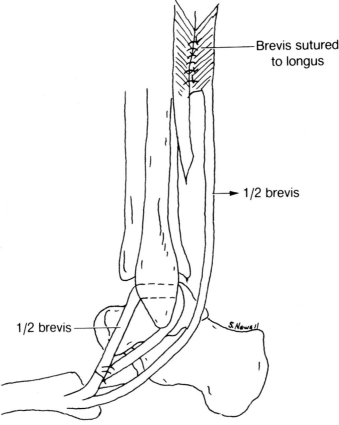

**Brevis sutured
to longus**

1/2 brevis

1/2 brevis

S. Newell

Figure 15C.10.   Peroneus brevis tenodesis (modified Chrisman-Snook). This figure shows one-half of the peroneus brevis being separated from the muscle aspect and the lower one-third of the leg. This half of the tendon is left attached at the styloid process of the fifth metatarsal. It is drawn from anterior to posterior through a drill hole in the wide flair of the fibula and then brought back down and sutured into itself. This allows for appropriate repair of the anterior lateral collateral ligament. The remaining peroneus brevis is sutured into the peroneus longus at its detachment in the lower one-third of the leg with nonabsorbable sutures.

cations can be caused by too tight a repair. When this occurs, prolonged physical therapy is necessary to stretch the ligament.

When a lateral stabilization is performed for chronic instability, an Evans procedure is recommended for a relatively non-athletic, middle-aged patient. This procedure is simply a peroneus brevis tenodesis utilizing the entire peroneus brevis through an oblique fibular drill hole (Fig. 15C.10). The tenodesis should be performed with the calcaneus taken from full eversion into 4° of inversion. If this is not performed, the patient may complain of persistent sinus tarsi syndrome secondary to excessive eversion

and compression, and medial capsulitis about the ankle joint and/or posterior tibial tendonitis may be an unwanted sequella. Post-operative care for this procedure is 4 weeks immobilization in a below-knee walking cast.

Inasmuch as lateral stabilization procedures of the ankle appear to work quite well, it appears appropriate to reserve immediate repair of ruptured collateral ligaments for the serious or the professional athlete. Surgical repair of acute ankle ruptures lead to a stable ankle with rapid return to activity. Likewise, cast immobilization for short periods of time followed by

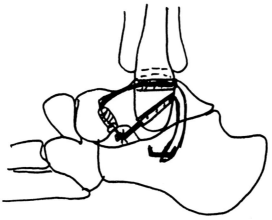

Figure 15C.11. Lateral stabilization of the ankle joint with woven dacron—synthetic ligament (after the method of Park). A woven dacron synthetic ligament is placed through three drill holes. It is first anchored to the calcaneus with a staple in the event that the middle collateral ligament is ruptured. One arm is then taken through a superior drill hole about 1.5 cm from the distal tip of the fibular malleolus. The second arm is taken from posterior to anterior through an inferior drill hole angled from posterior superior to anterior inferior. The ligament going through the superior drill hole is then taken from superior to inferior through a talar neck drill hole. The subtalar and ankle joints are held in a neutral position with the heel neutral as well and the synthetic ligament tightened. It must be tightened at each passage through the drill hole to allow for proper security and guard against lateral instability at the ankle and subtalar joints. The dacron graft should be moistened with copious amounts of normal saline before pulling it through the drill hole. Once the subtalar joint is held in a neutral or 1–2° inverted position, the two free ends of the ligament are tied in a square knot. The knot is reinforced, utilizing nonabsorbable suture tied through the knot. Tenodesis can be further enhanced, utilizing nonabsorbable suture at the entrance and exit sites of the drill holes. It is important that when the ankle joint is stressed, only 1–2° degrees of eversion is present. Neutral to 2° valgus is permissible. More valgus than 2° will result in limited range of motion and may compromise the end result with this procedure.

a well planned physical therapy program leads to full return of functional activity. There may be some chronic stretching of the collateral ligaments which may lead to instability. If this is the case, there very well may be a second sprain and, if this occurs, primary repair of the ligaments is suggested. If the ligaments are severely stretched, then the bifurcate ligament can be utilized to help repair the anterior collateral ligament. When there has been chronic instability of the ankle joint and, at the time of surgery, the anterior collateral ligament is found to be atrophic and inadequate for primary repair, a lateral stabilization should be carried out. Although the bifurcate ligament stabilizing procedure may be adequate for a relatively inactive patient, it is inadequate for an athlete.

Failure with the peroneus brevis tenodesis procedure occurs secondary to excessive eversion stabilization, and failure to adequately tenodese the entrance and exit sites at the pivot drill holes. Excellent results exist when the patient is back to full activity 6 weeks following surgery. Moderately good results exist when the patient is participating in activities relatively pain free 10–12 weeks following surgery. Poor results exist when the patient is still having pain and disability 8 months following surgery. Poor results occur as a result of overcorrection with a very tight peroneus brevis tendon. Other complications include anesthesia to the lateral portion of the foot secondary to sectioning of the sural nerve. Incidences of excessively tight brevis tendons following Watson-Jones procedures, as well as modified Chrisman-Snook procedures, are also possible.

Lateral Ligamentous Reconstruction of the Unstable Ankle with Dacron

Park and associates (26) reported at a meeting of The American Orthopedic Society for Sports Medicine, on utilization of woven dacron grafts for the reconstruction of lateral collateral ligaments. A 2-year follow-up in 17 patients showing 11 patients having rates of grade 1 with full activity including strenuous sports, no pain, no swelling, or giving way of the ankle was presented. Four patients were grade 2 with occasional aching following strenuous exercise, but no giving way, but some remaining apprehension while walking on rough ground (Fig. 15C.11).

The authors have used dacron double velour, woven graft in coracoclavicular ligament substitution for third-degree acromicoclavicular separations with satisfactory results and have previously reported upon the results of this procedure. They note that animal studies have shown a marked fibrous ingrowth with maturation and organization of collagen throughout the graft, incorporating the dacron fibroles into the newly forming ligament. Fibrous ingrowth is associated with an increase of strength in a dacron template.

The authors contend that dacron graft reconstruction is a reliable procedure for treating chronic lateral ligamentous instability of the ankle without sacrifice of musculotendinous units or restriction of subtalar motion. They admit that it is a short-term study but the results, to date, are quite promising and state that they have no reason to believe that the results will diminish with time as the dacron template serves as a lattice for permanent fibrous ingrowth. The method they use is that after Sefton (27).

Grumbine (28) has also reported upon the utilization of Marlex synthetic ligamentous material for lateral stabilization of the ankle. He places one oblique anterior posterior drill hole through the fibula, then trephines into the calcaneous and the fibular neck completing the trephine hole with a Kirschner wire. He then utilizes the synthetic material in such a way that it passes through the fibular drill hole and then goes into the calcaneus, into the fibula, and, finally, is attached with dacron suture which is tied on to the free ends and then secured over a buttress on the medial aspect of the foot at the exit from the calcaneus and talus. Grumbine has also reported upon the utilization of free tendon graft on the peroneus brevis below the level of the ankle joint for a tenodesis procedure as described above.

CONCLUSION

Ankle joint surgical procedures may render the athlete asymptomatic for varying periods of time. These procedures may not be lasting due to the chronic repetitive stress of sports. Acute injuries to an ankle joint may undo even the best surgical results. A biomechanical understanding of the sports and forces involved may aid the surgeon in predicting the success of surgery and in properly planning surgical procedures. Biomechanical foot orthotics or various forms of ankle joint braces may be necessary in the post-operative course. It is emphasized that there is a need for full recovery of balance, flexibility, and strength. When an athlete returns to activity having gained these three essential functions, there is less likelihood of recurrent or repeat injuries.

Primary surgical procedures should be reserved for professional athletes or high-caliber college athletes who may become professionals. Ankle joint implants have yet to be perfected to such an extent that they are applicable to the young or athletic individual. Ankle joint arthroplasty is preferred for spurs about the ankle joint. The results may not be permanent. Fusion is reserved for severe arthritis and pain.

References

1. Inman, V. T. *Joints of the Ankle.* Williams & Wilkins, Baltimore, 1976.
2. Kleiger, B. The mechanism of ankle injuries. J. Bone Jt. Surg. 38A:969, 1956.
3. Subotnick, S. I. Anterior impingement exostosis of the ankle. JAPA 66:958–963, 1976.

4. Root, M. L., Orein, W., Weed, J. H., and Hughes, R. J. *Biomechanical Examination of the Foot.* Clinical Biomechanics Corporation., Los Angeles, 1971, vol. 1.

5. Sgarlato, T. E. *A Compendium of Podiatric Biomechanics.* California College of Podiatric Medicine, San Francisco, 1971.

6. Subotnick, S. I. *Podiatric Sports Medicine.* Futura, Mt. Kisco, New York, 1975.

7. Subotnick, S. I. Orthotic foot control and the overuse syndrome. *The Physician and Sports Medicine* 3:75–79, 1975.

8. Weil, L. S. Personal communication, 1980.

9. McMurray, T. P. Footballer's ankle. J. Bone Jt. Surg. 32B:68, 1950.

10. Berndt, A. L., and Harty, M. Transchondral fractures (osteochondritis desicans) of the talus. J. Bone Jt. Surg. 41A:988, 1959.

11. Jacobs, B Epidemiology of traumatic and nontraumatic osteonecrosis. Clin. Orthop. 130:51, 1978.

12. Martel, W., and Siterly, B. H. Roentgeologic manifestations of osteonecrosis. Am. J. Roentgenol. 106:509, 1969.

13. Wiltberger, B. R., and Mallory, T. H. Reconstruction of the deltoid ligament of the ankle: A new method. Audio-Visual Program, Annual Meeting, American Academy of Orthopedic Surgeons, 1972.

14. Subotnick, S. I. *Podiatric Sports Medicine.* Futura, Mt. Kisco, New York, 1975, pp. 173–175.

15. Earle, A. A., Moritz, J. E., and Tapper, E. H. Dislocation of peroneal tendons at the ankle: An analysis of 25 ski injuries. N. Engl. J. Med. 71:108, 1972.

16. Marti, R. Dislocation of the peroneal tendons. Am. J. Sports Med. 5:19, 1977.

17. Savastano, A. A. The Treatment of Recurrent Dislocations of the Common Peroneal Tendons. Presented at the Eighth Annual Meeting of the American Orthopedic Foot Society, Dallas, February, 1978.

18. Jones, E. Operative treatment of chronic dislocation of the peroneal tendons. J. Bone Jt. Surg. 14:547, 1932.

19. Kelly, R. E. An operation for chronic dislocation of peroneal tendons. Br. J. Surg. 7:502, 1920.

20. Garrick. Personal communication, 1981.

21. Bosien, W. Residual disability. J. Bone Jt. Surg. 37A:1237–1243, 1955.

22. Watson-Jones, R. *Fractures and Joint Injuries.* Williams & Wilkins, Baltimore, 1975, vol 2, pp. 112–116.

23. Anderson, K. J., and Le Cocq, J. F. Operative treatment of fibular collateral ligament. J. Bone Jt. Surg. 36A:825–832, 1954.

24. Chrisman, O. D., and Snook, F. A. Reconstruction of lateral ligament tears of the ankle. J. Bone Jt. Surg. 51A:904–1912, 1969.

25. Evans, D. L. Recurrent instability of the ankle: A method of surgical treatment. Proc. R. Soc. Med. 46:343–344, 1953.

26. Park, J. P., Arnold, J. A., Cocker, T. P., and Becker, D. A. Lateral Ligamentous Reconstruction of the Unstable Ankle with Dacron: A Preliminary Report. Presented at the American Orthopedic Society for Sports Medicine Meeting, City June 21–25, 1981.

27. Sefton, G. K., George, J., Fiton, J. N., McMullen, H. Reconstruction of anterior talofibular ligament for the treatment of the unstable ankle. J. Bone Jt. Surg. 61B: 821–829, 1973.

28. Grumbine, N. Personal communication, 1982.

POST-OPERATIVE

CHAPTER 16

Management of Infection

DONALD W. HUGAR, D.P.M.

Among surgeon's top priorities are the prevention, recognition, and treatment of infection. The principles of safe surgery include proper hemostatis, adequate anesthesia, and control of infection. Controlling infection requires close attention to basic principles. Early signs of infection must be recognized so that treatment will not be delayed. Therefore, the surgeon must instruct his patients in the recognition of symptoms.

It is important to stress, at this point, that many post-operative infections are the result of negligence on the part of the surgeon, negligence which usually occurs before or during the actual surgery.

An aseptic environment, mechanical cleanliness of the skin, atraumatic handling of tissues, minimal residual foreign body in the wound, avoidance of constricting sutures, satisfactory hemostasis, elimination of dead space, and careful post-operative observation are all factors that help to prevent the entry of bacteria and to control the development of conditions favorable to their growth.

PREDISPOSING FACTORS

The major components of post-operative wound infection are a receptive host, the presence of organisms, and a wound culture medium. The local and general immune response of the patient depends mainly on the type of tissue injured and its vascularity. The immune response mechanism of the body resides most particularly in the globulin fraction of the plasma, the cells of the reticuloendothelial system, and the protective action of the lymphatic system. The patient's general health must be evaluated.

Dehydration, shock, malnutrition, uncontrolled diabetes, and anemia can lower resistance sufficiently to allow bacterial invasion. Steroids and immunosuppressive agents may also render patients susceptible to infection.

The virulence, types and numbers of bacteria are critical factors. Infection is the unfavorable result of the equation of bacterial dose multiplied by virulence and divided by the resistance of the host. The presence of virulent bacteria does not mean that infection will result. The physiologic state of the tissue in the wound before and after treatment is more important than the mere presence of bacteria. All wounds are contaminated, but not all wounds become infected. Routine cultures of clean operative wounds at closure have been reported as positive in up to 85% of cases. This is not unusual, considering the normal flora of the skin. The skin is never sterile and cannot be made sterile by any practical means.

Surgical scrubbing with soap and water for 10 minutes removes about half the normal skin flora. Several hours of scrubbing with frequent alcohol dips will still not eliminate all organisms, some of which are inaccessible because of their position deep within the skin follicles. The skin surface is rich in fats, protein, nitrogenous substances, carbohydrates, and minerals, which allow microflora to thrive.

There are substantial differences in the microflora of individuals and in the skin flora of specific regions of the body. Intertriginous areas support a different spectrum of microflora from those found on glabrous skin. Climatic conditions, perspiration, upper respiratory infections, body hygiene, and other factors can influence the composition of skin flora. Resident flora may include *Microsporum flavius* and a variety of Corynebacteria. Also, common skin transients are present in varying degrees, including *Staphylococcus, Streptococcus, Escherichia coli* from the gastrointestinal tract, several species of diphtheroids, *Sarcinae,* and several of the gram-positive aerobic spore-formers.

The most important component in the development of infection is a wound culture medium, which may be created by any local destruction of tissue. Faulty surgical technique with unnecessary scalpel strokes can cause superfluous tissue necrosis. The longer the wound is open and exposed to the environment, the greater the tendency toward infection. Tissue necrosis may also be caused by oversized suture material, too much suture material, and tissue strangulation. Other causes include local ischemia due to prolonged tourniquet time and an excess of local anesthetic with epinephrine. Inadequate hemostasis can cause formation of a hematoma, which allows bacteria to thrive. In a patient with adequate circulation, it is the single most important factor leading to the development of wound infection. Wounds may also be contaminated by unscrubbed personnel, by the hands of the operating assistants, and by the use of inadequately sterilized equipment and instruments.

DIAGNOSIS

Although it is important to establish a provisional diagnosis based on clinical signs and symptoms, no final diagnosis of a specific organism is complete without detailed laboratory and microscopic studies. Virtually all wounds are contaminated by microorganisms, but not all microorganisms cause infection. The surgeon must determine whether a wound is infected.

An unusual amount of pain at the surgical site on the 2nd and/or 3rd postoperative day is a sign of the presence of infection. Along with pain, check for other signs such as an increase in temperature, edema, erythema, or cellulitis which usually extends from the primary site of contamination or abscess, and loss of function of the part. If the inflammation is greater than normally expected, then infection is highly probable. Realize, however, that at times it is difficult to distinguish infection from such things as normal wound healing, wound dehiscence, or hematoma formation.

If the patient's pulse is too rapid or his temperature is elevated (>100°F), if the degree of prostration is too great, or if the patient is excessively restless, infection may be the cause. Fever post-operatively can be caused not only by infection, but also by drugs, constipation, phlebitis at the site of an indwelling catheter, thrombophlebitis, urinary and respiratory infections, and anesthetic hepatitis. Pain away from the surgical site may be a sign of septicemia. Once infection is diagnosed in the wound, the microbial etiology must be established.

Note the characteristic features of the exudate and, under sterile conditions, remove two or three sutures and probe with a sterile blunt instrument, allowing for free drainage. A gram stain, together with culture and sensitivity, will aid in the final diagnosis.

TYPES OF INFECTION AND SEQUELAE

Micro-organisms and their by-products generally travel along anatomic pathways, which are: tissue spaces (subcutaneous), tendon sheaths, fascial spaces, muscles, bones, and lymphatic channels. The result is bacteremia or septicemia.

Tissue Spaces

These are the most common and vulnerable areas for infection. In many instances, infection of a superficial nature is confined here.

Tendon Sheaths

Inflammation of the tendon sheaths may originate when pathogens enter through the surgical wound, or it may already exist as a subcutaneous fascial infection. Tendon sheath infections tend to spread rapidly. Usually the sheath becomes infected throughout its entire length. The key sign is tenderness, which is sharply outlined and limited to the sheath's dimension and course. *When a toe is the site of a tendon sheath infection, the digit is rigid in a semiflexed state.* Movement causes severe pain. The swelling which generally occurs can extend to the dorsum of the foot. If hemolytic *Streptococcus* or *Staphylococcus* enter the sheath, tendon necrosis can ensue in the absence of prompt and effective therapy.

Muscle Infection

Muscles, which are frequently attacked by microorganisms, can be the site of acute or chronic infection. Myositis is the primary characteristic. Affected muscles exhibit inflammatory changes that vary from a barely discernible reaction to massive destruction as seen in a gas bacillus infection. Any of the pyogenic organisms can cause purulent myositis and, since muscle tissue forms an ideal substrate for bacterial growth, irreparable damage to the muscle belly may occur in the absence of proper treatment.

Aerobic organisms such as *Streptococcus* or *Staphylococcus* help to advance gas gangrene infections by devitalizing the muscle and utilizing the oxygen. The major organisms responsible for gas gangrene include the gram-positive bacilli; *Clostridium perfringens, Clostridium novyi,* and *Clostridium septicum.* The onset of gas gangrene is usually sudden, from 6 hours to a few days after surgery. The patient may exhibit marked prostration and systemic toxicity. Gas may be demonstrated by crepitus or palpation of the involved muscle belly or by radiolucent areas on x-ray. The exudate will be brown to blood-tinged.

Bone Infection

Infection reaches the bone via the exogenous or hematogenous route. A wound in-

fection is exogenous, while examples of the hematogenous type include a local spreading infection of the skin, infections of the throat, or pneumonia. Osteomyelitis can develop hematogenously with acute septicemia.

Some of the physical signs of local osteomyelitis are pyrexia, swelling, tenderness, limitation of joint motion, erythema, heat, fluctuation, effusion into nearby joints, and limited use of the limb. Although the differential diagnosis may be difficult at times, osteomyelitis differs from acute cellulitis in that it causes graver general disturbances, while cellulitis displays a possible septic focus on the overlying skin. Cellulitis is frequently associated with lymphangitis and lymphadenitis of the regional lymph nodes. Increasing numbers of gram-negative organisms are found to cause osteomyelitis. Once the osteomyelitis has burst through the periosteum, a secondary cellulitis will develop, and lymphangitis and lymphadenitis may ensue.

Radiographs can help in diagnosis, but bone changes are not visible in the early stages. Some characteristic findings include osteolysis, soft tissue swelling, periosteal elevation, eventual extensive reabsorption of bone, and fibrous replacement, which can spread over the shaft, while the infection may extend along the marrow cavity. The entire shaft can become necrotic, or the spread may be arrested at any point. Soon after the death of the bone, the periosteum, which has become separated from it, begins to lay down new bone. The necrotic bone separates from the surrounding living bone as a sequestrum. Through the involucrum—the tube of the new bone around the old shaft—there are openings in the sinuses called cloacae, through which pus escapes and communicates with the surface.

Some of the systemic manifestations of osteomyelitis are fever or chills, nausea, vomiting, general malaise with increased pulse rate, leukocytosis, and an elevated erythrocyte sedimentation rate (ESR).

Chronic osteomyelitis is generally resistant to conservative treatment because purulence in the venous sinusoids of the metaphysis progresses to granular tissue, which matures to dead scar. This avascular scar forms an impenetrable wall around the infected area. Excision or surgical curettage of bone is recommended. Closed irrigation—suction units utilizing a mixture of physiologic saline, urokinase, and appropriate antibiotics—have proved successful in the treatment of chronic bone and joint infections. Early diagnosis of bone infection and therapeutic controls can prevent its spread or prevent chronicity.

Fascial Spaces

Fascial space infection occurs more frequently than does infection of tendon sheaths. The fascial space in the toe webs follows the lumbricales muscle and leads into the spaces on the foot's plantar surface. Tenderness over the area may be indicative of the infection in the fascial space.

The three deep fascial spaces on the plantar aspect are the medial, central, and lateral. The medial and lateral are rarely infected, while the central is most susceptible. The presence of pus in the bottom compartment of the central plantar space is manifested by swelling on the dorsum and tenderness of the in-step. The tenderness distinguishes the condition from infection of the interdigital cutaneous space. But infection of the central plantar space can spread to the interdigital subcutaneous space along the tiny tunnel accommodating the interdigital nerve, vessels, and tendons of the lumbricales. Another sign is edema of the in-step, which assumes a convex formation.

When an infection is confined to the toe webs, the signs include pain over the infected space, inability to walk with comfort and pain between two metatarsals. In some instances, an abscess cavity lying within calloused skin or in the interdigital space is seen.

Infection of the fascial spaces of the heel is distinguished by throbbing pain that disrupts sleep, the inability to bear weight, and tissue swelling on one or both sides of the calcaneus. If edema of the ankle is also present with acute tenderness over the fascial space with fluctuation, infection is certain.

Lymphadenitis

This is inflammatory swelling of regional lymph nodes. Any organism that produces infection can produce lymphadenitis. The most common agents are *Streptococcus* and *Staphylococcus*. Lymphadenitis is generally secondary to the extension of another infectious process, although it may be primary in some instances.

Lymphadenitis is recognized by palpable, tender, painful regional nodes, with inflamed overlying skin. Voluntary inhibition of function of the adjacent structures, pronounced swelling of the surrounding tissues, and possible abscess formation with suppuration are common. Non-tender nodes may be present if the inflammatory process has persisted for a long time.

Septicemia

Bacteremia is simply the presence of bacteria in the blood. Septicemia is the presence of pathogenic bacteria and their toxins in the blood with accompanying physical signs and symptoms. Fever almost always accompanies septicemia, but temperature elevations vary. Most often the fever is intermittent, with septic spiking. Chills are experienced at the onset. Skin eruptions, which are frequent, can be petechial or purpuric. In some instances they may be papular, pustular, or vesicular lesions. Major signs are enlargement of the spleen and splinter hemorrhages under the nails.

Specific Organisms

The number and varieties of microorganisms found on the skin depend largely on personal hygiene and environmental conditions. Relatively few types multiply freely on the skin. Among those that do are the aerobic and anaerobic staphylococci. Sometimes aerobic Corynebacteria (e.g., *Cory-*

nebacterium acnes) and yeasts and fungi such as *Candida albicans,* cryptococci and mycobacteria are isolated. Areas adjacent to body openings are host to *Escherichia coli, Proteus* and other intestinal organisms. *Streptococcus pyogenes* is an occasional skin microorganism.

The skin and body-lining membranes are the first barriers between deep structures and microorganisms. Disturbance of the adequate functioning of these coverings enhances the opportunity for infection.

Microorganisms contaminating a wound depend to some degree on the tissue involved, the mode of infliction (whether traumatic or surgical), and the microbial contamination of adjacent areas perforated.

The risk of infection in a clean surgical site is slight. If it does occur, these infected wounds, depending on the site, yield *Staphylococcus aureus,* enterococci or gram-negative rods, but rarely *S. pyogenes,* Corynebacteria, pneumococci or *Bacillus subtilis.*

When surgery is conducted in a contaminated area, infection is to be expected. Frequently, microorganisms that are present in small numbers at the site enter the sterile tissue of the wound. Such microorganisms include *P. aeruginosa, Proteus, E. coli,* and the *Klebsiella-Enterobacter* group.

The risk of infection in a burn wound or a compound fracture, with crushing or laceration of the tissue, is high. The wound is likely to be contaminated by microorganisms close to the wound site, including those found on the skin and clothes, the soil, or other debris that comes in contact with the site of injury. The organisms found in such sites include *S. aureus, S. pyogenes,* enterococci, *E. coli, Proteus* species, *P. aeruginosa,* the anaerobic *Clostridium tetani,* the anaerobes of gas gangrene, *Clostridium perfringens* type A, *Clostridium septicum,* and *Bacteroides* species and other anerobic gram-negative rods.

Wounds may become infected without obvious clinical manifestations of disease, except perhaps prolonged healing time. Successive predominating organisms can infect a wound: first *S. aureus,* followed by *S. pyogenes, P. aeruginosa,* and just before healing, *Staphylococcus epidermidis* and diphtheroids. A wound must be protected against the risk of infection until fully healed.

Under the following specific circumstances, these infections should be suspected:

1. Bright red, poorly localized infection with little or no pus: streptococcal erysipelas (*S. pyogenes*);
2. Abscess with creamy yellow, odorless pus: *S. aureus;*
3. Immunosuppressed patient: bacteroides (foul odor);
4. Tissue crepitation: *Clostridium perfringens septicum* (gas gangrene, foul odor) or gas-producing *E. coli;*
5. Chronic skin infection with considerable induration and inflammation but little pus: blastomycosis, histoplasmosis, actinomycosis;
6. Relatively painless toe infection: secondary pyogenic sepsis in patients with neuropathy due to diabetes or leprosy;
7. Chronic suppuration with little or no erythema: fever and tenderness in submaxillary or subclavicular areas: tuberculosis;
8. Chronic paronychia: atypical *Mycobacterium* or fungus.

TREATMENT

Consider the cause of the infection, the organism involved, the general health of the patient, and the location and extent of involvement. Then decide on local or systemic treatment, or both.

Local

There are many measures available. Moist heat is a common form of treatment and often the best. It promotes localization of the infection and makes the patient comfortable. Apply moist heat by wrapping the area in a wet towel and enclosing the wrapped limb in a plastic bag. The moist, warm towel should be applied directly over the dressing, and never over the skin of a surgical wound.

The patient's activities should be drastically limited. Large dressings, splints, and gentle handling are essential to prevent mechanical disruption of tissue planes so that microorganisms are localized rather than disseminated.

Elevation will prevent unnecessary swelling and promote venous and lymphatic drainage. Watch for lymphangitis, which appears as an erythematous streak 3–5 cm wide, usually overlying the major veins. Lymphangitis indicates the presence of β-hemolytic streptococci and calls for systemic antibiotics.

The procedure of incision and drainage is the undisputed treatment of choice whenever infection is localized or abscessed in a closed space. Infection is localized when fluctuation is present.

Aspiration provides a guide to the depth of the abscess. The incision must be large enough, must follow the natural skin lines, and must be in the most dependent wound area. The drains used may be gauze, rubber, or polyethylene. Drains may be removed gradually at intervals of 24–48 hours.

Irrigation can begin 24–48 hours after incision and drainage are completed. Saline, 2% hydrogen peroxide, or hypochlorite solutions aid in breaking up residual abscesses and stimulate the formation of granular tissue.

Suture removal permits optimal drainage and irrigation. When sutures are removed prematurely, however, a slightly wider scar is produced, but if effective treatment is delayed, serious infection can develop. Therefore, try to remove only a few sutures, if possible, to minimize scarring.

When redressing infected wounds, betadine solution, usually half-strength, can be applied topically. Iodine is a much better antimicrobial agent than mercury (Mercurochrome®, Merthiolate®). A 1:20,000 solution of elemental iodine kills wet spores in 15 minutes. Organic mercurial antiseptics are primarily bacteriostatic, relatively ineffective in killing spores, and penetrate tissues poorly. As betadine-soaked gauze dries, it acts as a splint to immobilize the area and when removed gently debrides necrotic tissue.

Systemic

Chemotherapy frequently accompanies the local management of infected wounds. The results of the gram stain and the practitioner's experience should provide quick identification of the microorganism responsible for the infection. Table 16.1 provides a guide to identifying the bacteria and fungi that cause acute infections.

When a tentative diagnosis is made, select a drug that will be effective against the organism (Table 16.2). Always obtain specimens for laboratory examination. Change the antibiotic if the laboratory data so indicates, but lab results should not automatically override clinical judgment, especially if the patient demonstrates clinical recovery.

Prescribe adequate dosage to maintain proper blood levels. The age and weight of the patient, the rate of excretion of the agent, the time required to establish the desired blood levels, the duration of the effect of a single dose, and the ability of the agent to reach the infection all contribute in dosage determination.

Some infections require more time than others to resolve, but those commonly encountered in the lower extremities generally do not require antibiotic therapy for more than 10 days. Prolonged therapy invites adverse drug effects. Adverse reactions take several forms: (a) hypersensitivity, with fever and rashes; (b) direct toxicity with nausea, vomiting, and diarrhea. More serious reactions are impairment of renal, hepatic, or hematopoietic functions; (c) superinfection, which is caused by drug-resistant microorganisms.

Evaluate the severity of the reaction and choose between continuing the offending drug, changing the chemotherapeutic agent, or changing therapy. If the patient is responding favorably, treatment should

Table 16.1.
Bacteria and Fungi that Cause Acute Infections[a]

Skin and subcutaneous tissues	Traumatic and surgical wounds
1. Staphylococcus, coagulase-positive	1. Staphylococcus, coagulase-positive
2. *Streptococcus pyogenes* group A	2. *S. anaerobius*
3. Dermatophytes and *Candida albicans*	3. Gram-negative bacilli
4. Gram-negative bacilli	4. Clostridium
5. *Treponema pallidum*	5. *S. pyogenes,* group A

Burns	Bones (osteomyelitis)
1. Staphylococcus, coagulase-positive	1. Staphylococcus, coagulase-positive
2. *S. pyogenes,* group A	2. Salmonella or other gram-negative bacilli
3. *Pseudomonas aeruginosa* and other gram-negative bacilli	3. *Neisseria gonorrheae*
	4. *S. anaerobius* (chronic)

Decubitus wound infections	Joints
1. Staphylococcus, coagulase-positive	1. Staphylococcus, coagulase-positive
2. *Escherichia coli* or other gram-negative bacilli	2. *S. pyogenes,* group A
3. *S. pyogenes,* group A	3. *Neisseria gonorrheae*
4. *Streptococcus anaerobius*	4. Gram-negative bacilli
5. Clostridium	5. *Diplococcus pneumoniae*
6. Enterococcus	6. *Neisseria meningitidis*
	7. Fungi
	8. *Mycobacterium tuberculosis*

[a] From *The Medical Letter-Handbook of Antimicrobial Therapy*, Issue 340, Jan. 1972.

be discontinued quickly to minimize the possibility of adverse reaction. Appropriate clinical and laboratory findings are the best guide to the withdrawal of antibiotics. Parenteral administration affords a high concentration of the antibiotic at the site of infection and therefore is the method of choice.

The effectiveness of antibiotic therapy can be established by improving the patient's general health and reducing the local signs of infection. The body temperature should fall to normal within 12 hours after administration of the proper antibiotic. The white blood count will gradually normalize, and the erythema, infectious exudate, and edema will recede.

If the patient is not responding to the antibiotic, then consider the following: 1) Is the isolated organism really the etiologic agent? 2) Is a previously unsuspected infection present? 3) Is adequate antimicrobial therapy being given in appropriate doses? 4) Is the antibiotic penetrating the body space in which the infection is located? 5) Have resistant organisms emerged? 6) Is a superinfection present? 7) Is the fever due to a drug reaction?

Routine administration of antimicrobial agents must be avoided unless the patient's natural resistance to bacterial invasion has been lowered or if an extensive procedure is planned. Antibiotics, if used, should be administered before surgery as a prophylactic measure. Antibiotics administered during the operation are usually not effective in preventing infections. Administration of antibiotics should begin one day before the surgical procedure and be continued for a proper length of time after surgery.

A systemic drug has a direct effect on how quickly the infection will be alleviated. An ideal agent should:

1. Exhibit selective and effective activity against a broad range of organisms
2. Be bacteriocidal and not bacteriostatic
3. Not induce bacterial resistance
4. Not act as a sensitizing agent or disrupt vital organs or function

For each pathogenic organism causing an infection, there is one drug or combination of drugs that will be most effective.

Suffice it to say that the outpatient control of a surgical infection prior to culture and sensitivity findings can be best man-

Table 16.2.
Antimicrobial Drugs of Choice[a]

Infecting Organism	First Choice	Alternatives
Gram-positive cocci		
Streptococcus pyogenes. groups A, B, B, and G	Penicillin G	Erythromycin, lincomycin, clindamycin
Viridans group of Streptococcus	Penicillin G with or without streptomycin	Cephalosporin; vancomycin; erythromycin with streptomycin
Streptococcus, anaerobic	Penicillin G	Erythromycin, a tetracycline
Staphylococcus aureus (nonpenicillinase producing)	Penicillin G	Lincomycin, clindamycin, cephalosporin, gentamicin, vancomycin
Penicillinase-producing	A penicillinase-resistant penicillin	Some alternate drugs for nonpenicillinase-producing strains
Gram-negative cocci		
Neisseria gonorrheae	Penicillin G	Tetracycline, ampicillin, spectinomycin
Gram-negative bacilli		
Salmonella	Chloramphenicol	Ampicillin; sulfamethoxazole-trimethoprim
Shigella	Ampicillin	
Gram-negative bacilli		Oral kanamycin, tetracycline; oral polymyxin; chloramphenicol
Escherichia coli, enteropathogenic	Oral polymyxin	Oral kanamycin
Sepsis		
Community acquired	Ampicillin	Tetracycline, kanamycin, gentamicin; a cephalosporin
Hospital acquired	Kanamycin	Kanamycin, tetracycline, carbenicillin; cephalosporin; polymyxin
Proteus mirabilis	Ampicillin	Kanamycin, gentamicin; cephalosporin
Spirochetes		
Treponema pallidum (syphilis)	Penicillin G	Tetracycline; erythromycin

[a] From *The Medical Letter-Handbook of Antimicrobial Therapy*, Issue 340, Jan. 1974.

aged by oral erythromycin. *S. aureus* is the primary contaminant in most infections, and usually is penicillin-resistant. Erythromycin affords excellent protection against this form of *S. aureus,* as well as most gram-positive cocci. A dosage of 500 mg immediately followed by 250 mg q.i.d. is usually sufficient.

Other forms of treatment may be necessary. If tissue necrosis is present, antibiotics may be ineffective until debridement is performed, since the necrosis divorces the infected area from its blood supply. Abscesses that become established produce marked tissue necrosis, and immediate drainage is required. Drainage for more than 2 weeks may indicate an inadequate incision, the presence of a foreign body, involvement of the bone, tuberculosis, fungal infection, neoplasm, or an underlying debilitating chronic disease.

PREVENTION

Central to the prevention of the transmission of infection is a sanitary operating suite. Clean equipment, sterile instrumentation, and draping, demand attention to detail and adherence to strict regulations.

Materials are sterilized by thermal or chemical treatment. Thermal means are more effective than chemical. Steam under pressure is recommended, as bacteria and their spores are destroyed in the autoclave.

Sterile draping of the patient should cover all non-sterile areas within a reasonable distance of the area undergoing surgery.

The manner of surgery and the quality of follow-up care are as important as the pre-operative preparations in eliminating opportunities for infection.

One week preceding surgery, the patient should follow a sensible diet, exercise properly, and obtain sufficient rest. One or two days prior to hospital or office surgery, the patient should undergo appropriate lab tests and physical examination to determine his ability to undergo surgery.

Just prior to surgery, the foot and ankle should be shaved. The foot should then be prepared in a routine manner, using warm water, brushes or pads, and a suitable cleansing agent for 10 minutes. Rinse with an aqueous solution from the toes proximally. Do not use alcohol. Blot the foot dry with a sterile towel and encase it in a sterile stockinette.

The surgeon must be mindful of the fact that every operation is an exercise in surgical bacteriology. Infection is prevented only if the surgeon is vigilant. Bacteria in the wound do not make infection a certainty, but prevention is much easier than treatment. Asepsis combined with antisepsis helps prevent post-operative infection.

Suggested Readings

American College of Surgeons. *Manual of Pre-operative and Post-operative Care.* W. B. Saunders, Philadelphia, 1973.

Burnet, F. M. *Natural History of Infectious Disease,* Cambridge, 3rd ed. Cambridge University Press, Cambridge, 1962.

Charlton, M. A., and Krupp, M. A. *Current Diagnosis and Treatment.* Lange, Los Altos, 1971.

Cohen A., and Yourofsky, R. Gangrene: A post-operative complication. J. Foot Surg. 19: 202–206, 1980.

Cole, W. A., and Elmon, R. *Textbook of General Surgery,* 6th ed. Appleton-Century-Crofts, New York, 1952.

Condon, E., and Nyhus, L., with Department of Surgery, University of Iowa and University of Illinois. *Manual of Surgical Therapeutics.* Little, Brown and Co., Boston, 1973.

Department of Medicine, Washington University School of Medicine, St. Louis, Missouri. *Manual of Medical Therapeutics.* Little, Brown and Co., Boston, 1977.

Elmon, R. *Surgical Care—A Practical Physiologic Guide.* Appleton-Century-Crofts, New York, 1951.

Estersohn, H. S., and Fuerstman, R. The local use of antibiotics to prevent wound infection. JAPA 69: 127–130, 1979.

Giannestros, N. H. *Foot Disorders: Medical and Surgical Management.* Lea & Febiger, Philadelphia, 1967.

Goodman, L. S., and Gillman, A. *The Pharmacologic Basis of Therapeutics.* Macmillan, New York, 1968.

Hill, G. J. *Outpatient Surgery.* W. B. Saunders, Philadelphia, 1971.

Inman, V. T., ed. *DuVries' Surgery of the Foot,* 3rd ed. C. V. Mosby, St. Louis, 1973.

Kawashima, M., et al. The treatment of pyogenic bone and joint infections by closed irrigation—Suction. Clin. Orthop. 148: 240–242, 1980.

Kippax, P. W., and Thomas, E. T. Surgical wound sepsis in a general hospital. Lancet 2: 1297–1300, 1966.

Pelczar, M. J., and Ried, R. D. *Microbiology,* 2nd ed. McGraw-Hill, New York, 1965.

Pulaski, E. J. *Common Bacterial Infections.* W. B. Saunders, Philadelphia, 1954.

Robbins, S. L. *Pathology* W. B. Saunders, Philadelphia, 1969.

Rosenburg, R. *Microorganisms Indigenous to Man.* McGraw-Hill, New York, 1961.

Rubinstein, E. Soft tissue infections. Prog. Surg. 16:25–37, 1979.

Schwartz, S. I. *Principles of Surgery.* McGraw-Hill, New York, 1969.

Smith, D. T., Conant, N. F., and Willet, H. F. *Zinsser Microbiology,* 14th ed. Appleton-Century-Crofts, New York, 1968.

Stein, J. M. Infections of wounds and soft tissues. Comp. Ther. 5:38–43, 1979.

Vargish, T. Prophylactic use of antibiotics in surgery. J. Iowa Med. Soc. 70:14–15, 1980.

Weinstein, F. *Principles and Practice of Podiatry.* Lea & Febiger, Philadelphia, 1968.

Wilson, G. S., and Miles, A. A., eds. *Topley and Wilson's Principles of Bacteriology and Immunity,* 5th ed. Williams & Wilkins, Baltimore, 1964.

CHAPTER 17

Osteomyelitis and Wound Complications

STANLEY R. KALISH, D.P.M.
MARLA JASSEN, D.P.M.

WOUND COMPLICATIONS

Major problems occurring in the post-operative phase are usually a result of poor recognition of predictable factors of wound infection and dehiscence in the pre-operative phase. Very simply, the absence of blood, the presence of edema and diabetes mellitus, and the lack of surgical skill will create a suitable environment for post-operative infection. The insensitive foot, pre-existing infection, including osteomyelitis, are also significant factors which can create post-operative wound complications (Fig. 17.1).

In predicting factors of failure, one must carefully look at the insensitive foot before surgery to determine the pros and cons of an elected procedure. Diabetes mellitus, spina bifida and myelomeningocele, traumatic neurotmesis, leprosy, syphilis, and yaws are diseases which must be recognized and dealt with prior to surgical intervention.

Patients with poor blood supply secondary to diabetes mellitus will predictably have greater rates of infection since the small vessel disease which occurs creates a tissue hypoxia during the post-operative convalescence. These fragile vessels can often be occluded by simple gravitational pressure which occurs in the operating suite. Patients with spina bifida and myelomeningocele have an inability to cope with normal trauma following surgery. A similar situation will occur in patients with traumatic neurotmesis secondary to peroneal nerve injury or sciatic nerve damage. In all of these situations, with predictable factors of failure, one must be reasonably sure that the post-operative result warrants the risk of surgery.

Another situation, in which the surgeon can create unexpected problems, occurs in the pre-operative edematous foot (Fig. 17.2). Edema, whether it be unilateral or bilateral, creates a state that disturbs the normal homeostasis of healing. It is expected, after a surgical operation, for there to be a certain amount of post-operative edema. If one enters the surgical theater with a patient in an edematous state, then we can be assured of greater complications. Unilateral edema can be caused by trauma (Fig. 17.3), venous disease, tumor, infection, or underlying autoimmune diseases. Generally speaking, bilateral edema often involves cardiovascular disease, liver disease, kidney disease, or bilateral lymphatic and venous disease (Fig. 17.4). It is important to note that patients who have cardiovascular disease, who are brought into an operating theater undiagnosed, not only have a greater risk of infection due to edema, but can present themselves with life-threatening anesthetic situations. Consultations with cardiologists, internists, and anesthesiologists are imperative and are the usual protocols in hospitals prior to podiatric surgery.

Of great importance, are those special situations in which patients have a loss of

1. **No Blood**

2. **Edema**

Before 3. **Diabetes**

4. **Surgeon's Skill**

5. **The Insensitive Foot**

6. **Pre-existing Infection**

Figure 17.1.   "The big problems."

Edema

1. **Unilateral**
   a. **Trauma**
   b. **Venous**
   c. **Tumor**
   d. **Infection**
   e. **Autoimmune**

2. **Bilateral**
   a. **Heart**
   b. **Liver (loss of colloid oncotic pressure)**
   c. **Kidneys**
   d. **Bilateral lymphatic or venous diseases**

Figure 17.2.   Predictable factors of failure.

colloid oncotic pressure. These conditions can be found especially in the alcoholic and malnourished patient. Patients with kidney disease of all types, whether it be acute or chronic glomerulonephritis or the nephrotic syndrome, have a greater incidence of edema as they are permitting a flow of colloid particles to the interstitium. The alcoholic or malnourished patient, on the other hand, creates a situation in which the intracellular colloid oncotic pressure is not great enough and allows a reverse osmosis to occur in the interstitium. This negative osmotic state, in which fluid is drawn from the intercellular space to the intracellular space, has disasterous results in elective foot surgery. Patients with pre-edematous or edematous states prior to surgery will have a naturally higher incidence of postoperative infection and wound dehiscence. Proper evaluation and cooperation with other specialists can avoid unnecessary complications. The statement "To thine own self be true," is especially pertinent in dealing with patients who enter the operating theater with potential problems. Again, the risks of surgery are great in a

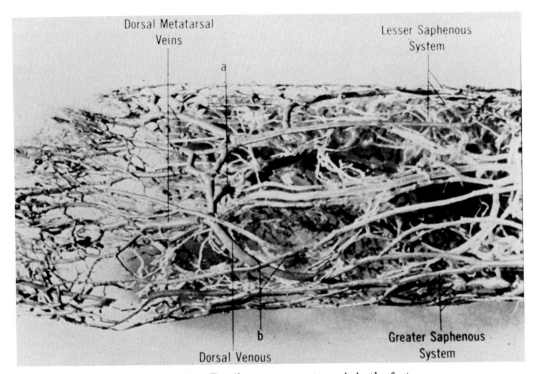

Figure 17.3.   Fragile venous anastomosis in the foot.

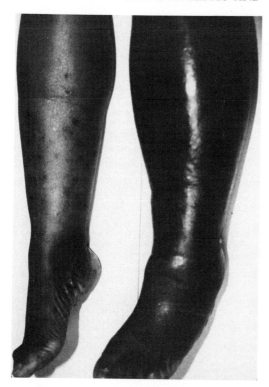

Figure 17.4. Chronic lymphedema.

normal patient and become even greater in patients with edema.

Vascular disease, including arteriosclerosis obliterans, thromboangiitis obliterans, Raynaud's syndrome and disease, varicosities, thrombophlebitis and lymphedema of all causes, create situations which also lead to a higher incidence of wound complications. Obesity in itself can provide diasterous thromboembolic phenomenon, especially in females over 40 years of age. Patients who fit into this category should be routinely anticoagulated with low-dose heparin, using 5000 units of aqueous heparin every 12 hours. One might elect to utilize a regimen of aspirin, 10 grains q.i.d., for 2 days prior to surgery. Patients with arteriosclerosis obliterans should be evaluated pre-operatively with a comprehensive vascular examination. In some cases, the vascular physiologist and vascular surgeon should be called in for consultation. Arteriosclerosis obliterans itself occurs in the 5th and 6th decades of life and manifests itself with pathological atherosclerotic

plaques. Ischemic neuritis secondary to Wällerian degeneration is seen. Diabetics have an accelerated rate of arteriosclerosis obliterans and should be evaluated with special care and concern.

Patients with Raynaud's disease and Raynaud's syndrome elicit a spastic reaction to cold and often will react to the trauma and stresses of surgery by severe vasoconstriction (Fig. 17.5). Raynaud's syndrome is generally associated with autoimmune disease and one must be quite selective in diagnosing and evaluating the patient prior to an elective procedure. A typical patient with Raynaud's syndrome will elicit in early stages an intolerance to cold, with blanching and hyperemia. A simple test is to take the patient with Raynaud's syndrome and immerse the hands in cool water to evaluate the amount of erythema and blanching which occurs. The use of epinephrine in local anesthetics is strongly dissuaded in these patients.

Patients with superficial and deep varicosities are also in the category of dangerous pre-operative candidates and should be evaluated through vascular consultation.

A phenomenon more commonly found in the northern climates is pernio (Fig. 17.6). Patients who have had pernio have a change in cellular constituency and tissue damage secondary to freezing and cooling. Patients with cryoglobulinemia and cryoprecipitates should also be evaluated prior to any foot surgery. Confusing as it may seem, a history of pernio may also be misdiagnosed and falls into the category of Raynaud's or autoimmune type diseases. The recognition and treatment of all vascular diseases are of extreme importance. Diagnosing patients with vascular afflictions prior to surgical procedures will save you a great deal of post-operative diasters.

"Know thy patient well" (Fig. 17.7) is an important and sometimes overlooked diagnostic feature in predicting post-operative failure. Metabolic and vascular diseases are situations of extreme importance. A history of keloid formation and severe emotional disease are two conditions which are often missed in evaluating patients for surgery.

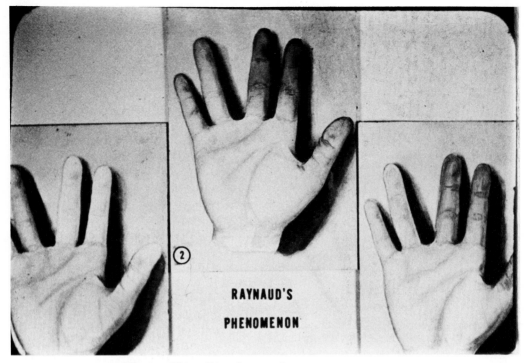

Figure 17.5. Blanching and cyanosis in Raynaud's.

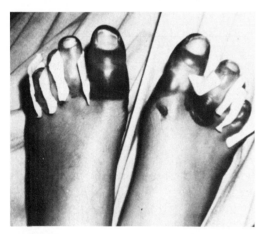

Figure 17.6. Pernio following immersion exposure.

1. **Metabolic disease**

2. **Vascular disease**
   a. **Arterial**
   b. **Venous & lymphatic**

3. **Compliance impossible**

4. **Keloid history**

5. **Emotional disease history**

Figure 17.7. "Know thy patient well."

A comprehensive questionnaire can be provided by most psychological services and psychiatric services in patients who may prove to be unreasonable and unable to cope with the normal post-operative stresses of convalescence. Keloid formation in a routine surgical procedure can provide a severe complication and lead the patient to a painful condition far greater than the original pathology (Fig. 17.8). Black patients are especially prone to keloid formation and this history must be elicited prior to an elective procedure.

The Surgeon's Skill

The surgeon's skill is dependent on limitations, training, and surgical planning (Fig. 17.9). A physician who attempts to perform an operation for which he is untrained creates an environment which will lead to failure. It seems very fashionable to

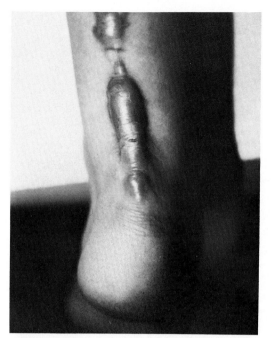

Figure 17.8.   Keloid following tendo-Achilles lengthening.

discuss and "try out" various methods of fixation for osteotomies. One should avoid the temptation to become fashionable "at the risk of becoming incompetent."

Significant, predisposing factors in wound healing intra-operatively, in addition to the surgeon's skill, include those situations which determine the proficiency of the surgeon himself. Inappropriate and rough tissue handling, excessive undermining or retraction, improper or tight suture placement, and tissue hypoxia secondary to massive dissection will create wound dehiscence and infection (Fig. 17.10). Tissue hypoxia secondary to increased tourniquet time may also lead to severe problems. A tight surgical dressing can compromise arterial supply and, in some cases, even produce peripheral gangrenous changes. We must be especially careful in evaluating these situations in patients with metabolic and arterial disease.

Wound Dehiscence

Wound dehiscence is an unfortunate and sometimes disastrous complication which occurs following surgery. Patients who have

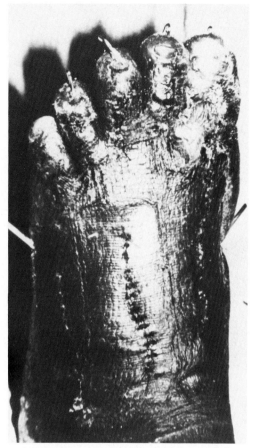

Figure 17.9.   Post-surgical edema and tissue trauma.

1. **Sterile technique (infection)**
2. **Poor incision planning**
3. **Undermining of skin**
4. **Layer loss**
5. **Over-zealous retraction**
6. **Dehydration & bone-burning**
7. **Ligation and electrocautery**
8. **Over-zealous suture technique**
   a. **where and how?**
9. **Dead space and hematoma**
10. **No drain**

Figure 17.10.   Surgical wound complications.

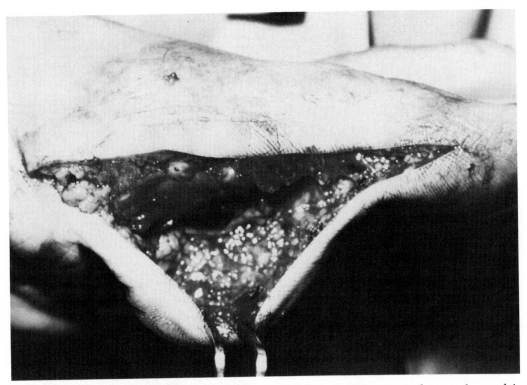

Figure 17.11. Potential dead space, fifth metatarsal area. This area and type of wound is amenable to small closed suction drainage systems.

an increase in post-operative pain, following an operation, must be carefully observed for post-operative infection and subsequent dehiscence. Patients with intolerable pain in one foot versus a normal asymptomatic post-operative foot can have a post-operative infection. Factors such as hyperpraxia, leukocytosis, and the other cardinal signs of infection, including localized heat, pain, and redness, will allow one to determine during the post-operative course whether the patient is developing a post-operative infection and bacteremia.

Suture Material

The overzealous use of large or inappropriate volumes of suture material can lead to tissue strangulation and wound slough. Patients with a history of keloid formation should be exposed to the most inert forms of skin closure. A stainless steel pull-out suture is advocated.

Wound Drainage

Patients with an excessive amount of bleeding, who have post-operative "dead space" (Fig. 17.11), should receive proper intra-operative wound drainage. The TLS closed suction wound drainage system developed at Doctors Hospital, Tucker, Georgia, has a #10 and #7 French gauge catheter attached to two sterile microvac tubes which provide an atmosphere to reduce post-operative hematoma and infection. A large closed suction drain apparatus such as the Hemovac® is also available.

Differentiating between Wound Infection and Wound Slough

Because both are unfortunate and miserable cousins of each other, infection can produce slough, and slough can produce infection (Fig. 17.12). It is important to

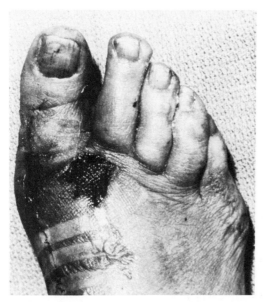

Figure 17.12. First interspace hematoma leading to slough and subsequent split-thickness grafting.

realize that infections involving the joints are generally staphylococcal and gonococcal in origin. Infections involving the skin are generally *Staphylococcus aureus*, anaerobic or aerobic *Streptococcus* (*Streptococcus* Group A). Furuncles and abscesses are generally *S. aureus*. We realize, unless otherwise proven, that all *S. aureus* infections are penicillinase-producing and must be treated with an appropriate antibiotic.

Antibiotic Failure

The failure of patients to respond to appropriately chosen and administered antimicrobial agents is a common problem. The following list recounts the most frequent causes of failure:

1. Drug fever or drug reaction
2. Deep seated, non-draining abscess
3. Obstruction to natural drainage (i.e., implant)
4. Presence of exogenous or endogenous foreign body
5. Antagonism between antibiotics administered simultaneously: bactericidal versus bacteriostatic (i.e., erythromycin and lincomycin)

Patients who have a displaced implant or an implant that may be in its normal functional position, but has infection around it, must be removed before there is a chance for the infection to be resolved. Classical cases of implant removal will be arthroereisis (Fig. 17.13), silastic implantation for forefoot surgery, and total ankle replacement (Fig. 17.14). Surgical wound complications can occur naturally by breach of sterile technique. This may occur anywhere in the operating theater and may even occur prior to the patient entering the theater. Poor incision planning, undermining the skin, loss of layer formation, overzealous retraction, dehydration, and bone burning are intra-operative complications which can also produce wound infection. Surgical wound complications are especially prevalent in our era of high-speed bone cutting instruments. These instruments have made foot surgery an exacting science by allowing us to precisely cut bone surfaces and create osteotomies that were otherwise impossible with larger orthopedic instrumentation. However, these instruments can create secondary wound infection by bone burning if the following situations exist:

1. Dull blades
2. Excessive nonhydrated bone cutting
3. Contamination of instrumentation

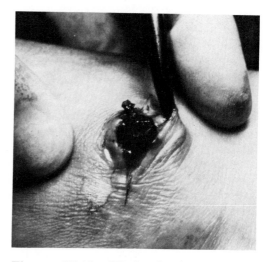

Figure 17.13. Displaced arthroeresis implant.

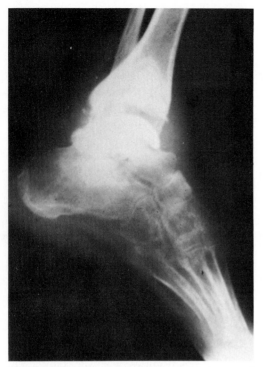

Figure 17.14. Osteomyelitis following total ankle replacement.

The use of chilled saline, as suggested, with careful and frequent lavage can provide the surgeon with a cooling lubricant which avoids bone burning. A more subtle determination in the creation of post-operative wound complications involves dehydration. Dehydration of the wound can frequently occur in environments where there is low humidity and hot penetrating lights.

Summary

Predictable factors of failure include metabolic, vascular, and surgical skill, including poor technique, poor tissue mobilization, poor incision planning, and poor post-operative convalescence. A careful understanding of all the ramifications that will lead the surgeon down the path of destruction can often be found and eliminated in the pre-operative phase.

OSTEOMYELITIS

Osteomyelitis is defined as an inflammation of bone secondary to an infection.

The infection may be due to bacteria, fungi, parasites, or a virus. The manifestations of osteomyelitis are varied and dependent upon the anatomic site of involvement, the infecting organism, initiating event, and previous treatment, as well as the particular point in the cause of the disease. Successful therapy may require collaboration with several medical disciplines. Early diagnosis and treatment are imperative to prevent major complications.

Classification

Osteomyelitis may be classified several ways. Traditionally, it has been defined as either acute, subacute, or chronic, depending upon the clinical course of pathological findings. In actuality, the disease process is more of a gradual blending, and distinction among the above classifications is difficult.

It is possible to categorize osteomyelitis on the basis of the route of contamination. These include hematogenous osteomyelitis, direct inoculation as spread from a contiguous source, and post-operative infection. Hematogenous osteomyelitis, more common in children than adults, is the result of a blood-borne infection. The long bones of the lower extremity, particular the femoral and tibial metaphysis are most commonly affected (Fig. 17.15). The invading organisms settle in the terminal capillary loops, causing bone destruction. Although it is well known that the mere presence of bacteria in bone is not enough to cause disease, these areas are believed to be susceptible to infection due to the slowing and turbulence of blood flow secondary to tortuous vessels, as well as diminished phagocytic ability of the cells lining the vessels. The clinical, radiological, and pathologic features of osteomyelitis differ according to the age of the patient. In the infant, hematogenous osteomyelitis begins in the metaphysis of bone, but may extend to the epiphysis by penetration of vessels through the growth plate. This can lead to epiphyseal and cartilage damage producing disturbances or arrest in growth. The childhood form of the disease rarely spreads to the epiphysis due to the inability of vessels

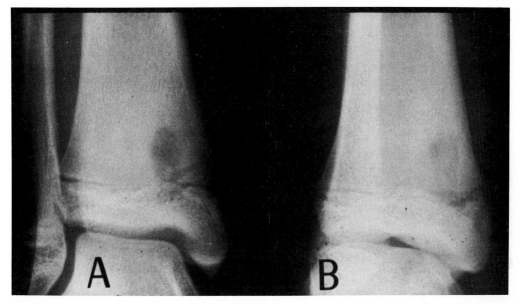

Figure 17.15. Hematogenous osteomyelitis. *A*, pre-antibiotic treatment. *B*, 6 weeks post-treatment.

to penetrate the open epiphyseal plate. Instead, infection spreads through the marrow cavity of the diaphysis.

ADULT DIAPHYSIS

Adult hematogenous osteomyelitis, similar to that of the infant, can cross the closed growth plate. Involvement of the spine, pelvis, and small bones in the hands and feet are not common.

It must be emphasized that hematogenous osteomyelitis begins within the bone. The inflammatory process causes changes in pH levels, edema, stasis, and ischemia leading to necrosis. The necrotic tissue then serves as a media for further infection and a cystic process is instituted. Osteomyelitis via direct inoculation as spread from a contiguous source is more commonly seen by the podiatrist. This is defined as an infection arising from an exogenous source or extension of a soft tissue infection to bone. Post-operative infections can be included in this category, although they will be considered separately. Sinus cavity disease, felons, burns, puncture wounds, poor oral hygiene, ulcerations, radiation therapy, foreign bodies, and trauma may also progress to severe osteomyelitic infection.

There are several routes available to organisms which become lodged in the soft tissues of the foot. Either the infection is contained and resolves, or it may spread through tendon sheaths, lymphatics, or fascial planes. The plantar aspect of the foot is especially vulnerable, as well as anatomically complex. Vascular as well as neurologic disease further complicates the situation. The plantar aspect of the foot is divided into three main compartments by a medial and lateral intramuscular septum extending from the plantar fascia to the overlying osseous structures. Transverse septa further divide these compartments. Spread of infection may occur within these compartments and appear as a bone infection distant from the original source. More importantly, dissemination of infection may occur from the foot into the lower leg.

Few puncture wounds of the foot can result in osteomyelitis or even elicit a clinically significant response. When a problem does arise, it usually presents in the following manner. The patient will give a history of stepping on a sharp object two or three weeks prior to hospital admission (Fig. 17.16). Initially, therapy should include tetanus prophylaxis, foot soaks, elevation of

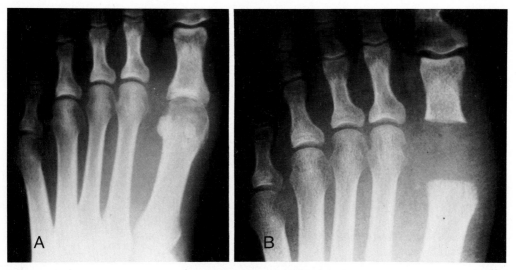

Figure 17.16. Post-puncture wound. *A*, early osteomyelitis, first metatarsal. (note diminished joint space). *B*, resection of proximal phalangeal base and first metatarsal head.

the extremity, rest and antibiosis. Initial improvement is seen, but after a short interval of time the foot becomes edematous, erythematous and symptomatic. Systemic symptoms may or may not be present. Unlike hematogenous osteomyelitis where Staphylococcus aureus is the most common etiologic agent, puncture wounds show a high incidence of gram-negative organisms such as Pseudomonas. The indolent nature of this infection emphasizes the need for early diagnosis and treatment.

Post-operative osteomyelitic infections, although rare, are a common concern to all physicians. It may result from direct inoculation, spread from soft tissue or hematogenous dissemination. Clinical symptoms and laboratory evaluation is difficult and often confused with a normal post-operative course. The symptoms of the disease process can be masked by normal postoperative pain, the body's response to surgical trauma as well as routine post-operative medications, especially analgesics and antibiotics. No matter what the route of infection, early diagnosis and initiation of appropriate therapy cannot be overemphasized. Clinical symptoms are often vague. Pain and edema are the most common. Constitutional complaints such as fever

and malaise may not be present. If the infection is localized, laboratory studies such as a complete blood count (CBC) and the ESR (erythrocyte sedimentation rate) may be normal.

RADIOGRAPHIC INTERPRETATION

Radiographic changes associated with bone infection are often of limited diagnostic value especially in the initial phase of osteomyelitis. Osseous destruction followed by the formation of new bone can occur. Lytic processes are not recognized radiographically until 50 to 65% of the mineral content of bone is lost. There is also a delay in visualization of new bone formation. Therefore, the inflammatory response is well established before radiographic changes become evident, approximately 10 to 14 days later. Changes in medullary bone are virtually invisible on radiographs and most often soft tissue edema as well as obliteration of soft tissue planes are the initial presenting signs. The treatment regimen should be well established prior to the radiographic diagnosis of osteomyelitis.

The classical radiographic signs of osteomyelitis, although seen less frequently today include sequestrum, involucrum and cloaca. A sequestrum is a fragment of dead bone devoid of a blood supply. Radiographically, it appears as an area of increased density due to the hyperemic changes occurring in the surrounding bone secondary to the infection. Involucrum is the layer of new bone and represents the body's response to an attempt to wall off the infection. Involucrum develop holes termed cloacae, which sometimes form sinus tracts to the skin surface.

Radiographic changes are delayed during the healing phase of osteomyelitis and therefore should not be initially used as an indication of successful treatment. If proper antibiosis is administered, radiographic evidence of healing may lag behind clinical improvement. The physician should not overreact to this and alter therapy. If the patient is improving clinically, radiographic findings may be ignored.

Because of the above mentioned limitations of laboratory and radiographic findings, additional diagnostic tests have been developed to aid in the early recognition and treatment of osteomyelitis. Abnormal bone scans occur prior to osseous radiographic changes. These generally appear within 24 hours following clinical symptoms. Unfortunately, scans are sensitive to metabolic changes occurring within the bone but are not very specific. Increased uptake of radioactive material is seen in bone tumors, areas of growth, Paget's disease, trauma, arthritis or any inflammatory disease. Technetium Phosphate and Gallium are the most common radioisotopes used for evaluation of musculoskeletal disorders. The mechanism by which the isotopes are incorporated into bone is not completely understood. Technetium has an affinity for the hydroxyapatite crystals and its concentration is dependent upon new bone formation and blood flow. Gallium is less dependent on blood flow due to its affinity for polymorphonuclear leukocytes and therefore, more specific for an infectious process.

Acute osteomyelitis may initially present as a cold technetium scan on area of decreased activity. One must remember that in the early stages of osteomyelitis, ischemia and thrombosis are present due to increased pressure within the bone. This may be followed by a transitional period showing a normal scintigraphic evaluation prior to the hyperemic stages of infection. Gallium will not present as a cold spot with an acute infection. By performing both the Technetium and Gallium scan, additional information is available. A Technetium scan, both after initial injection and delay of 3–5 hours, will show an area of increasing activity in the process of osteomyelitis. If a cellulitic rather than an osseous process is present, the delay will show a gradual decrease in activity. Successful therapy cannot be determined by a Technetium scan because this will remain hot long after the infection has resolved. Gallium accumulation decreases with time, which has led to its use in guiding therapy.

Tomography is occasionally performed to determine the extent of osseous involvement. It also gives better visualization of sequestra and aids the surgeon in determining the exact location as well as whether or not surgical debridement is necessary. When surgical intervention is being considered, a thorough knowledge of sinus tracts is important. By injecting a contrast media through the tract, the course and extent of the fistula and its possible communications with bone can be determined. Computerized tomography may soon have a role in the diagnosis and treatment of osteomyelitis. Increased intramedullary densities are noted in the presence of an infection. This may be due to edema and vascular congestion. The scan can differentiate between cortical, periosteal, intramedullary and soft tissue involvement. Due to the non-specific nature of these changes, further evaluation of this modality is necessary.

Treatment

The most important therapeutic measures for osteomyelitis are surgical debridement and administration of intravenous antibiotics. Both are dependent upon the location of the infection, the virulence of the organism, and stage of the disease process.

The antibiotic of choice should be determined by culture and sensitivity taken from the site of the infection. Blood cultures are also taken but are negative in greater than 50% of patients with osseous infection. If a causative organism is not determined, antibiosis should be instituted on the basis of high probability. Some physicians feel that with hematogenous osteomyelitis, due to the high incidence of *Staphylococcus aureus* a penicillinase resistant penicillin should be given parenterally. When dealing with post-operative infections as well as spread from a contiguous source, a broad-spectrum antibiotic is begun initially due to increased incidence of gram-negative infections.

There is much controversy over the in-

dications for surgical debridement. Acute osteomyelitis generally responds well to appropriate antibiotic treatment, although surgery is sometimes necessary for evacuation of abscess and biopsy to ascertain the etiologic agent. Chronic osteomyelitis, which usually implies vascular compromise, is an indication for surgical saucerization (Fig. 17.17). Adequate antibiotic levels at the site are difficult to achieve under the above circumstances. As stated earlier, sequestra found in chronic osteomyelitis represent necrotic bone walled off from the circulation (Fig. 17.18). Antibiotics cannot penetrate dead bone and organisms may become trapped, serving as the source of continuous infection. Therefore, surgical debridement to remove the necrotic tissue is recommended. As mentioned previously, osteomyelitis and infec-

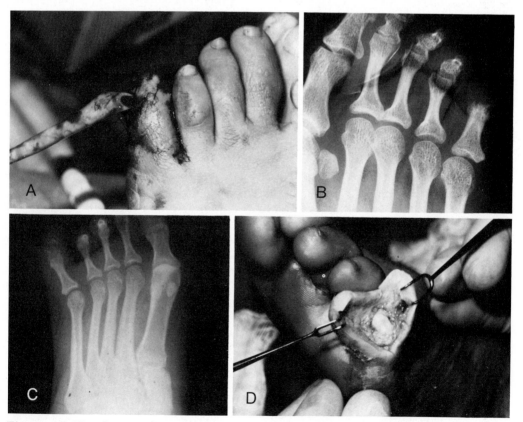

Figure 17.17. Osteomyelitis of fifth toe. *A*, pre-op radiograph of fifth toe osteomyelitis. *B*, amputation of distal phalanx, fifth toe. *C*, Penrose drainage in osteomyelitis of fifth toe. *D*, amputation of fifth toe, distal phalanx. (Photos courtesy of Dr. John Ruch.)

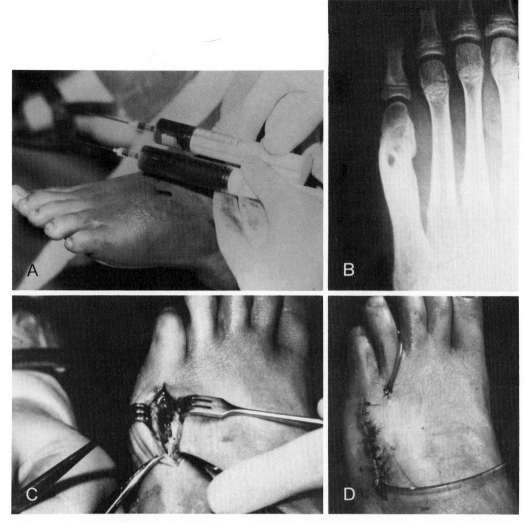

Figure 17.18. Treatment of osteomyelitis (fifth metatarsal). *A*, evacuation of abscess cavity, dorsal aspect, fifth metatarsal (courtesy of Dr. John Ruch). *B*, Fifth metatrsal, osteomyelitis, pre-op. *C*, osteomyelitis, fifth metatarsal, surgical exposure. *D*, ingress and egress antibiotic closed suction drainage for fifth metatarsal osteomyelitis.

tion in the presence of an implant necessitates the removal of the implant.

Another form of therapy, performed in conjunction with surgical debridement, is closed suction irrigation. This system reduces hematoma formation and dead space following debridement as well as cross contamination from open packing. First, radical debridement is essential. Then, two sets of tubes are placed intramedullary and extramedullary, depending on the location and severity of the infection. The flow rate must be high enough to provide optimal mechanical irrigation. Irrigating solutions consist of physiologic saline combined with an antibiotic, maintained at a high flow rate and cool temperature to create an osmotic pressure in the wound. This favors the flow of fluid and organisms into the wound cavity. Determining the duration necessary for closed suction irrigation is controversial. Usually, negative cultures are present after a few days of irrigation with an antibiotic solution and therefore,

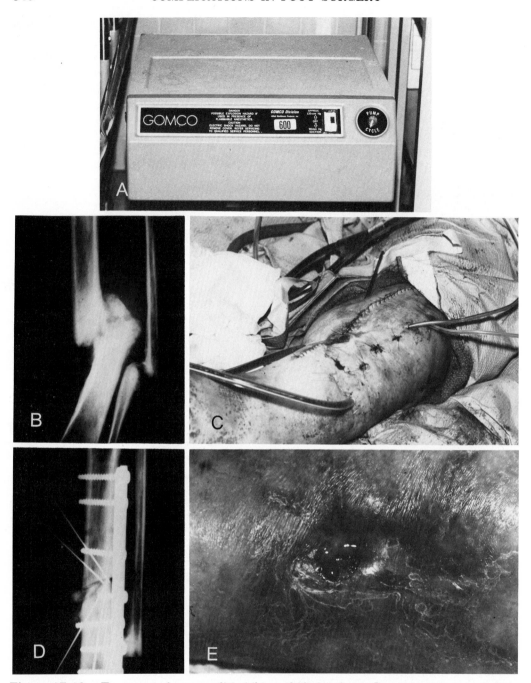

Figure 17.19. Treatment of osteomyelitis (tibia and fibula). Gomco® suction apparatus. *B*, tibia and fibula pseudoarthrosis with osteomyelitis. *C*, insertion of ingress and egress antibiosis. *D*, fixation of pseudoarthrosis tibia and fibula, with electrical bone stimulators. *E*, granulating wound following osteomyelitis of tibia and AO plate fixation. (Figures 17.19, *B–E* courtesy of Dr. Nathan Schwartz.)

the criteria for three consecutive negative cultures are unreliable. Some authors recommend leaving the irrigation system in place for one week following negative cultures. Others recommend culturing after physiologic saline has been used for 24 to 48 hours. Ideally, irrigation should be maintained until the dead space is eliminated and the blood flow is re-established. Painful edema results if inflow exceeds outflow (Fig. 17.19).

Summary

Osteomyelitis rarely presents as a classically described infection. The frequency of failures as well as complications are due to difficulty in diagnosing the infection process which ultimately delays treatment. Complications such as permanent deformity, residual pain, loss of function, chronic infection and carcinoma must be avoided by early diagnosis and appropriate therapy.

Suggested Readings

Boda, A. Antibiotic irrigation with perfusion treatment for chronic osteomyelitis. Arch. Orthop. Trauma Surg. 95:1–2, 41–35, 1979.

Brock, J. G., et al. A case report—102 cases rof osteomyelitis of the hallux sesamoid. Skeletal Radiol. 4:2369, 1929.

Butt, W. P. The radiology of infection. Clin. Orthop. Relat. Res. 96:20–30, 1973.

Capitanio, M. A., and Kirkpatrick, J. A. Early roentgen observation in acute osteomyelitis. Clin. Orthop. 108:488–496, 1970.

Cartildge, I. J., et al. Hematogenous osteomyelitis of the metatarsal sesamoid cartilage. Br. J. Surg. 66:214–216, 1979.

Chusid, M. J., Jacobs, W. N., and Sty, J. R. Pseudomonas arthritis following puncture wounds of the foot. J. Pediatr. 94:429–431, 1979.

Davis, L. A. Antibiotic modified osteomyelitis. Clin. Orthop. 103:602–610, 1968.

Gilday, D. L., Paul, D. J., and Patterson, J. Diagnosis of osteomyelitis in children by blood pool and bone imaging. Radiology 117:331–335, 1975.

Gilday, D. L. Problems in the scintigraphic detection of osteomyelitis. Radiology 135:79, 1980.

Green R., et al. A suction irrigation technique utilizing a hemovac system in the treatment of osteomyelitis. J. Foot Surg. 17:22–27, 1978.

Hagen, R. Osteomyelitis after operative traction and treatment—A report of 62 cases treated with radical surgery and lincomycin. Acta Orthop. Scand. 49:542–548, 1978.

Harris N. W., and Kirkaldy, W. H. Primary pyogenic osteomyelitis. J. Bone Surg. 47B: 526–532, 1965.

Hemingway, D. C., et al. Bone scan findings with radiographic clinical and surgical correlation in extensive osteomyelitis. Clin. Nucl. Med. 5:29–30, 1980.

Jequeira, F. W., and Smith, W. L. Seldinger sinography. Radiology 137:238–239, 1980.

Jones, D. C., and Cody, R. B. Cold bone scans in acute osteomyelitis. J. Bone J. Surg. 63B:376–378, 1981.

Kahn, D. J., and Pritzker, K. P. N. Pathofeld's physiology of bone infection. Clin. Orthop. Relat Res. 96:12–19, 1973.

Kelly, P. J., Martin, W. J., Coventry, N. B. Chronic osteomyelitis treatment with closed irrigation suction. JAMA 213:1843–1848, 1970.

Kolyuas, E., et al. Serial 67 bacitrate imaging during treatment for subacute osteomyelitis in childhood. Clin. Nucl. Med. 3:461–466, 1978.

Kuhn, J. P., et al. Computer tomography diagnosis of osteomyelitis. Radiology 130:503–506, 1979.

Lispona, R., and Rosenthal, L. Observations on the sequential use of 99 technetium phosphate complex and gallium imaging in osteomyelitis, cellulitis and septic arthritis. Radiology 123:123–129, 1977.

Martin, B. F. Observation of the muscles and tendons of the medial aspect of the sole of the foot. J. Anat. 98:437–453, 1964.

Medoff, G. Current concepts in the treatment of osteomyelitis. Postgrad. Med. 58:157–161, 1975.

Miller, E. H., and Seniar, S. W. Gram-negative osteomyelitis following puncture wounds of the foot. J. Bone Surg. 57A: 535–537, 1975.

Miller, W. B., Jr., et al. Brodie's abscess with reappraisal. Radiology 132:15–23, 1979.

Mitra, R. N. Experimental osteomyelitis in rabbits. Orthop. Surv. 41:171–181, 1964.

Morrey, D. F., et al. Hyperbaric oxygen and chronic osteomyelitis. Clin. Orthop. 144:121–127, 1979.

Murray, R. A. Importance of soft tissue to treatment of chronic osteomyelitis. JAMA 180:198–203, 1962.

Nelson, H. T., et al. Bone scanning in the diagnosis of acute osteomyelitis. J. Nucl. Med. 3:267–269, 1980.

Rosen, R. A., Sorchouse, H. T., and Karp, H. J. Intracortical fissuring in osteomyelitis. Radiology 141:17–20, 1981.

Schurman, D. J., et al. Gram-negative bone and joint infection: 60 patients' treatment with amikacin. Clin. Orthop. 134:268–274, 1978.

Septimus, E. J., et al. Osteomyelitis—Recent clinical and laboratory aspects. Orthop. Clin. North Am. 10:347–359, 1979.

Sontowski, E. T., and Sonn, A. W., Treatment of osteomyelitis by debridement and closed suction wound irrigation. Clin. Orthop. 3:215–231, 1965.

Sudmanne, Treatment of chronic osteomyelitis by trace grafts of cancellous autogenous bone tissue—A preliminary report. Acta Orthop. Scand. 50:145–150, 1979.

Torgerson, W. R., and Hammond, G. Osteomyelitis of the sesamoid bones of the first metatarsophalangeal joint. J. Bone Jt. Surg. 51A: 1420–1422, 1969.

Tructa, J. Three types of acute hematogenous osteomyelitis. J. Bone Jt. Surg. 41B:671–680, 1959.

Waldvogel, F. A., Medoff, G., and Swartz, M. N. Osteomyelitis: A review of clinical features, therapeutic considerations, and unusual aspects (first of three parts). N. Engl. J. Med. 282:198–206, 1970.

Waldvogel, F. A., Medoff, G., and Swartz, M. N. Osteomyelitis: A review of clinical features, therapeutic considerations, and unusual aspects (second of three parts). N. Engl. J. Med. 282:260–266, 1970.

Waldvogel, F. A., Medoff, G., and Swartz, M. N. Osteomyelitis: A review of clinical features, therapeutic considerations, and unusual aspects (third of three parts). N. Engl. J. Med. 282:316–322, 1970.

West, W. F., Kelly, P. J., and Martin, W. J. Chronic osteomyelitis: Factors affecting the result and treatment in 186 patients. JAMA 213:1837–1842, 1970.

Index

Page numbers in *italics* denote figures; those followed by "t" or "f" denote tables or footnotes, respectively.